PSYCHOBIOLOGY OF POSTTRAUMATIC STRESS DISORDER

ANNALS OF THE NEW YORK ACADEMY OF SCIENCES
Volume 821

PSYCHOBIOLOGY OF POSTTRAUMATIC STRESS DISORDER

Edited by Rachel Yehuda and Alexander C. McFarlane

The New York Academy of Sciences
New York, New York
1997

Cover: Peter Breughel's *Fall of Icarus* appears on the softcover version of this volume. For an explanation of its significance, please see the Introduction.

Library of Congress Cataloging-in-Publication Data

Psychobiology of posttraumatic stress disorder / edited by Rachel
    Yehuda and Alexander C. McFarlane.
        p.   cm. — (Annals of the New York Academy of Sciences : 821)
    Includes bibliographical references and index.
    ISBN 1-57331-078-6 (cloth : alk. paper). — ISBN 1-57331-079-4
(paper : alk. paper)
        1. Post-traumatic stress disorder—Pathophysiology—Congresses.
    2. Biological psychiatry—Congresses.   3. Psychobiology—Congresses.
    I. Series.
        [DNLM: 1. Stress disorders, Post-traumatic—congresses.
    2. Biological psychiatry—congresses.]
    Q11.N5   vol. 821
    [RC552.P67]
    500 s—dc21
    [616.85'21]
    DNLM/DLC
    for Library of Congress   97-21354
                                                                       CIP

PCP
Printed in the United States of America
ISBN 1-57331-078-6 (cloth)
ISBN 1-57331-079-4 (paper)
ISSN 0077-8923

ANNALS OF THE NEW YORK ACADEMY OF SCIENCES

Volume 821
June 21, 1997

PSYCHOBIOLOGY OF POSTTRAUMATIC STRESS DISORDER[a]

Editors and Conference Organizers
RACHEL YEHUDA and ALEXANDER C. MCFARLANE

CONTENTS

[a]This volume is the result of a conference entitled **Psychobiology of Posttraumatic Stress Disorder** sponsored by the New York Academy of Sciences and held on September 7–10, 1996 in New York, New York.

Part 5. How Basic Research Informs the Clinical Observations of the Biology of PTSD

Part 6. Psychobiology of Treatment

Poster Papers

Financial assistance was received from:

Supporters
- Eastern Paralyzed Veterans Association, Inc.
- Pfizer Inc

Contributors
- Ambulatory Monitoring Inc.
- Novartis Pharmaceuticals

Introduction

RACHEL YEHUDA [a] AND
ALEXANDER C. McFARLANE [b]

[a]*Traumatic Stress Studies Program*
Mount Sinai School of Medicine
New York, New York 10021

Posttraumatic Stress Disorder Program
Bronx Veterans Affairs
Bronx, New York 10468

[b]*The University of Adelaide*
Department of Psychiatry
The Queen Elizabeth Hospital
Woodville, South Australia

Less than 20 years ago the field of mental health did not have the language or a paradigm to describe the long-term consequences of traumatic stress. In retrospect, historical attempts to bring the plight of trauma survivors to the attention of the mental health community probably failed in part because of the lack of specific biological markers that could substantiate claims of long-term psychological scars. In the absence of a discrete biology, the psychological symptoms of trauma survivors could easily be subsumed under the umbrella of neurotic and even psychotic disorders and the etiology of these symptoms be attributed to causes other than trauma exposure.

Posttraumatic stress disorder (PTSD) became a diagnosis in 1980 as a culmination of over a century of clinical observations. However, although the diagnosis provided a descriptive nomenclature for the long-term effects of trauma, nothing was known about the biological concomitants of this condition at the time it was described. In the last decade, biological findings have provided objective validation that PTSD is more than a politically or socially motivated conceptualization of human suffering. Indeed, biological observations have delineated PTSD from other psychiatric disorders and have allowed a more sophisticated description of the long-term consequences of traumatic stress.

This volume summarizes the major findings and themes that have emerged. Perhaps the greatest challenge is that the biological findings suggest that PTSD is a different disorder from the one original conceptualized. In particular, it appears that the biology of PTSD is not simply the biology of stress. This point really must be emphasized because it has major implications in the choice of biological models that could potentially explain the onset of PTSD as well as its maintenance or reemergence. Indeed, one of the major points highlighted in this volume concerns the biological or pathophysiological differences between PTSD, stress, and other psychiatric disorders. On the other hand, Dr. Pitman's call for caution in the interpretation of biological research militates against exaggerated causal assumptions.

The first section of this volume deals with the epidemiological and phenomenological studies that objectified the important clinical observations on the prevalence of trauma and its manifestations. A discussion of these studies is critical to an analysis of biological findings, because without clinical observations there is no appropriate context for evaluating the meaning of biological alterations. One of the reasons that the field of PTSD has been so successful in its exploration of the biological basis of this illness is its insistence in relating biological information to clinical complexities. For example, the relative infrequency of PTSD following trauma discussed by Dr. McFarlane, the frequent co-occurrence of PTSD with other psychiatric disorders discussed by Drs. Keane and Kaloupek, and most importantly, the presence of familial and possibly genetic risk factors for PTSD mentioned by Dr. Pitman and Drs. Connor and Davidson are phenomenological observations that have led the field to understand PTSD as more than a simple stress response and accordingly have uncovered a series of important challenges for biological observations. As such, the findings have compelled researchers to yield to clinical observation rather than allow biological findings in the field of stress to dominate the conceptual development of biological models in PTSD. In turn, clinical paradigms of PTSD must continue to be reconceptualized on the basis of the biology of traumatic stress and its aftermath. Some of the clinical observations and conundrums that continue to shape our understanding of the field of trauma are further highlighted in Dr. Green's overview.

The second section represents the core of the psychobiological studies of chronic PTSD in adults. Indeed, there have been tremendous gains in our understanding of the neuroendocrinology (reviewed by Dr. Yehuda), brain neuroanatomy (reviewed by Dr. Stein *et al.*), functional brain activity (reviewed by Drs. Rauch and Shin and Dr. van der Kolk *et al.*), psychophysiology (discussed by Dr. Orr), neurochemistry (Dr. Southwick *et al.*), and sleep architecture (Dr. Mellman) of PTSD. Because these findings represent biological disturbances in chronic PTSD, one of the major challenges is how to link these observations with the acute stress response and how to describe the transitional incubation process that transduces the various acute responses into chronic ones. An additional challenge involves delineating the interaction between the biological changes observed following a trauma and the preexisting neurobiological phenotypes and genotypes. Because of the limited prevalence of PTSD in trauma survivors, it has become increasingly important to differentiate between biological changes in trauma survivors with and those without PTSD in the acute as well as in chronic stages.

The third section introduces an important framework that is becoming increasingly recognized in trauma studies – the developmental perspective. Indeed, when thinking about trauma from this angle, it is important to go beyond the scope of PTSD and explore the way trauma, or environmental information in general, can modify the neurobiological reactivity of individuals to heighten or modify their responses to subsequent events. This approach is clearly delineated by Dr. Putnam and Dr. Trickett. Indeed, the younger trauma survivor is more vulnerable to a myriad of consequences that are far less circumscribed than are those experienced by adult trauma survivors, because the changes in neurobiological reactivity actually alter the developmental experience. A knowledge of neurobiological plasticity and other factors is critical to understanding the rather diffuse effects of adverse events. Dr. Teicher *et al.* examine this issue in the context of exploring the biological changes occurring following abuse. Dr. Pynoos and colleagues consider the complex interrelationship of trauma and developmental progression and the essential linkage between disrupted and normal development. Dr. Nemeroff and colleagues describe how early adverse experiences can be linked to dysfunction later in life.

The fourth section deals with the biology of normal and traumatic memories in both animals and humans. The first two papers in this section present a neuropsychological assessment of subjects with PTSD from two different approaches. Dr. Wolfe and Dr. Schlesinger consider the cognitive and information-processing disorders that neuropsychological testing has identified in PTSD. Dr. McNally's discussion of the explicit and implicit memory of traumatic events looks at cognitive functioning from the perspective of traumatic memories. One clinical challenge in the field of PTSD is the relationship between disruptions in nontraumatic and traumatic information processing, a complexity infrequently acknowledged. Dr. Spiegel delineates a neurobiological approach to understanding the different types of memory states and distortions (e.g., dissociation, amnesias, and intrusive recollections) associated with PTSD and reaction to traumatic experience. This requires an independent understanding of how traumatic material may be processed in different states of arousal in humans (as reviewed by Dr. Cahill) and animals (as reviewed by Drs. Roozendahl and colleagues). Finally, it is essential to link these states with the neuroanatomical structures that modulate arousal, memory, and conditioning, as illustrated by Dr. Armony and Dr. LeDoux.

In the fifth section, eminent scientists provide theoretical models to explain the way that traumatic experiences might be potentiated to pathological states as well as provide information from basic science that might address some of the difficult paradoxes that have emerged from psychobiological studies. The complexity of the cellular transformations associated with hippocampal morphology are highlighted by Dr. McEwen and Dr. Magarinos who provide a sophisticated model for understanding hippocampal atrophy in light of the psychobiological observations of low cortisol levels. Indeed, it has been necessary to search for explanations other than glucocorticoid toxicity, which is not present in PTSD, to account for hippocampal atrophy in this disorder. Another important issue in the field of trauma is how a brief event can be transformed into a chronic and debilitating disorder, but only in some people. Dr. Post *et al.* and Dr. Antelman *et al.* offer slightly different models from studies of sensitization in animals that are useful in understanding how brief events can sometimes have lifelong consequences. Dr. Davis and colleagues discuss how animal studies of fear and anxiety have already been applied to PTSD in understanding startle reflexes and conditioned fear responses. Finally, Drs. Rasmusson and Charney provide an overview of the types of animal models that can be helpful in understanding the clinical manifestations of PTSD. Dr. Murburg presents a synthesis and overview of biological findings in PTSD and how they may be informed by basic science studies.

The sixth section provides an analysis of how biological studies must influence the treatment of PTSD. Indeed, an important reason for delineating the psychobiology of PTSD is that it may provide some important clues about treatment, particularly pharmacotherapy. However, as pointed out by both Dr. Friedman and Dr. Shalev, psychopharmacological studies performed to date have not provided a clear answer to the question of how to medicate in PTSD. Both chapters provide cogent, but somewhat different, discussions of the reasons for drug treatment failure in PTSD. It is clear from both chapters that pharmacotherapeutic success in PTSD depends on applying our understanding of the unique biology and phenomenology of PTSD to the treatment of this disorder. To date, the rationale for most medications in PTSD has been their efficacy in mood and anxiety disorders that may be related to PTSD phenomenologically but not biologically. Griffin and colleagues describe a novel approach to the treatment of PTSD that utilizes biological measures as outcome variables in the nonbiological treatment of PTSD. Indeed, such an approach contributes to our understanding of the psychobiology of PTSD by delineating which biological alterations, if any, would change following symptom improvement. This type of information might prove to be a critical informant for psychopharmacological observations. Finally, Dr. Foa provides a thoughtful synthesis of how nonbiological treatments can be efficacious in biological disorders and analyzes the significance of treatment efficacy of cognitive-behavioral therapy in understanding both psychological and neurobiological processes in PTSD.

In the aggregate then, this volume demonstrates the value of linking psychobiology with clinical knowledge to further our understanding of posttraumatic disorders. One of the most important contributions of psychobiology is that it provides a structure for understanding clinical observations. However, an understanding of PTSD will undoubtedly require a synthesis of many models, each targeting various components of the complex response to trauma. This volume also underscores the fact that although much progress has been made in understanding the psychobiology of PTSD, many questions about the role and function of neurobiological systems in the acute and chronic aftermath of stress remain unanswered.

Finally, in the age of the information superhighway, there is the constant task of separating relevant from irrelevant information. There is a need to acquire the meticulous details that define biological models without losing the overview of the salient questions being asked. It is imperative to continue to have meetings between colleagues of different disciplines who are investigating the same problems but from very different perspectives so that ultimately we can develop paradigms specifically relevant to PTSD that are framed in the larger context of basic science and clinical psychiatry.

About the cover. The *Fall of Icarus* by Peter Breughel provides a succinct metaphor for how easy it has been for all of society to walk by and fail to notice traumatic events and their devastating impact. According to Greek mythology, Icarus was the son of Daedalus who built waxen wings with which to fly to the sun. He chose not to listen to the warnings of his father that if he flew too close to the sun his wings would melt. Alas, Icarus did fly too close to the sun, his wings melted, and he dropped swiftly to his death. The right side of the painting depicts Icarus's traumatic fate, his mangled limbs visible above the water, barely disturbing the peaceful village scene. About this painting, the poet W. H. Auden wrote: "About suffering, the masters were never wrong. . . ."

> About suffering they were never wrong.
> The Old Masters: how well they understood
> Its human position: how it takes place
> While someone else is eating or opening a window
> or just walking dully along.

The clarity of the findings of biological studies in trauma survivors with PTSD has made it that much harder to ignore and dismiss the persistent and devastating effects of traumatic events in the lives of those who experience them. Although many of the observations described in this volume are somewhat different from what might have been predicted when PTSD was initially described as a diagnosis, their presence offers a concrete validation of human suffering and a legitimacy that does not depend on arbitrary social and political forces. Establishing that there is a biological basis for psychological trauma is an essential first step in allowing the permanent validation of human suffering.

Many thanks to the conference speakers for their thoughtful contributions to this volume and to the conference and editorial staff of the New York Academy of Sciences.

Overview of Biological Themes in PTSD[a]

ROGER K. PITMAN [b]

VA Medical Center
Manchester, New Hampshire 03103

Department of Psychiatry
Harvard Medical School
Boston, Massachusetts

Biology is truly a land of unlimited possibilities. We may expect it to give us the most surprising information and we cannot guess what answers it will return in a few dozen years to the questions we have put to it. They may be of a kind which will blow away the whole of our artificial structure of hypotheses (Sigmund Freud, 1920).

The Decade of the Brain is seeing an end to the dominance of the mind-body dichotomy. The fourth edition of the "Diagnostic and Statistical Manual of Mental Disorders" (DSM-IV)[1] has eliminated the distinction between so-called "organic" and "functional" mental illness, recognizing that all mental disorders have important functional and organic aspects. Nowhere in psychiatric research is the collapse of the mind-body dichotomy better illustrated than in posttraumatic stress disorder, or PTSD. (TABLE 1 summarizes the DSM-IV diagnostic criteria for PTSD.)

When PTSD first appeared in DSM-III,[2] it was viewed as a disorder with almost exclusively psychological symptoms, most of which were based on self-report. As such, it met with substantial skepticism both within and outside the psychiatric community. Many laymen viewed PTSD as little more than a political concession to disgruntled Vietnam veterans. Many psychiatrists thought PTSD lacked valid standing apart from already recognized anxiety and depressive disorders.

Results of biological research into PTSD have changed all this. TABLE 2 presents a partial list of biological abnormalities reported in PTSD. This table is neither authoritative nor exhaustive but merely illustrative. Importantly, not all of these findings have been replicated, and sometimes opposite findings have emerged from different laboratories or even the same laboratory. Some abnormalities that have especially been plagued by inconsistent or opposite results were omitted from TABLE 2. Much more empirical research is needed to resolve the contradictions in the data and to establish the factual biological status of PTSD. This must be the first priority in PTSD investigation.

[a] This work was supported by the VA Medical Research Service, US Public Health Service (grant RO1MH54636), and the US Army (grant DAMD17-94-J-4365). This work was performed by an employee of the US Government during the course of official duties and is in the public domain.

[b] Address for correspondence: 228 Maple Street, Manchester, NH 03103 (tel: (603) 626-6565; fax: (603) 668-6574; e-mail: PITMAN@WARREN.MED.HARVARD.EDU).

1

TABLE 1. Abbreviated DSM-IV Criteria for Posttraumatic Stress Disorder

A. 1. Experiencing, witnessing, or being confronted by event(s) that threaten physical integrity (e.g., death or serious injury) of self or others
    2. Response of intense fear, helplessness, or horror
B. Reexperiencing criteria (one required)
    1. Recurrent, intrusive, distressing recollections
    2. Recurrent, distressing dreams
    3. Flashbacks
    4. Intense psychological distress at exposure to events that symbolize or resemble the traumatic event
    5. Physiological reactivity to cues that symbolize or resemble the traumatic event
C. Avoidance criteria (three required)
    1. Avoidance of associated thoughts and feelings
    2. Avoidance of associated activities or situations
    3. Inability to recall an important aspect of the trauma
    4. Markedly diminished interest in significant activities
    5. Feelings of detachment or estrangement from others
    6. Restricted range of affect (numbing)
    7. Sense of foreshortened future
D. Arousal criteria (two required)
    1. Insomia
    2. Irritability or outbursts of anger
    3. Difficulty concentrating
    4. Hypervigilance
    5. Exaggerated startle response
E. Duration at least 1 month
F. Clinically significant distress or impairment

Nevertheless, as revealed in other chapters in this volume, consensus is building on the robustness and internal inconsistency of some PTSD biological abnormalities. Some of these are specific to PTSD because they are conceptually linked to the traumatic event. For example, PTSD patients show increased physiological responses to cues that symbolize or resemble an aspect of the traumatic event, an abnormality that is not shared by trauma victims with non-PTSD anxiety disorders. When PTSD patients are challenged with lactate and yohimbine, like panic disorder patients, they are more likely to have a panic attack, but unlike panic disorder patients, they are also likely to have flashbacks. Other biological abnormalities in PTSD, such as enhanced suppression of serum cortisol by low doses of the synthetic corticosteroid dexamethasone, are not readily linked to the traumatic event conceptually but empirically have been found to distinguish PTSD from other mental disorders such as depression.

Just as advances in the biological understanding of schizophrenia and affective disorder have refuted the once popular suggestion that mental illness is a myth, the demonstration of biological changes in PTSD patients has refuted the suggestion that PTSD is a scam. Indeed, since its faltering beginnings, the PTSD diagnosis has steadily grown in popularity to the point that it may now be threatened more by

TABLE 2. Partial List of Biological Abnormalities Reported in Posttraumatic Stress Disorder

Increased
  Baseline (or anticipatory) heart rate and blood pressure
  Lymphocyte glucocorticoid receptors
  Cerebrospinal fluid corticotropin-releasing hormone (CRH)
  Hypothalamic-pituitary-adrenal (HPA) axis negative feedback
  Blood triiodothyronine (T3)
  Physiologic (autonomic, electromyographic, catecholaminergic) responses to trauma-related stimuli
  Physiologic responses to trauma-unrelated stimuli, such as loud tones
  Naloxone-reversible analgesia to trauma-related stimuli
  Yohimbine-potentiated startle
  Sleep movements, disruptions, and awakenings
  REM density

Reduced
  Blood and urinary cortisol
  Platelet alpha$_2$-adrenergic receptor binding
  Platelet serotonin uptake
  Platelet monoamine oxidase activity
  Blood adrenocorticotropin (ACTH) response to corticotropin-releasing hormone (CRH)
  Sleep time, efficiency
  Inhibitory modulation of startle response
  P3 event-related potential response to target stimuli
  P1 event-related potential habituation
  Hippocampal volume

Other
  "Reduction" pattern of P2 event-related potential responses
  Yohimbine- and lactate-induced panic attacks and flashbacks
  Traumatic memory-induced right electroencephalographic (EEG) shift

overuse than by neglect. The word "trauma" is becoming equally applied to genocide and tongue lashing. Objective biological measurement has the potential to redeem PTSD from the subjectivity of self-report and separate the wheat from the chaff in the evaluation of PTSD claims.[3]

The central principle of modern medical science is the correlation of function with structure. Historically, medicine has advanced by characterizing disease entities in terms of their signs and symptoms, that is, coherent disturbances in physiological function, and then discovering the pathological structural changes that underlie them. The principle of correlation of function with structure has been most elegantly exemplified in the clinical neurosciences, where the identification of signs on neurological examination has been followed by the pinpoint anatomical localization of their source in lesions in the brain. For a long time psychiatry was excluded from this tradition. The most important mental disorders were characterized as functional, a euphemism to connote lacking in identified structural correlates.

TABLE 3. Partial List of Biological Models of Posttraumatic Stress Disorder

Learned helplessness/inescapable shock
Stress-induced sensitization to subsequent stressors
Neurobiological sensitization, such as kindling, emotive biasing
Hormonally mediated memory overconsolidation
Conditioned fear
Paradoxical enhancement (incubation) of conditioned response
Dysregulated central monoamine, opioid, neuropeptide, or glutamatate activity or responsivity
Neuronal injury or death

Having so long refused to reveal their secrets to traditional neuropathological investigation, such classic mental disorders as schizophrenia and obsessive compulsive disorder are now yielding to the high technology of neuroimaging. Psychiatry is finally assuming its rightful place among the medical neurosciences. In PTSD, neuroimaging is identifying structural brain abnormalities associated with this diagnosis[4–7] as well as allowing the neuroanatomical localization of psychological phenomena such as traumatic reexperiencing.[8,9] This PTSD research epitomizes the dissolution of the mind-brain dichotomy.

In a sense, a case can be made for PTSD as the ultimate functional mental disorder. PTSD is by definition caused by an external, psychologically (rather than physically) stressful event. Whereas it is not difficult to imagine how potential etiological agents such as inborn errors of metabolism, intrauterine infections, or autoimmune reactions might produce structural nervous system changes that are accompanied by mental signs and symptoms, it requires a greater leap to contemplate how psychological stress could do so. Nevertheless, the ultimate explanation of the role played by environment in psychopathology must be made at the cellular level.[10] Although many investigators have focused on the effects of environmental events on the mind, until recently little attention was given to their impact on the brain. PTSD may represent the most extreme example of the ability of external events to induce lasting brain alterations, in a manner parallel to artificial electrical or pharmacological stimulation; for example, PTSD may illustrate the ability of experience to "kindle" the human brain.[11] TABLE 3 presents a partial list (illustrative, not exhaustive) of biological models of PTSD, each of which explicitly involves or implies an alteration in the central nervous system. The possibility that traumatic stress changes the brain, alarming as it is, offers intriguing possibilities for the pharmacological prevention and treatment of this disorder.

The capacity of biology to inform psychopathology is well recognized. Less appreciated, however, is the reverse. Because psychopathological phenomena often represent extreme forms of ordinary human behavior, species-typical biological mechanisms may be cast in higher relief in the mentally disordered. Although Darwin was aware of this fact more than 100 years ago,[12] useful data provided by psychiatric patients are often overlooked by basic behavioral scientists. Information presented in this volume illustrates how research findings in PTSD may shed light on central evolutionary biobehavioral mechanisms of memory and emotion.

TABLE 4. Possible Origins of an Association between a Biological Abnormality and Posttraumatic Stress Disorder

1. The abnormality was preexisting and increased the risk of the individual's being exposed to a traumatic event.
2. The abnormality was preexisting and increased the individual's vulnerability to develop PTSD upon the traumatic exposure.
3. The traumatic exposure caused the abnormality, and the abnormality caused the PTSD.
4. The traumatic exposure caused the PTSD, and the PTSD caused the abnormality.
5. The traumatic event independently caused both the abnormality and the PTSD.
6. The traumatic exposure caused PTSD, the PTSD caused a sequel or complication, and the sequel or complication caused the abnormality.

As an example, evolution appears to have endowed mammalian species with a hormonally regulated memory storage mechanism that provides a means by which the importance of an experience modulates the strength of the memory for it.[13] The origin of this mechanism is assumed to have been natural selection of the ability to learn quickest and best that which is most essential for survival. Recent research has demonstrated the terrible durability of traumatic emotional memories, or conditioned responses, in PTSD. PTSD may represent the best human illustration of the ability of "significance" to facilitate "remembrance."[13] Indeed, PTSD may represent an unhappy human confirmation of the proposition that "emotional memory may be forever."[14]

Although the study of PTSD may demonstrate the operation of certain theoretical biological mechanisms, it challenges others. A long tradition of research into the role of the hypothalamic-pituitary-adrenal (HPA) axis in stress[15] suggests that a chronic stress disorder such as PTSD ought to be characterized by hypercortisolism. However, an unintuitive yet increasingly robust literature now indicates that cortisol may actually be reduced in stress victims[16] and PTSD sufferers[17] and that the HPA axis in PTSD may be hypersensitive to cortisol negative feedback. This is perhaps the best example in empirical PTSD research of the ability of data to "blow away our artificial structure of hypotheses." The "HPA paradox" in PTSD has yet to be explained, but it has the potential for opening new vistas in the understanding of the human stress response.

Because PTSD is defined in DSM-IV[1] as the result of a traumatic event, it is tempting to conclude that any biological abnormality found in PTSD patients must have resulted from this event. Indeed, in popular psychological lingo, the phrase "trauma" has come to signify all sorts of damaging effects of life events ranging from the trivial to the extreme. Assumption of traumatic causation, however, represents a pitfall that readers should keep in mind throughout their study of this volume. Almost all studies of biological abnormalities in PTSD to date have been correlative, and correlation does not necessarily imply causation. TABLE 4 presents a half dozen hypothetical origins of a biological abnormality in PTSD, only one of which is causation by the traumatic event.

An example of competing explanations for the origin of a biological abnormality in PTSD is provided by the recent interesting finding of diminished hippocampal volume in this disorder.[4–7] Animal studies indicate that stress can damage the hippocampus.[18,19] A straightforward interpretation of diminished hippocampal volume in PTSD is that the traumatic event that leads to the PTSD also produces the hippocampal damage; this explanation would correspond to origin 5 in TABLE 4. It might also be that chronic, repeated stress induced by persistent psychological reexperiencing of the traumatic event eventually comes to damage the hippocampus; this explanation would correspond to origin 4.

Along a different line, persons with smaller hippocampi to begin with might have a relative insufficiency of memorial aptitude that reduces their ability to learn from experience and avoid traumatic events. Thus, it is possible that diminished hippocampal volume represents a risk factor for exposure to trauma, corresponding to origin 1 in TABLE 4. In addition to its well-recognized role in memory, the hippocampus has been implicated in internal inhibition and extinction.[20] Consistent with origin 2, preexisting hippocampal compromise might confer a relative failure to extinguish traumatically acquired conditioned responses, increasing the likelihood of the PTSD outcome. Hippocampal damage that was not preexisting but was acquired as the result of the traumatic event still could interfere with extinction of conditioned responses associated with that event and increase the likelihood of the individual's developing PTSD, corresponding to origin 3.

Finally, alcoholism is a common comorbid disorder of PTSD. Some evidence suggests that alcohol may preferentially damage the hippocampus.[21] This combination could conceivably lead to origin 6 in TABLE 4 of the association between diminished hippocampal volume and PTSD. Resolution of competing hypothetical origins of biological abnormalities in PTSD necessarily awaits properly controlled prospective studies, which are methodologically challenging but ultimately essential to the advancement of the field.

Twin studies are a next-best strategy for elucidating the origin of biological abnormalities in mental disorders. Compelling twin data now argue that a portion of the biological abnormalities found in PTSD may antedate the traumatic event. Studies of subjects from the Vietnam Era Twin Registry have demonstrated a genetic component to the individual's propensity to experience a traumatic event[22] and a genetic component to the individual's vulnerability to develop PTSD following such an event.[23] The genes that contribute to PTSD must be represented by phenotypes, and some of the biological abnormalities found in PTSD (TABLE 2) may represent such phenotypes.

Alternately, abnormalities in PTSD that predate the traumatic event may have been acquired as the result of earlier life experiences. Histories taken from veterans with PTSD suggest higher pre-combat incidences of neurodevelopmental abnormalities such as delayed onset of walking and speech, learning disabilities, and enuresis.[24] Data such as these blow away an "artificial structure of hypotheses" that simplistically attributes all the manifestations of a mental disorder to a single environmental event, however traumatic. PTSD patients have complex biopsychosocial histories that include more than the obvious traumatic event(s) that may preempt clinical and research attention. Ultimately, the nature-nurture dichotomy, like the mind-brain dichotomy, must break down in favor of an interactive approach. PTSD may become a model psychiatric disorder for studying the interaction of genes and environment.

In an example of alternative explanations of etiology, it has been suggested that child abuse is typically committed by individuals with poor self-control, lability, and impulsivity, and that children abused by such family members could subsequently show the symptoms of mental disorders on a genetic rather than (traumatically) acquired basis.[25] Some might be inclined to regard this as "blaming the victim." Although we have to be sensitive to the personal issues that often motivate such concerns, scientists must put aside political correctness and regard such a viewpoint, and others like (and opposite to) it, as hypotheses capable of refutation or confirmation by appropriately collected data. Recent research results indicate that women with childhood sexual abuse-related PTSD show significantly increased physiological responses to cues that symbolize or resemble an aspect of their sexual abuse events, but not to cues of their other stressful life experiences.[26] Such data support a critical role for the traumatic event in the pathogenesis of PTSD that would ring true with most clinicians. More data, however, are needed.

Because traumatic events are often perpetrated by human beings, PTSD has become a political lightning rod among mental disorders. Currently, the validity of the PTSD diagnosis is threatened by the so-called "false memory syndrome," which disputes not the pathological effect of trauma but its very existence in the patient's life history. The true extent of this phenomenon remains to be elucidated by research. However, some of the responsibility for this dilemma belongs to PTSD clinicians who have allowed their political zeal to run ahead of their scientific objectivity. Biological investigation has become more important than ever to PTSD because the kinds of "hard" data it collects are relatively resistant to political influences.

The chapters to follow in this volume, which supplements and extends a recent New York Academy of Sciences conference on stress,[27] present the latest advances not only in the psychobiology of PTSD but also in the basic neurosciences of human memory and emotion. The astute reader should savor the insights offered but at the same time question in which of them lie the "artificial structure of hypotheses" to be blown away by surprising information still to come from the study of PTSD in the years ahead.

REFERENCES

1. AMERICAN PSYCHIATRIC ASSOCIATION. 1994. Diagnostic and Statistical Manual of Mental Disorders, 4th Ed. American Psychiatric Association. Washington, DC.
2. AMERICAN PSYCHIATRIC ASSOCIATION. 1980. Diagnostic and Statistical Manual of Mental Disorders, 3rd Ed. American Psychiatric Association. Washington, DC.
3. PITMAN, R. K. & S. P. ORR. 1993. Psychophysiologic testing for post-traumatic stress disorder: Forensic psychiatric application. Bull. Am. Acad. Psychiatry & Law 21: 37–52.
4. BREMNER, D., P. RANDALL, T. N. SCOTT, R. A. BRONEN, J. P. SEIBYL, S. M. SOUTHWICK, R. C. DELANEY, G. MCCARTY, D. S. CHARNEY & R. B. INNIS. 1995. MRI-based measurements of hippocampal volume in combat-related posttraumatic stress disorder. Am. J. Psychiatry 152: 973–981.
5. GURVITS, T. V., M. E. SHENTON, H. HOKAMA, H. OHTA, N. B. LASKO, M. W. GILBERTSON, S. P. ORR, R. KIKINIS, F. A. JOLESZ, R. W. MCCARLEY & R. K. PITMAN. 1996. Magnetic resonance imaging study of hippocampal volume in chronic, combat-related post-traumatic stress disorder. Biol. Psychiatry 40: 1091–1099.

6. BREMNER, J. D., P. RANDALL, E. VERMETTEN, L. STAIB, R. A. BRONEN, C. MAZURÉ, S.
    CAPELLI, G. MCCARTHY, R. B. INNIS & D. S. CHARNEY. 1997. Magnetic resonance
    imaging-based measurement of hippocampal volume in posttraumatic stress disorder
    related to childhood physical and sexual abuse. A preliminary report. Biol. Psychiatry
    41: 23-32.
7. STEIN, M. B., C. HANNAH, C. KOVEROLA & G. MCCLARTY. 1995. Neuroanatomic and
    cognitive correlates of early abuse. Am. Psychiatric Assoc. Syllabus & Proc. Summary
    148: 113.
8. RAUCH, S. L., B. A. VAN DER KOLK, R. E. FISLER, N. M. ALPERT, S. P. ORR, C. R. SAVAGE,
    A. J. FISCHMAN, M. A. JENIKE & R. K. PITMAN. 1996. A symptom provocation study
    of posttraumatic stress disorder using positron emission tomography and script driven
    imagery. Arch. Gen. Psychiatry 53: 380-387.
9. SHIN, L. M., S. M. KOSSLYN, R. J. MCNALLY, N. M. ALPERT, W. L. THOMPSON, S. L.
    RAUCH, M. A. MACKLIN & R. K. PITMAN. 1997. Visual imagery and perception in
    posttraumatic stress disorder: A positron emission tomographic investigation. Arch.
    Gen. Psychiatry 54: 233-241.
10. HESTON, L. 1987. What about environment? Paul Hoch Award Lecture. 77th Annual
    Meeting of the American Psychopathological Association. New York, NY.
11. PITMAN, R. K., S. P. ORR & A. Y. SHALEV. 1993. Once bitten, twice shy: Beyond the
    conditioning model of PTSD. Biol. Psychiatry 33: 145-146.
12. DARWIN, C. 1965. The Expression of the Emotions in Man and Animals. University of
    Chicago Press. Chicago, IL. (Reprinted from John Murray. London, 1872).
13. MCGAUGH, J. L. 1990. Significance and remembrance: The role of neuromodulatory
    systems. Psychol. Sci. 1: 15-25.
14. LEDOUX, J. E. 1990. Information flow from sensation to emotion: Plasticity in the neural
    computation of stimulus value. In Learning Computational Neuroscience: Foundations
    of Adaptive Networks. M. Gabriel & J. Moore, Eds.: 3-51. MIT Press. Cambridge, MA.
15. SELYE, H. 1946. The general adaptation syndrome and the diseases of adaptation. J. Clin.
    Endocrinol. 6: 117-230.
16. BOSCARINO, J. A. 1996. Post-traumatic stress disorder, exposure to combat, and lower
    plasma cortisol among Vietnam veterans: Findings and clinical implications. J. Consult.
    Clin. Psychol. 63: 191-201.
17. YEHUDA, R., M. H. TEICHER, R. L. TRESTMAN, R. A. LEVENGOOD & L. J. SIEVER. 1996.
    Cortisol regulation in posttraumatic stress disorder and major depression: A chronobio-
    logical analysis. Biol. Psychiatry 40: 79-88.
18. UNO, H., R. TARARA, J. ELSE, M. SULEMAN & R. M. SAPOLSKY. 1989. Hippocampal damage
    associated with prolonged and fatal stress in primates. J. Neurosci. 9: 1705-1711.
19. WATANABE, Y., E. GOULD & B. S. MCEWEN. 1992. Stress induces atrophy of apical
    dendrites of hippocampal CA3 pyramidal neurons. Brain Res. 588: 341-345.
20. DOUGLAS, R. J. 1972. Pavlovian conditioning and the brain. In Inhibition and Learning.
    R. A. Boakes & M. S. Halliday, Eds.: 529-553. Academic. London.
21. ESKAY, R. L., T. CHAUTARD, T. TORDA, R. I. DAOUD & C. HAMELINK. 1995. Alcohol,
    corticosteroids, energy utilization, and hippocampal endangerment. Ann. N.Y. Acad.
    Sci. 771: 105-114.
22. LYONS, M. J., J. GOLDBERG, S. A. EISEN, W. R. TRUE, J. MEYER, M. T. TSUANG &
    W. G. HENDERSON. 1993. Do genes influence exposure to trauma?: A twin study of
    combat. Am. J. Med. Genet. (Neuropsyschiatr. Genet.) 14: 22-27.
23. TRUE, W. R., J. RICE, S. A. EISEN, A. C. HEATH, J. GOLDBERG, M. J. LYONS &
    J. NOWAK. 1993. A twin study of genetic and environmental contributions to liability
    for posttraumatic stress symptoms. Arch. Gen. Psychiatry 50: 257-264.
24. GURVITS, T. V., N. B. LASKO, S. C. SCHACHTER, A. A. KUHNE, S. P. ORR & R. K. PITMAN.
    1993. Neurological status of Vietnam veterans with chronic post-traumatic stress disor-
    der. J. Neuropsychiatry Clin. Neurosci. 5: 183-188.

25. HUESSY, H. R. 1989. PTSD and sexually abused children. J. Am. Acad. Child Adolesc. Psychiatry **29:** 298.
26. ORR, S. P., N. B. LASKO, L. J. METZGER, N. J. BERRY, C. E. AHERN & R. K. PITMAN. 1997. Psychophysiologic assessment of PTSD in adult female victims of childhood sexual abuse. Ann. N.Y. Acad. Sci., this volume.
27. CHROUSOS, G. P., R. MCCARTY, K. PACÁK, G. CIZZA, E. STERNBERG, P. W. GOLD & R. KVETŇANSKÝ. 1995. Stress: Basic mechanisms and clinical implications. Ann. N.Y. Acad. Sci. Vol. 771.

The Prevalence and Longitudinal Course of PTSD

Implications for the Neurobiological Models of PTSD

ALEXANDER C. McFARLANE

Department of Psychiatry
University of Adelaide
Queen Elizabeth Hospital
Woodville
South Australia, 5011, Australia

Posttraumatic stress disorder (PTSD) cannot just be looked at from a cross-sectional perspective. It progresses and changes with the passage of time.[1,2] This suggests that the neurobiology should be viewed as being in a progressive state of modification in the different stages of the disorder. This issue needs to be considered against the background of a series of observations that have emerged which were not anticipated two decades ago.[3] First, PSTD is the exception rather than the rule following exposure to trauma. The disorder is not a normal response to an abnormal experience, because many studies have shown the existence of risk factors other than trauma as predictors of PTSD. The biological data suggest the atypical rather than normative nature of the posttraumatic stress response. The prevalence of posttraumatic comorbidity does not confirm the uniqueness or the independence of PTSD following exposure to trauma. It is one of a number of disorders that emerge in this context.

These findings have not been without controversy. There is an uneasy tension between those who wish to normalize the status of victims and those who wish to define and characterize PTSD as a psychiatric illness. The future of the traumatic stress field depends on acknowledgment of the contradictions that will drive the formulation of the next generation of conceptual issues. These concerns have a general relevance to psychiatry as PTSD is a prototypical illness; it can contribute to a broader understanding of mental illness. It allows a characterization of the effects of environmental factors in psychiatric illness and their interaction with the underlying neurobiology.

This highlights the way in which naturalistic observations about the prevalence, onset, and course of PTSD can inform the theoretical formulations about PTSD. In this paper, the prevalence and longitudinal course of PTSD are summarized as they are the template onto which emerging neurobiological findings need to be superimposed. One of the main issues that emerges is that PTSD involves a series of transitional states and that there is the progressive modification of the phenomenology of the disorder with the passage of time.

THE PREVALENCE OF TRAUMA

There has been a general reluctance to acknowledge just how frequent experiences are in people's lives that create such haunted preoccupation. When PTSD were first included in the DSM-III in 1980,[4] the diagnostic criteria proposed that traumatic events were characterised as being *outside the range of usual human experience.* This seemed to be confirmed by the first epidemiological study of PTSD which found that it was a relatively rare disorder with a prevalence of 1%.[5] However, using more sophisticated methods, recent studies demonstrated an alarming prevalence of traumatic events which suggests that the original definition that these experiences were outside the province of most people's lives was erroneous. Correspondingly, the definition of the events that lead to PTSD has been changed with DSM-IV,[6] proposing that such events should involve actual physical injury or threat to an individual's integrity. ICD 10[7] describes these events as *exceptionally threatening or catastrophic* and likely to cause distress to almost everyone. There is little doubt that many people experience the threat and distress of these events without being disabled or developing long-term psychological symptoms. Kessler *et al.*[8] as part of the recently conducted US National Comorbidity Study, found that the most common causes of PTSD in men are combat and witnessing death or severe injury, whereas rape and sexual molestation are the most common in women. Amongst the men in this representative sample, 60.3% had experienced a qualifying trauma and a further 17% had been exposed to a trauma that produced intrusive recollections but was not covered by the stressor criterion. In contrast, 50.3% of women had experienced a traumatic stressor. There were significant sex differences in the types of event experienced. For example, 25% of men had had an accident in contrast to 13.8% of women, and 9.2% of women had been raped in contrast to 0.7% of men. The capacity of these events to produce PTSD varied significantly, ranging from 48.4% of female rape victims developing PTSD to 10.7% of men witnessing death or serious injury.

Norris,[9] in a study of 1,000 adults in southern United States which was not a strict random sample, found 69% of the sample had experienced a traumatic stressor in their lives, and this included 21% in the last year alone. The most common trauma was tragic death, with sexual assault again leading to the highest rates of PTSD and motor vehicle accidents presenting the most adverse combination of frequency and impact. In both of these studies there were important age, racial, and sex effects on exposure to trauma. For example, Norris[9] found that black men had the highest rates of exposure and young people had the highest rates of PTSD. Kessler *et al.*[8] found that women had twice the risk of developing PTSD following trauma as men. In contrast to men where increasing age was associated with increased prevalence, there was no age effect in women. This lack of relationship existed because of the increased traumatization of younger women. Given the prevalence of these trauma in these US studies, there is a need to examine these issues in other cultures.

It is now nearly two decades since PTSD was included in DSM-III.[9] Reviewing the implications of the research that has emerged during this period is timely. This paper examines the issues that emerge from studies of the prevalence and longitudinal course of PTSD and how these clinical and epidemiological observations have important implications for understanding the neurobiology of PTSD. In particular, they provide the template on which neurobiological observations need to be fitted.

Where we find ourselves at this point is rather different from what might have been anticipated in 1980. In summary, these findings suggest that the prevalence of traumatic stress is greater than anticipated. On the other hand, PTSD only emerges in a minority of the individuals exposed. This has a series of implications. First, it highlights the importance of issues of resilience and vulnerability in determining both the onset of the acute disorder and the establishment of chronicity. It also raises the important question about whether exposure in itself to severely traumatic incidents may modify a person's subsequent neurobiology. In this regard, our understanding of the prevalence of such traumatic incidents may have wider implications for the onset of other psychiatric disorders, such as major depression and panic disorder, and not just PTSD. The first task to which these prevalence studies point is the need to carefully characterize the acute patterns of response to traumatic incidents and the extent to which the differential responses at this time may account for why some individuals develop PTSD, whereas others appear able to cope without sustaining prolonged and severe psychological disruption.

THE ONSET OF PTSD

When PTSD was first included in DSM-III, the individual had to have symptoms for at least 1 month before the diagnosis could be made. Also, there was no diagnostic category for an acute stress reaction other than an adjustment disorder. The relation between acute psychological symptoms and subsequent posttraumatic morbidity has been of particular interest in armed services. The significant rates of morbidity in intense combat[2] have had an important historical impact on the conceptualization of PTSD.[10] In fact, this has led to confusion about whether those individuals who develop PTSD respond with intense panic at the time of the incident which, particularly in World War I, led to these people being labeled as cowards. This highlights the importance of investigating this question in a more systematic way.

The 1980s produced a significant volume of research on the nature of acute stress reactions. Much of the work on PTSD during this period involved studying populations that had been involved in incidents such as disasters. These populations were generally identified in close proximity to the event and were often followed up. This led to the reformulation in DSM-IV[6] that the experience of helplessness and powerlessness was a central aspect of the acute response to the traumatic event if the individual was going to develop PTSD. This has now been incorporated in the stressor-A criteria. This formulation was in part encouraged by the reemergence of interest in dissociation as one of the main components of the phenomenology of PTSD.[11] Van der Kolk[12] particularly highlighted how the fragmentation of the laying down of memory and the inadequate construction of a narrative at the time of trauma are critical in the traumatic stress response. This question has been investigated empirically by several groups of researchers who concluded that dissociation during of trauma predicts PTSD.[13,14] Other studies by Bremner et al.[15,16] looked at this issue in Vietnam veterans. These studies, however, were concluded more than 20 years after exposure of the trauma, which raises important questions as to whether the symptoms of the disorder may modify the retrospective recall of the nature of the traumatic experience. Several studies[17–19] investigated this issue in closer proximity to the event and again highlighted the importance of peritraumatic dissociation. Shalev et al.'s study[17] was particularly noteworthy because the subjects were studied within 2 weeks of the accident. However, Malt et al.[20] and Malt and Olafsen,[21] studied accident victims, interviewing them on hospital admission, and did not confirm this finding. In fact, London et al.[22] (at the Jerusalem conference) found that peritraumatic dissociation protected people from the subsequent onset of psychiatric morbidity.

In a recent study my research group has looked at the acute patterns of reaction within 24 hours of subjects being admitted to the hospital following motor vehicle accidents. These data demonstrated that subjects who develop PTSD or major depression cannot be differentiated from subjects who have no disorder according to the nature of their symptomatic reactions on Day 2. On Day 2 the full range of symptoms, including intrusions, avoidance, hyperarousal, and dissociation, were examined. This contrasts with reexamination of this population 10 days after the accident. By this time, all of these symptoms had begun to differentiate the groups. Examination of the acute dissociative symptoms also highlighted that dissociation should not be seen as an independent variable simply describing the nature of the individual's reaction at the time of the event. Dissociative symptoms were higher in those who had a family history and also a past history of psychiatric disorder. Also, dissociative reactions at the time of the traumatic event can lead to individuals behaving in a way that might increase their exposure to the traumatic incident because of their inability to behave in an adaptive way.

In contrast to the lack of prediction according to the Day 2 psychological reactions, a cortisol sample was taken from blood drawn to measure the individual's blood alcohol immediately following the accident. This sample taken within a mean of 2 hours after the accident found that the PTSD group had the lowest cortisol rise and the group who developed major depressive disorder had the highest. Thus, the acute neurobiological stress response in contrast to the acute psychological state, seemed able to predict the onset of psychiatric disorders 6 months later.

These preliminary data highlight the need to better characterize the nature of the acute stress response and its transition into the range of psychiatric disorders which emerge following traumatic exposure. It may be that the response to the traumatic event may not be the critical issue; rather, it may be the individual's ability to modulate the acute stress response and to restore psychological and biological homeostasis which is the critical issue. Thus, PTSD may be a disorder of transition rather than a specific stress disorder. In other words, it is not that these persons have a greater acute stress responses; it is their inability to modulate this reaction that is the critical issue. The impact of family psychiatric history, prior psychiatric disorder, and peritraumatic dissociation on this transitional process are of particular importance to the further understanding of the neurobiology of PTSD. Also, the preliminary finding that subjects who developed PTSD had a lower cortisol rise emphasizes the need for greater understanding of the nature of the traumatic stress response that leads to PTSD. Interest in hypocortisolemia as a possible factor leading to decreased hippocampal volume in PTSD highlights the need for more careful systematic research around this question.[15,16] Furthermore, these data emphasize the importance of looking at the progression and changes in PTSD with the passage of time.

THE LONGITUDINAL COURSE OF PTSD

PTSD has a significant rate of natural remission in a number of cases. This emphasizes the importance of understanding those factors that might influence the timing of the remission and also those that might exacerbate the symptoms or modify them in the course of the disorder. Furthermore, with the passage of time it is important to consider whether these constellations of symptoms may change. The different subcategories of symptoms may in fact have different trajectories.

Breslau et al.[23] suggested that the type of traumatic experience may have a major impact on the long-term course of PTSD. Somewhat surprisingly, brief and circumscribed traumas such as accidents may have more enduring effects than combat.[9] However, the small numbers and limited range of traumas documented in these two studies limit the capacity to generalize from their findings. Kessler et al.[8] suggest that if a PTSD has not resolved within 72 months, it has a very substantial probability of remaining chronic. Most remissions occur in the first year in approximately 60% of cases. Treatment only appears to increase the rate of remission rather than the proportion who do remit.

The Vietnam readjustment study, one of the benchmark studies of trauma, found that 19 years after combat exposure 15% of veterans still suffered from PTSD.[24] Solomon et al.[2] suggested that soldiers who become acutely distressed at the time of combat have a much higher risk of PTSD and that this emerges from combat stress reactions. On the other hand, the rates of PTSD among those who cope at the time of the combat are significantly lower. This body of work also provided valuable insights into the patterns of symptom emergence. In this population, the prominence of intrusive symptoms decreased over a 2-year period while avoidance increased.[25]

The longitudinal study of disaster victims suggests a similar picture in which delayed PTSD is uncommon and the typical course of PTSD begins in the immediate aftermath of the trauma and continues. A study of 469 firefighters who had intense exposure to a major Australian bushfire disaster[26] found that in the majority with a chronic course the symptoms fluctuated significantly with the passage of time. This variable impact of different traumatic experience on the symptomatic outcome is suggested when these data are compared with a recent study of 188 motor accident victims who were assessed soon after the accident and followed for up to 1 year.[27] Eighteen percent were found to have an acute distress syndrome characterized by anxiety and depression together with "horrific" intrusive memories of the accident. Only 15% of these 31 victims did not have persistent psychiatric complications at the end of 1 year with 13 having a mood or anxiety disorder, 13 travel phobia, and 9 PTSD. This suggests that in this setting even when the initial reaction has the typical features of an acute traumatic reaction, PTSD accounts for only a minority of the psychopathological outcomes. These findings also indicate the enduring nature of the distress in those who develop acute traumatic reactions. They also indicate that horrific memories are not ubiquitously associated with PTSD as one third complained of these in the immediate aftermath of their accident but only 7% had a PTSD at 1 year.

The longest follow-up of persons with PTSD was conducted after the 1972 Buffalo Creek Dam collapse which caused a devastating flood disaster. Grace et al.[28] conducted a 14-year follow-up of the victims which included 121 (32%) of the original sample of 381 who participated in the study. This rate of participation highlights one of the central problems of conducting long-term follow-ups of trauma victims and is therefore examined in more detail. Of the 44% who had PTSD in 1974, this prevalence rate had decreased to 28% in 1986.

The health database kept on Norwegian citizens provided a longitudinal record of the effects of the Alexander Kielland oil rig disaster in which 123 men were killed.[13] The insurance records of the 73 survivors were compared with those of 89 oil rig workers not exposed to the disaster. Predisaster data showed no differences between the populations. Increased rates of both psychiatric and physical disorders were observed throughout the 8-year follow-up. The rates were greatest for the psychiatric diagnoses being 12.3 per 100 and 1.5 per 100 for the exposed and control populations, respectively. Two cohorts of the Epidemiological Catchment Area study were subsequently subjected to a disaster, which provided a unique opportunity for the prospective longitudinal effects to be studied. The Times Beach area was found to have been built on a dioxin dump and also floods occurred in the region. Following the disaster, the exposed population had greater symptoms of depression, somatization, phobia, generalized anxiety, PTSD, and alcohol abuse. However, when the symptoms that existed before the disaster were taken into account, the differences were less dramatic, with the differences for only depression and PTSD being significant. In contrast to the symptoms of PTSD were the de novo symptoms; the depressive symptoms were a recurrence of previous symptoms. Many of these symptoms had resolved within a year of the disaster. The Puerto Rico cohort experience a hurricane which involved loss of life and property and demonstrated similar findings.[29]

The early clinical literature about traumatic neurosis emphasized its chronic course and the progressive social decline it caused in its more severe forms.[1] Kardiner,[30] whose pioneering work with World War I veterans had a major impact on our current formulation of PTSD, wrote that the disorder included "a deterioration that is not dissimilar to that in schizophrenia. . . . The diminution of interest and intelligence is due to the continuous shrinkage of the field of effective functioning and the gratifications derived therefrom." The question arises as to whether this is a typical outcome, what is the range of other adaptations, and whether these are modified by the nature of the stressor.

Thus, the longitudinal effects of trauma are complex and involve the initiation of new symptoms, particularly those of PTSD, but also the emergence of symptoms of depression and anxiety which represent both the onset of new symptoms and the reactivation of prior affective distress and hyperarousal. However, the trauma may further increase the probability that these symptoms will become autonomous. PTSD is a syndrome that appears to have a variable course, and this is affected both by the nature of the precipitating event, the characteristics of the traumatized individual, and the recovery environment.

Range of the Long-Term Effects of Trauma

The long-term effects of events that cause extreme distress are central to understanding the psychological adjustment that PTSD has brought into focus. While PTSD has been a valuable conceptualization of the trauma response, it is insufficient to describe the full-range of the effects of trauma. This has important implications for planning the treatment services for traumatized populations such as those in Kuwait.

Physical Health

The impact of trauma on physical health is a neglected topic. The Grant Study, which followed the health of a group of sophomores recruited at Harvard University until the age of 65, recently examined the impact of combat.[3] These men were selected for their physical and psychological health and high levels of achievement at university. Although 72 had a high level of combat exposure, only one satisfied the diagnostic criteria for PTSD in 1946 with another 4 having a PTSD-like syndrome. Two of these men committed suicide, one became withdrawn and dropped out of the study, and another was murdered. This suggests that PTSD is the exception among a group of highly resilient individuals. However, combat exposure predicted early death independent of PTSD. Fifty-six percent of those men who had experienced heavy combat were dead or chronically ill by the age of 65.[31]

Similarly, mortality of concentration camp victims was much higher than that of control populations and was most marked in the youngest age groups. The death rate was highest in those in the death camps. The duration of imprisonment had no influence on mortality, perhaps as survival over time reflected a positive selection factor. Initial deaths were due to infectious diseases whereas in the later period coronary arterial disease, lung cancer, and violent death were especially marked.[32] Similar long-term health effects were observed among the merchant seamen who manned the convoys in the North Atlantic in the Second World War, an effect particularly noted in later life.[33]

Comorbid Disorders

The current tendency to focus exclusively on PTSD may prevent the adequate assessment and treatment of comorbid disorders such as depression and substance abuse in traumatized populations. Recently the range of specific trauma-related disorders has received more attention than has the nonspecific role of trauma as a trigger for a range of psychiatric disorders. There is a consistent finding across a range of traumatic events that PTSD is only one of many psychiatric disorders that occur in such settings. In fact, in most cases, even in community samples, PTSD is usually accompanied by another disorder such as major depression, anxiety, or substance abuse.[24,26]

The question arises as to the longitudinal relation between the experience of traumatic events and these other disorders. Moreover, some victims of trauma do not develop PTSD, but a range of other disorders such as depression, and in others the PTSD may go into remission but the other disorder remains. In general psychiatric patient populations, the role of the traumatic event in the latter group is easily underestimated because of the apparent dominance of a disorder that is not typically associated with a traumatic precipitant. This is particularly the case when there is a considerable time period between trauma and presentation for treatment.

The relation between traumatic stressors and general vulnerability to psychiatric disorder may differ significantly between different populations. For example, the Grant study found that the occurrence of PTSD was unrelated to the variables that predicted poor psychological health on a range of other parameters. This contrasts with studies that have not examined such an elite population. For example, Schnur et al.[34] found that MMPI scores prior to combat predicted subsequent PTSD. The National Comorbidity Study[8] and Breslau et al.[35] have shown the role of prior disorders and family history as predictors of PTSD.

Multiple Forms of PTSD

Blank[25] has highlighted that the longitudinal course of PTSD has multiple varia-tion, namely, acute, delayed, chronic, intermittent, residual, and reactivated patterns. In addition, the NVVRS study[24] suggests the need to define a posttraumatic syndrome in which full PTSD criteria are not met. An issue that has not been explored in depth is whether there are significant variations in the presentations of PTSD with time, such as the interpersonal dysfunction becoming more prominent with the passage of time. This is a critical question particularly among those subjected to prolonged and recurrent trauma especially in childhood.

Trauma can also have a series of longitudinal consequences other than the onset of psychological disorders. The experience of such events can modify an individual's vulnerability to subsequent traumatic events in the absence of a symptomatic response. In particular, the meaning of a threat or traumatic loss can lead to a major shift in an individual's internal perceptual sensitivities.[36] Equally, such experiences can become powerful sources of motivation for some individuals, indicating that trauma can have positive effects on those who survive the ordeal without an enduring sense of demoralization or having been damaged. The role of the memory of traumatic experi-ences as a source of motivation and a determinant of human behaviour is one of the major preoccupations of literature and art. This indicates that the impact of these experiences on values and beliefs has important implications for both individuals and society. The accommodation to the possibility of loss and the threat of danger plays a central role in molding many social attitudes and responses.

In understanding the longitudinal consequences of trauma, it is important that information be derived from a range of victim groups because the outcome of different types of trauma may vary substantially. For example, clinical experience suggests that the long-term consequences of child abuse are very different from the experience of a natural disaster or other circumscribed trauma in adult life.[37] The victims of abuse are more likely to have amnesia of the trauma and a range of dissociative symptoms.[38] Thus, conclusions about the longitudinal course of PTSD may not be as readily generalizable across different groups of trauma victims as is generally accepted.

General psychiatric patient populations have had surprisingly little research to examine the extent to which trauma plays a role in the onset and maintenance of the patients' disorders. However, now a series of investigations into the prevalence of child abuse in clinical samples found rates of 18-60%.[38] Davidson *et al.*[39] and McFar-lane[40] also found that in general patient samples the rates of PTSD are also significantly underestimated, which suggests that with further investigation the role of trauma in the initiation of a range of psychiatric disorder will be found to be greater than previously anticipated. These findings suggest that the relation between life event stress and psychiatric disorders may need to be reexamined, investigating the differen-tial impact of traumatic life events from that of the more general range of life experience.

Modified Vulnerability

In medico-legal circles in which the prognosis of PTSD and its long-term outcome are of particular relevance, it is assumed that once the symptoms of PTSD have resolved, the disorder does not recur. This is based on the idea that PTSD is an adaptational response to an event.[3] This process begins in the setting of an acute stress reaction which then follows a predictable course that eventually resolves without sequelae. However, emerging evidence suggests that this may not be the case. In particular, Solomon et al.[41] described 35 soldiers with multiple episodes of PTSD who had several exposures to combat. There was support for both the concept that the original PTSD was reactivated in some soldiers, whereas in others the second episode may have been substantially independent of the first.

Both clinical and biological data suggest that a significant number of individuals undergo a series of psychological and neurobiological changes in PTSD that have permanent sequelae, even when the disorder remits. These may include permanent modification of the individual's vulnerability to a range of psychiatric disorders, which may or may not be triggered by subsequent adverse life experience. Mellman et al.[42] suggested that the comorbid disorders triggered by PTSD, particularly panic disorder, major depressive disorder, and phobias, become increasing autonomous in their pattern of recurrence. This propensity of the concurrent disorder to have a recurrent course may, in fact, be one of the critical long-term consequences of trauma.[26] A further issue is whether the constellation of symptoms in PTSD changes with the passage of time. For example, interpersonal estrangement and emotional detachment may dominate the picture as intrusive memories become less dominant. This may have important implications for treatment as the effectiveness of different strategies may change according to the stage of the disorder.[40]

Implications for Neurobiology

This summary of the longitudinal course of PTSD highlights the complexity of the matrix onto which any neurobiological studies are superimposed. First, the differential course of PTSD in different subjects suggests that a range of different modifying factors could be reflected in the individual's neurobiological profile. Second, the differential course of the intrusive, avoidant, and hyperarousal subcategories of symptoms suggests that in fact there may not be a unifying neurobiology of this disorder; rather, the neurobiology should be investigated in relation to each of these symptom subcategories. The importance of this issue is further highlighted by the frequency of comorbidity with other psychiatric disorders. Whatever neurobiological abnormalities are thought to underpin PTSD must also be congruent with the existing neurobiological theories, particularly those of disorders such as major depression and panic.

The difference in characterization between the extremely chronic forms of PTSD after World War I and the more recent formulations that have emerged since the flourishing of research in 1980 suggest that it is important not to lose sight of the negative symptoms of this disorder. The neurobiology of the withdrawal and the intolerance of environmental stimuli is an issue that is very poorly addressed by treatment and has had little specific investigation of its neurobiology. Such research may also make an important contribution to the understanding of these phenomena and illnesses such as schizophrenia, given the many clinical commonalities and the recent documentation of posttraumatic phenomena in over 50% people who have an acute psychotic episode.[43]

Finally, a great deal of attention has been paid to the role of memory in PTSD. The observation that the intrusive phenomena are relatively nonspecific and become less dominant in the phenomenology of the disorder with the passage of time suggests that this emphasis should not be exclusive of a consideration of the other dimensions of the disorder. As will be discussed, it is possible[44] that in the chronic disorder the intrusive memories may be a secondary consequence of the disturbance of selective attention and working memory in the disorder, rather than solely a primary imprinting of the traumatic memories and the underlying biological concomitance. This suggests that one of the challenges of understanding the neurobiology of PTSD is to grapple with these counterintuitive relationships.

Neural Networks and PTSD

The complexity of the biological matrix underpinning PTSD and its trajectory on time suggests the need to have some theoretical model to underpin these apparently contradictory observations. There needs to be a constant interplay between the development of theory and research findings as an on-going process. As Kuhn[45] said, "the road to a firm research consensus is extraordinarily arduous. . . . in the absence of a paradigm or candidate paradigm, all of the facts could possibly pertain to the development of a given science are likely to seem equally relevant" (p15). One possible paradigm that may help integrate these divergent observations are neural network models. They provide a way of conceptualizing the transition across time of the phenomenological and neurobiological changes in this disorder. In particular, they address one of the critical questions.

This leads to one of the fundamental questions about PTSD, namely, how the acute response to what is often a single stressor of brief duration merges into the constellation of PTSD symptoms. A neural network model provides one hypothesis for the process by which the intrusive and distressing recollections following a trauma could potentially drive the biological and psychological dimensions that give rise to the disorder. This hypothesis is derived from the knowledge of how complex associated networks can be trained and modified and, as a result, how the brain processes, utilizes, and is modified by information[46] and is an adaptation of neural network models which have been usefully applied to other psychiatric disorders such as schizophrenia, obsessive compulsive disorder, and dissociative disorders. This is based on the proposition that intrusive thoughts occurring immediately following a traumatic event may modify neural networks in the brain through a series of predictable biological events and mechanisms, and lead to the more complex biobehavioral syndrome of PTSD. Thus, it is proposed that an individual's cognitive and affective adaptability is actually impaired by the dominance of his/her own internal memories. This model further proposes that the process of symptom exacerbation reflects the behavior of modified neural networks as a consequence of "pruning" and "top down activation." This, in turn, interferes with the development of more flexible meaning networks to explain and integrate the trauma, and it leads to other syndromal features of the disorder.

Thus, the catecholamines may both set the gain of the cortical association networks and thereby facilitate the processing of the traumatic stimuli but also secondarily be regulated by the affective valence of the memory via the amygdala and their conceptual representations in the cortex. The central noradrenaline system is one of the few systems in which the afferents have widely dispersed projections. Therefore, it stands in contrast to other neurotransmitter systems which are more localized and which generally carry specific information to circumscribed regions. The function of the noradrenergic system is that it sets the "signal-to-noise" ratio of the brain.[47] Thus, this system carries relatively nonspecific information to many areas, and in this capacity can influence and integrate the activity of other neurotransmitters and brain regions in a coordinated way. If this noradrenergic system is functionally altered, this will have consequences for the responsiveness and coordination of the brain. The neuroanatomical origin of the noradrenergic system is the locus coeruleus, a nucleus thought to be important in modulating cortical information processing. Evidence for this function comes from neuroanatomical lesion studies.

Abnormalities of this system are central to most biological theories of PTSD; however, debate about their exact nature and consequences is on-going.

Furthermore in primates, in particular, the noradrenergic terminal domains exhibit regional and laminar enervation patterns.[48] This distribution indicates that although locus coeruleus afferents provide nonspecific information to the cortex, their terminal fields are pattern-specific, that is, they modulate cortical information processing. Examination of these targets shows that they coincide with many of the regions forming the widely distributed cortical networks described by Goldman-Rakic.[49] This is a more complex process which was suggested by Kolb, escape from higher controls leading to the alarm reactions typical of PTSD. Similarly, it indicates that the animal model of inescapable electric shock is a paradigm that does not take into account the dynamic process involved in the early integration of traumatic memories. Activation of the dopamine and noradrenergic systems may be a consequence of both the intense arousal and fear experienced during the traumatic event and also the secondary process of reworking trauma-related memories. This secondary process may be more vulnerable to destabilization in humans than the initial reaction during the traumatic event.

CONCLUSION

In the last few years it has become apparent that the syndrome of PTSD is far more than a simple extension of the normative stress response. First, PTSD only develops in a proportion of individuals who are exposed to a traumatic event, whereas in most individuals the acute stress response symptoms typically abate within weeks following the traumatic event. Second, in some individuals PTSD symptoms first emerge months, years, or even decades after exposure to a traumatic event. In others, there may be a lifelong pattern of oscillating between active PTSD and remitted symptoms. These examples illustrate that PTSD may involve a complex set of antecedents as well as a cascade of biobehavioral changes. Thus, realistic models for the development of PTSD must account for a modification of a range of biological systems. These modifications may or may not be fully manifest over time and may in turn be affected by multiple variables.

REFERENCES

1. ARCHIBALD, H. & R. TUDDENHAM. 1965. Persistent stress reaction after combat: A twenty year follow up. Arch. Gen. Psychiatry **12:** 475-481.
2. SOLOMON, Z., N. LAOR & A. C. MCFARLANE. 1996. Acute posttraumatic reactions. *In* Traumatic Stress: The Effects of Overwhelming Experience on Mind, Body and Society. B. Van der Kolk, A. C. McFarlane & L. Weisaeth, Eds., Guilford. New York.
3. YEHUDA, R. & A. C. MCFARLANE. 1995. Conflict between current knowledge about PTSD and its original conceptual basis. Am. J. Psychiatry **152:** 1705-1713.
4. AMERICAN PSYCHIATRIC ASSOCIATION. 1980. Diagnostic and Statistical Manual of Mental Disorders (DSM-III), 3rd Ed. American Psychiatric Press. Washington, DC.
5. HELZER, J. E., L. N. ROBINS & L. MCEVOY. 1987. Post-traumatic stress disorder in the general population: Findings of the Epidemiologic Catchment Area survey. N. Engl. J. Med. **317:** 1630-1634.
6. AMERICAN PSYCHIATRIC ASSOCIATION. 1994. Diagnostic and Statistical Manual of Mental Disorders (DSM-IV), 4th Ed. American Psychiatric Press. Washington, DC.
7. WORLD HEALTH ORGANISATION. 1992. ICD-10 Classification of Mental and Behavioural Disorders: Clinical Descriptions and Diagnostic Guidelines. World Health Organization. Geneva.
8. KESSLER, R., A. SONNEGA, E. BROMET & C. B. NELSON. 1995. Posttraumatic stress disorder in the National Comorbidity Survey. Arch. Gen. Psychiatry **52:** 1048-1060.
9. NORRIS, F. H. 1992. Epidemiology of trauma: Frequency and impact of different potentially traumatic events on different demographic groups. J. Consult. Clin. Psychol. **60:** 409-418.
10. MCFARLANE, A. C. 1996. Attitudes to victims: Issues for medicine, the law and society. *In* Int. Victimology: Selected Papers from the 8th International Symposium. C. Sumner, M. Israel, M. O'Connell & R. Sarre, Eds.: 259-275. Australian Institute of Criminology. Canberra.
11. ATCHISON, M. & A. C. MCFARLANE. 1994. A review of dissociation and dissociative disorders. Aust. NZ J. Psychiatry **28:** 591-599.
12. VAN DER KOLK, B. A. 1996. Trauma and Memory. *In* Traumatic Stress: The Effects of Overwhelming Experience on Mind, Body and Society. B. Van der Kolk, A. C. McFarlane, & L. Weisaeth, Eds. Guilford. New York.
13. HOLEN, A. 1990. A long term study of survivors from a disaster. The Alexander L. Kielland Disaster in Perspective. Oslo University Press. Oslo.
14. SPIEGEL, D. 1990. Dissociation and trauma. *In* Review of Psychiatry, Vol 10. A. Tasman & S. M. Goldfinger, Eds. American Psychiatric Press. Washington, DC.
15. BREMNER, J. D., J. H. KRYSTAL, S. M. SOUTHWICK & D. S. CHARNEY. 1995. Functional neuroanatomical correlates of the effects of stress on memory. J. Traumatic Stress **8:** 527-553.
16. BREMNER, J. D., P. RANDALL, T. M. SCOTT, R. A. BRONEN, J. P. SEIBYL, S. M. SOUTHWICK, R. C. DELANEY, G. MCCARTHY, D. S. CHARNEY & R. B. INNIS. 1995. MRI-based measurement of hippocampal volume in patients with combat-related posttraumatic stress disorder. Am. J. Psychiatry. **152:** 973-981.
17. SHALEV, A. Y., T. PERI, L. CANETTI & S. SCHREIBER. 1996. Predictors of PTSD in injured trauma survivors: A prospective study. Am. J. Psychiatry **153:** 219-225.
18. KOOPMAN, C., C. CLASSEN & D. SPIEGEL. 1994. Predictors of posttraumatic stress symptoms among survivors of the Oakland/Berkeley, Calif., Firestorm. Am. J. Psychiatry **151:** 888-894.
19. WEISS, D. S., C. R. MARMAR, T. J. METZLER & H. M. RONFELDT. 1995. Predicting symptomatic distress in emergency services personnel. J. Consult. Clin. Psychol. **63:** 361-368.
20. MALT, U., S. KARLEHAGEN, H. HOFF, U. HERRSTROMER, K. HILDINGSON, E. TIBELL & H. LEYMANN. 1993. The effect of major railway accidents on the psychological health

of train drivers. I. Acute psychological responses to accident. J. Psychosom. Res. **37:** 793–805.

21. MALT, U. F. & O. M. OLAFSEN. 1992. Psychological appraisal and emotional response to physical injury: A clinical, phenomenological study of 109 adults. Psychiatric Med. **10:** 117–134.

22. LUNDIN, T. 1996. Psychological morbidity after the Estonia Ferry Disaster. Presented at the 2nd World Conference ISTSS. Jerusalem, June 1996.

23. BRESLAU, N., G. C. DAVIS, P. ANDERSKI & E. PETERSON. 1991. Traumatic events and posttraumatic stress disorder in an urban population of young adults. Arch. Gen. Psychiatry **48:** 216–222.

24. KULKA, R. A., W. E. SCHLENGER, J. A. FAIRBANK & R. HOUGH. 1990. Trauma and the Vietnam War Generation: Report of Findings from the National Vietnam Veterans Readjustment Study. Brunner/Mazel. New York.

25. BLANK, A. S. 1993. The longitudinal course of posttraumatic stress disorder. *In* Post Traumatic Stress Disorder: DSM IV and Beyond. J. R. T. Davidson & E. Foa, Eds. American Psychiatric Association Press. Washington, DC.

26. MCFARLANE, A. C. & P. PAPAY. 1992. Multiple diagnoses in posttraumatic stress disorder in the victims of a natural disaster. J. Nerv. Ment. Dis. **180:** 498–504.

27. MAYOU, R., B. BRYANT & R. DUTHIE. 1993. Psychiatric consequences of road traffic accidents. Br. Med. J. **307:** 647–651.

28. GRACE, M. C., B. L. GREEN, J. D. LINDY & A. C. LEONARD. 1993. The Buffalo Creek Disaster: A 14-Year Follow-up. *In* International Handbook of Traumatic Stress Syndromes. J. P. Wilson & B. Raphael, Eds.: 441–449 Plenum Press. New York.

29. SOLOMON, S. D. & G. J. CANINO. 1990. Appropriateness of DSM-III-R criteria for posttraumatic stress disorder. Comp. Psychiatry **31:** 227–237.

30. KARDINER, A. 1941. The Traumatic Neuroses of War. P. Hoeber. New York.

31. LEE, K. A., G. E. VAILLANT, W. C. TORREY & G. H. ELDER. 1995. A 50-year prospective study of the psychological sequelae of World War II combat. Am. J. Psychiatry **152:** 516–522.

32. EITINGER, L. & A. STROM. 1973. Mortality and Morbidity after Excessive Stress: A Follow-up Investigation of Norwegian Concentration Camps Survivors. Humanities Press. New York.

33. ASKEVOLD, F. 1980. The war sailor syndrome. Danish Med. Bull. **27:** 220–224.

34. SCHNURR, P. P., M. J. FRIEDMAN & S. D. ROSENBERG. 1993. Premilitary MMPI scores as predictors of combat-related PTSD symptoms. Am. J. Psychiatry **150:** 479–483.

35. BRESLAU, N. & G. C. DAVIS. 1992. Posttraumatic stress disorder in an urban population of young adults: Risk factors for chronicity. Am. J. Psychiatry **149:** 671–675.

36. VAN DER KOLK, B. A. 1989. The compulsion to repeat the trauma: Re-enactment, revictimization, and masochism. Psychiatr. Clin. N. Am. **12:** 389–411.

37. HERMAN, J. 1992. Trauma and Recovery. Basic Books. New York.

38. SAXE, G. N., B. A. VAN DER KOLK, R. BERKOWITZ, G. CHINMAN, K. HALL, G. LIEBERG & J. SCHWARTZ. 1993. Dissociative disorders in psychiatric inpatients. Am. J. Psychiatry **150:** 1037–1042.

39. DAVIDSON, J. R., D. HUGHES, D. G. BLAZER & L. K. GEORGE. 1991. Posttraumatic stress disorder in the community: An epidemiological study. Psychol. Med. **21:** 713–721.

40. MCFARLANE, A. C. 1994. Individual psychotherapy for posttraumatic stress disorder. Psychiatr. Clin. N. Am. **17:** 393–408.

41. SOLOMON, Z., R. GARB, A. BLEICH & D. GRUPPER. 1987. Reactivation of combat-related posttraumatic stress disorder. Am J. Psychiatry **144:** 51–55.

42. MELLMAN, T. A., C. A. RANDOLPH, O. BRAWMAN-MINTZER, L. P. FLORES & F. J. MILANES. 1992. Phenomenology and course of psychiatric disorders associated with combat-related posttraumatic stress disorder. Am. J. Psychiatry **149:** 1568–1574.

43. SHAW, K., A. C. MCFARLANE & C. B. BOOKLESS. 1997. The phenomenology of traumatic reactions to psychotic illness. J. Nervous Mental Dis. In press.

44. McFarlane, A. C., D. Weber & C. R. Clark. 1993. Abnormal stimulus processing in posttraumatic stress disorder. Biol. Psychiatry. **34:** 311-320.
45. Kuhn, T. S. 1962. The Structure of Scientific Revolutions. University of Chicago Press. Chicago.
46. Cohen, J. D. & D. Servan-Schreiber. 1992. Introduction to neural network models in psychiatry. Psychiatr. Ann. **22:** 113-118.
47. Harley, C. W. 1987. A role for epinephrine in arousal, emotion and learning? Progr. Neuropsychopharmacol. Biol. Psychiatry **11:** 419-458.
48. Clark, C. R., G. M. Geffen & L. B. Geffen. 1987. Catecholamines and attention. II. Pharmacological studies in normal humans. Neurosci. Biobehav. Rev. **11:** 353-364.
49. Goldman-Rakic, P. S. 1990. Topography of cognition. Ann. Rev. Neurosci. **11:** 137-156.

Comorbid Psychiatric Disorders in PTSD

Implications for Research

TERENCE M. KEANE AND DANNY G. KALOUPEK

Department of Veterans Affairs Medical Center
150 S. Huntington Ave.
Boston, Massachusetts 02130

Boston University School of Medicine
Boston, Massachusetts 02118

Problems associated with high rates of comorbidity in posttraumatic stress disorder (PTSD) were initially identified by Fairbank et al.[1] who conducted an empirical study of the psychological characteristics of Vietnam veterans with PTSD, comparing them to veterans with other psychiatric disorders and veterans who were well adjusted. High rates of depression and anxiety were found to be associated with a clinician's diagnosis of PTSD. The authors recognized the importance of elevations in concurrent psychiatric conditions for both research and treatment in the area of PTSD and suggested that future research should specify the precise nature of comorbidity among individuals with PTSD.

In a subsequent study, Keane et al.[2] identified high rates of substance abuse among individuals with PTSD. Veterans with PTSD reported problems with alcohol and drug abuse and also high rates of intake of nicotine and caffeine. These projects were among the first to collect objective data using diagnostic interviews on the problem of comorbidity in PTSD.

This paper organizes the extant information on the high rates of comorbidity observed in PTSD. We evaluate the extent to which the high rates of comorbidity are a function solely of concurrent problems in military veterans or if they are a more pervasive finding, and we suggest methodological strategies that may improve and enhance the quality of biological and psychological research conducted in this area.

LITERATURE REVIEW ON COMORBIDITY

Clinical Studies

In addition to the studies conducted in our laboratory, other groups were noticing the same trend of high rates of comorbidity in veterans with PTSD. Sierles et al.[3] examined a group of 25 inpatients with PTSD at the North Chicago VA Medical Center and learned that 84% of these patients met criteria for another disorder. Using the schedule for affective disorders and schizophrenia (SADS) they found that patients with PTSD frequently met criteria for alcoholism (64%) and antisocial personality disorder (48%). In addition, 72% of the patients reported a history of depression, although they did not meet criteria for formal diagnosis at the time of the study. Unfortunately, no comparison group was included in this study and so it was impossible to determine if the rates of comorbidity observed among veterans were greater for PTSD than for any other psychological disorder. Nonetheless, this was the first study to employ a comprehensive structured diagnostic interview for measuring both PTSD and the collateral disorders.

In a follow-up study, Sierles et al.[4] employed the same method with a sample of 25 PTSD outpatients. Their findings, also utilizing the SADS, indicated that 76% of these patients met criteria for alcoholism, 64% for an antisocial personality disorder, and 84% for at least one other disorder in addition to PTSD. Major affective disorder was found in 84% of the patients either at the current time or throughout lifetime. Again, the absence of a specific comparison group of patients with disorders other than PTSD limited the conclusions drawn in this study; however, clearly these investigations solidified the evidentiary base upon which future studies examining comorbidity were conducted.

Using the NIMH-Diagnostic Interview Schedule (DIS; Robins et al.[5]), Escobar and his colleagues[6] examined Hispanic veterans receiving care at the Los Angeles VA Outpatient Clinic. Studying 20 patients, all of whom were clinically diagnosed with PTSD, they found that PTSD patients had an average of 3.5 DSM-III lifetime diagnoses. The leading comorbid diagnosis was alcohol dependence (65%), followed by social phobia (50%), drug dependence (40%), major depression (35%), and schizophrenia (35%). While this study found high rates of comorbidity in patients with PTSD, the use of the DIS in clinical settings may present problems of reliability and validity. This is particularly problematic for diagnoses such as PTSD and schizophrenia where many symptoms appear to be overlapping and further intensive follow-up questioning is not possible. Yet these data are consistent with findings from other studies that used different diagnostic instruments. The high rates of comorbid schizophrenia are a likely result of the use of the DIS.

In a study designed to examine the interrelationship of substance abuse and PTSD, Keane et al.[7] interviewed 25 Vietnam veterans seeking treatment at the Boston VA Medical Center using a multimethod procedure that included clinician interviews, psychological tests, and psychophysiological assessment (cf, Keane et al.[8]; Malloy et al.[9]). Doctoral level clinicians using the Structured Clinical Interview for the DSM-III-R (SCID; Spitzer and Williams[10]) observed that 44% of PTSD patients met current diagnostic criteria for either drug abuse or drug dependence. In addition, 64% met criteria for alcohol abuse or dependence, and a total of 80% of the sample met diagnostic criteria for some form of substance abuse or dependence at the time that they sought treatment. Unfortunately, the focus of this study was on substance abuse and did not, therefore, include a more comprehensive range of psychiatric diagnoses.

Keane and Wolfe[11] selected randomly 50 outpatients seeking psychological treatment for PTSD. In this study, SCIDs were administered to all subjects so that a more complete view of comorbidity rates among help-seeking veterans with PTSD could be determined. This study found high rates of alcoholism (84%), drug abuse (42%), depression (68%), dysthymia (34%), and personality disorders, typically antisocial personality disorder (26%). The mean number of diagnoses in this sample was 3.8 including the PTSD diagnosis. The findings regarding the presence of personality disorders were replicated and extended by Southwick *et al.*[12] who found extensive evidence for borderline personality disorder in their patients. While these studies replicated the findings of Sierles and his colleagues[3,4] who found high rates of comorbidity among samples of veterans with PTSD, they still did not provide any comparative information on comorbidity across diagnoses other than PTSD. The strengths of these studies clearly were in the use of structured diagnostic clinician-administered interviews for determining both the PTSD diagnosis and the rates of comorbidity.

Evidence for high rates of comorbidity also comes from Keane *et al.*[13] who examined 1,328 outpatient Vietnam theater help-seeking veterans using the SCID. This project also confirmed the high rates of comorbidity in PTSD and, importantly, these rates were found across 15 different medical centers in the United States employing nearly 30 different doctoral level diagnosticians. In this study, rates of major depressive disorder were high (36%) as were those of alcoholism (24%), drug abuse (12%), borderline personality disorder (18%), and antisocial personality disorder (ASPD) (11%).

It is clear from these preliminary studies that at least among patients who are seeking treatment for PTSD, the overwhelming majority of them present with a wide range of symptoms other than those directly associated with PTSD criteria. In fact, these individuals, who are primarily Vietnam veterans with PTSD, meet criteria for an additional three DSM diagnostic categories. The data, however, are limited by the fact that they have included only male, combat-related PTSD patients who are seeking help. Naturally, these characteristics might potentially yield biased conclusions that differ in important ways from PTSD secondary to other traumatic events and PTSD in women. Even more fundamentally, veterans with combat-related PTSD, but who are not help seeking at VA medical centers, may also present a different diagnostic picture from that of veterans seeking treatment.

Field Survey Studies

Data from population-based surveys might provide important new information to assist us in determining the true rates of comorbidity among individuals with PTSD. Given that all the preceding studies involved subjects obtaining treatment, field surveys may provide important new and different information regarding comorbidity. Perhaps those subjects who are seeking help differ fundamentally from those with the disorder, but who are not seeking help.

The Vietnam Experience Study[14] evaluated the psychological characteristics of 2,490 Vietnam Army veterans and 1,972 Vietnam era veterans using the DIS. Among Vietnam veterans, 15% had a lifetime diagnosis of PTSD and 2.2% had the disorder within 1 month of the interview. Among those who met criteria for PTSD during the last month, 66% also met criteria for another anxiety or depressive disorder and 39% fulfilled criteria for alcohol abuse or dependence. Thus, in a community-based sample of veterans, PTSD is frequently associated with anxiety, depression, and substance abuse. Although this particular study relied on the DIS for diagnosing PTSD, its findings still supported the concept of high rates of comorbidity among non-help-seeking Vietnam veterans with PTSD.

In possibly the most comprehensive and thorough psychiatric epidemiological study conducted to date of Vietnam veterans' psychological adjustment, Kulka *et al.*[15] evaluated 3,016 Vietnam veterans, Vietnam era veterans, and civilian controls. Veterans were randomly selected from military records with women, blacks, Hispanics, and physically disabled veterans oversampled intentionally. High rates of comorbidity were observed among those veterans with PTSD. Substance abuse (73%) was easily the most prevalent accompanying disorder, with antisocial personality disorder (31%) and major depression (28%) also co-occurring with some frequency. Most impressive was the finding that 98.9% of all those diagnosed with PTSD met criteria for at least one other diagnosis. These findings from a field study confirm the high rates of comorbidity of PTSD with other conditions in combat-related PTSD.

Clearly, PTSD in Vietnam theater veterans is associated with meeting criteria for other disorders whether the samples were drawn from the clinic or the community or when comprehensive diagnostic interviews were used to evaluate veterans. Studies of clinical patients and community subjects also found a consistent association of PTSD with alcohol and drug abuse, major depressive disorder, dysthymia, and ASPD. Information regarding comorbidity rates needs to be obtained from other samples of traumatized patients and, in particular, from women with PTSD.

Studies of Female Subjects

In a study of 277 female victims of a recent sexual or nonsexual assault, Cashman *et al.*[18] presented information on the high rates of comorbidity among those subjects who developed acute PTSD as well as those subjects who developed a chronic form of the condition. With respect to Axis I disorders, both the acute and chronic cases of PTSD developed high rates of major depressive disorder (approximately 60% of the cases). In addition, substance abuse was present in approximately 25% of the cases and was represented equally in both the acute and chronic forms of PTSD. In terms of Axis 2 personality disorders, Cashman *et al.*[16] found high rates of paranoid personality disorder nearing 30% in both the acute and chronic forms of PTSD. Rates of borderline personality disorder and avoidant personality disorder were nearly 15% in the chronic cases of PTSD, findings that distinguished the acute and chronic forms of the condition.

Similarly, Resick *et al.*[17] presented comorbidity rates in women who developed rape-related PTSD. Among this outpatient help-seeking sample, 58% met diagnostic criteria for major depressive disorder, 39% for a substance abuse disorder, 12% for panic disorder, 12% for simple phobia, and 12% for social phobia. Data from these two research laboratories studying female victims of violent crimes indicate that rates of comorbidity, while not of the same magnitude as those found in veterans, are nonetheless quite high. In addition, the disorders typically associated with combat veterans also appear at high rates in assault victims with PTSD (i.e., depression, substance abuse, anxiety disorders). In the Resick *et al.*[17] study, 76% of female sexual assault victims with PTSD carried a current comorbid psychiatric condition, whereas only 24% of those who had been sexually assaulted but who did not develop PTSD carried a current comorbid condition.

Studies of PTSD and Trauma in Substance Abusers

Further information on the interrelationship of substance abuse and PTSD in women comes from studies of prevalence rates of PTSD among substance abusers seeking treatment. Brown *et al.*[18] examined the prevalence of PTSD among a sample of treatment-seeking, substance-abusing males and females. Approximately one quarter of the sample presented with significant PTSD symptoms. Women had histories of physical and sexual abuse and they also reported experiencing more traumatic life events. These trauma-exposed women, compared to the men, were more likely to have been diagnosed with possible PTSD. In addition, the PTSD group reported more hospitalizations and greater utilization of services than did the non-PTSD cohort.

Similarly, Fullilove *et al.*[19] examined the association of violent events, trauma, and PTSD among female drug users. Of 105 women in the sample, 104 subjects reported one traumatic event or more and 59% of these reported symptoms consistent with the diagnosis of PTSD. Violent assault including sexual and physical assault was the most common precipitant to the development of PTSD. The more traumatic events to which a woman was exposed, the more likely she was to develop PTSD in this substance-abusing population.

National Comorbidity Study

In the National Comorbidity Study, Kessler *et al.*[20] found that, among males, rates of comorbidity with PTSD were approximately 88%, with alcoholism (52%) depression (48%), conduct disorder (43%), drug abuse (35%), and simple phobias (31%) representing the bulk of the concurrent disorders observed. In this premier study, 59% of the PTSD subjects had more than three diagnoses. In contrast, for female subjects Kessler *et al.*[20] found that 79% had an accompanying disorder of one type or another including depression (49%), alcoholism (30%), drug abuse (27%), phobia (29%), and conduct disorder (15%). Among women, 44% had more than three diagnoses associated with PTSD. Interestingly, the Kessler *et al.*[20] epidemiological data suggest that at least among women the occurrence of trauma was more likely to precede the development of substance abuse. This particular finding is supportive of a self-medication model for the comorbidity of substance abuse (alcohol and drug abuse) and PTSD. Yet other studies have not found this particular temporal relationship.

Davidson *et al.*[21] and Bremner *et al.*[22] suggest that PTSD and substance abuse in their samples of combat veterans are initiated concurrently. In addition, it appears from the Bremner *et al.*[22] study that PTSD symptoms and substance abuse track each other in a parallel course (i.e., waxing and waning) over the measurement time period employed in the study.

Interestingly, in a reanalysis of the Epidemiologic Catchment Area study data from St. Louis, Cottler *et al.*[23] found that drug and alcohol abuse preceded the development of PTSD symptoms and presumably the traumatic events; however, the findings of this study are not conclusive because of the way in which data on temporal parameters were collected. This particular study, however, does support the notion that alcohol and drug use can be risk factors for exposure to traumatic events as well as for the development of PTSD, clearly a logical and viable hypothesis.

Summary of Literature Findings

From the foregoing review of the literature on comorbidity in PTSD it seems eminently reasonable to conclude that high rates of comorbidity have been found with respect to PTSD across populations (i.e., males, females, veterans, sexual assault victims, criminal assault victims, and the general population), stressors (i.e., military combat, rape, physical assault, childhood sexual abuse, and violence), patient and nonpatient status (help-seeking patients vs community-residing subjects), diagnostic measures (i.e., SCID, DIS, and self-report measures), and the level of interviewer training (lay interviewers vs doctoral level clinicians). These high rates of comorbidity appear to be most salient in the following disorders: (a) alcohol abuse, (b) drug abuse, (c) depression, (d) anxiety disorders (e.g., phobias and panic disorders), and (e) personality disorders, especially antisocial and borderline.

To explain these levels of comorbidity, clinicians and researchers have relied on various hypotheses including the self-medication hypothesis wherein individuals who develop PTSD on exposure to traumatic events ultimately begin to use substances to alleviate their emotional pain (e.g., Conger[24]). This self-medication or negative reinforcement model of comorbidity clearly explains some of the variance in predicting the rates of substance abuse in PTSD. Given that PTSD is characterized by elevations in arousal, reactivity, and sleep problems, it is not surprising that for a subsection of the PTSD population alcohol and drug use may provide immediate short-term relief from their symptoms.

Others have hypothesized different reasons for the great amount of comorbidity observed in PTSD. Keane and Wolfe[11] pointed out that there is considerable symptom overlap between PTSD and major depression and that symptoms such as arousal, reactivity, and avoidance are often associated with several other key disorders frequently observed in PTSD patients. This high degree of symptom overlap may in fact be responsible for some of the comorbidity observed. Further, Saladin et al.[25] found that symptoms of withdrawal from alcohol and drugs can mimic symptoms of PTSD which may contribute to the overwhelming evidence of comorbidity between these two problems. Furthermore, some researchers have proposed that the belief that alcohol and drugs will alleviate stress or tension (i.e., expectancies) is actually the operative variable in the high levels of alcohol and drug use in PTSD patients (e.g., Brown[26]). Thus, the question raised is whether the high levels of comorbidity observed in epidemiological and clinical studies may simply be an epiphenomenon of the diagnostic criteria employed for all these disorders.

A second possible explanation for high levels of comorbidity was offered by Hyer et al.[27] who found consistently that individuals with PTSD tend to report higher levels of symptoms than do individuals with other disorders. Is this high level of comorbidity between PTSD and other diagnostic categories simply a function of symptom overreporting? Or is it a function of global levels of distress that are apparent in PTSD? The extent to which these factors are responsible for or contribute to the levels of comorbidity in PTSD has not been addressed to date. It is clearly worthy of empirical testing.

Others have promoted the idea that the high levels of comorbidity in PTSD patients are actually a risk factor for the development of PTSD and that these disorders were present prior to trauma exposure. Indeed, the Kessler et al.[20] study provided some evidence that the substance abuse diagnoses appear to follow in a systematic way exposure to trauma and the development of PTSD. However, it is also clear from many studies in the literature that individuals who have a history of psychological or behavioral problems are at elevated risk for the development of PTSD (e.g., Kulka *et al.*[15]). Undoubtedly, a subsection of individuals carry either genetic, social, or familial vulnerabilities that are risk factors for the development of major psychiatric disorders following exposure to high magnitude stressors. It is also, indeed, likely that many individuals who develop PTSD on exposure to one or more traumatic events are inclined to have used alcohol simply because of its availability, the expectancies associated with alcohol and drug use, and the immediate short-term relief often experienced upon intoxication.

Other studies have challenged the relationship of PTSD and substance abuse by relying on measures of early childhood conduct problems and adolescent drug abuse to predict the development of long-term drug and alcohol problems. Reifman and Windle,[28] reexamining the Vietnam Experience Study, found that drug use in the Army was the single best predictor of current levels of drug use. Similarly, Boscarino[29] failed to find any relation between combat exposure and drug use. Premorbid variables such as conduct disorder and juvenile delinquency emerged as the strongest predictors of current alcohol and drug use. Clearly more research is needed to untangle these close interrelationships, but it should be clear to clinicians and researchers alike that there is a subpopulation of individuals with PTSD who have major psychological problems or predispositions prior to exposure to traumatic events which make it likely that they will subsequently develop PTSD. It should also be clear that for at least some individuals with one or multiple traumatic events and with serious psychological sequelae attendant to these events, these factors can unleash a cascade of psychological and social problems that continue to complicate their lives over time.

RESEARCH IMPLICATIONS OF HIGH LEVELS OF COMORBIDITY

With the relative explosion of research in the area of PTSD, several caveats must be highlighted to alert researchers to possible problems in the interpretation of findings. One primary concern that is particularly relevant for biological and psychosocial research is that PTSD may in fact be a marker variable for other ongoing factors that are more directly responsible for findings on various objective indices. For example, several research studies have found that PTSD is associated with elevations in risk factors for a variety of health-related behavioral problems. Litz *et al.*[30] found differences between PTSD and non-PTSD subjects on a wide range of health risk behaviors. These differences included items such as (a) nutritional differences, (b) differences in exercise regimens practiced, (c) elevated smoking rates, (d) elevated caffeine intake, (e) distinctions in available housing and homelessness, and, of course, (f) high rates of alcohol and drug use.

Each of these factors individually or collectively may directly influence findings in biological and psychological research. Efforts to rule out the contributions of each of these variables may help us to understand what is uniquely a function of PTSD and what is a function of disorganized life styles and addictive practices. Future research should consider measuring as many of these variables as possible in order to covary the relationships of these confounding factors from the objective measures of interest (e.g., Keane *et al.*[13]).

There are additional research implications of finding high rates of comorbidity among PTSD patients. Clearly, the PTSD population is relatively heterogeneous.

Patients with four diagnoses differ from patients with solely the PTSD diagnosis probably on multiple variables of importance and interest in research. Clearly these differences could be the result of greater symptom severity or else the presence of preexisting risk factors for developing the disorder once an individual is exposed to a traumatic event. In either case, PTSD appears to be a heterogeneous disorder with multiple subpopulations. Examining these subtypes of patients in biological or psychological studies without identifying them in data analyses may lead to erroneous conclusions. Rejecting the null hypothesis when it should not be rejected (a Type I error) is one possibility, but probably more likely is accepting the null hypothesis when in fact differences do exist but they are clouded by population heterogeneity. It seems reasonable to conclude that the biology of PTSD may vary if one has a single psychological disorder rather than multiple psychological conditions. It also seems likely that the biology of PTSD might vary if one is traumatized when these already are existing psychological conditions (e.g., major depressive disorder). Identifying, labeling, and analyzing for these differences may promote a more coherent understanding of the biological and psychological factors associated with PTSD.

The findings of high rates of comorbidity in PTSD lead us to make several discrete recommendations for research on biological and psychological factors and the evaluations of treatment interventions. First, and perhaps foremost, is the need for the use of critical or key comparison groups. Employing groups of subjects that carry only the PTSD diagnosis and comparing them to groups of subjects with PTSD and a major depressive disorder, for instance, may help us to disentangle any confounding effects of the presence of major depression, a commonly associated condition. Similarly, comparing subjects with comorbid substance abuse and PTSD to a PTSD only group will help us to understand the contribution of substance abuse to any findings observed. This type of design may complement the more typical studies that look at PTSD groups versus trauma exposure without PTSD versus individuals with other psychological traumas versus groups with no trauma exposure at all. Simply comparing PTSD to normal controls will not help us to disentangle the effects of the high rates of comorbidity and may further contribute to false leads in our understanding of PTSD.

An additional strategy to be employed in research is to ensure that levels of comorbidity are known and measured for both presence and absence of comorbid conditions, but perhaps even more importantly in terms of overall severity. This will provide key information for employing statistical methods such as covariance to control for the contributions of these concurrent conditions. To use statistical control has a long history in psychological research and is now being introduced more frequently in biological research in mental health. This trend needs to be supported and continued particularly as it applies to the study of PTSD.

A third recommendation is to employ psychometric methods in efforts to understand what is associated with PTSD and what is associated with other existing conditions. The use of methods developed for convergent and discriminant validity may help in this regard. Convergent validity recommends the use of multiple measures that should agree with one another when certain constructs are measured. Discriminant validity methods also use multiple measurement tools that should diverge when certain known conditions are met. The use of convergent and discriminant validity will assist in understanding what factors are due to PTSD predominantly and what factors might be a function of the levels of comorbidity in a given group of patients.

One final strategy that may help us to understand the role of comorbidity is to insure the measurement of functioning for all subject groups contained within a particular study. Utilizing a measure such as the Global Assessment of Functioning from Axis 5 of the DSM-IV may provide one index upon which subjects differing in levels of comorbidity are compared. In this way various biological or psychological variables found to be different in a particular research study can, through statistical means, be attributed to factors other than differences in overall levels of functioning.

SUMMARY

It is clear from the existing data that PTSD often occurs in the context of other major psychological conditions. Evidence to support this comes from clinical studies, epidemiological studies, and studies of PTSD among substance abusers. Clearly, probably several different subgroups of PTSD patients exist including those who had psychological or behavioral problems before exposure to traumatic events (e.g., substance abuse), those who developed other problems concurrent with exposure to the traumatic events, and those who developed problems secondary to the development of PTSD, perhaps in efforts to cope with the intensely debilitating symptoms of PTSD.

With this knowledge, research on PTSD must begin to contend with the comorbidity issue in systematic ways. The use of comparison groups that are carefully selected is one key way in which conclusions about PTSD can be most conservatively drawn. The use of statistical procedures to control for difference in levels of comorbidity is another responsible way in which to approach the problem. Finally, efforts to employ global measures of functioning such as the Global Assessment of Functioning to equate subjects within a study on minimally this characteristic may be the most economical method for trying to rule out the role of comorbidity and severity of condition in conclusions drawn in research studies. All these solutions presuppose the careful measurement of comorbidity in studies of PTSD, a recommendation that requires serious consideration for researchers operating in this field.

REFERENCES

1. FAIRBANK, J. A., T. M. KEANE & P. F. MALLOY. 1983. Some preliminary data on the psychological characteristics of Vietnam veterans with posttraumatic stress disorders. J. Consulting Clin. Psychol. **51:** 912–919.
2. KEANE, T. M., J. M. CADDELL, B. W. MARTIN, R. T. ZIMERING & J. A. FAIRBANK. 1983. Substance abuse among Vietnam veterans with posttraumatic stress disorders. Bull. Soc. Psychologists Addict. Behav. **2:** 117–122.
3. SIERLES, F. S., J. CHEN, R. E. MCFARLAND & M. A. TAYLOR. 1983. Post-traumatic stress disorder and concurrent psychiatric illness. Am. J. Psychiatry **140:** 1177–1179.
4. SIERLES, F. S., J. CHEN, M. L. MESSING, J. K. BESYNER & M. A. TAYLOR. 1986. Concurrent psychiatric illness in non-Hispanic outpatients diagnosed as having posttraumatic stress disorder. J. Nerv. Ment. Dis. **174:** 171–173.

5. ROBINS, L. N., J. E. HELZER, J. L. CROUGHAN, J. B. W. WILLIAMS & R. L. SPITZER. 1981. NIMH diagnostic interview schedule. Version III (Publication No. ADM-T-42-# [5-81, 8-81]). NIMH, Public Health Service. Rockville, MD.

6. ESCOBAR, J. I., E. T. RANDOLPH, G. PUENTE, F. SPIWAK, J. K. ASAMEN, M. HILL & R. L. HOUGH. 1983. Posttraumatic stress disorder in Hispanic Vietnam veterans: Clinical phenomenology and sociocultural characteristics. J. Nerv. Ment. Dis. 171: 585-596.

7. KEANE, T. M., R. J. GERARDI, J. A. LYONS & J. WOLFE. 1988. The interrelationship of substance abuse and posttraumatic stress disorder. In Recent Developments in Alcoholism. M. Galanter, Ed. Vol. 6: 27-48. Plenum. New York.

8. KEANE, T. M., J. WOLFE & K. L. TAYLOR. 1987. Posttraumatic stress disorder: Evidence for diagnostic validity and methods of psychological assessment. J. Clin. Psychol. 43: 32-43.

9. MALLOY, P. F., J. A. FAIRBANK & T. M. KEANE. 1983. Validation of a multimethod assessment of posttraumatic stress disorders in Vietnam veterans. J. Consult. Clin. Psychol. 51: 488-494.

10. SPITZER, R. L. & J. B. WILLIAMS. 1985. Structured clinical interview for DSM-III-R. Patient version. Biometrics Research Department of New York State Psychiatric Institute. New York.

11. KEANE, T. M. & J. WOLFE. 1990. Comorbidity in post-traumatic stress disorder: An analysis of community and clinical studies. J. Applied Soc. Psychol. 20: 1776-1788.

12. SOUTHWICK, S. M., R. YEHUDA & E. L. GILLER. 1993. Personality disorders in treatment-seeking combat veterans with posttraumatic stress disorder. Am. J. Psychiatry 150: 1020-1023.

13. KEANE, T. M., L. COLB, D. KALOUPEK, S. ORR, E. BLANCHARD, R. THOMAS, F. HSIEH & P. LAVORI. 1996. A psychophysiological study of chronic combat-related PTSD: Results from a Department of Veteran Affairs cooperative study. Unpublished manuscript.

14. CENTERS FOR DISEASE CONTROL. 1988. Vietnam Experience Study: Psychological and Neuropsychological Evaluation. Vol. 4. C.D.C. Atlanta, GA.

15. KULKA, R. A., W. E. SCHLENGER, J. A. FAIRBANK, R. L. HOUGH, B. K. JORDAN, C. R. MARMAR & D. S. WEISS. 1988. National Vietnam veterans readjustment study (NVVRS): Description, current status, and initial PTSD prevalence estimates. Final Report. Veterans Administration. Washington, DC.

16. CASHMAN, L., C. MOLNAR & E. B. FOA. 1995. Comorbidity of DSM-III-R Axis I and II disorders with acute and chronic post-traumatic stress disorder. Paper presented at the 29th annual convention of the Association for the Advancement of Behavior Therapy. Washington, DC.

17. RESICK, P., M. GRIFFIN & M. MECHANIC. 1996. PTSD assessment study. Unpublished manuscript.

18. BROWN, P. J., P. R. RECUPERO & R. STOUT. 1995. PTSD substance abuse comorbidity and treatment utilization. Addict. Behav. 20: 251-254.

19. FULLILOVE, M. T., R. E. FULLILOVE, M. SMITH, K. WINKLER, C. MICHAEL, P. G. PANZER & R. WALLACE. 1993. Violence, trauma, and post-traumatic stress disorder among women drug users. J. Traumatic Stress 6: 533-543.

20. KESSLER, R. C., A. SONNEGA, E. J. BROMET, M. HUGHES & C. B. NELSON. 1995. Posttraumatic stress disorder in the National Comorbidity Survey. Arch. Gen. Psychiatry 52: 1048-1060.

21. DAVIDSON, J. R. T., H. S. KUDLER, W. B. SAUNDERS & R. D. SMITH. 1990. Symptom and comorbidity patterns in World War II and Vietnam veterans with posttraumatic stress disorder. Compr. Psychiatry 31: 162-170.

22. BREMNER, J. D., S. M. SOUTHWICK, A. DARNELL & D. S. CHARNEY. 1996. Chronic PTSD in Vietnam combat veterans: Course of illness and substance abuse. Am. J. Psychiatry 153: 369-375.

23. COTTLER, L. B., W. M. COMPTON, D. MAGER, E. L. SPITZNAGEL & A. JANCA. 1992. Posttraumatic stress disorder among substance users from the general population. Am. J. Psychiatry **149:** 664-670.
24. CONGER, J. J. 1956. Alcoholism: Theory, problem, and challenge II. Reinforcement theory and the dynamics of alcoholism. Q. J. Stud. Alcohol **17:** 296-305.
25. SALADIN, M. E., K. T. BRADY, B. S. DANSKY & D. G. KILPATRICK. 1995. Understanding comorbidity between PTSD and substance use disorders: Two preliminary investigations. Addict. Behav. **20:** 643-655.
26. BROWN, S. A. 1985. Reinforcement expectancies and alcoholism treatment outcome after a one-year follow-up. J. Studies Alcohol **46:** 304-308.
27. HYER, L., J. H. FALLON, W. R. HARRISON & P. A. BOUDEWYNS. 1987. MMPI overreporting by Vietnam combat veterans. J. Clin. Psychol. **43:** 79-83.
28. REIFMAN, A. & M. WINDLE. 1996. Vietnam combat exposure and recent drug use: A national study. J. Traumatic Stress **9:** 557-568.
29. BOSCARINO, J. A. 1995. Post-traumatic stress and associated disorders among Vietnam veterans: The significance of combat exposure and social support. J. of Traumatic Stress. **8:** 317-336.
30. LITZ, B. T., T. M. KEANE, L. FISHER, B. MARX, *et al.* 1992. Physical health complaints in combat-related post-traumatic stress disorder: A preliminary report. J. Traumatic Stress **5:** 131-141.

Familial Risk Factors in Posttraumatic Stress Disorder[a]

KATHRYN M. CONNOR AND
JONATHAN R. T. DAVIDSON

Department of Psychiatry and Behavioral Sciences
Duke University School of Medicine
Durham, North Carolina 27710

Patient, a shoemaker, aged 37, was partially buried by the detonation of a high-explosive shell; short loss of consciousness followed, and later he became stupid, shaky, and weak. He had terrifying dreams, was very fearful of the dark, and twice attacked his companions with murderous intent whilst in a dazed state. He had no recollection of these attacks. He had always possessed a violent temper, the outbursts usually being followed by attacks of petit mal. He was always afraid of the dark. Patient is married, one child has "fits", three others are hysterical and have fits of impulsive temper. The patient's father is now in an insane hospital, likewise his brother and sister. Three others are very irritable, one has convulsions. Three sisters are very "nervy". One other sister is an exceptional musician. His paternal grandfather was very excitable, and died in a "passion of temper". An uncle was a rebel leader, very excitable and brilliant, and had a child with an intolerable temper, and another with "St. Vitus' dance". Another uncle was a rogue and a crook and his son was a crook. A normal aunt had six children, one of whom is insane and five very excitable. His great grandfather had an intolerable temper and died in an insane hospital. One great-uncle with an intolerable temper had an insane son. Another aunt by her own brother begot three children, one of whom became a prostitute and the two others were imbeciles.

Captain J. M. Wolfsohn, M.S., M.D., M.R.C.[1]

The importance of heredity as a risk factor for disease has been well documented in numerous conditions. In psychiatry, the role of familial inheritance in the development of psychopathology has been studied in a variety of illnesses including major depression, bipolar disorder, anxiety disorders, schizophrenia, personality disorders, and alcoholism. Familial transmission may represent genetic, environmental, or combined mechanisms of transmission. The study of familial aspects of disease provides a means for distinguishing genetic and nongenetic factors. Studying family factors in disease also provides evidence for the validation and understanding of the entity, promotes the development of new methods of disease classification, and has implications for prevention of illness.

[a]This work was supported by National Institute of Mental Health grant 1 R01-MH44749-01A3 and 2 R01-MH47448-04 to the second author.

In this chapter, the authors examine the role of familial risk factors in the development of posttraumatic stress disorder (PTSD). The importance of familial psychopathology and the family methods approach to data collection are discussed. Early published accounts of familial aspects of combat neurosis are described. A review of the current literature on familial features of PTSD is then presented. Finally, the multipathogenic aspects and inherent diagnostic heterogeneity of PTSD are discussed in relation to the topic of this chapter.

IMPORTANCE OF FAMILIAL PSYCHOPATHOLOGY

The study of family psychopathology represents one important method for validating a disease, understanding its diagnostic position, and elaborating its characteristics.[2] Familial transmission may signify either a genetic, an environmental, or a combined influence of inheritance. A practical implication of familial loading for a disorder is that it can be expected to serve as a risk factor, increasing the likelihood that the particular disease will emerge under stressful or provoking circumstances. Many studies have demonstrated familial and/or genetic influences for alcoholism,[3] affective disorder,[4–14] schizophrenia,[15] generalized anxiety disorder,[16,17] panic disorder,[16–22] obsessive compulsive disorder,[23,24] social phobia,[25,26] and other phobias.[27,28] Studies suggesting the role of familial determinants in PTSD are reviewed below.

The two most widely used approaches to collecting family data are the family history method and the family study method. The family history technique involves obtaining information from the patient or a relative about all family members. With the family study method, relatives are interviewed directly concerning their own past and present symptoms. Each technique has its inherent advantages and disadvantages.

The family history method provides a simple and efficient mechanism to collect information about the genetic and nongenetic familial transmission of disorders. This strategy is effective in screening large populations to select particular families for further study. Although the specificity is high, the sensitivity of the family history method is generally low.[29–32] The information is obtained secondhand, and the accuracy of the data often varies as a function of the subject and the characteristics of the illness.[31,33] In addition, the frequencies of psychiatric disorders in relatives are often underreported, resulting in the underestimation of the prevalence of disorders.[29–31] This point is especially likely to apply in the case of anxiety disorders, which are not always as apparent to relatives, in comparison with more obvious disorders such as psychosis and alcohol abuse.

In contrast, the family study method provides more precise, accurate, firsthand data with good sensitivity. This technique, however, tends to be more costly and time consuming. The accuracy of the data collected is also limited by the availability of the family members, often making this method of study impractical.[33,34]

The data collected in both family history and family study methods are subject to potential biases. Family history data are prone to a recall bias, as not all psychiatric disorders will be observed and reported by family members. These data are also subject to a selection bias, as a result of a proband's ability, willingness, or unwillingness to participate. Family study data are also vulnerable to a selection bias, as determined by the availability (limited by geography, mortality, or proband refusal) and willingness of relatives to participate.[34-37] For example, in the case of certain kinds of disorders, such as incest-induced PTSD, serious doubts have to be raised as to the accuracy of reporting when parents are interviewed. Findings from studies of other psychiatric disorders suggest that the inclusion of data from multiple informants can increase the sensitivity, thereby increasing the accuracy of diagnostic estimates and reducing an information bias.[38] Although the studies are limited in number, these issues should be considered when evaluating family data in studies of PTSD.

FAMILIAL ASPECTS OF COMBAT NEUROSIS

The first medical references to the traumatic stress response date back to Civil War accounts of veterans and female civilians. Since that time, traumatic stress states have been well documented, primarily in military populations, under a wide variety of names including: anxiety neurosis; battle fatigue; bomb happy; cardiac neurosis; combat fatigue; Da Costa's syndrome; debility; disordered action of the heart; effort syndrome; hysteria; irritable heart; neurocirculatory asthenia; neurasthenia; neurotic illness in soldiers; psychoneurosis; shell shock; somatization reaction general; somatization reaction psychogenic asthenic reaction; somatization reaction psychogenic cardiovascular reaction; vasomotor instability; vasomotor neurosis; and war neurosis. All of these conditions shared essentially the same three symptom clusters now represented in the Diagnostic and Statistical Manual of Mental Disorders, fourth edition (DSM-IV),[39] description of PTSD, notably recurrent intrusive features, avoidance behaviors, and autonomic arousal. Little data are available on familial aspects of these conditions, and this information is largely limited to survey statistics. A summary of published findings from studies conducted during World War I and World War II is provided in TABLE 1.

The majority of these investigations represent survey studies of military personnel. Family history data were collected along with other information to examine factors impacting on a soldier's response to traumatic stress from such experiences as flying, combat, and other war-related exposures.[1,40-48] In each study, the rate of familial psychopathology was greater in affected individuals: between 48% and 74% of cases reported a positive family psychiatric history contrasted with 0% to 10% of controls. These authors concluded that familial psychoneurotic factors contribute to a predisposition for neurotic breakdown in individuals exposed to war trauma. They suggested that these factors be considered in assessing the stability of recruits to the military in an effort to reduce the proportion of men who break down under the stress of war.

One study of neurocirculatory asthenia in civilians utilized family study methods to examine the familial aspects of this condition.[49] Wheeler and colleagues identified individuals who had been diagnosed with neurocirculatory asthenia 20 years previously and interviewed adult children of these individuals, comparing them with the children of adults not previously diagnosed with neurocirculatory asthenia. The prevalence of neurocirculatory asthenia was 48.6% in the sons and daughters of parents with neurocirculatory asthenia compared to 5.6% in offspring in the control group, a highly significant difference. The authors note, however, that these results do not reveal whether the disorder is hereditary or acquired through environmental exposure, a point of particular importance in the case of PTSD.

TABLE 1. Family Findings in Studies of World War I and World War II Military Personnel and Civilians with Combat Neuroses

Study	Population	Subjects	Findings
Wolfsohn,[1] 1918	WWI soldiers, Maudsley Extension, 4th Extension London General Hospital	100 cases of war psychoneuroses 100 cases of war-related somatic injuries	74% of psychoneurotic cases had a family history of psychoneurosis including insanity, epilepsy, alcoholism, and nervousness; no family histories of neuropathic or psychopathic stigmas were reported in controls.
Oppenheimer et al.,[40] 1918	WWI soldiers, Military Heart Hospital, Colchester	100 cases from the British Expeditionary Force	56% of subjects reported a family history of psychoneurotic factors, including nervousness, alcoholism, teetotaling, irritability of temper, insanity, epilepsy, tuberculosis, and stigmas.
Robey et al.,[41] 1918	WWI soldiers, Camp McClellan, Alabama	89 patients in the base hospital	Most patients gave a family history of nervous disorder. The father, mother, or some of the siblings are nervous and irritable and are easily upset.
Swan,[42] 1921	WWI veterans	58 men referred to the US PHS group internist for evaluation	52% reported a family history of nervous disease, including insanity, suicide, cerebrospinal syphilis, alcoholism, meningitis, melancholia, and diabetes.
Curran et al.,[43] 1940	WWII soldiers, Royal Naval auxiliary hospital	100 patients admitted to neuropsychiatric unit 50 controls from surgical unit	45% of cases had a positive family history.[a] Efforts were made to predict the number of breakdowns by performing more thorough physical and psychiatric assessments, and the authors found that 26 of 45 represented cases that were unpredictable, suggesting that the prognostic importance of a positive family history had been underestimated.

Wood,[44] 1941	Patients in an emergency hospital in London	210 militiamen (75 organic heart disease cases, 85 cases of DaCosta's syndrome, and 50 normals) 175 patients at an emergency hospital	56% of cases of DaCosta's syndrome and 35% of EMS patients reported a family history of nervousness or "cardiac neurosis," compared with 8% of normals and 11% of cases of organic heart disease. It was rare to find siblings with similar complaints unless these were also noted in the parents.
Cooper et al.,[45] 1942	WWII soldiers, war neurosis clinic in an underground concrete shelter, Tobruk	207 patients	A family history of neurotic traits was noted in 50% of patients.
Symonds,[46] 1943	WWII flying personnel, assessed by neuropsychiatric specialists, Royal Air Force	2,000 cases exposed to flying stress	More than 66% reported a family or personal predisposition to neurosis.
Slater,[47] 1943	WWII service service personnel, Sutton Emergency Hospital	2,000 patients admitted to a neuropsychiatric ward	56% reported a positive family history of neurotic illness, psychosis, epilepsy, or some form of psychopathy. Positive family history was positively associated with psychopathic personality and bad outcome and negatively associated with military stress and organic syndromes. Positive family history was more prevalent in patients undergoing trifling vs. moderate or severe military stress (57% vs 56% vs 45%, respectively).
Cohen et al.,[48] 1948	WWII service personnel, patients in service hospitals	144 cases of neurocirculatory asthenia 105 healthy controls 25 controls with healing infected war wounds 23 soldiers convalescing from infectious hepatitis	Of 67 families of cases and 54 families of healthy controls, a history of neurocirculatory asthenia was noted in 58% of mothers, 18.5% of fathers, and 12.6% of siblings of families of cases and in none of the families of controls. Of 15 direct interviews of family members, the patient's history was corroborated 100%.

TABLE 1. Family Findings in Studies of World War I and World War II Military Personnel and Civilians with Combat Neuroses (*Continued*)

Study	Population	Subjects	Findings
Wheeler et al.,[49] 1948	Civilians	50 patients, in 22 families, diagnosed with NCA[b] 20 years earlier 234 controls	Of 37 children from 18 case families, 48.6% of offspring reported NCA, in contrast with 5.6% of control offspring who reported NCA.

[a] Family history: considered positive when a near blood-relative (parent, aunt, sibling) had been in a mental hospital or attempted suicide; when more than one such relative had shown evidence of psychiatric disorder though not resulting in mental hospital treatment (shell-shock, obvious psychopathy as shown by chronic alcoholism or a very bad work record).
[b] NCA = neurocirculatory asthenia.

FAMILY DATA FROM STUDIES OF PTSD

In contrast to studies conducted prior to 1980, which did not use specified diagnostic criteria for PTSD or similar disorders, studies since that date have adopted DSM-III[50] or DSM-III R[51] criteria for PTSD. The published literature on familial aspects of PTSD is small and primarily limited to family history data. Populations studied have included at risk groups such as combat veterans, prisoners of war (POWs), firefighters, abused children, and rape survivors as well as community samples of adults and twin studies. Results from these investigations regarding the heritability of PTSD are varied. A summary of these studies is detailed TABLE 2 and the findings are reviewed below.

Trauma Related to Wartime Experience

Family history findings in investigations of veterans and POWs with PTSD are inconclusive. In a study of inpatient and outpatient male combat veterans, Davidson and colleagues[52] observed that two thirds of individuals with PTSD reported a family history of psychopathology, noting primarily alcoholism, anxiety, and depressive disorders. In another investigation of outpatient veterans, Davidson et al.[53] reported that individuals with PTSD did not differ significantly from controls on the basis of family history; however, greater familial anxiety was noted in the PTSD group when compared to a diagnostically mixed control group who had all been exposed to combat trauma. In the same study, comparing World War II and Vietnam veterans, the latter group exhibited increased morbidity risks for substance abuse and for chronic psychiatric disorders among siblings/parents and children, respectively. Attention deficit hyperactivity disorder was also observed in the offspring of Vietnam veterans with PTSD.[53] In a study of POWs, Speed and colleagues[54] found that a family history of mental illness was weakly correlated, at best, with persistent PTSD and that any risk associated with heritable factors was superseded by the overwhelming nature of the trauma. This is an important point, entirely in line with observations by Slater[46] and Foy et al.,[55] which suggest that heritability factors are important within a certain range of trauma severity and that it takes proportionately more trauma to produce PTSD in less predisposed individuals. In other words, extreme levels of trauma, such as POW and holocaust experiences, may bring out PTSD in the hardiest.

Trauma Related to Civilian Experiences

Data from studies of civilian populations at risk for PTSD are varied as well. McFarlane[56] examined Australian firefighters exposed to a devastating bushfire and observed that family psychiatric history was one of several premorbid risk factors significantly associated with the development of chronic PTSD. This result is supported by findings from a family study of mothers and their children who presented to a juvenile/family court for assessment of child abuse. Famularo and associates[57] found that 36% of these children met diagnostic criteria for PTSD, and this group was significantly overrepresented among mothers with PTSD and other disorders as well. In a family study of rape survivors, familial aggregation of neither anxiety nor

TABLE 2. Studies Reporting Familial Risk Factors for PTSD[a]

Study	Population	Subjects	Findings
Davidson et al.,[52] 1985 (FH)	Inpatient and outpatient veteran males Nonveteran males	36 patients with combat-related stress and chronic PTSD 13 GAD controls 19 depression controls	A positive family history of psychopathology was noted in 66% of patients, with alcoholism, depression, and anxiety noted most commonly. Probands with PTSD more closely resembled probands with generalized anxiety than probands with depression with respect to proportion of familial anxiety to familial depression.
McFarlane,[56] 1988 (FH)	Volunteer firefighters exposed to bushfire disaster	469 subjects determined to be at high risk for PTSD at 4 months after the trauma	In 50 randomly selected subjects 8 months after the disaster, a family history of psychiatric illness was noted in 55% of subjects with PTSD and 20% of subjects without PTSD.
Davidson et al.,[53] 1989 (FH)	Outpatient male veterans	108 MHC cases with PTSD 21 nonpsychiatric controls 24 depressed controls 15 alcoholic controls	Siblings and parents of depressed controls had a greater morbidity risk for depression and children a greater risk for generalized anxiety than did families of PTSD probands. In combat-exposed veterans only, PTSD was associated with greater familial anxiety than in controls. In Vietnam veterans with PTSD, higher morbidity risks were noted for substance abuse and other chronic psychiatric disorders in siblings/parents and children, respectively.

Study	Sample	Sample size	Findings
Speed et al.,[54] 1989 (FH)	WWII POWs	31 diagnosed with PTSD 31 never diagnosed with PTSD	Family history of mental illness, including alcoholism, was weakly correlated with persistent PTSD symptoms and superseded by the severity of the trauma.
Breslau et al.,[59] 1991 (FH)	Adult members of a large health maintenance organization	1,007 respondents	394 reported exposure to trauma that fit the DSM-IIIR PTSD stressor definition, 24% of whom had PTSD. Vulnerability to the effects of traumatic events was significantly increased in respondents with a family history of anxiety (including nervousness, panic, and phobia), depression, psychosis, and antisocial behavior.
Davidson et al.,[60] 1991 (FH)	Community sample	39 PTSD respondents 2946 non-PTSD respondents	PTSD respondents were 3 times more likely to report a family history of mental illness.
True et al.,[61] 1993 (TW)	Vietnam veterans	2224 MZ twin pairs 1818 DZ twin pairs	After adjusting for combat exposure in pairs, significant genetic influence on symptom liability was observed in each symptom cluster. The development of PTSD was not associated with shared environment.
Skre et al.,[16] 1993 (TW)	Norwegian same-sex twin pairs	20 MZ and 29 DZ co-twins of anxiety disorder probands 12 MZ and 20 DZ co-twins of nonpsychotic mental disorder probands	PTSD was significantly more prevalent in co-twins of anxiety disorder probands and was more prevalent in MZ than in DZ co-twins.

TABLE 2. Studies Reporting Familial Risk Factors for PTSD[a] (*Continued*)

Study	Population	Subjects	Findings
Famularo et al.,[57] 1994 (FI)	Women and children in juvenile/family court	109 maltreated children 109 mothers of these children	16% of mothers met criteria for current PTSD, whereas 37% had a history of PTSD; 36% of the children met criteria for PTSD and these cases were significantly overrepresented among mothers with PTSD. The onset of maltreatment was also significantly earlier in children of mothers with PTSD.
Davidson et al.,[58] unpublished (FI)	Advertisement-recruited sample of women	56 rape survivors with chronic PTSD 25 rape survivors without chronic PTSD 31 depression controls 20 anxiety disorder controls 39 healthy, nonpsychiatric controls	A weakly increased morbidity risk for anxiety was noted in family members of rape survivors. Morbidity risk for major depression was strongly increased.

Abbreviations: FH = family history study; FI = family interview study; GAD = generalized anxiety disorder; MHC = Durham Veterans Administration Mental Health Clinic; TW = twin study; MZ = monozygotic; DZ = dizygotic.

[a] Studies utilizing DSM-III and DSM-III-R diagnostic criteria.

PTSD was noted in rape survivors, whereas increased rates of major depression were observed.[58] Unlike the studies of military personnel, the variation noted in these data may, in part, reflect the heterogeneity in the samples studied.

Community-Based Studies

Familial aspects of PTSD have been addressed in two community studies. Breslau and colleagues[59] examined young, urban adults in a health maintenance organization to assess the prevalence of PTSD and associated risk factors. Among their observations, they found that a family history of psychiatric disorder or substance abuse was a risk factor for exposure to traumatic events in probands. Family history of an anxiety disorder, sociopathy, or depression was also identified as a risk factor for the development of PTSD. Davidson and associates[60] studied PTSD in the Piedmont region of North Carolina using data from the Epidemiologic Catchment Area study. They also reported significantly higher rates of psychiatric illness, but not alcohol abuse, in families of individuals with PTSD.

Twin Studies

Results from twin studies support the hypothesis that, in many cases, there is a genetic contribution to the etiology of PTSD, or more specifically in the following study, to the symptoms of PTSD. In an investigation of 4,042 Vietnam era veteran monozygotic (MZ) and dizygotic (DZ) male twin pairs, True and colleagues[61] applied quantitative genetic analyses and found significant genetic influences on symptom liability. After adjusting for differences in combat exposure, genetic factors were determined to account for 13-30% of variance in liability of reexperiencing symptoms, 30-34% for avoidance symptoms, and 28-32% for arousal symptoms. Of note, symptoms in the reexperiencing cluster and one symptom in the avoidance cluster (e.g., avoided activities that might remind you of things that happened to you while in the military) were strongly associated with combat exposure, and MZ pairs were more highly concordant for combat exposure than DZ pairs. There was, however, no evidence that shared environment contributes to the development of PTSD symptoms.

In a study of the prevalence of anxiety disorders, Skre and associates[16] compiled twin data from several sources, including the Norwegian Twin Register, the national register for mental disorders, a university-based psychiatric clinic, and other twin studies conducted by the authors to develop a database of 81 same sex twin pairs with one twin proband. PTSD was more prevalent in co-twins of anxiety probands as well as in MZ than DZ co-twins.

Summary

In each study reviewed, increased rates of psychiatric illness were observed in family members of probands with PTSD, lending further support for familial influence on the susceptibility to PTSD. The strength of these results, however, varied from statistically significant to weakly correlative at best. This variability may be explained, in part, by the data collection methods employed. In all but one family history study reviewed, elevated rates of mental illness were demonstrated, noting specifically anxiety disorders, affective disorders, sociopathy, and/or substance abuse in several studies. The study by Speed *et al.,*[54] however, reported a weak correlation between trauma and familial psychiatric illness, supporting the notion that the severity of the trauma experienced supersedes other vulnerabilities in the development of PTSD. By comparison, family interview studies provided firsthand data pertaining to the effects of traumatic stress in family members. The prevalence of PTSD was increased among first-degree relatives, including co-twins, of probands with PTSD in three of four family studies. An elevated morbidity risk for depression was observed in family members of individuals with PTSD in the fourth study. Do these differences reflect the biases inherent in these two study methods or are they related to the severity of trauma experienced or to other environmental influences? These issues warrant further investigation.

CLASSIFICATION OF PTSD

The diagnosis of PTSD requires the presence of symptoms from each of three symptom categories, along with exposure to a traumatic event. PTSD is distinct from other psychopathologic entities in its requirement of an external, environmental influence. As noted in the DSM-IV diagnostic criteria, this traumatic event must have involved a threat to self or others and elicited a response of fear, helplessness, or horror in the exposed individual.[39] Therefore, in examining the development of PTSD, multipathogenic features of the trauma as well as characteristics of the individual's response to that trauma need to be considered.

The heterogeneity of PTSD is also reflected in the symptom criteria outlined in DSM-IV. These symptoms of reexperiencing, avoidance, and autonomic arousal are unique to PTSD as a constellation of symptoms in the setting of a traumatic exposure. Elements of these groupings, however, are common to many other psychiatric conditions (TABLE 3). For example, recurrent and intrusive recollections are features of obsessive compulsive disorder. Fear and avoidance are characteristic of several anxiety disorders, notably agoraphobia, simple phobia, and social phobia. Increased autonomic arousal is noted in generalized anxiety and in combination with psychic and/or physiologic numbing in panic disorder. Symptoms of withdrawl and detachment, numbing, guilt, and a foreshortened future may be observed in major depression. Reexperiencing phenomena and avoidance behaviors are noted in dissociative conditions. The poor impulse control exhibited by some individuals with PTSD is also a feature of certain personality structures, as noted in antisocial and borderline personality dynamics.

Consideration of PTSD in this light opens the possibility of different forms of predisposition, according to the predominance of the symptom picture. For example, it is conceivable that those with prominent dissociative tendencies and marked impulse dyscontrol may have a different family history than those with marked obsessive compulsive symptoms or comorbid obsessive compulsive disorder even though both share the same diagnosis. In a family study of obsessive compulsive disorder, Black and colleagues[62] suggested that an anxiety diathesis is transmitted in families with

TABLE 3. Features of Axis I and Axis II Disorders and Corresponding DSM-IV PTSD Diagnostic Criteria

Diagnostic Features	Corresponding DSM-IV PTSD Diagnostic Criteria
Obsessions and compulsions	B.1. Recurrent and intrusive recollections of the event, including images, thoughts, or perceptions B.2. Recurrent, distressing dreams of the event
Phobic avoidance	C.1. Efforts to avoid thoughts, feelings, or conversations associated with the trauma C.2. Efforts to avoid activities, places, or persons that arouse recollections of the trauma
Generalized anxiety (tonic hyperarousal)	D.1. Difficulty falling or staying asleep D.2. Irritability or outbursts of anger D.3. Difficulty concentrating D.4. Hypervigilence D.5. Exaggerated startle response
Panic (phasic hyperarousal)	B.4. Intense psychological distress at exposure to internal or external cues that symbolize or resemble an aspect of the traumatic event B.5. Psychological reactivity on exposure to internal or external cues that symbolize or resemble an aspect of the traumatic event
Depression	C.4. Markedly diminished interest or participation in significant activities C.5. Feelings of detachment or estrangement from others C.6. Restricted range of affect C.7. Sense of foreshortened future
Dissociation	B.3. Acting or feeling as if the traumatic event were recurring (includes sense of reliving the experience, flashbacks, illusions, and hallucinations) C.3. Inability to recall an important aspect of the trauma D.3. Difficulty concentrating
Poor impulse control	B.4. Intense psychological distress at exposure to internal or external cues that symbolize or resemble an aspect of the traumatic event D.2. Irritability or outbursts of anger

obsessive compulsive disorder, however with variability in expression. A similar argument may be made for PTSD, whereby any of a variety of diatheses (i.e., anxiety, depression, and phobic avoidance) may be passed on, with the variability of expression impacted by the nature of the trauma and other individual vulnerabilities. This raises the possibility that the trauma itself interacts with a predisposition to produce a factor for the development of PTSD (e.g., PTSD after rape is different from that after accident in salience of self-blame, depression, and suicide).[63]

These observations support the concept that PTSD is multipathogenic and raise the issue of where PTSD should be classified as a diagnostic entity. Since its inclusion in DSM-III in 1980, PTSD has been classified as an anxiety disorder, primarily because of the predominance of anxiety symptoms included in the diagnostic criteria. This categorization, however, has generated much debate with opponents arguing that PTSD should be included under another diagnostic heading.[64] Alternatively, as noted in other heterogeneous conditions, PTSD may be conceptualized as consisting of etiologically homogeneous subgroups, such as a depressive subtype, a phobic avoidant subtype, an obsessive-compulsive subtype, etc. A better understanding of familial influences and individual predispositions would help to clarify these issues.

CONCLUSION

Heritability is complicated by heterogeneity, and it is this heterogeneity that distinguishes PTSD from other anxiety disorders. This presents a challenge to the family method of study. Studies to date support a role for familial influences in the development of PTSD, although it remains unclear what vulnerabilities are inherited and how these may or may not interact with the trauma experienced. Although family study data may help to define specific PTSD subtypes, obtaining this information is often impractical or impossible. In individuals with a predisposition for the development of PTSD, understanding which vulnerabilities are inherited and which patients are at risk would further clarify questions of diagnostic classification and provide direction for therapeutic interventions.

REFERENCES

1. WOLFSOHN, J. M. 1918. The predisposing factors of war psycho-neuroses. Lancet **1:** 177-180.
2. ROBINS E. & S. B. GUZE. 1970. Establishment of diagnostic validity in psychiatric illness: Its application to schizophrenia. Am. J. Psychiatry **126:** 107-111.
3. PITTS, F. N. & G. WINOKUR. 1966. Affective disorder. VII. Alcoholism and affective disorder. J. Psychol. Res. **4:** 37-50.
4. WEISSMAN, M. M., E. S. GERSHON, K. K. KIDD et al. 1984. Psychiatric disorders in the relatives of probands with affective disorders: The Yale University National Institute of Mental Health Collaborative Study. Arch. Gen. Psychiatry **41:** 13-21.
5. CORYELL, W., J. ENDICOTT, T. REICH et al. 1984. A family study of Bipolar II Disorder. Br. J. Psychiatry **145:** 49-54.
6. ASHBY, H. B. & R. R. CROWE. 1978. Unipolar depression: A family study of a large kindred. Compr. Psychiatry **19:** 415-417.
7. BLAND, R. C., S. C. NEWMAN & H. ORN. 1986. Recurrent and nonrecurrent depression: A family study. Arch. Gen. Psychiatry **43:** 1085-1089.

8. Cassano, G. B., L. Musetti & G. Perugi. 1992. Family history and stressors in subtypes of depression. Clin. Neuropharmacol. **15S:** 570-571.
9. Gershon, E. S., M. M. Weissman, J. J. Guroff et al. 1986. Validation of criteria for major depression through controlled family study. J. Affect. Dis. **11:** 125-131.
10. Klein, D. N. 1990. Symptom criteria and family history in major depression. Am. J. Psychiatry **147:** 850-854.
11. Kupfer, D. J., E. Frank, L. L. Carpenter et al. 1989. Family history in recurrent depression. J. Affect. Dis. **17:** 113-119.
12. McGuffin, P., R. Katz & P. Bebbington. 1987. Hazard, heredity, and depression. A family study. J. Psychiat. Res. **4:** 365-375.
13. Leckman, J. F., M. M. Weissman, B. A. Prusoff et al. 1984. Subtypes of depression: Family study perspective. Arch. Gen. Psychiatry **41:** 833-838.
14. Winokur, G., W. Coryll, M. Keller et al. 1995. A family study of manic-depressive (bipolar I) disease. Arch. Gen. Psychiatry **52:** 367-373.
15. Kendler, K. S., A. M. Gruenberg & M. T. Tsuang. 1985. Psychiatric illness in first-degree relatives of schizophrenic and surgical control patients: A family study using DSM-III criteria. Arch. Gen. Psychiatry **42:** 770-779.
16. Skre, I., S. Onstad, S. Torgensen et al. 1993. A twin study of DSM-IIIR anxiety disorders. Acta Psychiatr. Scand. **88:** 85-92.
17. Noyes, R., C. C. Clarkson, R. R. Crowe et al. 1987. A family study of generalized anxiety disorder. Am. J. Psychiatry **144:** 1019-1024.
18. Crowe, R. R., R. Noyes, D. L. Pauls et al. 1983. A family study of panic disorder. Arch. Gen Psychiatry **40:** 1065-1069.
19. Maier, W., D. Lichtermann, J. Minges et al. 1993. A controlled family study of panic disorder. J. Psychiat. Res. **27S:** 79-87.
20. Weissman, M. M., P. Wickamaratne, P. B. Adams et al. 1993. The relationship between panic disorder and major depression. Arch. Gen. Psychiatry **50:** 767-780.
21. Goldstein, R. B., M. M. Weissman, P. B. Adams et al. 1991. Psychiatric disorders in relatives of probands with panic disorder and/or major depression. Arch. Gen. Psychiatry **51:** 383-394.
22. Hopper, J. L., F. K. Judd, P. L. Derrick et al. 1987. A family study of panic disorder. Genet. Epidemiol. **4:** 33-41.
23. Pauls, D. L., J. P. Alsobrook, W. Goodman et al. 1995. A family study of obsessive-compulsive disorder. Am. J. Psychiatry **152:** 76-84.
24. Riddle, M. A., L. Scahill, R. King et al. 1990. Obsessive compulsive disorder in children and adolescents: Phenomenology and family history. J. Am. Acad. Child Adolesc. Psychiatry **29:** 766-772.
25. Fyer, A. J., S. Mannuzza, T. F. Chapman et al. 1993. A direct interview family study of social phobia. Arch. Gen. Psychiatry **50:** 286-293.
26. Reich, J. & W. Yates. 1988. Family history of psychiatric disorders in social phobia. Compr. Psychiatry **29:** 72-75.
27. Fyer, A. J., S. Mannuzza, M. S. Gallops et al. 1990. Familial transmission of simple phobias and fears. Arch. Gen. Psychiatry **47:** 252-256.
28. Fyer, A. J., S. Mannuzza, T. F. Chapman et al. 1995. Specificity of familial aggregation of phobic disorders. Arch. Gen. Psychiatry **52:** 564-573.
29. Andreasen, N. C., J. Endicott, R. L. Spitzer et al. 1977. The family history method using diagnostic criteria: Reliability and validity. Arch. Gen. Psychiatry **34:** 1229-1235.
30. Mendlewicz, J., J. L. Fleiss, M. Cataldo et al. 1975. Accuracy of the family history method in affective illness: Comparison with direct interviews in family studies. Arch. Gen. Psychiatry **32:** 309-314.
31. Thompson, W. D., H. Orvaschel, B. A. Prusoff et al. 1982. An evaluation of the family history method for ascertaining psychiatric disorders. Arch. Gen. Psychiatry **39:** 53-58.
32. Heun, R., J. Hardt, M. Burkhart et al. 1996. Validity of the family history method in relatives of gerontopsychiatric patients. Psych. Res. **62:** 227-238.

33. ORVASCHEL, H., W. D. THOMPSON, A. BELANGER et al. 1982. Comparison of the family history method to direct interview: Factors affecting the diagnosis of depression. J. Affect. Disord. **4:** 49-59.

34. ANDREASEN, N. C., J. RICE, J. ENDICOTT et al. 1986. The family history approach to diagnosis: How useful is it? Arch. Gen. Psychiatry **43:** 421-429.

35. CHAPMAN, T. F., S. MANNUZZA, D. F. KLEIN et al. 1994. Effects of informant mental disorder on psychiatric family history data. Am. J. Psychiatry **151:** 574-579.

36. NORDEN, K. A., D. F. KLEIN, T. FERRO et al. 1995. Who participates in a family study? Compr. Psychiatry **36:** 199-206.

37. WEISSMAN, M. M., K. R. MERIKANGAS, P. WICKRAMARATNE et al. 1986. Understanding the clinical heterogeneity of major depression using family data. Arch. Gen. Psychiatry **43:** 430-434.

38. KENDLER, K. S. & M. A. ROY. 1995. Validity of a diagnosis of lifetime major depression obtained by personal interview versus family history. Am. J. Psychiatry **152:** 1608-1614.

39. AMERICAN PSYCHIATRIC ASSOCIATION, COMMITTEE ON DSM-IV TASK FORCE. 1994. Diagnostic and Statistical Manual of Mental Disorders, fourth edition. American Psychiatric Association. Washington, DC.

40. OPPENHEIMER, B. S. & M. A. ROTHSCHILD. 1918. The psychoneurotic factor in the irritable heart of soldiers. JAMA **70:** 1919-1922.

41. ROBEY, W. H. & E. P. BOAS. 1918. Neurocirculatory asthenia. JAMA **71:** 525-529.

42. SWAN, J. M. 1921. An analysis of ninety cases of functional disease in soldiers. Arch. Int. Med. **28:** 586-602.

43. CURRAN, D. & W. P. MALLINSON. 1940. War-time psychiatry and economy in man-power. Lancet **2:** 738-743.

44. WOOD, P. 1941. Aetiology of Da Costa's syndrome. Br. Med. J. **1:** 845-851.

45. COOPER, E. L. & A. J. M. SINCLAIR. 1942. War neuroses in Tobruk: A report on 207 patients from the Australian Imperial Force Units in Tobruk. Med. J. Australia **2:** 73-77.

46. SLATER, E. 1943. The neurotic constitution: A statistical study of two thousand neurotic soldiers. J. Neurol. Psychiatry **6:** 1-16.

47. SYMONDS, C. P. 1943. The human response to flying stress. Br. Med. J. **30:** 703-706.

48. COHEN, M. E., P. D. WHITE & R. E. JOHNSON. 1948. Neurocirculatory asthenia, anxiety neurosis or the effort syndrome. Arch. Int. Med. **81:** 260-281.

49. WHEELER, E. O., P. D. WHITE, E. REED et al. 1948. Familial incidence of neurocirculatory asthenia ("Anxiety Neurosis," "Effort Syndrome"). Proceedings of the 40th Annual Meeting of the American Society for Clinical Investigation, Atlantic City, NJ.

50. AMERICAN PSYCHIATRIC ASSOCIATION, COMMITTEE ON DSM-III TASK FORCE. 1980. Diagnostic and Statistical Manual of Mental Disorders, third edition. American Psychiatric Association. Washington, DC.

51. AMERICAN PSYCHIATRIC ASSOCIATION, COMMITTEE ON DSM-III R TASK FORCE. 1987. Diagnostic and Statistical Manual of Mental Disorders, third edition, revised. American Psychiatric Association. Washington, DC.

52. DAVIDSON, J., M. SWARTZ, M. STORCK et al. 1985. A diagnostic and family study of posttraumatic stress disorder. Am. J. Psychiatry **142:** 90-93.

53. DAVIDSON, J., R. SMITH & H. KUDLER. 1989. Familial psychiatric illness in chronic posttraumatic stress disorder. Compr. Psychiatry **30:** 339-345.

54. SPEED, N., B. ENGDAHL, J. SCHWARTZ et al. 1989. Posttraumatic stress disorder as a consequence of the POW experience. J. Nerv. Ment. Dis. **177:** 147-153.

55. FOY, D. W., H. S. RESNICK, R. C. SIPPRELLE et al. 1987. Premilitary, military, and postmilitary factors in the development of combat-related posttraumatic stress disorder. Behav. Therapist **10:** 3-9.

56. McFARLANE A. C. 1988. The aetiology of post-traumatic stress disorders following a natural disaster. Br. J. Psychiatry **152:** 116-121.

57. FAMULARO, R., T. FENTON, R. KINSCHERFF et al. 1994. Maternal and child posttraumatic stress disorder in cases of child maltreatment. Child Abuse & Neglect **18:** 27-36.

58. DAVIDSON, J. R., L. A. TUPLER & W. H. WILSON. A family study of chronic posttraumatic stress disorder. Submitted for publication.
59. BRESLAU, N., G. C. DAVIS, P. ANDRESKI et al. 1991. Traumatic events and posttraumatic stress disorder in an urban population of young adults. Arch. Gen. Psychiatry **48:** 216-222.
60. DAVIDSON, J. R., D. HUGHES, D. BLAZER et al. 1991. Posttraumatic stress disorder in the community: An epidemiological study. Psychol. Med. **21:** 713-721.
61. TRUE, W. R., J. RICE, S. A. EISEN et al. 1993. A twin study of genetic and environmental contributions to liability for posttraumatic stress symptoms. Arch. Gen. Psychiatry **50:** 257-264.
62. BLACK, D. W., R. NOYES, R. B. GOLDSTEIN et al. 1992. A family study of obsessive-compulsive disorder. Arch. Gen. Psychiatry **49:** 362-368.
63. DAHL, S. 1989. Acute stress respones to rape—a PTSD variant. Acta Psychiatr. Scand. **80**(355S): 56-62.
64. BRETT, E. A. 1993. Classifications of posttraumatic stress disorder in DSM-IV: Anxiety disorder, dissociative disorder or stress disorder. In J. R. T. Davidson & E. B. Foa, eds.: 191-206. Posttraumatic Stress Disorder: DSM-IV and Beyond. American Psychiatric Press. Washington DC.

Comments on the "Empirical Basis for Biological Studies of PTSD"

BONNIE L. GREEN

Department of Psychiatry
Georgetown University
Washington, DC 20007

The papers presented in this section give us an excellent backdrop for the remainder of the papers addressing the psychobiology of posttraumatic stress disorder (PTSD). They set the stage by proposing potential relationships among exposure to traumatic events, the psychology of PTSD, and the biology of PTSD, by describing what is known about family history of PTSD as well as about its comorbid occurrence with other psychiatric disorders and its longitudinal course. Globally, these papers describe a very complex disorder that does not lend itself to simple paradigms, research designs, or answers in either the psychological or biological realm. They indicate that research must proceed cautiously and conservatively to sort out the impact of multiple factors, some of which may be central, others peripheral, and still others obstructive or confounding.

Connor and Davidson summarized the extant research addressing family history findings associated with the diagnosis of PTSD. Family history studies usually are unable to separate out genetic versus environmental transmission, but at the very least can explicate important nonexposure variables that may play a critical role in the development of PTSD following exposure to traumatic events. Furthermore, they may suggest subgroups of subjects (i.e., those with and those without a family history) that might be hypothesized to differ in biological features or that might help explain or reconcile seemingly divergent findings. Unfortunately, family studies of PTSD are in their infancy and as yet have not produced definitive or consistent outcomes.

These types of studies have usually indicated more psychopathology in family members of individuals with PTSD than in those without PTSD; however, the nature of the psychopathology, including a history of major depression, substance abuse, and anxiety disorders, varies from study to study. Studies that have examined family history of PTSD specifically have had mixed findings with regard to the prediction of PTSD in probands.[1,2] At best, these studies indicate a general risk for PTSD among children of parents with Axis I pathology, but they do not easily suggest specific mechanisms for transmission.

Twin studies offer an opportunity to differentiate the genetic and environmental components of the association, but complicate matters further by demonstrating that different clusters of PTSD symptoms may be differentially determined. For example, True and colleagues[3] found a higher genetic loading for avoidance/numbing symptoms and for arousal symptoms than for intrusion symptoms among Vietnam veteran twin pairs. However, they found no evidence of the effects of a shared environment on PTSD symptoms. Further studies are clearly needed before genetic and developmental contributions to PTSD can be sorted out. Connor and Davidson raise the issue of comorbidity of PTSD with other disorders as a complicating factor in family studies of PTSD. From their own work they highlight the finding that the increased depression in proband relatives in their family study of rape victims was limited to those with comorbid depression.

Keane and Kaloupek make this issue of comorbidity the focus of their paper, offering compelling evidence that PTSD is usually comorbid with other disorders, especially when lifetime diagnoses are studied. For example, nearly all veterans with PTSD in the National Vietnam Veterans Readjustment study had other lifetime disorders.[4] In two chronic populations in the community (Vietnam veterans and disaster survivors at 14 years postevent), Green and colleagues found that 95% of individuals with current PTSD had other concurrent psychiatric disorders.[5] In the general population, lifetime PTSD occurs alone in only about 12% of men and 21% of women.[6] Few studies exist which have examined community samples with recently acquired PTSD, but even these populations may have high comorbidity rates. For example, McFarlane and Papay[7] found that 77% of firefighters with PTSD had other diagnoses. It is not clear if these disorders are really distinct clinical entities or the extent to which symptom overlap accounts for some of the findings. However, this situation clearly makes it imperative that comorbidity be taken into account in all studies of PTSD, psychological as well as biological. It also suggests that it is unlikely that biological findings will be easily categorized as applying to PTSD alone. As Keane and Kaloupek point out, it is also not clear if PTSD precedes or follows other disorders chronologically. The study by Kessler and colleagues[6] suggests that about half the time, PTSD seems to be the primary disorder, but this varies depending on the particular diagnosis and whether men or women are being studied. All of the studies addressing the chronology of comorbidity to date have been retrospective, however, and can only suggest various paths. Only prospective studies can answer questions about primary and secondary disorders with regard to PTSD. Assuming, however, that such studies would mirror those already completed, it can be hypothesized that PTSD is primary in some cases and secondary (i.e., other disorders may serve as a risk factor or vulnerability factor for PTSD) in others, perhaps again suggesting subtypes that may have different biological manifestations or associated features.

The suggestions of Keane and Kaloupek to address this issue in research are generally useful. However, the suggestion to find groups of individuals with only PTSD to compare to those with PTSD and other single disorders may not be practical given the epidemiology. Only a small portion of trauma survivors with PTSD have that diagnosis alone, and it may be difficult to isolate enough cases to study. Furthermore, cases of PTSD alone are likely atypical of PTSD cases in general. They may also represent a stage of the disorder rather than a distinct subtype associated with specific individuals. An important point made by these authors is that PTSD and its associated disorders are predictive of other behavioral factors that are likely to affect biology, such as smoking, caffeine intake, and exercise, in addition to those that would come up in an assessment of comorbidity (e.g., alcohol abuse).

In addition to the heterogeneity of the disorder with regard to family history and comorbidity, it is also becoming established that PTSD is an intermittent disorder with a variable course, as illustrated by McFarlane, further complicating its study. Adding to the discussion by Keane and Kaloupek, McFarlane's work with motor vehicle accident victims indicates that PTSD is only one of several outcomes associated with traumatic exposure. This work suggests that biological studies in this area should begin by examining the biology of individuals who are exposed to extreme stressors immediately following exposure. These individuals need to be followed longitudinally to evaluate not only PTSD outcomes, but also other outcomes and comorbidities along with their associated biological changes and the ways in which the biological findings diverge over time and are associated with psychopathological changes. Fortunately, in addition to McFarlane's study, other studies of this nature are being conducted.[8]

Pitman's introductory paper provides an excellent overview of the work to date on the physiology and biology of PTSD. He points out, however, that the extant work on biological abnormalities in PTSD has largely been correlational, leaving unanswered questions about causality. He suggests at least six different ways in which traumatic exposure, psychological symptoms, and biological findings might be related, reminding us that we are only just beginning to examine these complex issues.

The papers in this section suggest a number of themes and approaches to the study of PTSD and its biology. One is that we should perhaps be studying the *biology of trauma* rather than the biology of PTSD per se. If PTSD is not the only outcome related to trauma exposure, if it is almost never found alone, and if its course is intertwined with those of other disorders, it is unlikely that a biology of PTSD alone will be possible. Furthermore, if we were able to isolate cases of PTSD that were not comorbid with other disorders, they would not be representative of PTSD cases in general, and the generalizability of findings with these individuals would be limited. As just noted, the most promising work is likely to include studies in which subjects are identified immediately following a traumatic event, and their biology, physiology, and psychology are tracked over time. These studies would undoubtedly identify subjects who did show PTSD as their initial disorder, and the building of comorbidity over time might become clearer. Such studies would also allow better study of associated risk and protective factors that might attenuate or enhance a pathological response, as underlined by McFarlane.

Biological studies to date have been conducted almost exclusively on hospitalized male combat veterans with chronic disorders. These individuals are only a small subset of those who develop PTSD. They may be atypical psychologically and biologically. Work with this population has provided the extremely important information that has initiated the study of biological findings in PTSD and has provided important underpinnings to the psychopathology that has been described for a longer period. However, studies must move from hospitalized, chronic samples of men to more representative samples in the community, particularly those including women. Although women represent two thirds of those diagnosed with PTSD, they have barely begun to be studied from a biological perspective. Yet, biological correlates of PTSD and biological moderators of the response to trauma could conceivably differ between men and women. Women have somewhat different comorbidities associated with the diagnosis of PTSD as well.[6] All PTSD research, including that which focuses on psychological and clinical findings, has the problem that men and women, on average, are exposed to different types of stressor experiences. Men are more often the victims of war and physical assault, and women are more often the victims of sexual assault and abuse. They develop PTSD at different rates following the same types of events (e.g., 2% of men, but 21% of women, developed PTSD following a physical attack[6]). It is therefore difficult to directly compare men and women because they tend to be studied separately and to be recruited from groups exposed to different stressors. The exception to this is the disaster literature, which has always encompassed both. Yet, disasters are in some ways the most difficult events to study, because by definition they cannot be anticipated and planned for. In studies of motor vehicle accidents the possibility exists to directly compare men and women, and a number of investigators have turned their attention to this type of event. However, traumatic events of human design are thought to be the most pathogenic by some investigators[9] and clearly need to be studied as well. Although the epidemiology of traumatic exposure will continue to dictate to some extent what we are able to study, some attempt must be made to directly compare the responses of men and women to the same event at the same point in time.

A final area that requires study is the exposure of the research subject to other traumas prior to the one being targeted for investigation. Some studies have shown that prior trauma is a risk factor for PTSD, suggesting that those individuals with PTSD are statistically likely to have had multiple trauma exposure. Other work has indicated that prior exposure indeed *alters* the biology of the trauma response.[10] Yet, none of the papers has focused on the importance of evaluating multiple trauma exposure. Furthermore, research findings also indicate that childhood trauma, especially that of human design, may have a more pervasive impact on psychopathology than do events occurring in adulthood.[11] Childhood trauma also increases the risk for later exposure.[12] Therefore, careful evaluation of multiple exposures in trauma subjects is crucial, as the event that serves as the recruitment avenue for PTSD studies may not be the one that is actually critical in the development of biological abnormalities. The prospective study of children who are traumatized, as well, would help to sort out issues of course and causality.[13,14]

In conclusion, the papers in this section provide an excellent background for developing studies of the biology of PTSD. They clarify that PTSD is a complex, multifaceted disorder that does not lend itself to simple research designs or hypotheses. It rarely occurs alone, the extent of its genetic or even familial component is unclear, and it is not the only outcome associated with traumatic exposure. Biological studies to date have focused on hospitalized samples of men with chronic war-related PTSD and have relied on retrospective information to evaluate exposure variables. Nor have these studies focused on women, although women are twice as likely to develop the diagnosis. And careful evaluation of prior trauma exposure and comorbidity has only begun, even though they are likely to be crucial to understanding the biological response to trauma. It is proposed that we may have to shift our focus to the study of the biological response to *trauma,* rather than to PTSD per se. Although these issues make our task daunting, they also make it exciting in that if carefully done, they have the opportunity to elucidate non-PTSD adaptations to trauma as well and to contribute more fully to the study of psychopathology and resilience in general. Studies now underway include those of rape survivors, women war veterans from the Persian Gulf (and men as well), and motor vehicle and disaster victims, all with designs that identify trauma-exposed individuals early and track their psychology and biology over time. All have excellent potential to contribute new information about the biological response to extreme events.

REFERENCES

1. FAMULARO, R., T. FENTON, R. KINSCHERFF, C. AYOUB & R. BARNUM. 1994. Maternal and child posttraumatic stress disorder in cases of child maltreatment. Child Abuse & Neglect **18**: 27-36.
2. DAVIDSON, J., L. TUPLER & W. WILSON. 1997. A family study of chronic posttraumatic stress disorder. Submitted.
3. TRUE W., J. RICE, S. EISEN, A. HEATH, J. GOLDBERG, M. LYONS & J. NOWAK. 1993. A twin study of genetic and environmental contributions to liability for posttraumatic stress symptoms. Arch. Gen. Psychiatry **50**: 257-264.
4. KULKA, R., W. SCHLENGER, J. FAIRBANK, R. HOUGH, K. JORDAN, C. MARMAR & D. WEISS. 1990. Trauma and the Vietnam War Generation. Brunner/Mazel. New York.
5. GREEN, B., J. LINDY, M. GRACE & A. LEONARD. 1992. Chronic posttraumatic stress disorder and diagnostic comorbidity in a disaster sample. J. Nerv. Ment. Dis. **180**: 760-766.
6. KESSLER, R., C. SONNEGA, E. BROMET, M. HUGHES & C. NELSON. 1995. Posttraumatic stress disorder in the National Comorbidity Survey. Arch. Gen. Psychiatry **52**: 1048-1060.
7. MCFARLANE, A. & P. PAPAY. 1992. Multiple diagnoses in posttraumatic stress disorder in the victims of a natural disaster. J. Nerv. Ment. Dis. **180**: 498-504.
8. SHALEV, A., T. PERI, L. CANETTI & S. SCHREIBER. 1996. Predictors of PTSD in injured trauma survivors: A prospective study. Am. J. Psychiatry **153**: 219-225.
9. GREEN, B. 1993. Identifying survivors at risk: Trauma and stressors across events. *In* International Handbook of Traumatic Stress Syndromes. J. Wilson & B. Raphael, Eds.: 135-144. Plenum. New York.
10. RESNICK, H., R. YEHUDA, R. PITMAN & D. FOY. 1995. Effect of previous trauma on acute plasma cortisol level following rape. Am. J. Psychiatry **152**: 1675-1677.
11. VAN DER KOLK, B., D. PELCOVITZ, S. ROTH, F. MANDEL, A. MCFARLANE & J. HERMAN. 1996. Dissociation, somatization, and affect regulation: The complexity of adaptation to trauma. Am. J. Psychiatry **153** (Suppl. 7): 83-93.
12. WYATT, G., D. GUTHRIE & C. NOTGRASS. 1992. Differential effects of women's child sexual abuse and subsequent sexual revictimization. J. Consult. Clin. Psychol. **60**: 167-173.
13. DEBELLIS, M. & F. PUTNAM. 1994. The psychobiology of childhood maltreatment. Child & Adolesc. Clin. North Am. **3**: 663-678.
14. ORNITZ, E. & R. PYNOOS. 1989. Startle modulation in children with post-traumatic stress disorder. Am. J. Psychiatry **147**: 866-870.

Sensitization of the Hypothalamic-Pituitary-Adrenal Axis in Posttraumatic Stress Disorder[a]

RACHEL YEHUDA [b]

Traumatic Stress Studies Program
Psychiatry Department
Mount Sinai Medical School
Bronx Veterans Affairs
New York, New York 10029

Posttraumatic stress disorder (PTSD) is a psychiatric condition that can occur in individuals who have experienced traumatic events. The symptoms of PTSD were initially conceptualized as reflecting a natural process of adaptation to extraordinarily adverse life events.[1-5] However, in recent years prevalence studies have clarified that PTSD only occurs in a percentage of those exposed to trauma.[6-9] Furthermore, among trauma survivors who develop this disorder, a substantial proportion appear to show full remission of their symptoms over time.[6] This observation demonstrates that chronic PTSD represents a specific type of adaptation to trauma, which may not necessarily reflect typical or even normative stress responsiveness.[10]

Because PTSD is clearly precipitated by a traumatic event, and because of the original conceptions that this disorder described normative consequences of trauma, initial theories about the biologic underpinnings of PTSD posited that neurobiological alterations in PTSD would be similar to those observed in stress.[11-13] However, as reviewed in this chapter, the descriptions of actual neurobiologic alterations in PTSD suggest a very different profile in trauma survivors with PTSD from that observed in classical stress studies. Furthermore, trauma survivors with PTSD show different biologic alterations from those of trauma survivors without PTSD. Thus, many of the biologic findings, particularly the neuroendocrine observations, also support the idea that PTSD is a specific type of adaptation to stress that does not necessarily reflect classic or typical responses to stress.

This chapter specifically describes findings of hypothalamic-pituitary-adrenal (HPA) axis alterations in PTSD and contrasts these findings with the well-documented observations of HPA axis dysfunction after stress and in psychiatric disorders such as major depression. It is suggested that rather than the classic profile of increased adrenocortical activity and resultant dysregulation of this system described in studies of stress and other psychiatric disorders, trauma survivors with PTSD show evidence

[a] This work was supported by National Institute of Mental Health-49555 and a Veterans Administration merit grant (both awarded to R.Y.).

[b] Address for correspondence: Rachel Yehuda, PhD, Psychiatry 116/A, Bronx VA, 130 West Kingsbridge Road, Bronx, NY 10468 (tel: (718) 584-9000, ext. 6964; Yehuda.Rachel@Bronx. VA.gov).

of a highly sensitized HPA axis characterized by decreased basal cortisol levels and increased negative feedback regulation. The significance of the sensitization paradigm for explaining clinical phenomenology in PTSD is also discussed.

HYPOTHALAMIC-PITUITARY-ADRENAL ALTERATIONS IN STRESS

The hypothalamic-pituitary-adrenal axis is one of the major biological systems involved in coordinating the body's response to stress. During stress, neuropeptides in the brain stimulate the release of corticotrophin-releasing factor (CRF) and other secretagogues, such as arginine vasopressin, from the hypothalamus, which in turn initiate the release of adrenocorticotropic hormone (ACTH) from the pituitary and cortisol from the adrenals.[14,15] The major function of cortisol is to manage or contain the body's biologic stress response by stimulating the termination of the neural defensive reactions that have been activated by stress.[14] As these stress-activated biological reactions begin to shut down, HPA axis activity is suppressed by the negative feedback inhibition of cortisol on the pituitary, hypothalamus, and other sites.

High cortisol levels have traditionally been associated with stress,[15] so much so that in both human and animal literature, the magnitude of a stress response is often defined by the level of cortisol secreted. In fact, high levels of cortisol are typically considered de facto proof that stress has occurred. In the early 1970s, for example, Sacher and his colleagues[16] noted that depressed patients had significantly higher levels of cortisol than did nonpsychiatric controls. This finding was widely replicated and led investigators in the late 1970s and early 1980s to more formally consider the role of negative life events and stress in the etiology of major depression.

CORTISOL LEVELS IN PTSD

Because of the strong association between cortisol levels and stress,[17] and because high cortisol levels were widely observed in depression (which is a frequent comorbid condition with PTSD), it was initially hypothesized that cortisol levels would be elevated in PTSD. However, the first exploration of cortisol levels in PTSD demonstrated that the 24-hour urinary excretion of cortisol was actually lower in combat veterans with PTSD than in hospitalized VA patients with other psychiatric diagnoses such as major depression, schizoaffective disorder, bipolar disorder, and schizophrenia.[18] Most published studies have confirmed this initial observation.

Urinary Cortisol Levels in PTSD

To date, four[18-21] of six studies[18-23] have demonstrated that urinary cortisol levels are lower in trauma survivors with PTSD than in similarly exposed trauma survivors without PTSD and/or nonpsychiatric comparison subjects. The other two studies demonstrated that cortisol levels were significantly increased in PTSD subjects than in trauma survivors without PTSD[22,23] and normals. The findings are summarized in TABLE 1.

The discrepancies observed across the six studies can easily be rationalized if some basic facts about cortisol secretion in humans with and without psychiatric disorder are considered. First, it should be established that the normal range of urinary cortisol excretion over a 24-hour period in man is estimated to be between 20 and 90 μg/day.[24] Values that are at either extremes of this range—either above or below this range—may indicate endocrinologic abnormality. It is important to note that cortisol levels in psychiatric disorder have generally not been considered to be in the endocrinologically abnormal range. For example, in studies of major depression, cortisol levels are described as being elevated compared to those in appropriately matched controls, but not elevated beyond the normal range of cortisol release or to the extent seen in endocrinopathies such as Cushing's disease. In fact, in most studies, the mean urinary free cortisol excretion in depressed patients is well under 90 μg/day.[18, 20, 25] So too, in four of the six studies of PTSD,[18–21] cortisol levels were lower than those in other groups, but these levels were still well within the normal endocrinologic range (i.e., well above 20 μg/day).

From the mean cortisol levels in TABLE 1, it can be seen that the cortisol values for the control subjects in the Pitman and Orr[22] and Lemieux and Coe[23] studies are in the very high range of normal and more within the range of what was reported for very hypercortisolemic depressed patients. The most parsimonious explanation for the high cortisol values in the Pitman and Orr and Lemieux and Coe studies is the presence of methodologic artifacts in the collection of urine or the radioimmunoassay of cortisol (because it is unlikely that the normal or PTSD subjects in these studies had abnormally high cortisol levels in the endocrinologic sense). In the Pitman and Orr study,[22] for example, urine was collected at room temperature in a bottle containing acid preservative (to prevent degradation of catecholamines, which were also measured). Acidification of the urine may promote hydrolysis of the unconjugated cortisol, yielding artificially high cortisol values.[18] Furthermore, acid treatment can interfere with the antibody antigen reaction in the radioimmunoassay procedure and therefore result in artificially higher cortisol values. Failure to perform extraction of steroids with methylene chloride before radioimmunoassay can yield estimates of cortisol that may be as much as threefold higher than those obtained when steroids are extracted before assay.[26] In the Lemieux and Coe study,[23] information on assay characteristics was not provided, and it is difficult to know which if any of these issues may have contributed to the results. In evaluating the results of urinary cortisol studies, it is essential to first determine if the raw cortisol levels for the comparison group are within the normal range of urinary cortisol excretion. Evaluating group differences in the context of unreliable cortisol estimates may be futile.

Differences in results between studies may be due to differences in sampling populations and in control groups. In our studies, we tried to carefully control for artifacts such as substance abuse, medications, hospitalization status, and psychiatric and medical comorbidity. Our studies demonstrated that cortisol is low in combat veterans regardless of whether they met the diagnostic criteria for past substance dependence or for current major depressive disorder.[19] Cortisol levels were also low whether the subjects were inpatients, outpatients, or nontreatment-seeking, community-dwelling subjects.[19–21] We also observed that cortisol levels are equally low in

TABLE 1. Summary of Urinary Cortisol[a] Levels across All PTSD Studies

Study/Year	Trauma Survivors with PTSD		Trauma Survivors without PTSD		Normal Controls		Psychiatric Controls		Classification
	X̄ ± SD	(n)	X̄ ± SD	(n)	X̄ ± SD	(n)	X̄ ± SD	(n)	
Mason et al., 1986	33.3 ± 3.2[b]	(9)	—		—		49.6 ± 5.9	(8)	Depression
							62.7 ± 6.7	(8)	Mania
							50.1 ± 8.9	(7)	Schizophrenia
							37.5 ± 3.9	(12)	Paranoia schizophrenia
Yehuda et al., 1990	40.9 ± 12.3[b]	(16)	—		62.8 ± 22.2	(16)			
Pitman & Orr, 1990	107.3 ± 37.0	(20)	80.5 ± 25.9	(15)	—				
Yehuda et al., 1993	38.6 ± 5.8[b]	(8)	—		—		84.3 ± 29.6	(10)	Depression
							81.5 ± 38.1	(7)	Mania
							55.4 ± 24.6	(9)	Psychotic disorder
							51.5 ± 20.1	(6)	Panic
Lemieux & Coe, 1994	111.8 ± 55.8	(11)	83.1 ± 28.9	(8)	87.8 ± 21.2	(9)	—		
Yehuda et al., 1995	32.6 ± 17.0[b]	(22)	62.7 ± 25.3	(25)	51.9 ± 23.7	(15)	—		

[a] Cortisol is expressed as µg/24 hours.
[b] Mean cortisol levels in PTSD significantly lower than those in comparison subjects.

men and women with PTSD.[21] Furthermore, because we were able to study more than one type of subject population, we were able to conclude that low cortisol levels are present in PTSD subjects regardless of the actual type of trauma, the age at traumatization, the duration (in years) of symptoms, and the age of subjects at the time of biologic assessment.

Plasma Cortisol Levels

Cortisol levels that are measured from a single blood draw are not generally thought to provide reliable estimates of basal cortisol release, because the stress of venipuncture or stressors occurring immediately before blood withdrawal may lead to transient fluctuations in basal cortisol levels. Probably for this reason, studies estimating basal cortisol levels from a single plasma sample have produced a wide range of results ranging from increases,[27] decreases,[28] or no differences,[29,30] in cortisol levels in PTSD than in controls. Nonetheless, when the timing of blood withdrawal and other experimental conditions (e.g., fasting) is carefully standardized, it is possible to increase the reliability of single sample estimates. Furthermore, it is possible to decrease some of the variance from transient fluctuations by studying large samples. A particularly noteworthy study is a recent epidemiologic study conducted on a sample of over 2,000 Vietnam veterans, which showed lower morning plasma cortisol levels in 293 veterans with PTSD than in veterans without PTSD.[31]

The recent use of salivary cortisol methods also may increase the reliability of single sample estimates of cortisol by eliminating anticipatory or actual stress associated with needle sticks. In two studies, salivary cortisol levels were lower in individuals with PTSD symptoms than in those with fewer or no symptoms. Goenjian et al.[32] demonstrated that basal salivary cortisol levels were lower in children who had been close to the epicenter of the Armenian earthquake 5 years earlier and who still had substantial PTSD symptoms than in children who had been further away from the epicenter and who, as a group, had fewer symptoms. Heim et al.[33] demonstrated lower basal salivary cortisol levels in a sample of women presenting with chronic pelvic pain who had a high prevalence of sexual trauma and PTSD than in normal women presenting with infertility, but who did not have a high prevalence of sexual trauma and PTSD. (See also this volume; Heim has a poster.)

The ideal way to estimate basal plasma cortisol levels is to obtain repeated samples over a long time from subjects who are in a controlled environment. In a recent study, we examined the circadian release of cortisol over the 24-hour diurnal cycle.[34] Following an overnight stay in the clinical research center, the subject had blood samples withdrawn through an iv every 30 minutes for a 24-hour period while on bedrest and in a fasted state (until 6:00 PM). Under these conditions, basal plasma cortisol release was significantly lower, primarily in the late evening and very early morning hours, in combat veterans with PTSD than in both depressed patients and normal controls.[34] Chronobiologic analysis of raw cortisol levels using multioscillator cosinor modeling revealed a greater degree of circadian rhythm and a higher signal-to-noise ratio of cortisol release in subjects with PTSD than in the other two groups. That is, relative to lower cortisol excretion, PTSD patients tended to show high cortisol fluctuations. The data indicate that important differences may exist in the central regulation of cortisol that account for the low basal levels. To date, the extent to which this regulation facilitates or attenuates the HPA axis response to environmental stressors is unknown and constitutes an important area for future research.

In summary, the results of our studies suggest that cortisol levels are low in trauma survivors with PTSD than in trauma survivors without PTSD. Therefore, it may be concluded from our research that cortisol levels do not reflect an adaptation that directly results from the experience of trauma, but rather they reflect a measure related to the presence of symptoms. Indeed, in our studies of both combat veterans[19] and Holocaust survivors,[21] cortisol levels were significantly associated with the severity of PTSD symptoms.

Other Instances of Low Cortisol Levels in Response to Chronic Stress and Trauma in Man

Low cortisol levels in man have also been observed more generally in other instances involving chronic or traumatic stress. For example, lower than normal urinary cortisol levels have been observed in parents of chronically, fatally ill children,[35] in persons exposed to highly stressful, chronic, occupational tasks,[36] and in nurses subjected to particularly stressful work-related responsibilities.[37] Low cortisol levels have also been observed in soldiers subjected to chronic combat exposure, who were studied while stationed in Vietnam during a threat of imminent enemy attack.[38,39] A recent report documented unusually low cortisol levels in a Croatian soldier with PTSD after being exposed to heavy artillery fire at the frontline for several days.[40] Low plasma cortisol levels were also observed in a sample of 29 recently liberated detainees from a prisoner of war camp in Bosnia[41] and in a group of 84 refugees who had fled from East to West Germany who were still symptomatic 6 weeks after their arrival in West Berlin.[42] In most of these investigations, the events sustained would have qualified as traumatic events that could produce PTSD. However, inasmuch as PTSD was not specifically addressed in these studies, it is difficult to know for sure if the findings are related to stress exposure or the presence of symptoms. Regardless, the findings substantially support the idea that low cortisol levels may represent a type of stress response.

GLUCOCORTICOID RECEPTORS IN PTSD

The physiological and behavioral effects of cortisol depend on the ability of cortisol to bind to glucocorticoid receptors.[43] Alterations in the sensitivity of glucocorticoid receptors can therefore influence the dynamic functioning of the HPA axis. For example, in major depression,[25] both the number and sensitivity of lymphocyte glucocorticoid receptors are reduced compared with those in normal subjects.[44,45] Therefore, although high cortisol levels are present in major depression, the decreased sensitivity of the receptor may actually result in an attenuation of the normal biobehavioral effects of steroids. This phenomenon is sometimes referred to as ''glucocorticoid resistance.''[46] The occurrence of glucocorticoid resistance explains why, for example, depressed patients with very high cortisol levels do not show stigmata of Cushing's syndrome.

In PTSD, the number of basal glucocorticoid receptors is larger than normal. Three studies of combat veterans[20,28,47] and one study of adult survivors of childhood sexual abuse[48] demonstrated that glucocorticoid receptor numbers are higher in PTSD than in nontraumatized subjects without psychiatric disorders. To date, it is unclear whether glucocorticoid receptors regulate or are regulated by hormone levels in PTSD. Based on the findings that glucocorticoid receptors mediate the strength of negative feedback,[46] we hypothesized that increases in glucocorticoid receptor activity constitute a primary deficit in PTSD that results in the secondary alteration of low cortisol levels.[49] On the other hand, however, it is well known that low circulating levels of a hormone result in an upregulation or increased number of receptors.[43] For example, glucocorticoid receptors become "downregulated" or decreased in number in response to both cortisol administration and stress.[50]

Theoretically, if alterations in glucocorticoid receptors constituted a primary deficit in PTSD, receptor alterations would not be expected in trauma-exposed individuals who do not develop PTSD. Although preliminary observations suggest that trauma-exposed individuals without PTSD do have a somewhat higher number of receptors than do normals (TABLE 2), it is difficult to determine if trauma exposure per se is responsible for these alterations, because some of the individuals studied in the non-PTSD condition may have met criteria for past PTSD. More data are needed before this issue can be resolved.

Sensitivity of the lymphocyte glucocorticoid receptor in man has primarily been achieved by measuring the number of cytosolic glucocorticoid receptors in response to exogenous steroid administration (i.e., dexamethasone treatment). The number of cytosolic glucocorticoid receptors after dexamethasone therapy reflects the migration of receptors from the cell body to the cell nucleus. Because genomic activity is accomplished after translocation of the steroid-receptor complex into the cell nucleus, the number of receptors following dexamethasone administration provides an estimate of receptor sensitivity.[28,51] In major depression, the number of cytosolic glucocorticoid receptors after dexamethasone administration is higher than that of normals, which suggests that fewer bound receptors successfully translocated into the cell nucleus. This translates into less protein synthesis and less biological activity. In contrast, the cytosolic glucocorticoid receptor number was decreased after dexamethasone treatment in combat veterans with PTSD than in trauma survivors without PTSD or normal controls.[28] The decreased number of cytosolic glucocorticoid receptors suggests greater translocation of the steroid-receptor complex into the nucleus, resulting in a greater degree of protein synthesis.

CORTISOL RESPONSE TO DEXAMETHASONE IN PTSD

Consistent with both low cortisol and increased glucocorticoid receptor number, the cortisol response to dexamethasone is enhanced in PTSD. An augmented cortisol response to dexamethasone in PTSD is opposite the classic nonsuppression of cortisol (8:00 AM postdexamethasone cortisol levels at or above 5.0 μg/dl) reported in about half the depressed patients.[42,43] Nonsuppression of cortisol results from a reduced

TABLE 2. Percent Increase in Lymphocyte Glucocorticoid Receptor Number between Trauma Survivors with PTSD and Other Subjects

Study/Year	Trauma without PTSD	Percent Greater Than Normals	Psychiatric Controls
Yehuda et al., 1991	—	63%	—
Yehuda et al., 1993	—	—	113%
Yehuda et al., 1995	25%	91%	—
Stein et al., 1997	14%	33%	—
Average Increase across Studies	20%	62%	113%

TABLE 3. Cortisol Low-Dose (0.5 mg) Dexamethasone Suppression Test Using Plasma and Saliva Cortisol Estimates

Study/Year	Trauma with PTSD		Trauma without PTSD		Normal Subjects	
	$\bar{X} \pm SD$	(n)	$\bar{X} \pm SD$	(n)	$\bar{X} \pm SD$	(n)
Yehuda et al.,* 1993	1.4 ± 0.6	(21)	—		4.8 ± 2.9	(12)
Yehuda et al.,* 1995	1.1 ± 0.6	(14)	3.9 ± 3.5	(12)	3.9 ± 2.9	(14)
Stein et al.,* 1997	1.5 ± 1.4	(12)	2.0 ± 1.2	(6)	3.2 ± 3.2	(21)
Heim et al.,** 1997	0.39 ± 0.32	(4)[a]	0.96 ± 1.16	(8)[b]	2.03 ± 1.42	(9)[c]

Note: Values represent $\bar{X} \pm SD$ for 8:00 AM postdexamethasone cortisol expressed as μg/dl.
[a] Women with chronic pelvic pain and PTSD.
[b] Women with chronic pelvic pain and no PTSD.
[c] Infertile women presenting to OB/GYN clinic for infertility.
* Plasma.
** Saliva.

ability of dexamethasone to exert negative feedback inhibition on the release of CRF and ACTH.[53] Reduced negative feedback inhibition is likely a consequence of reduced glucocorticoid receptor activity.

The initial dexamethasone suppression test (DST) studies in PTSD used the 1.0 mg dose of dexamethasone, because these studies were conducted in the absence of information about that cortisol and glucocorticoid receptor number. Furthermore, investigators were interested in examining the hypothesis that PTSD would show similar types of HPA axis alterations to those observed in stress and major depression, and they did not consider the possibility of hypersuppression to dexamethasone.[54-58] Contrary to the initial hypotheses, these studies unanimously failed to find compelling evidence for nonsuppression of cortisol after dexamethasone in nondepressed PTSD patients. Most studies also failed to demonstrate nonsuppression in depressed PTSD patients. The exception is the study by Kudler et al.[54] who found a 50% rate of nonsuppression in depressed PTSD patients.

Our findings of low cortisol levels and an increased number of glucocorticoid receptors led us to hypothesize that PTSD patients would show enhanced suppression, rather than the classic nonsuppression, to dexamethasone. Testing this hypothesis required administering lower doses of dexamethasone to cause partial suppression of cortisol in the comparison group and to determine whether PTSD subjects would show significantly lower postdexamethasone cortisol levels. Indeed, augmented suppression was observed in PTSD patients than in nonexposed subjects.[28,29] This effect was dose dependent and was accompanied by a decline in cytosolic lymphocyte glucocorticoid receptor number.[28] The hyperresponsiveness to dexamethasone was also present in combat veterans with PTSD who met the diagnostic criteria for concurrent major depression, and importantly, was not present in combat veterans without PTSD. The finding of enhanced cortisol suppression to 0.50 mg dexamethasone in veterans has now been independently replicated in adult survivors of childhood sexual abuse,[48] adult sexual abuse,[33] and children exposed to natural disasters.[32]

PITUITARY RELEASE OF ACTH IN PTSD

ACTH released from the pituitary directly stimulates the adrenal production of cortisol. Therefore, an understanding of pituitary activity is critical in evaluating HPA axis alterations. However, determining plasma ACTH levels using single routine venipuncture techniques has been problematic, because under basal conditions the normal negative feedback influences on the pituitary mask the true activity of this gland. The pituitary normally mediates between CRF stimulation from the hypothalamus and inhibition of ACTH release resulting from the negative feedback of cortisol. Therefore, baseline ACTH levels may appear "normal" even though the pituitary gland is receiving excessive stimulation from CRF. Indeed, two studies reported that ACTH levels in PTSD patients were comparable to those in nonexposed subjects.[27,99] Because ACTH is released in bursts rather than continuously, an accurate description of ACTH level requires repeated sampling over short periods of time. Alternatively, it is possible to estimate pituitary sensitivity as well as basal ACTH activity using neuroendocrine challenge tests such as the CRF and the metyrapone stimulation test, respectively.

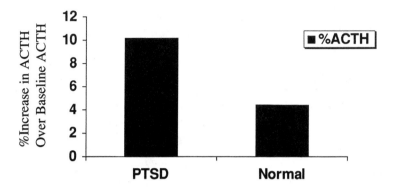

FIGURE 1. Percent rise in ACTH after metyrapone administration in posttraumatic stress disorder (PTSD) and normal control subjects.

The CRF challenge test, which measures ACTH and cortisol responses to the infusion of CRF, has been used to test pituitary sensitivity in PTSD.[59] Similar to observations in depressed patients,[60,61] the ACTH response to CRF is blunted in PTSD. However, it is critical to understand that a blunted ACTH response to CRF can reflect many different alterations such as downregulation of pituitary CRF receptors caused by hypothalamic CRF hypersecretion, increased negative feedback inhibition of the pituitary secondary to high cortisol levels, or increased glucocorticoid receptor number or sensitivity. In PTSD, increased glucocorticoid sensitivity may at least partially account for the blunted ACTH response to CRF.

The metyrapone stimulation test has been used to provide information about basal ACTH release in PTSD. Metyrapone temporarily blocks the synthesis of cortisol from its immediate precursor, 11-deoxycortisol, thereby removing negative feedback influences on the pituitary and brain.[62] Metyrapone prevents adrenal steroidogenesis by blocking the conversion of 11-deoxycortisol to cortisol, thereby unmasking the pituitary gland from the influences of negative feedback inhibition. Thus, metyrapone administration allows direct examination of pituitary release of ACTH without the potentially confounding effects of differing ambient cortisol levels or glucocorticoid receptor responsiveness. When metyrapone is administered in the morning, when HPA axis activity is relatively high, maximal pituitary activity can be achieved, making it possible to evaluate group differences in pituitary capability. If there are either chronic elevations in hypothalamic CRF release and/or increased glucocorticoid receptor sensitivity at the level of the pituitary, metyrapone administration would result in a relatively greater increase in ACTH release from the pituitary and an augmented accumulation of 11-deoxycortisol (i.e., hyperresponsiveness) compared to the normal increase (usually between two- and fivefold higher than baseline) typically observed in healthy and nonpsychiatric controls.[63] The reason is that in the absence of cortisol, the glucocorticoid receptors on the pituitary are rendered temporarily inert and cannot attenuate ACTH release via the normal negative feedback.

Indeed, the ACTH and 11-deoxycortisol response to metyrapone was more than fourfold higher in PTSD than in normal subjects (FIG. 1). This suggests that in the absence of negative feedback, the pituitary gland releases significantly more ACTH in individuals with PTSD.

HYPOTHALAMIC CRF RELEASE IN PTSD

There are now three lines of evidence that support the idea of increased CRF release in PTSD. First, there has now been an observation of elevated CRF in the cerebrospinal fluid of combat Vietnam veterans,[64] similar to that of depressed patients.[65] Although CSF levels of CRF may not necessarily reflect hypothalamic CRF release (since the CSF also reflects brain activity other than hypothalamic), this observation is certainly compatible with the idea of increased hypothalamic CRF release.

Other support for the idea of increased hypothalamic CRF release comes from the results of the aforementioned challenge studies. Relative increases in hypothalamic release of CRF in PTSD can be inferred from the results of the CRF challenge test. A blunted ACTH response to CRF in PTSD is consistent with the idea of CRF hypersecretion, because ACTH blunting might occur in response to a decreased number of CRF receptors on the pituitary gland.

However, the most definitive support for the idea of increased hypothalamic CRF release in PTSD is from the results of the metyrapone stimulation test, because it is unlikely that ACTH levels could be so much higher in PTSD than in normal subjects after metyrapone stimulation unless there was suprapituitary activation by CRF. The most likely source of this activation is CRF release (although other explanations such as alterations in vasopressin, somatostatin, or other neurotransmitters that modulate the pituitary gland might also be relevant). Thus, all studies to date support the idea that CRF hypersecretion is an important element in the pathophysiology of PTSD.

ENHANCED NEGATIVE FEEDBACK INHIBITION OF THE HPA AXIS IN PTSD: A PROTOTYPE OF BIOLOGICAL SENSITIZATION FOLLOWING TRAUMA

The findings just described are consistent with the idea of enhanced negative feedback inhibition of the HPA axis in PTSD. Under conditions of enhanced negative feedback inhibition, chronic increases in the release of hypothalamic and possibly extrahypothalamic CRF lead to altered responsiveness of the pituitary (e.g., hyporesponsiveness to CRF as evidenced by the blunted ACTH response and hyperresponsiveness to steroids as evidenced by the enhanced suppression to dexamethasone). However, because the glucocorticoid receptors are more responsive in this disorder (rather than less), there is attenuation in baseline cortisol levels and enhanced responsiveness to exogenous steroids (i.e., dexamethasone).

The model of enhanced negative feedback describes a sensitization of the HPA axis. This sensitization helps to explain why PTSD patients appear to be unusually responsive to stress (as opposed to being less responsive to stress, as would be indicated by models of glucocorticoid resistance). Indeed, PTSD patients often show exaggerated behavioral and biological response to environmental challenge. The maximally low background (i.e., low basal cortisol levels) and the ability to hyperrespond to the environment (e.g., by showing exaggerated responses to neuroendocrine challenges such as the DST and the metyrapone stimulation test) are consistent with symptoms of hypervigilence, increased startle, and physiological arousal or distress to reminders of the trauma.

Interestingly, studies of psychophysiologic,[66–69] electrophysiologic,[70,71] and neurochemical[72–74] alterations in PTSD have revealed similar abnormalities of the sympathetic nervous system and other neuromodulatory systems. Many of these studies have demonstrated that PTSD patients have exaggerated and more finely tuned biological responses to both stimuli that are reminders of the traumatic events and to perturbations, such as neuroendocrine challenge[72] and other laboratory stressors such as loud tones and exercise.[74,75]

In contrast, depressed patients have a less responsive negative feedback system which is more compatible with insensitivity to environmental stimuli. Indeed, the diminished ability of depressed patients to interact with the environment has repeatedly been demonstrated. For example, depressed patients who show nonsuppression to dexamethasone fail to dishabituate to tones and to discriminate between novel and familiar stimuli and therefore show an attenuated ability to perceive or respond to environmental change.[76]

WHAT DETERMINES BIOLOGICAL SENSITIZATION?

The studies just reviewed suggest that individuals with PTSD show a biological sensitization of the HPA axis. However, in considering the significance of these alterations it is imperative to consider when in the time course of trauma or PTSD are these changes manifest? The foregoing data have been collected on trauma survivors with chronic PTSD. Therefore, the studies just reviewed do not address the issue of whether the enhanced negative feedback phenomenon constitutes a chronic adaptation to trauma or PTSD symptoms or, rather, is an alteration observable in the early aftermath of trauma. A third possibility is that the alterations observed are predisposing risk factors that explain the emergence of PTSD following trauma. Although the answers to these questions are currently unknown, preliminary studies have begun to explore the acute biological response to trauma. These studies suggest that biological sensitization of the HPA axis may be observable in the acute aftermath of a trauma and may be related to the subsequent development of PTSD.

BIOLOGICAL STUDIES IN THE ACUTE AFTERMATH OF TRAUMATIC EVENTS: RELATIONSHIP TO THE BIOLOGY OF PTSD

Recent longitudinal studies have begun to examine whether differences in the acute biological response to trauma exist in those who subsequently do and those who do not develop PTSD. One study demonstrated that women who are most likely to develop PTSD had lower cortisol levels at the time of trauma. Low cortisol levels at the time of rape were associated with a history of rape, which was the strongest predictor of the subsequent development of PTSD.[77] Interestingly, the severity of the rape did not predict either cortisol levels or subsequent PTSD. However, rape severity was associated with MHPG responses immediately following rape. As would be predicted, the higher the rape severity, the higher the MHPG response. However, MHPG levels were not associated with the subsequent development of PTSD (H. Resnick and R. Yehuda, unpublished data).

In a second study, the cortisol response to motor vehicle accidents was examined in individuals who appeared in the emergency room in the immediate aftermath of the trauma. Six months later, subjects were evaluated for the presence or absence of psychiatric disorder. In subjects who had developed PTSD, the cortisol response immediately after the motor vehicle accident was lower and the cortisol response in those who developed major depression was higher than that in individuals who did not develop psychiatric disorder (McFarlane *et al.*, personal communication).

These two longitudinal studies demonstrate that the acute cortisol responses to trauma in individuals who develop PTSD may be different from those in individuals who do not develop PTSD in response to a similar trauma. As such, the low cortisol levels observed in chronic PTSD may reflect more than simply the state of having a chronic illness. The findings do not preclude the possibility that individuals who showed an attenuated cortisol response to a trauma may have had lower basal cortisol levels before the traumatic event. The resolution of this question necessitates prospective studies that assess cortisol levels in subjects before and after they experience traumatic events which, for obvious reasons, are difficult to perform. Nonetheless, the possibility that there may be biologic alterations prior to a traumatic event that influence the response to trauma is intriguing. It may be that PTSD reflects a biologic sensitization following stress due to preexisting risk factors. If so, perhaps it might be more appropriate to consider the symptoms and neurobiologic changes following trauma as reflecting a posttraumatic *sensitization* disorder rather than a posttraumatic *stress* disorder.

IMPLICATIONS OF HPA AXIS FINDINGS TO UNDERSTANDING FINDINGS OF REDUCED HIPPOCAMPAL VOLUME IN PTSD

One of the most fascinating biologic observations in PTSD is that of reduced hippocampal volume. (See Stein *et al.*, this volume, for a complete review.) This finding has now been replicated in four separate reports.[78–81] The initial impetus for investigating hippocampal atrophy in PTSD was based on evidence from numerous animal studies demonstrating the deleterious effects of stress and glucocorticoids in the hippocampus of laboratory animals. (See McEwen, this volume, for a review.) Because stress is the precipitant of PTSD, it was simply assumed that at some time during or after the traumatic event, cortisol levels would be high enough to damage the hippocampus, leading to permanent loss of neurons in this region. The data summarized in this chapter suggest that there is no evidence that cortisol levels were ever higher in individuals who develop PTSD than in those who do not either immediately after the trauma or in the chronic aftermath of the event. Rather, cortisol levels were found to be low during psychological trauma,[38,39] in the acute aftermath of trauma,[77] and chronically thereafter in individuals with PTSD. Therefore, it is unlikely that glucocorticoid toxicity explains the findings of hippocampal atrophy in PTSD. Rather, the HPA axis findings in PTSD compel researchers to consider other possible mechanisms as explanations for the hippocampal atrophy. (See McEwen, this volume, for a discussion of possible alternative mechanisms.)

Even in the absence of the recent empirical demonstrations of Resnick *et al.* and McFarlane *et al.* of the heterogeneous nature of the cortisol stress response in those who develop versus those who do not develop PTSD, the assertion of glucocorticoid toxicity as the causal mechanism for hippocampal atrophy in PTSD would be problematic. Primarily, if we assume that hippocampal damage occurs because of trauma exposure, then we would expect this lesion to be present in individuals who have sustained comparable levels of trauma, regardless of PTSD status. Gurvits *et al.*'s study clearly demonstrates that trauma-exposed individuals without PTSD do not have significantly smaller hippocampal volumes than do normal subjects. To explain the neuroanatomical observations in PTSD, one must consider that most trauma-exposed individuals will not develop this disorder. Therefore, alterations other than those specifically associated with stress exposure that are associated with PTSD are more reasonable alterations to consider in the context of hippocampal damage.

In this context, it might be that hippocampal atrophy is related to glucocorticoid receptor responsiveness. As reviewed in this chapter, trauma survivors with PTSD, but not those without PTSD, appear to have more sensitive glucocorticoid receptors. It has been hypothesized that the sensitivity of these receptors is associated with the enhanced negative feedback inhibition and overall sensitization of the HPA axis observed in PTSD. The enhanced sensitivity of glucocorticoid receptors in the hippocampus may cause the induction of NMDA receptors and other biologic events (usually attributed to hypercortisolism; see McEwen, this volume), which ultimately renders the hippocampus more vulnerable to atrophy. Indeed, the one study that actually examined hippocampal atrophy and glucocorticoid receptor responsiveness in tandem demonstrated an increased number of glucocorticoid receptors and enhanced cortisol response to dexamethasone in the trauma-exposed group with the reduced hippocampal volumes.[81]

Therefore, a consideration of the role of glucocorticoid receptor responsiveness in mediating hippocampal atrophy may be informative. As reviewed in this chapter, about half of those with major depressive disorder have hypercortisolism. However, despite this hypercortisolism, major depression has not been associated with hippocampal loss.[82] Although a recent study found decreased hippocampal volumes in remitted, nonhypercortisolemic depressed patients, these individuals were geriatric subjects, and other explanations (such as aging) more parsimoniously account for the neuroanatomical findings.[83] Despite the chronic hypercortisolism in depressed patients, hippocampi may not be smaller in this disorder, because hypercortisolism in depression is often associated with glucocorticoid resistance (i.e., glucocorticoid receptor sensitivity). If reduced glucocorticoid receptor sensitivity explains the lack of hippocampal atrophy in depression, then it is reasonable to consider the role of increased glucocorticoid receptor sensitivity in the hippocampal atrophy in PTSD.

CONCLUSIONS

An important conclusion from the just-reviewed neuroendocrine studies is that there is a distinct set of biological alterations that characterize the state of prolonged or persistent symptoms in response to a traumatic event. However, contrary to all initial expectations and hypotheses, the neuroendocrinology of PTSD does not resemble the neuroendocrine alterations observed in stress or those observed in psychiatric disorders such as major depression. The apparent uniqueness of the neuroendocrine constellation in PTSD is a paradox but one that affords an opportunity to explore the use of neuroendocrine measures as aids in the diagnosis of PTSD. Furthermore, because PTSD does develop in response to a traumatic event, the neuroendocrine alterations observed must represent a type of stress response, albeit atypical. Thus, the alterations allow us to more broadly expand our conceptions of stress responses.

REFERENCES

1. HOROWITZ, M. J. 1986. Stress Response Syndromes. Jason Aronson. New York.
2. FIGLEY, C. R. 1989. Helping Traumatized Families. Jossey-Bass. San Francisco.
3. GREEN, B. L., J. P. WILSON & J. D. LINDY. 1985. Conceptualizing posttraumatic stress disorder: A psychosocial framework. In C. R. Figley, Ed.: 53-69. Trauma and Its Wake. Brunner/Mazel. New York.
4. HERMAN, J. 1992. Trauma and Recovery. Basic Books. New York.
5. ANDREASEN, N. C. 1980. Posttraumatic Stress Disorder. In H. I. Kaplan, A. M. Freedman & B. J. Sadock, Eds. Comprehensive Textbook of Psychiatry, Third Edition. Vol. 2. Williams & Wilkins. Baltimore, MD.
6. KESSLER, R. C., A. SONNEGA, E. BROMET et al. 1995. Posttraumatic stress disorder in the national comorbidity survey. Arch. Gen. Psychiatry 52: 1048-1060.
7. DAVIDSON, J. R. T., D. HUGHES, D. BLAZER et al. 1991. Posttraumatic stress disorder in the community: An epidemiological study. Psychol. Med. 21: 1-9.
8. BRESLAU, N., G. C. DAVIS, P. ANDRESKI et al. 1991. Traumatic events and post traumatic stress disorder in an urban population of young adults. Arch. Gen. Psychiatry 48: 216-222.
9. KULKA, R. A., W. E. SCHLENGER, J. A. FAIRBANK et al. 1991. Trauma the Vietnam War Generation: Report of Findings from the National Vietnam Veterans' Readjustment Study. Brunner/Mazel. New York.
10. YEHUDA, R. & A. C. MCFARLANE. 1995. Conflict between current knowledge about posttraumatic stress disorder and its original conceptual basis. Am. J. Psychiatry 152: 1705-1713.
11. KRYSTAL, J. H., T. R. KOSTEN, B. D. PERRY et al. 1989. Neurobiological aspects of PTSD: Review of clinical and preclinical studies. Behav. Ther. 20: 177-198.
12. VAN DER KOLK, B., M. GREENBERG, H. BOYD et al. 1985. Inescapable shock, neurotransmitters, and addition to trauma: Toward a psychobiology of posttraumatic stress disorder. Biol. Psychiatry 20: 314-325.
13. KOLB, L. C. 1987. A neuropsychological hypothesis explaining the posttraumatic stress disorder. Am. J. Psychiatry 144: 989-995.
14. MUNCK, A., P. M. GUYRE & N. J. HOLBROOK. 1984. Physiological functions of glucocorticoids in stress and their relation to pharmacological actions. Endocr. Rev. 93: 9779-9783.
15. CHROUSOS, G. P. & P. W. GOLD. 1992. The concepts of stress and stress system disorders: Overview of physical and behavioral homeostasis. J. Am. Med. Assoc. 267: 1244-1252.
16. SACHAR, E. J., L. HELLMAN & H. P. ROFFWARG. 1973. Disrupted 24-hr patterns of cortisol secretion in psychotic depression. Arch. Gen. Psychiatry 28: 19-24.
17. SELYE, H. 1956. The Stress of Life. McGraw-Hill Book Co., Inc. New York.
18. MASON, J. W., E. L. GILLER, T. R. KOSTEN et al. 1986. Urinary-free cortisol levels in post-traumatic stress disorder patients. J. Nerv. Ment. Dis. 174: 145-159.

19. YEHUDA, R., S. M. SOUTHWICK, G. NUSSBAUM et al. 1990. Low urinary cortisol excretion in patients with PTSD. J. Nerv. Ment. Dis. **178:** 366-369.
20. YEHUDA, R., D. BOISONEAU, J. W. MASON et al. 1993. Relationship between lymphocyte glucocorticoid receptor number and urinary-free cortisol excretion in mood, anxiety, and psychotic disorder. Biol. Psychiatry **34:** 18-25.
21. YEHUDA, R., B. KAHANA, K. BINDER-BRYNES et al. 1995. Low urinary cortisol excretion in holocaust survivors with PTSD. Am. J. Psychiatry **152:** 7-12.
22. PITMAN, R. K. & S. ORR. 1990. Twenty-four hour urinary cortisol and catecholamine excretion in combat-related PTSD. Biol. Psychiatry **27:** 245-247.
23. LEMIEUX, A. M. & C. L. COE. 1995. Abuse-related posttraumatic stress disorder: Evidence for chronic neuroendocrine activation in women. Psychosom. Med. **57:** 105-115.
24. MEIKLE, A. W., H. TAKIGUCHI & S. MIZUTANI. 1969. Urinary cortisol excretion determined by competitive protein binding radioassay: A test of adrenal cortical function. J. Lab. Clin. Med. **74:** 803-812.
25. KATHOL, R. G., R. S. JAECKLE & W. F. LOPEZ. 1989. Pathophysiology of HPA axis abnormalities in patients with major depression: An update: Am. J. Psychiatry **1246:** 311-317.
26. YEHUDA, R., E. L. GILLER, S. M. SOUTHWICK et al. 1991. Hypothalamic-pituitary-adrenal dysfunction in PTSD. Biol. Psychiatry **30:** 1031-1048.
27. HOFFMAN, L., P. B. WATSON, G. WILSON et al. 1989. Low plasma b-endorphin in posttraumatic stress disorder. Aust. N. Z. J. Psychiatry **23:** 269-273.
28. YEHUDA, R., D. BOISONEAU, M. T. LOWY et al. 1995. Dose-response changes in plasma cortisol and lymphocyte glucocorticoid receptors following dexamethasone administration in combat veterans with and without posttraumatic stress disorder. Arch. Gen. Psychiatry **52:** 583-593.
29. YEHUDA, R., S. M. SOUTHWICK, J. M. KRYSTAL et al. 1993. Enhanced suppression of cortisol following dexamethasone administration in combat veterans with posttraumatic stress disorder and major depressive disorder. Am. J. Psychiatry **150:** 83-86.
30. SOUTHWICK, S. M., J. H. KRYSTAL, A. C. MORGAN et al. 1993. Abnormal noradrenergic function in post traumatic stress disorder. Arch. Gen. Psychiatry **50:** 266-274.
31. BOSCARINO, J. A. 1996. Posttraumatic stress disorder, exposure to combat, and lower plasma cortisol among Vietnam veterans: Findings and clinical implications. J. Clin. Consult. Psychol. **64:** 191-201.
32. GOENJIAN, A. K., R. YEHUDA, R. S. PYNOOS et al. 1996. Basal cortisol and dexamethasone suppression of cortisol among adolescents after the 1988 earthquake in Armenia. Am. J. Psychiatry **153:** 929-934.
33. HEIM, C., U. EHLART, J. REXHAUSEN, J. P. HANKER & D. H. HELLHAMER. Ann. N. Y. Acad Sci., this volume.
34. YEHUDA, R., M. H. TEICHER, R. L. TRESTMAN et al. 1996. Cortisol regulation in posttraumatic stress disorder and major depression: A chronobiological analysis. Biol. Psychiatry **40:** 79-88.
35. FRIEDMAN, S. B., J. W. MASON & D. A. HANBURG. 1963. Urinary 17-hydroxycorticosteroid levels in parents of children with neoplastic disease. A study of chronic psychological stress. Psychosom. Med. **25:** 364-376.
36. VERNIKOS DANELLIS, J., W. L. GOLDENRATH & C. B. DOLAS. 1975. The physiological cost of flight stress and flight fatigue. US Navy Med. J. **66:** 12-16.
37. HELLHAMMER, D. H. & S. WADE. 1993. Endocrine correlates of stress vulnerability. Psychother. Psychosom. **60:** 8-17.
38. BOURNE, P. B., R. M. ROSE & J. W. MASON. 1967. Urinary 17-OHCA levels. Data on seven helicopter ambulance medics in combat. Arch. Gen. Psychiatry **17:** 104-110.
39. BOURNE, P. B., R. M. ROSE & J. W. MASON. 1968. 17-OHCS levels in combat: Special forces "A" team under threat of attack. Arch. Gen. Psychiatry **19:** 135-140.

40. VRKLJAN, M., T. VILIBIC, B. VIZENER et al. 1994. Case report of a patient with posttraumatic stress disorder and pituitary apoplexy. Paper presented at the International Society for Psychoneuroendocrinology, Annual Meeting.
41. DEKARIS, D., A. SABIONCELLO, R. MAZURAN et al. 1993. Multiple changes of immunologic parameters in prisoners of war. JAMA 270: 595-599.
42. BAUER, M., S. PRIEBE, K. J. GRAF et al. 1994. Psychological and endocrine abnormalities in refugees from East Germany: Part II. Serum levels of cortisol, prolactin, luteinizing hormone, follicle stimulating hormone and testosterone. Psychiatry Res. 51: 75-85.
43. SVEC, F. 1985. Minireview: Glucocorticoid receptor regulation. Life Sci. 35: 2359-2366.
44. WHALLEY, L. J., N. BORTHWICK & D. COPOLOV. 1986. Glucocorticoid receptors and depression. Br. Med. J. 292: 859-861.
45. GORMLEY, G. J., M. T., LOWY, A. T. REDER et al. 1985. Glucocorticoid receptors in depression: Relationship to the dexamethasone suppression test. Am. J. Psychiatry 142: 1278-1284.
46. LOWY, M. T., G. J. GORMLEY & A. T. REDER. 1989. Immune function, glucocorticoid receptor regulation and depression. In Depressive Disorders and Immunity. A. H. Miller, Ed.: 105-134. APA Press. Washington, DC.
47. YEHUDA, R., M. T. LOWY, S. M. SOUTHWICK et al. 1991. Increased lymphocyte glucocorticoid receptor number in PTSD. Am. J. Psychiatry 149: 499-504.
48. STEIN, M. B., R. YEHUDA, C. KOVEROLA et al. 1997. HPA axis functioning in adult women who report experiencing severe childhood sexual abuse. Biol. Psychiatry. In press.
49. YEHUDA, R., E. L. GILLER, S. M. SOUTHWICK et al. 1995. Hypothalamic-pituitary-adrenal alterations in PTSD. In Neurobiological and Clinical Consequences of Stress: From Normal Adaptation to PTSD. M. J. Friedman, D. S. Charney & A. Y. Deutch, Eds. Raven Press. New York.
50. SAPOLSKY, R. M., L. C. KREY & B. S. McEWEN. 1984. Stress down regulates corticosterone receptors in a site specific manner in the brain. Endocrinology 114: 287-292.
51. LOWY, M. T., M. Y. REDER, G. J. GORMLEY et al. 1988. Comparison of in vivo and in vitro glucocorticoid sensitivity in depression: Relationship to the dexamethasone suppression test. Biol. Psychiatry 24: 619-630.
52. APA Task Force on Laboratory Tests in Psychiatry. 1987. The dexamethasone suppression test: An overview of its current status in psychiatry. Am. J. Psychiatry 144: 1253-1262.
53. CAROLL, B. J., M. FEINBERG, J. F. GREDEN et al. 1981. A specific laboratory test for the diagnosis of melancholia. Arch. Gen. Psychiatry 38: 15-22.
54. KUDLER, H., J. DAVIDSON & K. MEADOR. 1987. The DST and posttraumatic stress disorder. Am. J. Psychiatry 144: 1068-1071.
55. OLIVERA, A. A. & D. FERO. 1990. Affective disorders, DST, and treatment in PTSD patients: Clinical observations. J. Traumatic Stress 3: 407-414.
56. DINAN, T. G., S. BARRY, L. N. YATHAM et al. 1990. A pilot study of a neuroendocrine test battery in posttraumatic stress disorder. Biol. Psychiatry 28: 665-672.
57. HALBREICH, U., J. OLYMPIA, S. CARSON et al. 1989. Hypothalamic-pituitary-adrenal activity in endogenously depressed posttraumatic stress disorder patients. Psychoneuroendocrinology 14: 365-370.
58. KOSTEN, T. R., V. WAHBY, E. GILLER et al. 1990. The dexamethasone suppression test and thyrotropin-releasing hormone stimulation test in PTSD. Biol. Psychiatry 28: 657.
59. SMITH, M. A., J. DAVIDSON, J. C. RITCHIE et al. 1989. The corticotropin releasing hormone test in patients with PTSD. Biol. Psychiatry 26: 349-355.
60. GOLD, P. W., D. L. LORIAUX & A. ROY. 1986. Responses to corticotropin-releasing hormone in the hypercortisolism of depression and Cushing's disease. N. Engl. J. Med. 314: 1329-1335.
61. HOLSBOER, F., U. VON BARDELEBEN & A. GERKEN. 1984. Blunted corticotropin and normal cortisol responses to human corticotropin-releasing factor in depression. N. Engl. J. Med. 311: 1127-1131.

62. LISANSKY, J., G. T. PEAKE, R. J. STRASSMAN *et al.* 1989. Augmented pituitary ACTH response to a threshold dosage of CRH in depressives pretreated with metyrapone. Arch. Gen. Psychiatry **46:** 641–649.

63. YEHUDA, R., R. LEVENGOOD, J. SCHMEIDLER *et al.* 1996. Increased pituitary activation following metyrapone administration in PTSD. Psychoneuroendocrinology **21:** 1–16.

64. DARNELL, A., J. D. BREMNER, C. B. NEMEROFF *et al.* 1994. CSF levels of CRF in chronic PTSD. Neurosci. Abstr. **20:** 15:4.

65. NEMEROFF, C. B., E. WIDERLOV, G. BISSETTE *et al.* 1984. Elevated concentrations of CSF corticotropin-releasing factor-like immunoreactivity in depressed patients. Science **226:** 1342–1344.

66. PITMAN, R. K., S. P. ORR, D. F. FORGUE *et al.* 1987. Psychophysiologic assessment of posttraumatic stress disorder imagery in Vietnam combat veterans. Arch. Gen. Psychiatry **44:** 970–975.

67. SHALEV, A. & Y. ROGEL-FUCHS. Psychophysiology of the PTSD 1993. From sulfur fumes to behavioral genetics. Psychosom. Med. **55:** 413–423.

68. SHALEV, A. Y., F. P. ORR & R. K. PITMAN. 1993. Psychophysiologic assessment of traumatic imagery in Israeli civilian patients with posttraumatic stress disorders. Am. J. Psychiatry **150:** 620–624.

69. SHALEV, A. Y., S. P. ORR, P. PERI *et al.* 1992. Physiologic responses to loud tones in Israeli post-traumatic stress disorder patients. Arch. Gen. Psychiatry **40:** 870–975.

70. MCFARLANE, A. C., D. WEBER & R. CLARK. 1993. Abnormal stimulus processing in posttraumatic stress disorder. Biol. Psychiatry **34:** 311–320.

71. PAIGE, S. R., G. M. REID, M. G. ALLEN *et al.* 1990. Psychophysiological correlates of posttraumatic stress disorder in Vietnam veterans. Biol. Psychiatry **27:** 419–430.

72. RAINEY, J. M., A. ALEEM & A. ORTIZ. 1987. A laboratory procedure for the induction of flashbacks. Am. J. Psychiatry **144:** 1317–1319.

73. MURBURGH, M. M. 1994. Catecholamine Function in Posttraumatic Stress Disorder: Emerging Concepts. APA Press. Washington, DC.

74. MCFALL, M., M. MURBURG & G. KO. 1990. Autonomic response to stress in Vietnam combat veterans with post-traumatic stress disorder. Biol. Psychiatry **27:** 1165–1175.

75. HAMNER, M. B., B. I. DIAMOND & A. HITRI. 1994. Plasma norepinephrine and MHPG responses to exercise stress in PTSD. *In* Catecholamine Function in Posttraumatic Stress Disorder: Emerging Concepts. M. M. Murburg, Ed.: 221–232. Washington, DC. APA Press.

76. REUS, V. I., V. S. PEEKE & C. MINER. 1985. Habituation and cortisol dysregulation in depression. Biol. Psychiatry **20:** 980–989.

77. RESNICK, H. S., R. YEHUDA, R. PITMAN *et al.* 1995. Effect of previous trauma on acute plasma cortisol level following rape. Am. J. Psychiatry **152:** 1675–1677.

78. BREMNER, D., P. RANDALL, T. N. SCOTT, R. A. BRONEN, J. P. SEBYL, S. M. SOUTHWICK, R. C. DELANEY, G. MCCARTHY, D. S. CHARNEY & R. B. INNIS. 1995. MRI-based measurements of hippocampal volume in combat-related posttraumatic stress disorder. Am. J. Psychiatry **152:** 973–981.

79. GURVITS, T. V., M. E. SHENTON, H. HOKAMA, H. OHTA, N. B. LASKO, M. W. GILBERTSON, S. P. ORR, R. KIKINIS, F. A. JOLESZ, R. W. MCCARLEY & R. K. PITMAN. 1996. Magnetic resonance imaging study of hippocampal volume in chronic, combat-related posttraumatic stress disorder. Biol. Psychiatry **40:** 1091–1099.

80. BREMNER, J. P., P. RANDALL, E. VERMETTEN, L. STAIB, R. A. BRONEN, C. MAZURE, S. CAPELLI, G. MCCARTHY, R. B. INNIS & D. S. CHARNEY. 1997. MRI-based measurement of hippocampal volume in posttraumatic stress disorder related to childhood physical and sexual abuse: A preliminary report. Biol. Psychiatry **41:** 23–32.

81. STEIN, M. B. *et al.*, this volume.

82. AXELSON, D. A., P. M. DORAISWAMY, W. M. McDONALD, O. B. BOYKO, L. A. TUPLER, L. J. PATTERSON, C. B. NEMEROFF, E. H. ELLINWOOD & K. R. KRISHNAN. 1993. Hypercortisolemia and hippocampal changes in depression. Psychiatry Res. **47:** 163–173.
83. SHELINE, Y. I., P. O. WANG, M. H. GADO, J. G. CSERNANSKY & M. W. VANNIER. 1996. Hippocampal atrophy in recurrent major depression. Proc. Natl. Acad. Sci. USA **93:** 3908–3913.

Structural Brain Changes in PTSD

Does Trauma Alter Neuroanatomy?[a]

MURRAY B. STEIN,[b] CINDY HANNA,[c]
CATHERINE KOVEROLA,[c] MARK TORCHIA,[d] AND
BLAKE McCLARTY[d]

[b]Department of Psychiatry
San Diego Veterans Affairs Medical Center and
University of California, San Diego
3350 La Jolla Village Dr.
San Diego, California 92161

[c]Department of Psychology
University of Manitoba
Winnipeg, Manitoba, Canada

[d]St. Boniface General Hospital Research Centre
Winnipeg, Manitoba, Canada

Posttraumatic stress disorder (PTSD) was first codified in DSM-III to describe the range of syndromal responses to extreme stressors. In the 16 years since the publication of DSM-III and its evolution through DSM-III-R into DSM-IV, numerous studies have shown that PTSD frequently follows exposure to a variety of traumas such as combat, criminal victimization, sexual assault, natural disasters, motor vehicle accidents, and other events.[1–10] Moreover, we have come to appreciate that traumas of this nature are not rare and, accordingly, that rates of PTSD in the general population are much higher than we would have expected a mere decade ago.[11–16] The primary effect of this series of findings has been an enhanced professional and public awareness about the pervasiveness of PTSD. A secondary effect of these findings has been an increased interest in the pathophysiology of PTSD, with the hypothesis that it is a disorder characterized by dysfunction within specific brain systems.[17,18]

PRECLINICAL RATIONALE

Considerable preclinical research has shown that experimental stressors (e.g., restraint stress or social stress) can result in functional and morphological changes within the hippocampus in rodents and primates.[19–21] It is now generally accepted that stress-induced elevations of glucocorticoids augment the extracellular accumulation of excitatory amino acids (EAA) such as glutamate, resulting in hippocampal damage

[a]This work was supported in part by the St. Boniface General Hospital Research Foundation, Winnipeg, Manitoba, Canada (M.B.S. and B.M.) and by an Academic Senate Grant from the University of Manitoba (C.K.).

which is evident from both a cytoarchitectural (i.e., reduced cell sprouting and neuronal cell death, particularly in the CA3 region) and a functional (i.e., impaired learning and memory) perspective.[22-24] These findings have led clinical investigators to hypothesize that exposure to traumatic stress might analogously affect hippocampal morphology and functioning in humans and, moreover, that these effects might be mediated by the direct or indirect (e.g., NMDA-dependent mechanisms) effects of glucocorticoids.[25-28] In light of the well-established effects of hippocampal damage on explicit memory systems in humans and other primates,[29-32] recent research efforts have focused on determining whether or not patients with PTSD have explicit memory problems[33-39] and manifest corresponding neuroanatomic evidence of hippocampal pathology.[25,40,41]

NEUROPSYCHOLOGIC FUNCTIONING IN PTSD

Most studies published to date have found some evidence of short-term explicit verbal memory dysfunction in patients with PTSD.[33-38] However, the nature and extent of memory dysfunction have varied widely among the studies, from global memory deficits in some studies[33-36] to a highly circumscribed deficit manifested by the presence of excessive retroactive interference in another study.[37]

There are several weaknesses to the extant literature. First, substance abuse has not always been well-controlled for, even though this is probably the most likely alternative interpretation of the data given the well-established effects of chronic alcohol abuse on cognitive functioning.[42,43] Therefore, future studies should carefully control for alcohol abuse. Another criticism of certain studies[37] is that "a specific deficit in memory functioning" has been ascribed to the finding that the results in one out of a dozen or more memory tests or subtests are abnormal in patients with PTSD, whereas the rest are normal. In our opinion, a better explanation for this finding is a type I error resulting from multiple comparisons. Therefore, future studies should control for multiple comparisons by establishing clear *a priori* hypotheses and, when necessary, using analytic techniques that group together complementary measures of domain-specific (e.g., explicit verbal memory) functioning. A third weakness of these studies is that, with some exceptions,[33,36,38] the possibility that attentional dysfunction might be a more parsimonious explanation for the mnemonic findings in PTSD has received scant consideration.[44]

A primary disturbance in supervisory attentional control (sometimes referred to as "executive" functioning, a set of functions that is highly contiguous with the concept of "working memory")[44] may underly the so-called deficit in "short-term memory" seen in PTSD.[45] Future studies should include measures of selective attention and other aspects of supervisory attentional control which would allow this alternate hypothesis to be rigorously tested.

NEUROANATOMY IN PTSD: ASSESSING STRUCTURE WITH MRI AND ¹H-MRS

Bremner *et al.*[25] showed that 26 male combat veterans with PTSD had reduced MRI-derived right-sided hippocampal volume (8% less than that of 22 comparison subjects) and, moreover, that short-term verbal memory deficits were associated with the reduction in hippocampal volume.[25] Gurvits et al.[41] in a study of seven male combat veterans with PTSD, seven non-PTSD combat veterans, and eight normal volunteers found a bilateral reduction (26% on the left; 22% on the right) in hippocampal volume in the PTSD subjects. Bremner et al.[40] compared hippocampal volume in 17 adult survivors of childhood sexual abuse (who were inpatients or outpatients at a VA hospital) and 17 healthy subjects and found a 12% smaller volume in left-sided hippocampal volume in the abuse survivors.[40] In our own work,[40a] we found a small (5%) but statistically significant reduction in left-sided hippocampal volume in 21 women with severe childhood sexual abuse compared to 21 nonvictimized comparison subjects.

Taken together, these studies provide a strong rationale for further assessing hippocampal neuroanatomy in PTSD. They also pose several questions that should be further considered. In particular, the possibility that alcohol abuse (a common comorbid condition in PTSD)[46] is responsible for the findings has not been ruled out, even though most studies have attempted to use statistical approaches (e.g., covarying for years of alcohol abuse) to address this likelihood.[25,40] Therefore, future studies should systematically exclude subjects with histories of substantial alcohol abuse (e.g., > 2 years) and, for subjects with lesser alcohol abuse histories, match controls for years of abuse.

Another aspect of these studies that deserves further scrutiny is the finding that in three of the four extant studies the hippocampal volume reduction was small (5-12%), raising questions about the clinical significance and replicability of the finding. In this regard, it should be noted that considerable hippocampal "damage" may have occurred before an MRI-volumetric loss was detectable. Therefore, even though MRI-assessed hippocampal volume changes may correspond with loss of function (e.g., explicit verbal memory) when the structural damage is advanced and hippocampal loss is extreme,[47–49] this may not be the case when neuroanatomical changes are more subtle. It would therefore be useful if a more "sensitive" technique than MRI were available to assess structural change in the hippocampus and other regions of interest.

One such technique with ostensibly greater sensitivity than structural MRI for detecting hippocampal damage is proton magnetic resonance spectroscopy (^{1}H-MRS).[50–52] N-acetylaspartate (NAA), which is readily quantified using ^{1}H-MRS,[50–52] has been demonstrated to be a suitable marker of neuronal viability in a given region.[53,54] Moreover, in preliminary studies it was shown to indicate neuronal damage before structural changes are in evidence on MRI.[55] Therefore, future studies should include proton spectroscopic measurement of NAA in conjunction with high-resolution MR morphometry to maximize the likelihood of detecting neuronal damage.

Finally, to address the alternate hypothesis of attentional dysfunction in PTSD (and/or dissociative disorders),[45] it is important to also focus the neuroimaging efforts on regions of the frontal cortex that mediate supervisory attentional control ("executive function"). Although assigning a single neuroanatomic locus for this complex set of functions is overly simplistic, the anterior cingulate gyrus plays an integral role[56–59] and should be a focus of future studies.

SUMMARY

Although the impetus for studying hippocampal morphology and functioning in PTSD was the finding that stress could result in hippocampal damage in rodent and primate models, it is far from proven that the findings to date in PTSD represent defects that have been *caused* by trauma. It is equally possible that the findings represent a preexisting anomaly which might serve as a risk factor for the development of PTSD following trauma exposure. To resolve this dilemma, it is necessary to study persons at high risk for trauma (e.g., soldiers) *prior* to trauma exposure and again after exposure. Such methods will permit the determination not only of whether trauma alters hippocampal morphology, but also, if so, of whether this effect is limited to persons with PTSD.

At the present time, the field would be well advised to proceed vigorously but with appropriate caution along these lines of research. As just outlined, sample sizes have been small, and potentially confounding variables have abounded in most studies. The next few years of research may well continue to replicate the finding of abnormal hippocampal morphology in PTSD. However, it would not be surprising to find that other brain regions are also involved and that these represent part of a broader risk spectrum for the development of psychopathology under stress. Until these issues are clarified, the neuroanatomical findings to date in PTSD should be viewed as tentative, tantalizing, and in need of additional study.

REFERENCES

1. BRESLAU, N. & G. C. DAVIS. 1987. Posttraumatic stress disorder: The etiologic specificity of wartime stressors. Am. J. Psychiatry **144:** 578.
2. KULKA, R. A., W. E. SCHLENGER, J. A. FAIRBANK, R. L. HOUGH, B. K. JORDAN, C. R. MARMAR & D. S. WEISS. 1990. Trauma and the Vietnam War Generation. Brunner/Mazel. New York, NY.
3. KILPATRICK, D. G. & H. S. RESNICK. 1993. Posttraumatic stress disorder associated with exposure to criminal victimization in clinical and community populations. *In* Postraumatic Stress Disorder: DSM-IV and Beyond. J. R. T. Davidson & E. B. Foa, Eds.: 113-146. American Psychiatric Press. Washington, DC.
4. RESNICK, H. S., D. G. KILPATRICK, B. S. DANSKY, B. E. SAUNDERS & C. L. BEST. 1993. Prevalence of civilian trauma and posttraumatic stress disorder in a representative national sample of women. J. Consult Clin. Psychol. **61:** 984-991.
5. ASTIN, M. C., K. J. LAWRENCE & D. W. FOY. 1993. Posttraumatic stress disorder among battered women: Risk and resiliency factors. Violence & Victims **8:** 17-28.
6. NORTH, C. S., E. M. SMITH & E. L. SPITZNAGEL. 1994. Posttraumatic stress disorder in survivors of a mass shooting. Am. J. Psychiatry **151:** 82-88.
7. GIACONIA, R. M., H. Z. REINHERZ, A. B. SILVERMAN, B. PAKIZ, A. K. FROST & E. COHEN. 1995. Traumas and posttraumatic stress disorder in a community population of older adolescents. J. Am. Acad. Child Adolesc. Psychiatry **34:** 1369-1380.
8. TAYLOR, S. & W. J. KOCH. 1995. Anxiety disorders due to motor vehicle accidents: Nature and treatment. Clin. Psychol. Rev. **15:** 721-738.
9. DANCU, C. V., D. S. RIGGS, D. HEARST-IKEDA, B. G. SHOYER & E. B. FOA. 1996. Dissociative experiences and posttraumatic stress disorder among female victims of criminal assault and rape. J. Traumatic Stress **9:** 253-267.
10. SHARAN, P., G. CHAUDHARY, S. A. KAVATHEKAR & S. SAXENA. 1996. Preliminary report of psychiatric disorders in survivors of a severe earthquake. Am. J. Psychiatry **153:** 556-558.

11. HELZER, J. E., L. N. ROBINS & L. McEVOY. 1987. Post-traumatic stress disorder in the general population. N. Engl. J. Med. **317:** 1630-1634.
12. DAVIDSON, J. R. T., D. HUGHES, D. G. BLAZER & L. K. GEORGE. 1991. Post-traumatic stress disorder in the community: An epidemiological study. Psychol. Med. **21:** 713-721.
13. BRESLAU, N., G. C. DAVIS, P. ANDRESKI & E. PETERSON. 1991. Traumatic events and posttraumatic stress disorder in the community: An epidemiologic study. Arch. Gen. Psychiatry **48:** 216-222.
14. NORRIS, F. H. 1992. Epidemiology of trauma: Frequency and impact of different potentially traumatic events on different demographic groups. J. Consult. Clin. Psychol. **60:** 409-418.
15. VRANA, S. & D. LAUTERBACH. 1994. Prevalence of traumatic events and posttraumatic psychological symptoms in a nonclinical sample of college students. J. Traumatic Stress **7:** 289-302.
16. KESSLER, R. C., A. SONNEGA, E. BROMET, M. HUGHES & C. B. NELSON. 1995. Posttraumatic stress disorder in the national comorbidity survey. Arch. Gen. Psychiatry **52:** 1048-1060.
17. CHARNEY, D. S., A. Y. DEUTCH, J. H. KRYSTAL et al. 1993. Psychobiologic mechanisms of posttraumatic stress disorder. Arch. Gen. Psychiatry **50:** 295-305.
18. FRIEDMAN, M. J., D. S. CHARNEY & A. Y. DEUTCH, Eds. 1995. Neurobiological and Clinical Consequences of Stress: From Normal Adaptation to Post-Traumatic Stress Disorder. Lippincott-Raven. Hagerstown, MD.
19. SAPOLSKY, R. M. 1994. The physiological relevance of glucocorticoid endangerment of the hippocampus. Ann. N.Y. Acad. Sci. **743:** 294-304.
20. GOULD, E. 1994. The effects of adrenal steroids and excitatory input on neuronal birth and survival. Ann. N.Y. Acad. Sci. **743:** 73-92.
21. STEIN-BEHRENS, B., M. P. MATTSON, I. CHANG, M. YEH & R. SAPOLSKY. 1994. Stress exacerbates neuron loss and cytoskeletal pathology in the hippocampus. J. Neurosci. **14:** 5373-5380.
22. STEIN-BEHRENS, B., W.-J. LIN & R. M. SAPOLSKY. 1994. Physiological elevations of glucocorticoids potentiate glutamate accumulation in the hippocampus. J. Neurochem. **63:** 596-602.
23. MOGHADDAM, B., M. L. BOLINAO, B. STEIN-BEHRENS & R. SAPOLSKY. 1994. Glucocorticoids mediate the stress-induced extracellular accumulation of glutamate. Brain Res. **65:** 251-254.
24. BODNOFF, S. R., A. G. HUMPHREYS, J. C. LEHMAN, D. M. DIAMOND, G. M. ROSE & M. J. MEANEY. 1995. Enduring effects of chronic corticosterone treatment on spatial learning, synaptic plasticity, and hippocampal neuropathology in young and mid-aged rats. J. Neurosci. **15:** 61-69.
25. BREMNER, J. D., P. RANDALL, T. M. SCOTT, R. A. BRONEN, J. P. SEIBYL, S. M. SOUTHWICK, R. C., DELANEY, G. McCARTHY, D. S. CHARNEY & R. B. INNIS. 1995. MRI-based measurement of hippocampal volume in combat-related posttraumatic stress disorder. Am. J. Psychiatry **152:** 973-981.
26. YEHUDA, R., E. L. GILLER, JR., R. A. LEVENGOOD, S. M. SOUTHWICK & L. J. SIEVER. 1995. Hypothalamic-pituitary-adrenal functioning in post-traumatic stress disorder: Expanding the concept of the stress response spectrum. In Neurobiological and Clinical Consequences of Stress: From Normal Adaptation to Post-Traumatic Stress Disorder. M. J. Friedman, D. S. Charney & A. Y. Deutch, Eds. Lippincott-Raven. Hagerstown, MD.
27. KRYSTAL, J. H., L. P. KARPER, J. P. SEIBYL, G. K. FREEMAN, R. DELANEY, J. D. BREMNER, G. R. HENINGER, M. B. BOWERS, JR. & D. S. CHARNEY. 1994. Subanesthetic effects of the noncompetitive NMDA antagonist, ketamine, in humans. Arch. Gen. Psychiatry **51:** 199-214.
28. BREMNER, J. D., J. H. KRYSTAL, D. S. CHARNEY & S. M. SOUTHWICK. 1996. Neural mechanisms in dissociative amnesia for childhood abuse: Relevance to the current controversy surrounding the "False Memory Syndrome." Am. J. Psychiatry **153** (suppl): 71-82.

29. SQUIRE, L. R., J. G. OJEMANN, F. M. MIEZIN, S. E. PETERSEN, T. O. VIDEEN & M. E. RAICHLE. 1992. Activation of the hippocampus in normal humans: A functional anatomical study of memory. Proc. Natl. Acad. Sci. USA **89:** 1837–1841.

30. ZOLA-MORGAN, S. & L. R. SQUIRE. 1993. Neuroanatomy of memory. Annu. Rev. Neurosci. **16:** 547–563.

31. ALVAREZ, P., S. ZOLA-MORGAN & L. SQUIRE. 1995. Damage limited to the hippocampal region produces long-lasting memory impairment in monkeys. J. Neurosci. **15:** 3796–3807.

32. SCHACTER, D. L., N. M. ALPERT, C. R. SAVAGE, S. L. RAUCH & M. S. ALBERT. 1996. Conscious recollection and the human hippocampal formation: Evidence from positron emission tomography. Proc. Natl. Acad. Sci. USA **93:** 321–325.

33. SUTKER, P. B., D. K. WINSTEAD, Z. H. GALINA & A. N. ALLAIN. 1991. Cognitive deficits and psychopathology among former prisoners of war and combat veterans of the Korean conflict. Am. J. Psychiatry **148:** 67–72.

34. BREMNER, J. D., T. M. SCOTT, R. C. DELANEY, S. M. SOUTHWICK, J. W. MASON, D. R. JOHNSON, R. B. INNIS, G. MCCARTHY & D. S. CHARNEY. 1993. Deficits in short-term memory in posttraumatic stress disorder. Am. J. Psychiatry **150:** 1015–1019.

35. BREMNER, J. D., P. RANDALL, T. M. SCOTT, S. CAPELLI, R. DELANEY, G. MCCARTHY & D. S. CHARNEY. 1995. Deficits in short-term memory in adult survivors of childhood abuse. Psychiatry Res. **59:** 97–107.

36. SUTKER, P. B., J. J. VASTERLING, K. BRAILEY & A. N. ALLAIN. 1995. Memory, attention, and executive deficits in POW survivors: Contributing biological and psychological factors. Neuropsychology **9:** 118–125.

37. YEHUDA, R., R. S. E. KEEFE, P. D. HARVEY, R. A. LEVENGOOD, D. K. GERBER, J. GENI & L. J. SIEVER. 1995. Learning and memory in combat veterans with posttraumatic stress disorder. Am. J. Psychiatry **152:** 137–139.

38. UDDO, M., J. J. VASTERLING, K. BRAILEY & P. B. SUTKER. 1993. Memory and attention in posttraumatic stress disorder. J. Psychopathol. Behav. Assess. **6:** 33–41.

39. GURVITS, T. V., N. B. LASKO, S. C. SCHACHTER, A. A. KUHNE, S. P. ORR & R. K. PITMAN. 1993. Neurological status of Vietnam veterans with chronic post-traumatic stress disorder. J. Neuropsychiatry Clin. Neurosci. **5:** 183–188.

40. BREMNER, J. D., P. RANDALL, E. VERMETTEN, L. STAIB, R. A. BRONEN, C. MAZURE, S. CAPELLI, G. MCCARTHY, R. B. INNIS & D. S. CHARNEY. 1997. MRI-based measurement of hippocampal volume in posttraumatic stress disorder related to childhood physical and sexual abuse: A preliminary report. Biol. Psychiatry **41:** 23–32.

40a. STEIN, M. B., C. KOVEROLA, C. HANNA, M. TORCHIA & B. MCCLARTY. 1997. Hippocampal volume in women victimized by childhood sexual abuse. Psychol. Med. In press.

41. GURVITS, T. G., M. R. SHENTON, H. HOKAMA, H. OHTA, N. B. LASKO, M. W. GILBERTSON, S. P. ORR, R. KIKINIS, F. A. JOLESZ, R. W. MCCARLEY & R. K. PITMAN. 1996. Magnetic resonance imaging study of hippocampal volume in chronic, combat-related posttraumatic stress disorder. Biol. Psychiatry **40:** 1091–1099.

42. GOLDMAN, M. S., D. L. WILLIAMS & D. K. KLISZ. 1983. Recoverability of psychological functioning following alcohol abuse: Prolonged visual-spatial dysfunction in older alcoholics. J. Consult. Clin. Psychol. **51:** 370–378.

43. DE SCLAFANI, V., F. EZEKIEL, D. J. MEYERHOFF, S. MACKAY, W. P. DILLON, M. W. WEINER & G. FEIN. 1995. Brain atrophy and cognitive function in older abstinent alcoholic men. Alcohol Clin. Exp. Res. **19:** 1121–1126.

44. BADDELEY, A. D. 1993. Working memory or working attention? *In* Attention: Selection, Awareness and Control. A. D. Baddeley & L. Weiskrantz, Eds. Oxford University Press. New York.

45. KRYSTAL, J. H., A. L. BENNETT, J. D. BREMNER, S. M. SOUTHWICK & D. S. CHARNEY. 1995. Toward a cognitive neuroscience of dissociation and altered memory functions in posttraumatic stress disorder. *In* Neurobiological and Clinical Consequences of

Stress: From Normal Adaptation to Post-Traumatic Stress Disorder. M. J. Friedman, D. S. Charney & A. Y. Deutch, Eds. Lippincott-Raven. Hagerstown, MD.

46. PENICK, E. C., B. J. POWELL, E. J. NICKEL, S. F. BINGHAM, K. R. RIESENMY, M. R. READ & J. CAMPBELL. 1994. Co-morbidity of lifetime psychiatric disorder among male alcoholic patients. Alcohol Clin. Exp. Res. **18:** 1289-1293.

47. TRENERRY, M. R., C. R. JACK, JR., R. J. IVNIK, F. W. SHARBROUGH, G. D. CASCINO, K. A. KIRSCHORN, W. R. MARSH, P. J. KELLY & F. B. MEYER. 1993. MRI hippocampal volumes and memory function before and after temporal lobectomy. Neurology **43:** 1800-1805.

48. DEWEER, B., S. LEHERICY, B. PILLON, M. BAULAC, J. CHIRAS, C. MARSAULT, Y. AGID & B. DUBOIS. 1995. Memory disorders in probable Alzheimer's disease: The role of hippocampal atrophy as shown with MRI. J. Neurol. Neurosurg. Psychiatry **58:** 590-597.

49. TRENERRY, M. R., C. R. JACK, JR., G. D. CASCINO, F. W. SHARBROUGH & R. J. IVNIK. 1995. Gender differences in post-temporal lobectomy verbal memory and relationships between MRI hippocampal volumes and preoperative verbal memory. Epilepsy Res. **20:** 69-76.

50. DAGER, S. R. & R. G. STEEN. 1992. Applications of magnetic resonance spectroscopy to the investigation of neuropsychiatric disorders. Neuropsychopharmacology **6:** 249-266.

51. HENNIG, J., H. PFISTER, T. ERNST & D. OTT. 1992. Direct absolute quantification of metabolites in the human brain with *in vivo* localized proton spectroscopy. NMR Biomed. **5:** 193-199.

52. MICHAELIS, T., K.-D. MERBOLDT, H. BRUHN, W. HANICKE, D. MATH & J. FRAHM. 1993. Absolute concentrations of metabolites in the adult human brain *in vivo:* Quantification of localized proton MR spectra. Radiology **187:** 219-227.

53. URENJACK, J., S. R. WILLIAMS, D. G. GADIAN *et al.* 1992. Specific expression of *N*-acetylaspartate in neurons, oligodendrocyte type 2 astrocyte progenitors, and immature oligodendrocytes *in vitro.* J. Neurochem. **59:** 55-61.

54. EBISU, T., W. D. ROONEY, S. H. GRAHAM, M. W. WEINER & A. A. MAUDSLEY. 1994. *N*-acetylaspartate as an *in vivo* marker of neuronal viability in kainate-induced status epilepticus: ^{1}H magnetic resonance spectroscopic imaging. J. Cereb. Blood Flow Metab. **14:** 373-382.

55. CENDES, F., F. ANDERMANN, M. C. PREUL *et al.* 1994. Lateralization of temporal lobe epilepsy based on regional metabolic abnormalities in proton magnetic resonance spectroscopic images. Ann. Neurol. **35:** 211-216.

56. PARDO, J. V., P. J. PARDO, K. W. KANER & M. E. RAICHLE. 1990. The anterior cingulate cortex mediates processing selection in the Stroop attentional conflict paradigm. Proc. Natl. Acad. Sci. USA **87:** 256-259.

57. BENCH, C. J., C. D. FRITH, P. M. GRASBY, K. J. FRISTON, E. PAULESU, R. S. J. FRACKOWIAK & R. J. DOLAN. 1993. Investigations of the functional anatomy of attention using the Stroop test. Neuropsychologia **31:** 907-922.

58. PARDO, J. V., P. T. FOX & M. E. RAICHLE. 1996. Localization of a human system for sustained attention by positron emission tomography. Nature **349:** 61-64.

59. POSNER, M. I. & S. E. PETERSEN. 1990. The attentional system of the human brain. Ann. Rev. Neurosci. **13:** 182-196.

Functional Neuroimaging Studies in Posttraumatic Stress Disorder

SCOTT L. RAUCH [a] AND LISA M. SHIN [b]

[a]Departments of Psychiatry and Radiology
Massachusetts General Hospital and
Department of Psychiatry
Harvard Medical School
Boston, Massachusetts 01890

[b]Department of Psychology
Harvard University
Cambridge, Massachusetts 02138

Neuroimaging techniques provide some of the most powerful methods available for the study of brain structure and function *in vivo*. Functional neuroimaging entails constructing maps that reflect indices of gross neuronal activity (i.e., regional cerebral blood flow [CBF] or glucose metabolism), neuroreceptor binding capacity, or concentrations of specific chemical compounds. The various imaging modalities can be categorized on the basis of the type of energy utilized to generate the signals from which the maps are formed. Nuclear medical techniques (i.e., positron emission tomography [PET] and single photon emission computed tomography [SPECT]) rely on energy emitted via radioactive decay, whereas magnetic resonance techniques (i.e., functional magnetic resonance imaging [fMRI] and magnetic resonance spectroscopy [MRS]) rely on the energy released by brain tissue constituents when placed within a strong magnetic field and perturbed with radiowaves. Although a comprehensive discussion of functional imaging methods is beyond the scope of this review,[1,2] we provide a scheme for considering the various types of paradigms employed in psychiatric imaging research: neutral state (single session or pre-posttreatment), symptom provocation, cognitive activation, and neurochemical characterization studies. Within this framework, we present and summarize the current literature on functional neuroimaging studies in posttraumatic stress disorder (PTSD). Given that very few studies on this topic have been published to date, we have chosen to augment the extant peer-reviewed material with preliminary reports from other sources. Furthermore, we present the PTSD data against a backdrop of analogous studies pertaining to other anxiety disorders and normal emotional states. Finally, we discuss several critical considerations and the future of this field as it relates to PTSD research.

Although one hope is that psychiatric imaging research might ultimately lead to clinical applications that aid in diagnosis or treatment, initial studies of anxiety states and disorders have reflected intermediate goals. Functional neuroimaging studies of PTSD and other anxiety disorders have thus far focused on exploring pathophysiology and brain correlates of symptoms by mapping indices of gross neuronal activity. As with many areas of psychiatric neuroscience, surveying the literature can also help one to appreciate the evolution from naturalistic to hypothesis-driven experiments.

NEUTRAL STATE PARADIGMS

Neutral state paradigms are those in which subjects perform either a nonspecific task or no task during the period assayed by functional imaging. Thus, brain activity maps are generated with little attention to subtle aspects of the subject's state. When the PET-fluorodeoxyglucose method is used, the resulting maps reflect brain metabolism integrated over a 20–40-minute uptake period; when PET-oxygen-15 or SPECT-HMPAO methods are used, the resulting maps reflect rCBF over approximately 1–5 minutes. Single-session neutral state paradigms can be used in psychiatric research to contrast brain activity profiles in psychiatric patients vs control subjects. The results of such group comparisons graphically illustrate which brain territories exhibit differential activity between groups, thereby providing circumstantial evidence about the functional neuroanatomy of psychiatric disorders. Beyond such between-group contrasts, multiple session neutral state paradigms can also be employed in the context of pre-posttreatment studies. In this way, within-subject contrasts can be performed to illustrate which brain regions exhibit changes in activity associated with clinical improvement. Furthermore, inspection of pretreatment activity profiles, informed by subsequent clinical outcome, can yield information on predictors of treatment response. The following is a review of studies that have used neutral state paradigms to investigate obsessive compulsive disorder (OCD), panic disorder, and PTSD.

Obsessive Compulsive Disorder

Baxter *et al.*[3] studied resting cerebral glucose metabolic rates in three groups of subjects: 14 patients with OCD, 14 patients with major depressive disorder, and 14 healthy control subjects. Absolute glucose metabolic rates in bilateral head of caudate and orbital gyri were higher in the OCD group than in the normal and depressed control groups. Relative glucose metabolic rates in the left orbital gyrus (i.e., left orbital/left hemisphere ratios) were higher in the OCD group than in the normal control group. OCD subjects were then treated with trazodone hydrochloride, with or without a monoamine oxidase inhibitor; those who responded to this treatment showed significant bilateral increases in caudate/hemisphere ratios.

Nordahl *et al.*[4] measured glucose metabolic rates in 8 medication-free patients with OCD and 30 healthy control subjects. Subjects underwent PET scanning while they participated in an auditory continuous performance task involving the detection of low tones. Results revealed higher normalized regional metabolic rates in bilateral orbitofrontal cortex (including right anterior, right posterior, left anterior, and anterior medial orbitofrontal regions) in OCD subjects than in normal control subjects.

Benkelfat *et al.*[5] measured cerebral glucose metabolic rates in 8 OCD patients before and after treatment with clomipramine. After treatment, normalized glucose metabolic rates increased in the right putamen and decreased in the inferomedial orbitofrontal cortex and left caudate.

In a study of childhood-onset OCD, Swedo *et al.*[6] measured resting cerebral glucose metabolic rates in 18 patients with OCD and 18 healthy control subjects. Glucose metabolic rates in the following regions were higher in OCD subjects than in control subjects: bilateral prefrontal, left orbitofrontal, bilateral anterior cingulate, left premotor, right sensorimotor, right inferior temporal, right thalamus, left paracentral, and right cerebellar cortex. Ratios of regional glucose metabolic rates to mean cortical gray matter metabolism in the right prefrontal cortex and left anterior cingulate cortex were higher in OCD subjects than in control subjects. Furthermore, severity of OCD was correlated positively with both right orbitofrontal regional metabolism and the ratio of right orbitofrontal metabolism to mean cortical gray matter metabolism.

Swedo et al.[7] restudied a subset of the subjects from their earlier report[6] after treatment with clomipramine or fluoxetine for at least 1 year. In comparing posttreatment to pretreatment values, they found decreased normalized bilateral orbitofrontal metabolism. Subjects who responded to treatment showed greater decreases in normalized left orbitofrontal metabolism than did nonresponders. OCD severity was correlated with a normalized right prefrontal glucose metabolic rate.

In a SPECT study of OCD, Machlin et al.[8] measured resting rCBF in 10 OCD patients and 8 healthy control subjects. Normalized rCBF in the medial frontal cortex was higher in the OCD group than in the control group. The groups did not differ with regard to orbitofrontal rCBF. This research group also measured rCBF in six OCD patients before and during treatment with fluoxetine;[9] treatment was associated with reductions in normalized medial frontal rCBF.

Rubin et al.[10] used SPECT to measure resting rCBF in 10 patients with OCD and 10 healthy control subjects. Relative to control subjects, OCD patients had higher ^{99m}Tc-HMPAO uptake in bilateral dorsal parietal cortex, left posterofrontal cortex, and bilateral orbitofrontal cortex. OCD patients also had reduced ^{99m}Tc-HMPAO uptake in the head of caudate bilaterally.

Baxter and colleagues[11] used PET to study resting cerebral glucose metabolic rates in patients with OCD before and after treatment. Nine patients were treated with fluoxetine and nine with behavior therapy. After both types of treatment, right caudate/right hemisphere ratios decreased significantly. Decreases in right anterior cingulate gyrus/right hemisphere and left thalamus/left hemisphere ratios were seen in the fluoxetine group only. Within the fluoxetine group, percent change in OCD symptom ratings correlated significantly with percent change in the right caudate/ right hemisphere ratios; a trend for this effect was found in the behavior therapy group. Subsequently, these findings have been replicated.[12]

Together, these studies implicate orbitofrontal cortex, anterior cingulate cortex, and caudate nucleus in the functional neuroanatomy of OCD. This pattern of results combined with nonimaging data suggests involvement of paralimbic and corticostriatal systems in the pathophysiology of OCD.[13,14]

Panic Disorder

Reiman et al.[15] used PET to study blood flow, blood volume, metabolic rate for oxygen, and oxygen extraction ratio in 16 individuals with panic disorder and 25 healthy control subjects. All subjects were examined in a resting state. Eight of the subjects with panic disorder were vulnerable to lactate-induced panic; in these eight subjects, Reiman et al.[15] found abnormally low left/right ratios of parahippocampal blood flow, blood volume, and oxygen metabolism. In addition, these subjects had abnormally high whole brain oxygen metabolism.

Nordahl et al.[16] measured cerebral glucose metabolic rates during an auditory continuous performance task in 12 patients with panic disorder and 30 healthy control subjects. Patients with panic disorder had lower left/right hippocampal ratios and lower normalized glucose metabolic rates in the left inferior parietal lobule than did control subjects. The following trends were also found in the panic disorder group relative to the control group: higher metabolic rates in the right hippocampal region and medial orbitofrontal cortex and lower metabolic rates in anterior cingulate.

PTSD

Semple et al.[17] studied six male veterans with PTSD and seven nonveteran normal control subjects. Five of the six PTSD subjects had comorbid substance abuse or dependence. Blood flow was measured during a resting baseline and while subjects performed two different tasks: a word generation task and an auditory continuous performance task involving tone-volume discrimination. PTSD subjects had greater rCBF than did control subjects in orbitofrontal cortex during both cognitive tasks. Subjects with PTSD also showed a trend for smaller hippocampal left/right ratios than did control subjects in the word generation task. Semple et al.[18] also reported on related data from an overlapping cohort of eight PTSD subjects (four from the original study plus four new subjects). The PTSD cohort exhibited more errors on the continuous performance task, and this performance decrement was correlated with decreased right parietal rCBF. Unfortunately, interpretation of these results is confounded by the comorbid substance abuse/dependence in the PTSD group.

Summary

The results of neutral state paradigms converge to suggest that the paralimbic system plays a role in OCD, PTSD and panic disorder, whereas involvement of the caudate nucleus may be more specific to OCD. Although these findings are interesting, interpreting the results of neutral state paradigms is complicated by several considerations. "Resting" states are poorly controlled and therefore may lead to type II errors as a consequence of increased intersubject variability or may lead to type I error if some systematic state difference (e.g., some epiphenomenon of symptoms such as increased motor activity) is unaccounted for and perpetuated between groups. Although nonspecific tasks may help to standardize the neutral state, the mediating anatomy of such tasks may actually serve to obscure or minimize real differences or to produce artifactual ones rather than to enhance sensitivity to salient between-group brain activity differences of interest. Finally, findings from neutral state paradigms may present ambiguity as to whether observed differences truly reflect manifestations of trait or state. Many of these limitations can be overcome with the use of carefully designed cognitive activation paradigms (to be discussed).

SYMPTOM PROVOCATION PARADIGMS

The purpose of symptom provocation paradigms is to delineate the brain systems that mediate the symptoms of psychiatric disorders. In such paradigms, images are generated to reflect both symptomatic and control states. Then, within-subject contrasts provide graphic illustration of which brain systems are differentially active in association with the symptomatic vs some control state. Symptoms can be induced by exposure to individually tailored stimuli, generic stimuli, or other means including pharmacologic challenge. In some sense, this represents the converse approach to that of neutral state pre-posttreatment studies, although with greater attention to state variables.

Obsessive Compulsive Disorder

Using the xenon-133 technique, Zohar et al.[19] studied 10 OCD patients with washing compulsions in three conditions: relaxation, imaginal flooding, and in vivo exposure. Ratings of anxiety and OCD symptoms were significantly higher in the imaginal flooding and in vivo exposure conditions than in the relaxation condition. During imaginal flooding vs relaxation, rCBF increases occurred in the temporal cortex only. During in vivo exposure vs relaxation, rCBF decreases occurred in several cortical regions. Interpretation of these findings is limited by the xenon technique, which yields two-dimensional projections and does not allow for visualization of deep structures, including those principally implicated in OCD (i.e., orbitofrontal cortex, anterior cingulate cortex, and caudate nucleus).

Rauch et al.[20] measured rCBF in eight patients with OCD during symptomatic and control states. In separate scans, subjects were exposed to provocative (e.g., a "contaminated" glove) and control (e.g., a clean glove) stimuli. Results revealed increased ratings of subjective anxiety and OCD symptoms during the provoked vs control conditions. In addition, rCBF increases occurred in the right caudate nucleus, left anterior cingulate cortex, and bilateral orbitofrontal cortex in the provoked condition, relative to the control condition. A trend for increased rCBF occurred in the left thalamus. Furthermore, left anterior orbitofrontal activation correlated significantly with severity of the obsessional state achieved.

McGuire et al.[21] examined the relation between rCBF and symptom intensity in four OCD patients with contamination fears and hand-washing rituals. Serial PET scans were performed during exposure to 12 hierarchically graded provocative stimuli. Positive correlations were found between symptom intensity and rCBF in the following regions: inferior frontal gyrus, caudate, putamen, and thalamus on the right and hippocampus, posterior cingulate, and cuneus on the left.

Most recently, Breiter and colleagues[22] employed a noncontrast fMRI technique and symptom provocation to study 10 subjects with OCD and 5 normal controls. The findings in the OCD group were broadly convergent with the research team's previous PET study,[20] but with more prominent and widespread activation in paralimbic and limbic regions, including the amygdala. The authors suggested that this discrepancy might be attributable to the more severe nature of the stimuli used, which were purposely designed to be universally provocative in order to test for comparable activations in normal subjects. Therefore, it is noteworthy that the provoked vs neutral contrast did not yield any significant activations in the normal cohort. However, not surprisingly, normal subjects were not provoked into a symptomatic state comparable to that of OCD subjects.

Phobias

Rauch et al.[23] measured rCBF during symptom provocation in seven individuals with small-animal phobias. In separate conditions, subjects were confronted with provocative stimuli (e.g., a spider in a container) and control stimuli (e.g., an empty container). Heart rate, respiratory rate, and self-reported anxiety were measured for each condition; results showed that all three of these indices were higher in the provoked condition than in the control condition. In the provoked vs control condition, rCBF increases occurred in multiple paralimbic territories (i.e., right anterior cingulate cortex, left insular cortex, right anterior temporal pole, and left posterior orbitofrontal cortex) as well as left somatosensory cortex and left thalamus. These results suggest that paralimbic structures mediate some aspects of phobic symptoms. Interestingly, activation of the dominant somatosensory cortex may reflect tactile imagery, since all subjects reported prominent experiences of such phenomena (i.e., imagining what it might feel like for the feared animal to come in bodily contact with them).

Other PET studies of specific phobias have yielded different results. Mountz et al.[24] studied seven subjects with a simple phobia of small animals. Although the presentation of phobic stimuli increased the subjects' heart rate, respiratory rate, and self-reported anxiety, no global or rCBF differences between conditions were found after PCO_2 correction was made. This may reflect a less sensitive region-of-interest-based data analytic scheme or less robust provocation of symptoms.

Wik et al.[25] measured rCBF in six persons with snake phobias during exposure to videotapes containing neutral, aversive, and snake-related scenes. Heart rate and anxiety levels were higher in the snake condition than in the neutral condition. In the snake vs neutral condition, Wik et al.[25] found increased rCBF in secondary visual cortex and decreased rCBF in hippocampus, prefrontal cortex, orbitofrontal cortex, temporopolar cortex, and posterior cingulate cortex. Nearly identical results were reported by Fredrikson et al.,[26] who studied eight persons with spider phobias in a similar paradigm. Fredrikson et al.[27] also found increased rCBF in the secondary visual cortex during symptom provocation in persons with snake phobias. The disparity in results between these studies and those of Rauch et al.[23] may be explained in part by the fact that these studies were performed with the subjects' eyes open, whereas Rauch and colleagues' subjects had their eyes closed. Thus, one interpretation is that most of these studies show fear-potentiated activation of sensory in-flow systems, somatosensory and insular cortex with eyes closed[23] and visual cortex with eyes open.[25-27]

Panic Disorder

Reiman et al.[28] measured rCBF in 17 patients with panic disorder and 15 healthy control subjects during lactate infusions. In the 8 patients who experienced lactate-induced panic attacks, blood flow increases occurred in the bilateral temporopolar cortex and bilateral insular cortex/claustrum/putamen. None of these increases were found in nonpanicking patients or control subjects. However, the blood flow increases in the temporopolar cortex may have reflected extracranial artifacts of muscular origin.[29,30].

Woods et al.[31] used SPECT to examine the effects of yohimbine on rCBF in six patients with panic disorder and six healthy control subjects. In patients with panic disorder, yohimbine administration was associated with both increased anxiety and decreased rCBF in bilateral frontal regions. This pattern of results was not found in control subjects.

Posttraumatic Stress Disorder

Rauch et al.[32] used a script-driven imagery technique to explore the mediating neuroanatomy of PTSD symptoms. A mixed-gender cohort (two male and six female) was comprised of eight subjects with PTSD, screened as psychophysiologically responsive to imagery of their own traumatic events. In separate scans, subjects imagined neutral and traumatic autobiographical events (prompted by audiotaped narratives). Subjects also participated in a teeth-clenching control condition during which they imagined neutral events while clenching their teeth. Heart rate and subjective ratings of emotional intensity were recorded for each condition. Results revealed that heart rate and subjective ratings of anxiety, fear, sadness, disgust, anger, and guilt were higher in the traumatic condition than in the neutral condition. In the traumatic condition, relative to the neutral condition, rCBF increases occurred in the medial orbitofrontal cortex, insular cortex, anterior temporal pole, medial temporal cortex, and secondary visual cortex, all on the right. In addition, rCBF decreases were found in the middle temporal cortex and inferior frontal cortex (Broca's area) on the left. When the traumatic condition was compared to the teeth-clenching control condition, rCBF increases within the anterior cingulate cortex and right amygdala also achieved significance. The results of this study suggest that symptoms of PTSD may be mediated by right-sided limbic and paralimbic components. The finding of activation within the amygdala was consistent with a priori hypotheses and the concept that this structure might play a role in emotional memory. Visual cortical activation is consistent with visual imagery perhaps as one aspect of reexperiencing phenomena. Deactivation of left-sided structures including Broca's area have prompted speculation that such brain changes might be related to patients' difficulties cognitively structuring or verbally expressing the events of their precipitating traumatic experience. The findings of this initial PTSD symptom provocation study should be interpreted cautiously however, pending replication and comparison with appropriate control cohorts.

Preliminary data from several similar studies were recently presented. Eberly et al.[33] used script-driven imagery to evoke fear and dysphoria in combat veterans with and without PTSD. Preliminary data analyses ($n = 5$ per group) revealed increased rCBF in the orbitofrontal cortex and anterior cingulate cortex in the dysphoric condition for both groups. Blood flow increases in these regions also occurred during the fear condition in subjects without PTSD.

Chamberlain et al.[34] used SPECT to examine rCBF in veterans with PTSD and age- and sex-matched control subjects. In separate scans, subjects were exposed to combat sounds and white noise. Preliminary results showed increased rCBF in parahippocampal gyri, brain stem nuclei, and the left caudate in the PTSD group.

Bremner et al.[35] used PET and fluorodeoxyglucose to examine the effect of yohimbine on cerebral glucose metabolic rates in combat veterans with PTSD and healthy control subjects. Yohimbine, which is an alpha-$_2$ antagonist, activates noradrenergic neurons and induces PTSD symptoms, such as intrusive thoughts and flashbacks, in veterans with PTSD.[36] In subjects with PTSD, yohimbine administration was associated with a relative decrease in brain glucose metabolism in a wide variety of cortical areas.

In another ongoing project, Shin and colleagues are seeking both to replicate the results of Rauch et al.[32] and to test the specificity of their findings by studying a matched control group of trauma-exposed individuals without PTSD. All subjects are being screened psychophysiologically. During serial scans, subjects are being exposed to neutral and traumatic autobiographical scripts, counterbalanced for order. A teeth-clenching control condition is also being employed, and psychophysiologic data as well as subjective emotional ratings are being recorded during the scanning sessions. At the time of this writing, Shin et al. have studied 15 women with histories of childhood sexual abuse, 8 with PTSD and 7 without PTSD. Completion of the project is anticipated shortly, and the results are expected to clarify the interpretations of our earlier research.

Pooled Analysis across Three Anxiety Disorders

To identify the mediating neuroanatomy of anxiety symptoms across different anxiety disorders, Rauch et al.[37] combined data from their symptom provocation studies of OCD,[20] simple phobia,[23] and PTSD[32] contributing to a total sample of 23 subjects. Pooled over the entire cohort, the provoked vs control contrast yielded significant rCBF increases in the right inferior frontal cortex, right posterior medial orbitofrontal cortex, bilateral insular cortex, bilateral lenticulate nuclei, and bilateral brain stem. Subjective ratings of anxiety were positively correlated with rCBF in the left brain stem.

Emotion Induction Paradigms in Normal Subjects

Reiman et al.[38] examined rCBF changes associated with anticipatory anxiety in eight healthy volunteers. In the anticipatory anxiety condition, subjects were told that they would receive a painful electric shock. In the control condition, subjects were told that no shock would be delivered. In the anticipatory anxiety vs control condition, heart rate, electrodermal activity, and self-reported anxiety increased; furthermore, rCBF increases were observed in bilateral temporal poles. Although similar results were demonstrated in patients with panic disorder,[28] further analyses suggested that the temporopolar activations in both studies were attributable to extracranial artifacts from jaw muscle contraction.[29]

Pardo et al.[39] examined the neural correlates of dysphoria in seven subjects without histories of major psychiatric disorders. Blood flow was measured in two conditions with eyes closed. In the "control" condition, subjects rested, whereas in the "active" condition, subjects imagined or recalled situations that would make them very sad. In the active vs control condition, rCBF increased in the superior frontal gyrus, inferior frontal gyrus, and orbitofrontal cortex. Foci of activation were reported as bilateral in female subjects and left sided in male subjects; however, the very small number of subjects make inferences about gender differences tenuous in this case.

George et al.[40] examined changes in rCBF associated with transient happiness and sadness in 11 healthy women. In separate conditions, subjects were instructed to recall, with eyes open, the emotions they experienced during specific happy, sad, and neutral autobiographical events. During each scan, subjects were also shown affect-appropriate faces to help them reexperience the corresponding emotion. In the sad vs neutral condition, rCBF increased in the right medial frontal gyrus, left cingulate gyrus, right putamen, caudate, left cingulate/orbitofrontal cortex, and left thalamus. No significant rCBF increases were found in the happy vs neutral contrast.

Benkelfat et al.[30] examined rCBF in eight healthy volunteers after bolus injections of either saline solution or cholecystokinin tetrapeptide (CCK_4), a maneuver that has induced panic attacks in healthy subjects.[41] Blood flow was also measured in an anticipatory anxiety condition in which subjects expected to receive CCK_4 but actually received saline solution. Results showed that CCK_4 administration elicited panic symptoms and heart rate increases. In the anticipatory anxiety vs saline condition, rCBF increases were observed in the left orbitofrontal cortex and cerebellar vermis. In the CCK_4 vs anticipatory anxiety condition, rCBF increases occurred in the right cerebellar vermis, left anterior cingulate, bilateral claustrum-insula-amygdala, and bilateral temporal poles. Again, further analyses suggested that the apparent temporal pole activations were probably attributable to extracranial artifacts from jaw muscle contraction. The authors also cautioned that bilateral activations in the claustrum-insula-amygdala may have reflected blood volume changes in insular arteries.

Ketter et al.[42] studied both the effects of procaine on rCBF and the association between blood flow changes and emotional changes. Regional CBF was measured in 32 healthy subjects after single-blind intravenous injections of either saline solution or procaine. Emotional responses after procaine administration varied across subjects, ranging from fear to euphoria. In addition, some subjects reported visual hallucinations after receiving procaine injections. In the procaine vs saline condition, rCBF increases occurred in anterior paralimbic regions, including the anterior cingulate cortex, amygdala, hypothalamus, basal forebrain, insula, and orbitofrontal cortex. Subjects reporting fear had larger blood flow increases in the left amygdala than did subjects reporting euphoria. In addition, changes in left amygdalar blood flow correlated positively with fear intensity and negatively with euphoria intensity. Subjects who reported visual hallucinations had larger blood flow increases in the right mesial occipital cortex than did those who did not report visual hallucinations.

Cahill et al.[43] examined cerebral glucose metabolism in the amygdaloid complex during the encoding of emotionally arousing stimuli. In two separate PET scanning sessions, eight healthy subjects viewed emotionally arousing and emotionally neutral film clips. After viewing each film clip, subjects rated its emotional intensity on a 10-point scale. Three weeks later, subjects were asked to recall as many film clips as possible. Results confirmed that subjects gave higher intensity ratings to the emotionally arousing clips than to the neutral clips. In addition, subjects recalled more emotionally arousing clips than neutral clips. Although activity in the amygdaloid complex did not differ between conditions, right amygdaloid complex activity in the emotionally arousing condition was positively correlated with the number of emotionally arousing clips recalled 3 weeks later. Right amygdaloid complex activity in the neutral condition was not correlated with the number of neutral clips recalled.

Summary

Taken together, the symptom provocation data implicate anterior paralimbic structures in the functional anatomy of symptomatic states across a range of different anxiety disorders. Analogous studies involving the induction of emotions in normal subjects implicate the very same anterior paralimbic territories in anxiety as well as other normal intense adverse emotional states. We have proposed that this may reflect a core physiological system that is likewise recruited as part of pathological emotional states.[37] In addition to this core anterior paralimbic involvement, symptom provocation studies suggest a more specific role for certain structures in states associated with particular diagnoses. For instance, the caudate nucleus is specifically activated in conjunction with OCD symptoms. In PTSD, initial data implicate activation of the right amygdala and perhaps deactivation of left-sided brain structures. Finally, there is mounting evidence to support the contention that the right amygdala plays a role in emotional memory.

COGNITIVE ACTIVATION PARADIGMS

The purpose of cognitive activation paradigms is to examine specific brain systems implicated in psychiatric disorders by developing probes that selectively recruit those systems. Patients and control subjects are then studied while performing these tasks in order to determine if a given disorder is associated with a decrement in task performance, a decrement in normal brain system recruitment, and/or aberrant recruitment of collateral systems. Cognitive activation paradigms are desirable because they allow for more tightly controlled contrasts than do neutral state or symptom provocation paradigms. Moreover, the premise is that, akin to a cardiac stress test, this approach will offer heightened sensitivity by examining a system while stressed (i.e., under demand functionally), thereby accentuating its limitations and revealing dysfunction if present. Until recently, this approach had not been applied to the study of anxiety disorders.

Obsessive Compulsive Disorder

Rauch and colleagues[44] validated an implicit sequence learning paradigm for use in conjunction with PET as a probe of corticostriatal system functional integrity. Moreover, a modified version of this probe was also validated for use in fMRI.[45] An initial study of nine females with OCD and an equal number of age-and education-matched female control subjects was conducted using this PET probe of corticostriatal function.[46] Whereas the normal cohort exhibited inferior striatal activation consistent with that of previous studies,[44] patients with OCD failed to normally recruit this system despite showing no performance decrement on the learning task.[46] Furthermore, patients with OCD exhibited aberrant recruitment of bilateral medial temporal structures, suggesting that different brain systems were being accessed in the context of nonconscious information processing. Analogous studies are underway to replicate the findings in males and to extend investigation to fMRI and other obsessive-compulsive spectrum disorders (e.g., Tourette syndrome).

Posttraumatic Stress Disorder

Shin *et al.*[47] sought to determine whether similar patterns of limbic and paralimbic activation would occur in individuals with and without PTSD during a cognitive task that involved viewing and visualizing different types of stimuli. Subjects consisted of seven Vietnam combat veterans with PTSD and seven healthy Vietnam combat veterans. Regional CBF was measured in six different conditions. In three of these conditions, subjects viewed pictures and evaluated statements about them (perception conditions). In the remaining three conditions, subjects imagined pictures and evaluated statements about them (imagery conditions). Within the perception and imagery conditions, different types of pictures, neutral, negative, and combat-related, were used. Results revealed increased rCBF in the right amygdala and anterior cingulate cortex during combat imagery conditions in the PTSD group, but not in the control group. In the PTSD group, decreased rCBF was found in the left inferior frontal cortex (Broca's area) in the combat perception vs negative perception condition. These results, along with those of Rauch *et al.,*[32] further implicate right amygdala activation and left inferior frontal deactivation in the pathophysiology of PTSD.

Summary

The foregoing two examples herald the promise of cognitive activation paradigms for probing the functional integrity of specific systems implicated in the pathophysiology of different anxiety disorders. Convergent with the findings from the only published symptom provocation study of PTSD,[32] results from this first cognitive activation study of PTSD[47] implicate activation of the anterior cingulate cortex and right amygdala as well as deactivation of Broca's area. Given emerging models of PTSD, future cognitive activation studies will undoubtedly include probes of frontohippocampal and amygdala function.

NEUROCHEMICAL CHARACTERIZATION PARADIGMS

Emerging methods for characterizing neurochemical parameters have not yet been applied to the study of PTSD or other anxiety disorders. PET and SPECT allow investigators to make quantitative maps of binding capacity using radiolabeled ligands for receptors of interest. For example, such methods have been used to detect apparent striatal dopaminergic receptor abnormalities in Tourette syndrome.[48] Similar methods could be used to probe adrenergic and serotonergic receptor systems in PTSD.

MRS can be employed to measure the *in vivo* brain concentration of various compounds[49] including medications (e.g., fluoxetine), products of metabolism (e.g., phosphocreatine), or neuronal markers (e.g., *N*-acetyl aspartate). Although MRS provides very limited spatial resolution (typically involving macrovoxels of ≥ 8 cc), such methods might still be used to study neuronal integrity within medial temporal territories in PTSD.

DISCUSSION AND FUTURE DIRECTIONS

Functional neuroimaging research offers great potential, but also many pitfalls. The scientific community is just beginning to learn together how best to utilize these powerful yet expensive tools. The data first reviewed illustrate several important points. First, many of the design issues related to subject populations are the same for neuroimaging as for other types of clinical research; rigorous clinical characterization, adequate matching, attention to comorbidity, and considerations about appropriate control groups are all paramount. Other issues are magnified in imaging research; for instance, the numbers of subjects are often small (in part due to expense and scanner access), contributing to risks of type I and type II error as well as mitigating against generalizability of findings to subpopulations poorly represented within the study cohort. Finally, many issues are specific to imaging research; considerations regarding spatial and temporal resolution limits, spatial normalization of images to a standard atlas so that data can be averaged across cohorts, statistical treatment of data via region-of-interest vs pixel-by-pixel statistical mapping methods, as well as conventions surrounding statistical thresholds and accommodations for multiple comparisons all remain topics of ongoing methodological study, subject to debate, and as yet incompletely resolved.

We would hope that the reader comes away from this review with a healthy skepticism regarding the interpretations of any single functional imaging study. At best, the track record of neuroimaging research for successful replication has been modest. Therefore, and especially in light of rapidly evolving technology and methodology, current findings are compelling only in those areas where convergence across studies, paradigms, and laboratories has prevailed: anterior paralimbic activation appears to be a common but nonspecific state marker of intense adverse emotions in health and disease; with respect to PTSD, a more specific role for the amygdala and Broca's area remains to be confirmed.

As the field matures, we can hope for a more sophisticated movement that is fundamentally hypothesis driven and that seeks to integrate various paradigms and modalities. On the immediate horizon, we should expect a proliferation of functional imaging studies involving PTSD populations. The completion of several symptom provocation studies is imminent, and once distilled they will hopefully yield some consensus of results. We should expect that follow-up studies utilizing PET cognitive activation paradigms, perhaps together with structural MRI to enhance localization of findings, will enable investigators to directly test hypotheses regarding the functional integrity of specific brain systems. In particular, frontohippocampal systems and the amygdala should be prime targets of study. Although MRS may be employed to probe these same territories, we should also expect that receptor characterization studies will be performed to test hypotheses regarding serotonergic and adrenergic function. Pragmatically, pre-posttreatment studies may be most likely to provide data of clinical utility, if characteristic pretreatment profiles can be established as predictive of response to specific interventions.

Finally, advances in the functional neuroimaging of PTSD will be influenced and informed by other modes of inquiry, including not only structural neuroimaging, but also the full panoply of basic neuroscience and clinical research methods. This is why it is so essential that specialists from the various relevant disciplines communicate and collaborate, integrating the tools and information that are at our collective disposal.

REFERENCES

1. RAUCH, S. L. & P. F. RENSHAW. 1995. Clinical neuroimaging in psychiatry. Harvard Rev. Psychiatry **2:** 297-312.
2. TOGA, A. W. & J. C. MAZZIOTTA. 1996. Brain Mapping: The Methods. Academic Press. Boston, MA.
3. BAXTER, L. R., M. E. PHELPS, J. C. MAZZIOTTA, B. H. GUZE, J. M. SCHWARTZ & C. E. SELIN. 1987. Local cerebral glucose metabolic rates in obsessive-compulsive disorder: A comparison with rates in unipolar depression and in normal controls. Arch. Gen. Psychiatry **44:** 211-218.
4. NORDAHL, T. E., C. BENKELFAT, W. E. SEMPLE, M. GROSS, A. C. KING & R. M. COHEN. 1989. Cerebral glucose metabolic rates in obsessive compulsive disorder. Neuropsychopharmacology **2:** 23-28.
5. BENKELFAT, C., T. E. NORDAHL, W. E. SEMPLE, A. C. KING, D. L. MURPHY & R. M. COHEN. 1990. Local cerebral glucose metabolic rates in obsessive-compulsive disorder: Patients treated with clomipramine. Arch. Gen. Psychiatry **47:** 840-848.
6. SWEDO, S. E., M. B. SCHAPIRO, C. L. GRADY, D. L. CHESLOW, H. L. LEONARD, A. KUMAR, R. FRIEDLAND, S. I. RAPOPORT & J. L. RAPOPORT. 1989. Cerebral glucose metabolism in childhood-onset obsessive compulsive disorder. Arch. Gen. Psychiatry **46:** 518-523.
7. SWEDO, S. E., P. PIETRINI, H. L. LEONARD, M. B. SCHAPIRO, D. C. RETTEW, E. L. GOLDBERGER, S. I. RAPOPORT, J. L. RAPOPORT & C. L. GRADY. 1992. Cerebral glucose metabolism in childhood-onset obsessive compulsive disorder: Revisualization during pharmacotherapy. Arch. Gen. Psychiatry **49:** 690-694.
8. MACHLIN, S. R., G. J. HARRIS, G. D. PEARLSON, R. HOEHN-SARIC, P. JEFFERY & E. E. CAMARGO. 1991. Elevated medial-frontal cerebral blood flow in obsessive-compulsive patients: A SPECT study. Am. J. Psychiatry **148:** 1240-1242.
9. HOEHN-SARIC, R., G. D. PEARLSON, G. J. HARRIS, S. R. MACHLIN & E. E. CAMARGO. 1991. Effects of fluoxetine on regional cerebral blood flow in obsessive-compulsive patients. Am. J. Psychiatry **148:** 1243-1245.
10. RUBIN, R. T., J. VILLANUEVA-MEYER, J. ANANTH, P. G. TRAJMAR & I. MENA. 1992. Regional xenon 133 cerebral blood flow and cerebral technetium 99m HMPAO uptake in unmedicated patients with obsessive-compulsive disorder and matched normal control subjects. Arch. Gen. Psychiatry **49:** 695-702.
11. BAXTER, L. R., J. M. SCHWARTZ, K. S. BERGMAN, M. P. SZUBA, B. H. GUZE, J. C. MAZZIOTTA, A. ALAZRAKI, C. E. SELIN, H-K. FERNG, P. MUNFORD & M. E. PHELPS. 1992. Caudate glucose metabolic rate changes with both drug and behavior therapy for obsessive-compulsive disorder. Arch. Gen. Psychiatry **49:** 681-689.
12. SCHWARTZ, J. M., P. W. STOESSEL, L. R. BAXTER, K. M. MARTIN & M. E. PHELPS. 1996. Systematic changes in cerebral glucose metabolic rate after successful behavior modification. Arch. Gen. Psychiatry **53:** 109-113.

13. INSEL, T. R. 1992. Toward a neuroanatomy of obsessive-compulsive disorder. Arch. Gen. Psychiatry **49:** 739–744.
14. RAUCH, S. L. & M. A. JENIKE. 1997. Neural mechanisms of obsessive-compulsive disorder. Curr. Rev. Mood Anxiety Dis. **1:** 84–94.
15. REIMAN, E. M., M. E. RAICHLE, E. ROBINS, F. K. BUTLER, P. HERSCOVITCH, P. FOX & J. PERLMUTTER. 1986. The application of positron emission tomography to the study of panic disorder. Am. J. Psychiatry **143:** 469–477.
16. NORDAHL, T. E., W. E. SEMPLE, M. GROSS, T. A. MELLMAN, M. B. STEIN, P. GOYER, A. C. KING, T. W. UDHE & R. M. COHEN. 1990. Cerebral glucose metabolic differences in patients with panic disorder. Neuropsychopharmacology **3:** 261–272.
17. SEMPLE, W. E., P. GOYER, R. MCCORMICK, E. MORRIS, B. COMPTON, G. MUSWICK, D. NELSON, B. DONOVAN, G. LEISURE, M. BERRIDGE, F. MIRALDI & S. C. SCHULZ. 1993. Preliminary report: Brain blood flow using PET in patients with posttraumatic stress disorder and substance-abuse histories. Biol. Psychiatry **34:** 115–118.
18. SEMPLE W. E., P. F. GOYER, R. MCCORMICK, B. COMPTON-TOTH, E. MORRIS, B. DONOVAN, G. MUSWICK, D. NELSON, M. L. GARNETT, J. SHARKOFF, G. LEISURE, F. MIRALDI & S. C. SCHULZ. 1996. Attention and regional cerebral blood flow in posttraumatic stress disorder patients with substance abuse histories. Psychiatry Res. Neuroimaging **67:** 17–28.
19. ZOHAR, J., T. R. INSEL, K. F. BERMAN, E. B. FOA, J. L. HILL & D. R. WEINBERGER. 1989. Anxiety and cerebral blood flow during behavioral challenge. Arch. Gen. Psychiatry **46:** 505–510.
20. RAUCH, S. L., M. A. JENIKE, N. M. ALPERT, L. BAER, H. C. R. BREITER, C. R. SAVAGE & A. J. FISCHMAN. 1994. Regional cerebral blood flow measured during symptom provocation in obsessive-compulsive disorder using oxygen 15-labeled carbon dioxide and positron emission tomography. Arch. Gen. Psychiatry **51:** 62–70.
21. MCGUIRE, P. K., C. J. BENCH, C. D. FRITH, I. M. MARKS, R. S. J. FRACKOWIAK & R. J. DOLAN. 1994. Functional anatomy of obsessive-compulsive phenomena. Br. J. Psychiatry **164:** 459–468.
22. BREITER, H. C., S. L. RAUCH, K. K. KWONG, J. R. BAKER, R. M. WEISSKOFF, D. N. KENNEDY, A. D. KENDRICK, T. L. DAVIS, A. JIANG, M. S. COHEN, C. E. STERN, J. W. BELLIVEAU, L. BAER, R. L. O'SULLIVAN, C. R. SAVAGE, M. A. JENIKE & B. R. ROSEN. 1996. Functional magnetic resonance imaging of symptom provocation in obsessive-compulsive disorder. Arch. Gen. Psychiatry **53:** 595–606.
23. RAUCH, S. L., C. R. SAVAGE, N. M. ALPERT, E. C. MIGUEL, L. BAER, H. C. BREITER, A. J. FISCHMAN, P. A. MANZO, C. MORETTI & M. A. JENIKE. 1995. A positron emission tomographic study of simple phobic symptom provocation. Arch. Gen. Psychiatry **52:** 20–28.
24. MOUNTZ, J. M., J. G. MODELL, M. W. WILSON, G. C. CURTIS, M. A. LEE, S. SCHMALTZ & D. E. KUHL. 1989. Positron emission tomographic evaluation of cerebral blood flow during state anxiety in simple phobia. Arch. Gen. Psychiatry **46:** 501–504.
25. WIK, G., M. FREDRIKSON, K. ERICSON, L. ERIKSSON, S. STONE-ELANDER & T. GREITZ. 1993. A functional cerebral response to frightening visual stimulation. Psychiatry Res. Neuroimaging **50:** 15–24.
26. FREDRIKSON, M., G. WIK, P. ANNAS, K. ERICSON & S. STONE-ELANDER. 1995. Functional neuroanatomy of visually elicited simple phobic fear: Additional data and theoretical analysis. Psychophysiology **32:** 43–48.
27. FREDRIKSON, M., G. WIK, T. GREITZ, L. ERIKSSON, S. STONE-ELANDER, K. ERICSON & G. SEDVALL. 1993. Regional cerebral blood flow during experimental fear Psychophysiology **30:** 126–130.
28. REIMAN, E. M., M. E. RAICHLE, E. ROBINS, M. A. MINTUN, M. J. FUSSELMAN, P. T. FOX, J. L. PRICE & K. A. HACKMAN. 1989. Neuroanatomical correlates of a lactate-induced anxiety attack. Arch. Gen. Psychiatry **46:** 493–500.

29. DREVETS, W. C., T. O. VIDEEN, A. K. MACLEOD, J. W. HALLER & M. E. RAICHLE. 1992. PET images of blood flow changes during anxiety: A correction. Science 256: 1696.
30. BENKELFAT, C., J. BRADWEJN, E. MEYER, M. ELLENBOGEN, S. MILOT, A. GJEDDE & A. EVANS. 1995. Functional neuroanatomy of CCK₄-induced anxiety in normal healthy volunteers. Am. J. Psychiatry 152: 1180–1184.
31. WOODS, S. W., K. KOSTER, J. K. KRYSTAL, E. O. SMITH, I. G. ZUBAL, P. B. HOFFER & D. S. CHARNEY. 1988. Yohimbine alters regional cerebral blood flow in panic disorder. The Lancet 2: 678.
32. RAUCH, S. L., B. A. VAN DER KOLK, R. E. FISLER, N. M. ALPERT, S. P. ORR, C. R. SAVAGE, A. J. FISCHMAN, M. A. JENIKE & R. K. PITMAN. 1996. A symptom provocation study of posttraumatic stress disorder using positron emission tomography and script-driven imagery. Arch. Gen. Psychiatry 53: 380–387.
33. EBERLY, R., M. KUSKOWSKI, D. ZALD, B. ENGDAHL, J. PARDO & T. DIKEL. 1995. A PET study of fear and dysphoria in veterans with and without PTSD. Paper presented at the 11th Annual Meeting of the International Society for Traumatic Stress Studies. Boston, MA.
34. CHAMBERLAIN, K. R., T. D. JUNG, S. F. TAYLOR, L. M. FIG, I. LIBERZON, R. A. KOEPPE & S. MINOSHIMA. 1995. SPECT imaging in posttraumatic stress disorder patients and normal controls. Paper presented at the 11th Annual Meeting of the International Society for Traumatic Stress Studies. Boston, MA.
35. BREMNER, J. D., L. STAIB, J. KRYSTAL, R. SOLOMON, S. SOUTHWICK, R. BRONEN, R. INNIS. & D. CHARNEY. 1994. PET measurement of noradrenergic contributions to metabolism in PTSD. Paper presented at the 10th Annual Meeting of the International Society for Traumatic Stress Studies. Chicago, IL.
36. SOUTHWICK, S. M., J. H. KRYSTAL, A. MORGAN, D. JOHNSON, L. M. NAGY, A. NICOLAOU, G. R. HENINGER & D. S. CHARNEY. 1993. Abnormal noradrenergic function in posttraumatic stress disorder. Arch. Gen. Psychiatry 50: 266–274.
37. RAUCH, S. L., C. R. SAVAGE, N. M. ALPERT, M. A. JENIKE & A. J. FISCHMAN. 1995. Functional neuroanatomy of anxiety: A study of three disorders using PET and symptom provocation [Abstr.] First International Conference on Functional Mapping of the Human Brain. Hum. Brain Mapping. (Suppl. 1): 398.
38. REIMAN, E. M., M. J. FUSSELMAN, P. T. FOX & M. E. RAICHLE. 1989. Neuroanatomical correlates of anticipatory anxiety. Science 243: 1071–1074.
39. PARDO, J. V., P. J. PARDO & M. E. RAICHLE. 1993. Neural correlates of self-induced dysphoria. Am. J. Psychiatry 150: 713–719.
40. GEORGE M. S., T. A. KETTER, P. I. PAREKH, B. HOROWITZ, P. HERSCOVITCH & R. M. POST. 1995. Brain activity during transient sadness and happiness in healthy women. Am. J. Psychiatry 152: 341–351.
41. DE MONTIGNY, C. 1989. Cholecystokinin tetrapeptide induces panic-like attacks in healthy volunteers: Preliminary findings. Arch. Gen. Psychiatry 46: 511–517.
42. KETTER, T. A., P. J. ANDREASON, M. S. GEORGE, C. LEE, D. S. GILL, P. I. PAREKH, M. W. WILLIS, P. HERSCOVITCH & R. M. POST. 1996. Anterior paralimbic mediation of procaine-induced emotional and psychosensory experiences. Arch. Gen. Psychiatry 53: 59–69.
43. CAHILL, L., R. J. HAIER, J. FALLON, M. ALKIRE, C. TANG, D. KEATOR, J. WU & J. L. McGAUGH. 1996. Amygdala activity at encoding correlated with long-term, free recall of emotional information. Proc. Natl. Acad. Sci. USA. 93: 8016–8021.
44. RAUCH, S. L., C. R. SAVAGE, H. D. BROWN, T. CURRAN, N. M. ALPERT, A. KENDRICK, A. J. FISCHMAN & S. M. KOSSLYN. 1995. A PET investigation of implicit and explicit sequence learning. Hum. Brain Mapping 3: 271–286.
45. RAUCH, S. L., C. R. SAVAGE, P. J. WHALEN, T. CURRAN, A. KENDRICK, H. C. BREITER, G. BUSH, H. D. BROWN & B. R. ROSEN. 1996. Development of a cognitive fMRI probe that reliably activates striatum [Abstr.]. Second International Conference on Functional Mapping of the Human Brain. Neuroimage 3 (suppl): S558.

46. RAUCH, S. L., C. R. SAVAGE, N. M. ALPERT, D. DOUGHERTY, A. KENDRICK. T. CURRAN, H. D. BROWN, P. MANZO, A. J. FISCHMAN & M. A. JENIKE. 1996. Probing striatal function in obsessive compulsive disorder using PET and a sequence learning task [Abstr.]. Second International Conference on Functional Mapping of the Human Brain. Neuroimage 3 (suppl): S507.

47. SHIN, L. M., S. M. KOSSLYN, R. J. MCNALLY, N. M. ALPERT, W. L. THOMPSON, S. L. RAUCH, M. L. MACKLIN & R. K. PITMAN. 1997. Visual imagery and perception in posttraumatic stress disorder: A positron emission tomographic investigation. Arch. Gen. Psychiatry 54: 233-241.

48. MALISON, R. T., C. J. MCDOUGLE, C. H. VAN DYCK, L. SCAHILL, R. M. BALDWIN, J. P. SEIBYL, L. H. PRICE, J. F. LECKMAN & R. B. INNIS. 1995. [^{123}I]B-CIT SPECT imaging of striatal dopamine transporter binding in Tourette's disorder. Am. J. Psychiatry 152: 1359-1361.

49. DAGER, S. R. & R. G. STEEN. 1992. Applications of magnetic resonance spectroscopy to the investigation of neuropsychiatric disorders. Neuropsychopharmacology 6: 249-266.

The Psychobiology of Traumatic Memory

Clinical Implications of Neuroimaging Studies

BESSEL A. VAN DER KOLK,

JENNIFER A. BURBRIDGE, AND JOJI SUZUKI

All these intrusive recollections only have an experiential quality to them: When I have these flashbacks they are not explainable, I can't make things sequential. Up till now they had very little outline to them. Now a tiny fraction of these torture experiences have become knowable to me, but when I come closer to them and stop warding them off, I start having all sorts of problems of a different kind: I become confused, I lose things and start getting into accidents. The tragedy is the loneliness: the inability to convey the inner experience, and knowing that I cannot get out of it without going through it again.

A patient with PTSD recounting her traumatic memories

William James noted that the power of the intellect is determined by the individual's perceptual processing style. The ability to comprehend (grasp, hold together, take hold of, from the Latin *cum-prendere*) depends on stimulus sampling, bias, and the formation of schematic representations of reality.[1] There seem to be qualitatively significant differences between the ways persons with posttraumatic stress disorder (PTSD) sample, bias, and categorize experience, and the ways in which nontraumatized persons do.[2,3] In recent years, systematic research has begun to confirm the clinical observation that failure to comprehend the experience (i.e., to dissociate) plays a critical role in making a stressful experience traumatic. Dissociation causes memories of the trauma to be organized, at least initially, as sensory fragments and intense emotional states that may have no linguistic components. This fragmentation is accompanied by subjective experiences of depersonalization and derealization.[4]

Whereas most patients with PTSD construct a narrative of their trauma over time, it is characteristic of PTSD that sensory elements of the trauma itself continue to intrude as flashbacks and nightmares, altered states of consciousness in which the trauma is relived, unintegrated with an overall sense of self. Because traumatic memories are so fragmented, it seems reasonable to postulate that extreme emotional arousal leads to failure of the central nervous system (CNS) to synthesize the sensations related to the trauma into an integrated whole. Earlier models for a biological substrate of these phenomena have become rapidly outdated with the availability of new information derived from neuroimaging studies of patients with PTSD. The emerging body of knowledge from these studies has stimulated a gradual shift in emphasis away from the neurochemicals involved in the organisms' response to overwhelming threat to a focus on the neuronal filters concerned in the *interpretation* of sensory information: the interactions between the various parts of the CNS that process and interpret the meaning of incoming information, such as the amygdala, hippocampus, corpus callosum, anterior cingulate, and prefrontal cortex.

THE APPARENT UNIQUENESS OF TRAUMATIC MEMORIES

The study of traumatic memories challenges several basic notions about the nature of memory: (1) that memory always is a constructive process and that memory traces are always contaminated by the attribution of meaning; (2) that memory is primarily declarative, that is, that people generally can articulate what they know in words and symbols; (3) that memory is generally present in consciousness in a continuous and uninterrupted fashion; and (4) that memory always disintegrates in accuracy over time. A century of study of traumatic memories shows that (1) they are primarily imprinted in sensory and emotional modes, although a semantic representation of the memory may coexist with sensory flashbacks;[5] (2) these sensory experiences often remain stable over time and unaltered by other life experiences;[6,7] (3) they may return, triggered by reminders, at any time during a person's life as vividly as if the subject were having the experience all over again;[8] (4) these sensory imprints tend to occur in a mental state in which victims may be unable to precisely articulate what they are feeling and thinking.[9,10]

While transformation of memories of day-to-day experiences is the norm, flashbacks and other sensory reexperiences of PTSD seem not to be updated or attached to other experiences. Triggered by a reminder, the past can be relived with an immediate sensory and emotional intensity that makes victims feel as if the event were occurring all over again. Patients with PTSD seem to remain embedded in their trauma as a contemporary experience and often become "fixated on the trauma."[11]

DISSOCIATION, AMNESIAS, AND HYPERMNESIAS

For well over a century psychiatrists and psychologists[9,11-15] have attempted to define and understand how traumatic memories are stored in the mind and continue to exert their effects on current attention and perception. After his visit to the psychological laboratories at the Salpêtrière Sigmund Freud, following Charcot and Janet, started out by claiming that the dissociation of traumatic memories was the key to understanding hysteria.[14] He claimed that, "Hysterics suffer mainly from reminiscences. In the great majority of cases it is not possible to establish the point of origin by a simple interrogation of the patient. . . . principally because he is genuinely unable to recollect it and often has no suspicion of the causal connection between the precipitating event and the pathological phenomenon."[17, p 12] Later in his career Freud claimed that if a person does not remember a trauma, he is likely to act it out: "he reproduces it not as a memory but as an action; he repeats it, without knowing, of course, that he is repeating, and in the end, we understand that this is his way of remembering" (1914).[14, p 150]

The psychiatrists who studied soldiers with "shell-shock" during World War I were struck with the similarity of these soldiers' symptoms and those of hysterical women. Myers, the British psychiatrist who coined the word "shell shock," described soldiers' reactions to traumatic experience as follows: "The recent emotional experiences of the individual have the upper hand and determine his conduct: the normal has been replaced by what we may call the 'emotional' personality. Gradually or suddenly an 'apparently normal' personality returns—normal safe for the lack of all memory of events directly connected with the shock [i.e., trauma], normal save for the manifestation of other ('somatic') hysteric disorders indicative of mental dissociation.''[16, p 67] Southard[18] compiled several hundred case reports of shell-shocked soldiers culled from the medical literature of the various belligerent nations. In it, he describes 23 cases of men with hysterical symptoms who lost all memories of their trauma. Similar observations were made during World War II. After the evacuation of Dunkirk, Sargant and Slater[19] observed amnesia for the trauma in 144 of 1,000 consecutive admissions to a field hospital. The DSM-III and IV recognize the issue of posttraumatic memory disturbances under the rubric of dissociative amnesia (300.12), which describes "reversible memory impairment in which memories of personal experience [related to traumatic or extremely stressful events] cannot be retrieved in a *verbal* form.''

During this last decade the validity of dissociative amnesia in adults with childhood sexual abuse histories has been called into question. However, every study, whether prospective or retrospective, of adults with histories of childhood sexual abuse has consistently found that dissociative amnesia is even more common in childhood victims of interpersonal violence than in combat soldiers and accident victims.[20–26] Amnesias for emotional and cognitive material seems to be age and dose related: the younger the age of the trauma and the more prolonged, the greater the likelihood of significant amnesia.[21,22,24,27]

LEVELS OF MEMORY

People possess a variety of complex and largely independent memory systems, most of which function outside of conscious awareness. These different categories of memory processing are known under several different names, including semantic, episodic, and procedural. Each of these memory systems has been associated with particular areas in the CNS.[28] Semantic memory is primarily symbolic in nature. It refers to the kinds of facts usually examined on IQ tests or college entrance examinations. Episodic memory refers to the specifics of autobiographical experiences, the location, colors and smells, mood and context of personal experiences. Typical examples of episodic memories are the details of specific emotion-laden events such as a death in the family or memories of love relationships. Such memories tend to be rich in specific perceptual content.[29] A third form of memory, procedural memory, refers to acquired skills and habits, emotional responses, reflexive actions, and classically conditioned responses, which generally have no verbal concomitant. People usually are unaware of how and where they learned to skate, enjoy particular pieces of music, or have averse physical reactions to certain sounds or physical sensations.

There never has been a question that semantic memory entails active and constructive processes and that even episodic memories tend to fade over time. Once an event or a particular bit of information becomes part of one's individual autobiography, it tends to be no longer available as a separate, immutable entity, but is liable to be altered by associated experiences, demand characteristics, and emotional frame of mind at the time of recall. As Schachtel[30, p 3] defined it, "Memory as a function of the living personality can be understood as a capacity for the organization and reconstruction of past experiences and impressions in the service of present needs, fears, and interests.''

The DSM definition of PTSD recognizes that trauma produces unusual memory phenomena and that it can lead to extremes of retention and forgetting; terrifying experiences may be indelibly etched into a person's memory or totally resist integration. In many instances, traumatized individuals report a combination of both. Although people seem to easily assimilate familiar and expectable experiences and although memories of ordinary events disintegrate in clarity over time, some aspects of traumatic events appear to get fixed in the mind, unaltered by the passage of time or by the intervention of subsequent experience. For example, in our own studies on posttraumatic nightmares, subjects claimed that they saw the same traumatic scenes over and over again without modification over a 15-year period.[31] It is intriguing that patients consistently claim that their perceptions are exact representations of sensations at the time of the trauma. For example, when Southwick and his group administered yohimbine to Vietnam veterans with PTSD, half their subjects reported trauma-related perceptions that they reported to be "just like it was" [in Vietnam].[32]

THE SENSORY ORGANIZATION OF TRAUMATIC EXPERIENCE

Although numerous authors have noted that trauma is organized in memory on a perceptual level, this issue has until recently received no systematic research attention. In a recent study we[5] designed an instrument, the Traumatic Memory Inventory (TMI), that allows for detailed examination of the nature of traumatic and nontraumatic memories, providing a structured way of recording whether and how memories of traumatic experiences are retrieved differently from memories of personally significant, nontraumatic events. To examine the retrieval of traumatic memories in a systematic way, we specifically inquired about the sensory modalities in which memories were experienced (a) as a story, (b) as an image (what did you see?), (c) in sounds (what did you hear?), (d) as a smell (what did you smell?), (e) as feelings in your body (what did you feel? where?), and (f) as emotions (what did you feel, what was it like?), about triggers for unbidden recollections of traumatic memories, and ways of mastering them.

We administered this instrument to 28 subjects with recent histories of trauma, such as physical or sexual assaults or motor vehicle accidents, and to 34 adults who had been physically or sexually assaulted as children. In addition to the traumatic incident, we asked our subjects about their recollections of a personally highly significant experience, such as a wedding or the birth of a child. Subjects considered most questions related to the nontraumatic memory nonsensical: none had olfactory, visual, auditory, kinesthetic reliving experiences related to their nontraumatic experiences. Subjects claimed not to have had periods in their lives when they had amnesia for any of these experiences. Environmental triggers did not suddenly bring back vivid and detailed memories, and none of the subjects felt a need to make special efforts to suppress memories of these events.

When asked about the traumatic memory, all of the childhood trauma subjects and 78% of the adult trauma subjects reported that they initially had no narrative memory of the event; they could not tell a story about what had happened, regardless of whether they always knew that the trauma had happened or whether they retrieved memories of the trauma at a later date. All these subjects, regardless of the age at

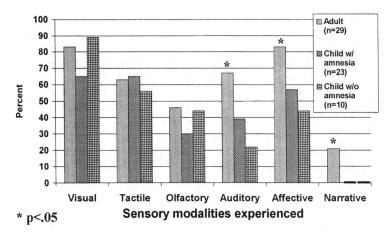

FIGURE 1. Initial sensory modalities experienced.

which the trauma occurred, claimed that they initially "remembered" the trauma in the form of somatosensory flashback experiences, as visual, olfactory, affective, auditory, or kinesthetic imprints (FIG. 1). As the trauma came into consciousness with greater clarity, more sensory modalities were activated, and a capacity to *tell* what actually had happened emerged over time (FIG. 2). These data support the notion that "memories" of a trauma tend, at least initially, to be experienced as fragments of the sensory components of the event that patients invariably seem to claim to be exact representations of elements of the original trauma.

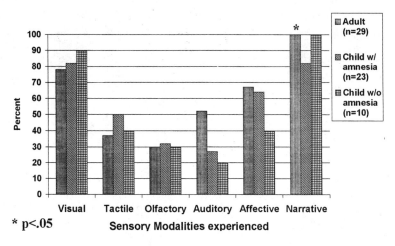

FIGURE 2. Current sensory modalities experienced.

These studies suggest that it is in the very nature of traumatic memory to be dissociated and to be initially stored as sensory fragments that have few or no linguistic components. It was surprising that this happened independent of the developmental level at which the trauma occurred; regardless of the age at which the trauma occurred, the experience initially was rarely reproduced as a personal narrative. Our subjects reported that as they became aware of more and more elements of the traumatic experience, they constructed a narrative that "explained" what happened to them. This process of weaving a narrative out of disparate sensory elements of an experience is probably not all that dissimilar from how people automatically construct a narrative under ordinary conditions. Like memories of day-to-day experience, the autobiography that the PTSD patient constructs out of the recall of the sensory elements of the trauma is likely to be contaminated by prior experience and by personal meaning schemes.

THE DIS-INTEGRATION OF EXPERIENCE

On the basis of these studies, I propose that the core issue that makes memories traumatic is the failure of the CNS to synthesize the sensations related to the traumatic memory into an integrated semantic memory; sensory elements of the experience are registered separately and are often retrieved independently of the context in which the experience occurred. This fragmentation or disorganization of memory interferes with the evaluation, classification, and contextualization of the experience. After a person develops PTSD, fragmented or misclassified sensations are reactivated in state-dependent fashion, in the form of flashbacks and nightmares. Lack of conscious recall of the trauma may coexist with flashback experiences or, alternatively, the (semantic) contents of their narratives may not match the (sensory) contents of their flashbacks.

Hence, when investigating the psychobiology of traumatic memories, we can expect to find abnormalities in areas in the CNS that are involved in the integration of ongoing experience. A variety of structures have been implicated in these integrative processes: (1) the parietal lobes are thought to integrate information between different cortical association areas,[33] (2) the hippocampus is thought to create a cognitive map that allows for the categorization of experience and its connection with other autobiographical information,[34] (3) the corpus callosum allows for the transfer of information by both hemispheres,[35] integrating emotional and cognitive aspects of experience, (4) the cingulate gyrus is thought to function as both amplifier and filter, helping to integrate the emotional and cognitive components of the mind,[36] and (5) the frontal lobes are thought to function as a "supervisory system" for the integration of experience.[37]

Recent neuroimaging studies of patients with PTSD suggest a role for most of these structures in the psychobiology of PTSD. These studies have opened up new avenues for understanding the various ways in which the CNS fails to integrate traumatic experiences and biases the traumatized individual to interpret subsequent sensory information in the direction of threat. It is against this background that I will interpret the first available neuroimaging studies of patients with PTSD.

TABLE 1. Neuroimaging Studies of Patients with PTSD, 1996

- Right-sided activation of amygdala and related structures
- Decrease in left inferior prefrontal activity at time of activation
- Decreased hippocampal size in chronic PTSD
- Decreased P300 activation in response to nontrauma-related stimuli
- Differential activation of the anterior cingulate in response to potentially threatening stimuli

NEUROIMAGING STUDIES IN PTSD

As of late 1996, there were four published neuroimaging studies of patients with PTSD[38-41] as well as two studies of Event Response Potentials (ERPs).[3,42] Two more studies have been completed and are in press,[43,44] whereas several other studies are currently underway. Three studies have used MRI to measure hippocampal volume in individuals with PTSD, and two studies have used positron emission tomography (PET)[38,44] to measure differential activation of the CNS in response to traumatic and nontraumatic scripts in patients with PTSD. Two studies have used SPECT: one[43] has looked at differential activation of the CNS in response to a traumatic versus a nontraumatic reminder in subjects with and without PTSD, and the other[44] has collected preliminary data on how the brain is differentially activated in response to a traumatic script before and after effective treatment (TABLE 1).

Hippocampal Volume

Three different studies done in three different laboratories have shown that persons with PTSD have decreased hippocampal volume compared with that of matched controls. Bremner and his colleagues[40] found that Vietnam combat veterans with PTSD had an 8% reduction in the volume of the right hippocampus compared with veterans who had no such symptoms. Stein *et al.*[41] found a 7% reduction in hippocampus volume in women with PTSD who had had repeated childhood sexual abuse. Gurvits and Pitman[39] found that Vietnam veterans with the most intense combat exposure and the most severe PTSD had an average shrinkage of 26% in the left hippocampus and 22% in the right hippocampus, compared with that of veterans who saw combat but had no symptoms. The severity of their PTSD was directly proportional to the degree of hippocampal shrinkage.

Event-Related Potentials (ERPs)

Paige *et al.*[42] reported significant differences in the pattern of cortical evoked potentials recorded in response to a stimulus pulse of white noise between PTSD patients and controls. The PTSD patients were more sensitive to sounds; they responded to sound intensities that were at or below threshold for most normal subjects. Furthermore, the pattern of cortical evoked potentials elicited by auditory stimuli in PTSD patients showed a reduced rather than the expected augmented electrical pattern.

Looking at the patterns of P300 and frontal cortical activation, McFarlane and his colleagues[3] found that persons with PTSD (1) were unable to differentiate relevant from irrelevant stimuli, (2) attended less to affectively neutral, but existentially relevant events, and (3) as a consequence of this relative lack of responsiveness, they needed to apply more effort than nontraumatized persons to respond to current experience (as reflected in a delayed reaction time).

Symptom Provocation Studies

Rauch and his colleagues[38] conducted a positron emission tomography (PET) scan study of patients with PTSD in which they were exposed to vivid, detailed narratives of their own traumatic experiences, e.g., a firefighter who had recovered the charred remains of bodies and a woman who accidentally caused the death of her own two children by going through a red light. For comparison, the patients were also exposed to narratives that invoked a neutral scene. During exposure to the script of their traumatic experiences these subjects demonstrated heightened activity only in the right hemisphere, specifically, in areas that are most involved in emotional arousal–the amygdala, insula, and medial temporal lobe. Activation of these structures was accompanied by heightened activity in the right visual cortex. When subjects were exposed to their traumatic scripts, there was a significant decrease in activation of the left inferior frontal area–Broca's area, which is thought to be responsible for translating personal experiences into communicable language. Shin et al's study,[45] utilizing a slightly different paradigm, essentially confirmed these findings in a different trauma population.

Liberzon and his colleagues[43] took SPECT images of Vietnam veterans with and without PTSD after exposing them to either the sounds of running water or to combat sounds. In the Vietnam veterans *without* PTSD, activation of the anterior cingulate was increased in response to the combat sounds, but not to the running water, whereas subjects with PTSD had no differential activation of this area.

Pre-Posttreatment Activation

We recently completed a pilot study utilizing eye movement desensitization and reprocessing (EMDR) in which the PTSD scores, as measured by the CAPS, dropped from an average of 84 to 36. After effective treatment, subjects registered increased activity in the anterior cingulate bilaterally and there was a suggestion of increased activation of the right prefrontal cortex. This suggests that recovery from PTSD may depend on the capacity of higher brain functions to override the input from limbic structures charged with the initial appraisal of the degree of threat posed by incoming sensory stimuli.

DISCUSSION

These early neuroimaging studies of patients with PTSD present a range of surprising findings that force us to reevaluate our previous concepts of the pathophysiology of PTSD. As we gain a deeper understanding of the meaning of these initial results and collect more data, these neuroimaging studies may force us to reevaluate appropriate therapeutic interventions as well.

Activation of the Amygdala and Related Structures

Of all the findings, seeing increased activation of the amygdala in response to traumatic scripts is the least surprising. After all, it has been well established that the amygdala is centrally involved in the interpretation of the emotional valence of the incoming information and that confrontation with feared stimuli activates the amygdala and related structures.[46] Exposure to traumatic scripts provokes autonomic activation of patients with PTSD,[47] and this is likely mediated by activation of the amygdala and related structures. It is well understood that the information evaluated by the amygdala is passed on to areas in the brain stem that control behavioral autonomic and neurohormonal response systems. By way of these connections, the amygdala transforms sensory stimuli into emotional and hormonal signals, thereby initiating and controlling emotional responses.[46]

Decrease in Hippocampal Volume

The twice replicated finding that persons with chronic PTSD have decreased hippocampal volume might explain some of the behavioral abnormalities in persons with chronic PTSD. The decreased size of the hippocampus in PTSD may, at least in part, be responsible for the ongoing dissociation and misinterpretation of information in the direction of threat, as noted in patients with PTSD. In animals, decreased hippocampal functioning has caused behavioral disinhibition.[48] It is thought that this plays a role in helping the animal define incoming stimuli in the direction of emergency (fight/flight) responses. If the same is true for people, this might explain why patients with PTSD have difficulties ''taking in'' and processing arousing information and learning from such experiences. Their altered biology would make them vulnerable to react to newly arousing stimuli as a threat and to react with aggression or withdrawal, depending on their premorbid personality.[49]

Aside from the putative relation between chronically high levels of cortisol and neurotoxicity to hippocampal cells (discussed elsewhere in this volume), research had shown that high levels stimulation of the amygdala can also interfere with hippocampal functioning.[49,50] Thus, high levels of emotional arousal may prevent the proper evaluation and categorization of experience by interfering with hippocampal function. I previously hypothesized that when this occurs, sensory imprints of experience are stored in memory, but because the hippocampus is prevented from fulfilling its integrative function, these various imprints are not united into a unified whole.[51] The experience is laid down, and later retrieved, as isolated images, bodily sensations, smells, and sounds that feel alien and separate from other life experiences. Some integrative function seems to break down, interfering with the localization of incoming information in time and space. It is possible that a less functional hippocampus plays a role in the continued fragmentation of experience in patients with PTSD.

TABLE 2. Properties of Left Hemisphere

- Organizes problem-solving tasks into well-ordered set of operations and processes information in sequential fashion
- Involved in perceiving and generating symbolic representation by breaking down a stimulus into categorical elements and combining them into novel images
- Manipulates words and symbols that transcribe personal experience into culturally shared meaning.
- Generativity is the distinguishing feature of left-hemisphere cognition.

Hemispheric Lateralization

The finding of marked hemispheric lateralization in subjects exposed to their personalized trauma scripts indicates that there is differential hemispheric involvement in the processing of traumatic memories. This finding has major implications for understanding the nature of PTSD. TABLES 2 and 3 summarize the relative functions of the two hemispheres. The right hemisphere, which developmentally seems to come "on-line" earlier than the left hemisphere, is involved in the expression and comprehension of global nonverbal emotional communication (tone of voice, facial expression, and visual/spatial communication). The early maturation of the right hemisphere is consistent with the importance of emotional communication early in life. The right hemisphere has a diffuse representational format, which allows for a dynamic and holistic integration across sensory modalities.[52]

The right hemisphere is thought to be particularly integrated with the amygdala which may mediate its involvement in assigning emotional significance to incoming stimuli and in regulating the autonomic and hormonal responses to that information. Although this hemisphere may be exquisitely sensitive to emotional nuances, it has, at best, a rudimentary capacity to think or communicate analytically, to employ syntax, or to reason.[52,53]

In contrast, the left hemisphere is thought to organize problem-solving tasks into a well-ordered set of operations and to process information in a sequential fashion. It is involved in perceiving and in generating symbolic representation by breaking

TABLE 3. Properties of the Right Hemisphere

- Involved in the expression and comprehension of global nonverbal emotional communication (tone of voice, facial expression, visual/spatial communication)
- Early maturation of right hemisphere consistent with importance of emotional communication early in life
- Diffuse representational format, allowing a dynamic and holistic integration across sensory modalities
- May be particularly integrated with the amygdala: emotional significance—fear and hostility
- Has, at best, a rudimentary capacity to think or communicate analytically, employ syntax, or reason

down a stimulus into categorical elements and combining them into novel images. It manipulates words and symbols that transcribe personal experience into culturally shared meaning. The labeling of perceptions is a left hemisphere function.[52] It is in the area of categorization and labeling of internal states that people with PTSD seem to have particular problems.[54,55]

It is conceivable that failure of left hemisphere function during states of extreme arousal is responsible for the derealization and depersonalization reported in acute PTSD.[56,57] In our brain scans we saw that during exposure to a traumatic script, Broca's area functioning was decreased. This would make it difficult for a traumatized individual to "understand" what is going on. They experience intense emotions without being able to label their feelings. Their bodies are aroused, and fragments of memories may be activated, but they often are unable to communicate what they are experiencing. A relative decrease in left hemispheric representation provides an explanation of why traumatic memories are experienced as timeless and ego-alien: the part of the brain necessary for generating sequences and for the cognitive categorization of experience is not functioning properly. Our research[38] indicates that during activation of the traumatic memory, the brain is "having" its experience. The person may feel, see, or hear the sensory elements of the traumatic experience, but he or she may be physiologically prevented from translating this experience into communicable language. When they are having their traumatic recall, victims may suffer from speechless terror in which they may be literally "out of touch with their feelings." Physiologically, they may respond as if they were being traumatized again, but this may be dissociated from subjective experience. If the victim experiences depersonalization and derealization, he cannot "own" what is happening and therefore cannot take steps to do anything about it.

Treatment Outcome (EMDR) Study

The small sample of patients on whom we have pre-posttreatment scans suggests that their improvement is reflected by increased activation of the anterior cingulate and the right prefrontal cortex. This seems to indicate that, at least in humans, the filter that ultimately interprets whether incoming stimuli are traumatic or not is set not only at the level of the amygdala, but also in more frontal regions of the brain. LeDoux *et al.*[58] demonstrated that emotional memories in animals seem to be indelible: they could not be modified over time. Improvement of PTSD symptoms may not be mediated by decreased activation of the amygdala, but by increased activation of the anterior cingulate and the prefrontal area which help the individual to become able to distinguish between real threats and traumatic reminders that are no longer relevant to current experience. Obviously, the processes and structures involved in such reinterpretation of traumatic reminders deserve a great deal more attention.

CONCLUSIONS AND TREATMENT IMPLICATIONS

When people receive sensory input, they ordinarily automatically synthesize this incoming information into the large store of preexisting information. If the event is personally significant, they generally transcribe these sensations into a narrative, without conscious awareness of the processes that translate sensory impressions into a personal story. Our research shows that in contrast with the way people seem to process ordinary information, traumatic experiences initially are imprinted as sensations or feeling states and are not collated and transcribed into personal narratives. The research presented here indicates that traumatic memories are retrieved as sensory and emotional representations, with impaired expression in communicable language. Failure to process information on a symbolic level, a prerequisite for proper categorization and integration with other experiences, seems to be at the very core of the pathology of PTSD.

Whereas the sensory perceptions reported in PTSD may well reflect the actual imprints of sensations that were recorded at the time of trauma, the narratives that weave sensory imprints into a socially communicable story are subject to condensation, embellishment, and contamination. Although trauma may leave an indelible sensory imprint, once people start talking about these sensations and try to make meaning of them, it is transcribed into ordinary memory and, like all ordinary memory, it is prone to distortion. Once people become conscious of intrusive elements of the trauma, they are liable to try to fill in the blanks and complete the picture: people seem to be unable to accept experiences that have no meaning; they will try to make sense of what they are feeling.

Because traumatic experiences appear to be stored primarily as somatic sensations and intense affect states, they may be least accessible to semantic processing. The apparently relative decrease in hemisphere functioning during reactivation of the trauma suggests that it is important to help persons with PTSD find a medium in which they can come to understand and communicate their experiences. In this process it may be important to compensate for a relative decrease in left hemispheric processes. It is possible that some of the newer therapies, such as dialectical behavior therapy or EMDR, may yield benefits that traditional insight-oriented therapies lack.

REFERENCES

1. PRIBRAM, K. H. 1987. The subdivision of the frontal cortex revisited. *In* The Frontal Lobes Revisited. E. Perecman, Ed.: 11-39. Lawrence Erlbaum. Hillsdale, NJ.
2. VAN DER KOLK, B. A. & C. DUCEY. 1989. The psychological processing of traumatic experience: Rorschach patterns in PTSD. J. Traumatic Stress **2:** 259-274.
3. MCFARLANE, A. C., D. L. WEBER & C. R. CLARK. 1993. Abnormal stimulus processing in PTSD. Biol. Psychiatry **34:** 311-320.
4. VAN DER KOLK, B. A., O. VAN DER HART & C. R. MARMAR. 1996. Dissociation and information processing in posttraumatic stress disorder. *In* Traumatic Stress: Effects of Overwhelming Stress on Mind, Body, and Society. B. A. van der Kolk, A. C. McFarlane & L. Weisaeth, Eds.: 303-330. Guilford Press. New York.
5. VAN DER KOLK, B. A. & R. FISLER. 1995. Dissociation and the perceptual nature of traumatic memories: Review and experimental confirmation. J. Traumatic Stress **8:** 505-525.
6. JANET, P. 1893. L'Amnesie continue. Rev. Gen. Sci. **4:** 167-179.
7. VAN DER KOLK, B. A. & O. VAN DER HART. 1991. The intrusive past: The flexibility of memory and the engraving of trauma. Am. Imago **48:** 425-454.
8. ELLIOT, D. M. & B. FOX. 1994. Delayed recall of child abuse memories: Prevalence and triggers to memory recall. Paper presented at the annual meeting of the International Society of Traumatic Stress Studies. Chicago, IL.

9. RIVERS, W. H. R. 1918. The repression of war experience. The Lancet, Feb. 2: 173-177.
10. BLANK, A. S. 1985. Irrational reactions to post-traumatic stress disorder. *In* The Trauma of War: Stress and Recovery in Vietnam Veterans. S. M. Sonnenberg, A. S. Blank & J. A. Talbott, Eds.: 69-98. American Psychiatric Press. Washington, DC.
11. KARDINER, A. 1941. The Traumatic Neuroses of War. Hoeber. New York.
12. CHARCOT, J. M. 1887. Leçons sur les maladies du systeme nerveux faites à la Salpêtrière [Lessons on the illnesses of the nervous system held at the Salpêtrière], Vol. 3. Progres Médical en A. Delahaye & E. Lecrosnie. Paris.
13. JANET, P. 1889. L'automatisme psychologique. Alcan. Paris.
14. FREUD, S. 1896/1962. The aetiology of hysteria. *In* The Standard Edition of the Complete Works of Sigmund Freud, Vol. 3. J. Strachey, Ed. and Trans.: Hogarth. 189-221. London.
15. PRINCE, M. 1910. The Dissociation of the Personality. Longmans, Green. New York.
16. MYERS, C. S. 1940. Shell Shock in France 1914-18. Cambridge University Press. New York.
17. BREUER, J. & S. FREUD. 1895/1955. Studies in hysteria. *In* The Standard Edition of the Complete Psychological Works of Sigmund Freud, Vol. 2. J. Strachy, Ed. & Trans. Horgarth Press. London.
18. SOUTHARD, E. E. 1919. Shell-shock and Other Neuropsychiatric Problems. W. W. Leonard. Boston.
19. SARGANT, W. & E. SLATER. 1941. Amnesic syndromes in war. Proc. Roy. Soc. Med. **34:** 757-764.
20. WILLIAMS, L. M. 1994. Adult memories of childhood abuse. J. Consult. Clin. Psychol. **62:** 1167-1176.
21. WILLIAMS, L. M. 1995. Recovered memories of abuse in women with documented child sexual victimization histories. J. Traumatic Stress **8:** 649-676.
22. HERMAN, J. E. & E. SHATZOW. 1987. Recovery and verification of memories of childhood sexual trauma. Psychoanal. Psychol. **4:** 1-14.
23. LOFTUS, E. F., S. POLENSKY & M. T. FULLILOVE. 1994. Memories of childhood sexual abuse: Remembering and repressing. Psychol. Women Q. **18:** 67-84.
24. BRIERE, J. & J. CONTE. 1993. Self-reported amnesia for abuse in adults molested as children. J. Traumatic Stress **6:** 21-31.
25. FELDMAN-SUMMERS, S. & K. POPE. 1994. The experience of 'forgetting' child abuse: A national survey of psychologists. J. Consult. Clin. Psychol. **62:** 636-639.
26. ELLIOT, D. M. & J. BRIERE. 1995. Posttraumatic stress associated with delayed recall of sexual abuse: A general population study. J. Traumatic Stress **8:** 629-648.
27. VAN DER KOLK, B. A., D. PELCOVITZ, S. ROTH, F. MANDEL, A. C. MCFARLANE & J. L. HERMAN. 1996. Dissociation, somatization, and affect dysregulation: The complexity of adaptation to trauma. Am. J. Psychiatry **153:** 83-93.
28. SQUIRE, L. R. 1994. Declarative and nondeclarative memory; Multiple brain systems supporting learning and memory. *In* Memory Systems. D. L. Schacter & E. Tulving, Eds. MIT Press. Cambridge, MA.
29. DONALD, M. 1991. Origins of the Modern Mind. Harvard University Press. Cambridge, MA.
30. SCHACHTEL, E. G. 1947. On memory and childhood amnesia. Psychiatry **10:** 1-26.
31. VAN DER KOLK, B. A., R. BLITZ, W. A. BURR & E. HARTMANN. 1984. Nightmares and trauma: Life-long and traumatic nightmares in Veterans. Am. J. Psychiatry **141:** 187-190.
32. SOUTHWICK, S. M., J. H. KRYSTAL, A. MORGAN, D. JOHNSON, L. NAGY, A. NICOLAOU, G. R. HENNINGER & D. S. CHARNEY. 1993. Abnormal noradrenergic function in posttraumatic stress disorder. Arch. Gen. Psychiatry **50:** 266-274.
33. DAMASIO, A. R. 1989. Time-locked regional retroactivation: A system level proposal for the neural substrate of recall and recognition. Cognition **33:** 25-62.

34. O'KEEFE, J. & L. NADEL. 1978. The Hippocampus as a Cognitive Map. Clarendon Press. Oxford.
35. JOSEPH, R. 1988. The right cerebral hemisphere: Emotion, music, visual-spatial skills, body-image, dreams, and awareness. J. Clin. Psychol. **44:** 630-673.
36. DEVINSKY, O., M. J. MORRELL & B. A. VOGT. 1995. Contributions of anterior cingulate cortex to behavior, Brain **118:** 279-306.
37. SHALLICE, T. 1988. From Neuropsychology to Mental Structure. Cambridge University Press. New York.
38. RAUCH, S., B. A. VAN DER KOLK, R. FISLER, N. ALPERT, S. ORR, C. SAVAGE, M. JENIKE & R. PITMAN. 1996. A symptom provocation study using Positron Emission Tomography and Script Driven Imagery. Arch. Gen. Psychiatry **53:** 380-387.
39. GURVITS, T., M. SHENTON, H. HOKAMA, H. OHTA, N. LASKO, M. GILBERTSON, S. ORR, R. KIKINIS, F. JOLESZ, R. MCCARLEY & R. PITMAN. 1996. Magnetic resonance imaging (MRI) study of hippocampal volume in chronic combat related posttraumatic stress disorder. Biol. Psychiatry **40:** 1091-1099.
40. BREMNER, J. D., P. RANDALL, T. M. SCOTT, R. A. BRONEN, J. P. SEIBYL, S. M. SOUTHWICK, R. C. DELANEY, G. MCCARTHY, D. S. CHARNEY & R. B. INNIS. 1995. MRI-based measured of hippocampal volume in patients with PTSD. Am. J. Psychiatry. **152:** 973-981.
41. STEIN, M. B. C. HANNAH, C. KOVEROLA, R. YEHUDA, M. TORCHIA & B. MCCLARTY. 1994. Neuroanatomical and neuroendocrine correlates in adulthood of severe sexual abuse in childhood. Paper presented at the 33rd Annual Meeting, American College of Neuropsychopharmacology, San Juan, PR, December 15.
42. PAIGE, S., G. REID, M. ALLEN & J. NEWTON. 1990. Psychophysiological correlates of PTSD. Biol. Psychiatry **58:** 329-335.
43. LIBERZON et al.
44. VAN DER KOLK, B. A., E. MATTHEW, T. HILL, J. A. BURBRIDGE, J. SUZUKI, S. LAZROVE, P. LEVIN & L. CALL. SPECT imaging before and after effective treatment of PTSD with EMDR. Presented at the 11th Annual Meeting, International Society for Traumatic Stress Studies. San Francisco, Nov. 1996.
45. SHIN, L. M., R. J. MCNALLY, S. M. KOSSLYN, W. L. THOMPSON, S. L. RAUCH, N. M. ALPERT, L. J. METZGER, N. B. LASKO, S. P. ORR & R. K. PITMAN. 1996. A positron emission tomographic study of symptom provocation in PTSD. Poster presented at the New York Academy of Sciences Conference on the Psychobiology of Posttraumatic Stress Disorder. New York, 1996.
46. LEDOUX, J. E. 1992. Emotion as memory: Anatomical systems underlying indelible neural traces. In Handbook of Emotion and Memory. S. A. Christianson, Ed.: 269-288. Lawrence Erlbaum. Hillsdale, N.J.
47. PITMAN, R. K., S. P. ORR, D. F. FORGUE, J. DE JONG & J. M. CLAIRBORN. 1987. Psychophysiologic assessment of posttraumatic stress disorder imagery in Vietnam combat veterans. Arch. Gen. Psychiatry. **17:** 970-975.
48. GRAY, J. F. 1982. The Neuropsychology of Anxiety: An Inquiry into the Functions of the Septo-hippocampal System. Oxford University Press. New York.
49. ADEMAC, R. E. 1991. Partial kindling of the ventral hippocampus: Identification of changes in limbic physiology which accompany changes in feline aggression and defense. Physiol-Behav. **49:** 443-454.
50. SQUIRE, L. R. & S. ZOLA MORGAN. 1991. The medial temporal lobe memory system. Science **153:** 2380-2386.
51. VAN DER KOLK, B. A. 1994. The body keeps the score: Memory and the evolving psychobiology of posttraumatic stress. Harvard Rev. Psychiatry **1:** 253-265.
52. DAVIDSON, R. J. & A. J. TOMARKEN. 1989. Laterality and emotion: An electrophysiological approach. In Handbook of Neuropsychology, Vol. 3. F. Boller & J. Grafman Eds.: 419-441. Elsevier. Amsterdam.

53. HENNINGER, P. 1992. Conditional handedness: Handedness changes in multiple personality disordered subject reflect shift in hemispheric dominance. Consciousness Cognit. **1:** 265-287.
54. KRYSTAL, H. 1978. Trauma and affects. Psychoanal. Study Child **33:** 81-116.
55. VAN DER KOLK, B. A. & A. C. MCFARLANE. 1996. The black hole of trauma. *In* Traumatic Stress: The Effects of Overwhelming Stress on Mind, Body, and Society. B. A. van der Kolk, A. C. McFarlane & L. Weisaeth, Eds.: 3-23. Guilford Press. New York.
56. MARMAR, C. R., D. S. WEISS, T. J. METZLER, H. M. RONFELDT & C. FOREMAN. 1995. Stress response of emergency services personnel to the Loma Prieta earthquake Interstate 880 freeway collapse and control traumatic incidents. J. Traumatic Stress **9:** 63-85.
57. SHALEV, A. Y., T. PERI, L. CANETI & S. SCREIBER. 1996. Predictors of PTSD in injured trauma survivors: A prospective study. Am. J. Psychiatry **153:** 219-225.
58. LEDOUX, J. E., L. ROMANSKI & A. XAGORARIS. 1991. Indelibility of subcortical emotional memories. J. Cognit. Neurosci. **1:** 238-243.

Psychophysiologic Reactivity to Trauma-Related Imagery in PTSD

Diagnostic and Theoretical Implications of Recent Findings[a]

SCOTT P. ORR

Veterans Affairs Research Service
228 Maple Street
Manchester, New Hampshire 03103

Department of Psychiatry
Harvard Medical School
Boston, Massachusetts 02115

According to the current version of the Diagnostic and Statistical Manual (DSM-IV),[1] establishing a diagnosis of posttraumatic stress disorder (PTSD) must include evidence that the traumatic event is persistently reexperienced (PTSD Category B). Included in the category of reexperiencing symptoms is that of "physiologic reactivity on exposure to internal or external cues that symbolize or resemble an aspect of the traumatic event" (Criterion B.5). The initial inclusion of this symptom (DSM-III-R)[2] was based on research evidence of heightened psychophysiologic reactivity to trauma-related cues in individuals diagnosed with PTSD. (For review see refs. 3-5.) The work comprising this literature has primarily used one of two methods for presenting trauma-related stimuli, either standardized stimuli or imaginal stimuli tailored to each individual's unique traumatic experience(s). A recent large multisite study combined these methods to examine combat-related PTSD in 1,328 Vietnam veterans.[6] Typically, when individuals with PTSD are exposed to internal or external cues representing their traumatic experience, they produce larger skin conductance, heart rate, blood pressure, or facial electromyogram (lateral frontalis) responses than do individuals without PTSD: Early research focused on PTSD resulting from trauma related to combat; recent studies have extended the findings of heightened physiologic reactivity to include PTSD resulting from civilian traumas such as motor vehicle accidents.[7-9]

Currently, the presence of physiologic reactivity to trauma-related cues is neither necessary nor sufficient for the diagnosis of PTSD. In fact, roughly one third of individuals meeting DSM criteria for PTSD do not show heightened physiologic reactivity on exposure to trauma-related cues. Diagnostic applications of psychophysiologic assessment have produced sensitivity values ranging from 60-90% and specificity values of 80-100%.[10-14] Results from the multisite study[6] of 1,328 Vietnam combat

[a] This project was supported by a Department of Veterans Affairs Merit Review Grant and National Institute of Mental Health grant RO1MH48559-01A2.

veterans, while replicating previous findings of heightened physiologic reactivity in individuals with PTSD, found lower sensitivity and specificity. The authors suggest that ascertainment and entrance requirements for inclusion in the study may have resulted in a PTSD sample with less severe symptoms than those characteristic of previously studied PTSD samples.

The failure of some individuals to show heightened physiologic reactivity when exposed to trauma-related cues could result from any, or a combination, of several factors.[5,6] First, physiologic responders and nonresponders might represent different subtypes of PTSD; the former group may experience emotional distress that has a strong physiologic component, whereas the latter's distress is more cognitive in nature. Second, the "menu approach" taken by the DSM and the categoric determination resulting from application of the criteria may tend to overdiagnose PTSD, that is, the specificity of the DSM criteria for PTSD may be low. An individual with pervasive and severe symptoms and an individual who meets the minimal requirements for the PTSD diagnosis will both be classified as having the disorder. Third, when some individuals are confronted with reminders of their traumatic experiences, as occurs in the laboratory, they may use defensive maneuvers that tend to reduce the emotional impact of trauma-related stimuli. Fourth, some individuals may exaggerate or overreport their symptoms as a means for generating helping behavior. Fifth, the psychophysiologic measures and methods commonly used in studies of PTSD might not be sufficiently sensitive to the full range of emotional expression and thereby miss the responses of some individuals.

Each of the aforementioned explanations for why some individuals with PTSD may not show heightened physiologic reactivity to trauma-related stimuli has particular diagnostic and/or theoretical implications. Currently there are few published data to support one explanation over another. However, a recent study of Operation Desert Storm (ODS) veterans found that individuals with PTSD failed to show heightened physiologic reactivity during imagery of experiences related to ODS and that the magnitudes of their responses were comparable to those of the non-PTSD group.[15] The authors noted that even though the ODS veterans met DSM criteria for PTSD, severity of the PTSD was fairly low; the mean Mississippi Scale score for the PTSD group was only 86. These results lend support to the possibility that classification of individuals solely on the basis of whether they meet DSM criteria for PTSD without regard for the severity of symptoms tends to overdiagnose the disorder, as reflected in a failure to show heightened emotional reactivity to trauma-related cues.

In addition to questions about the nature of the relation between physiologic reactivity and the presence, absence, and severity of current PTSD, little is currently known about the course of heightened reactivity as symptom severity declines. Limited evidence from treatment studies and case reports of PTSD suggest that physiologic reactivity declines with improvement in PTSD symptoms.[16-18] However, in the multisite study[6] of Vietnam combat veterans' physiologic responses to trauma-related cues, half of the 139 individuals with lifetime, but not current, PTSD were classified as physiologically reactive. This is an important finding because it suggests that physiologic reactivity can remain high even when the severity of self-reported symptoms declines.

RECENT FINDINGS FROM A PSYCHOPHYSIOLOGIC STUDY OF ADULT WOMEN SEXUALLY ABUSED DURING CHILDHOOD

A recent study[19] of physiologic reactivity in adult females with and without PTSD resulting from childhood sexual abuse provides additional insight into the relation between physiologic reactivity and a current or lifetime diagnosis of PTSD. This study used a script-driven imagery technique[9–12] to assess HR, SC, and facial EMG responses during recollection of two childhood sexual abuse experiences, as well as to other nonabuse-related events. Participants were classified on the basis of Structured Clinical Interview for DSM-III-R (SCID)[20] into Current ($n = 29$), Lifetime, but not current ($n = 24$), and Never ($n = 18$) PTSD groups. Results of univariate comparisons revealed larger HR responses in the Current than in the Lifetime and Never groups, and larger corrugator EMG responses in the Current than in the Never group during imagery of the abuse experiences. The Current PTSD group also showed a trend for larger lateral frontalis EMG responses. Responses of the Lifetime group tended to fall between those of the other two groups.

Physiologic data were pooled from previous script-driven imagery studies of civilian and combat-related PTSD ($n = 96$),[9–12] and a discriminant function was derived from the HR, SC, and lateral frontalis EMG responses during imagery of personal trauma-related experiences that maximally discriminated individuals with current PTSD from those who never had PTSD. Application of this function to physiologic responses generated during recollection of sexual abuse experiences correctly classified 19 of 29 Current (sensitivity = 66%) and 14 of 18 Never (specificity = 78%) participants in the childhood sexual abuse study.[19] When the discriminant function was applied to the responses of the Lifetime PTSD group, 10 of 24 (42%) participants were classified as physiologically reactive. This latter finding is consistent with results from the multisite study[6] of combat-related PTSD.

The 66% sensitivity observed in the study of childhood sexual abuse just noted is in line with previously reported sensitivities for physiologically based classification into dichotomous PTSD categories. In fact, it is quite respectable considering that the discriminant function was independently derived from the physiologic responses of mixed combat veteran and civilian trauma samples. Even so, the agreement between clinical and psychophysiologic assessment might be improved by incorporating an estimate of the severity of PTSD symptoms into the clinical diagnosis. To determine if a self-report based diagnostic instrument that assesses symptom severity might produce higher concordance with physiologic reactivity to trauma-related cues, we administered the Clinician-Administered PTSD Scale (CAPS)[21] to most ($n = 59$) participants in the childhood sexual abuse study. The Total CAPS score provides a continuous measure of overall severity (frequency and intensity) of PTSD symptoms in addition to allowing for a dichotomous diagnostic determination.

A scatter plot of posterior probabilities and Total CAPS scores is presented in FIGURE 1. The posterior probabilities were obtained by applying the discriminant function, derived from previously studied trauma samples, to the physiologic responses generated during imagery of the sexual abuse experiences. FIGURE 1 also

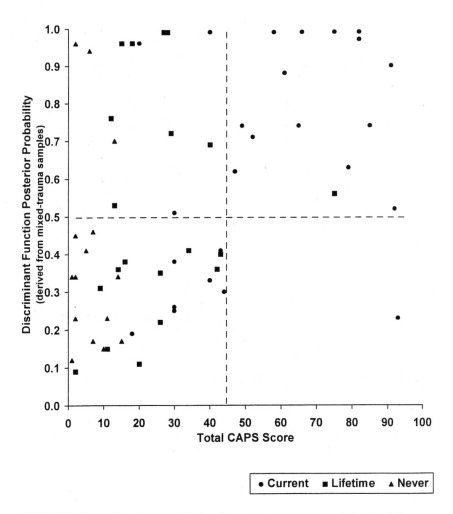

FIGURE 1. Scatter plot of physiologic-based posterior probabilities and Total CAPS scores.

identifies the SCID-based diagnostic classification (Current PTSD, Lifetime PTSD, and Never) for each individual. Overall, the Pearson product moment correlation was $r = 0.41$, $p = 0.001$, between physiologic posterior probability and Total CAPS score. Using a posterior probability > 1/2 to identify physiologically responsive individuals, several possible cutoff values for Total CAPS scores were explored and produced the following results:

Total CAPS Score $\geq$	% Responders	Total CAPS Score <	% Nonresponders
35	74	35	68
40	74	40	68
45	94	45	68
50	93	50	65
55	92	55	64

These computations included individuals with lifetime PTSD; because they have relatively low Total CAPS scores but a substantial number are physiologically responsive, the percentage of nonresponsive individuals (i.e., "sensitivity") tends to be low. A cutoff value $\leq$ 45 on the CAPS was selected as optimal for the present sample. As can be seen in FIGURE 1, 15 of 16 individuals with a Total CAPS score $\geq$ 45 were physiologically responsive. Only one individual had a total CAPS score > 45 and was not physiologically responsive. A posterior probability $\leq$ 1/2 identified 80% of individuals who had CAPS Total scores <45 and never met DSM criteria for PTSD according to the SCID as physiologically nonresponsive. Nearly all individuals who were physiologically responsive and had total CAPS score <45 had a diagnosis of lifetime or current PTSD according to the SCID.

Group means (and SDs) for severity ratings of the abuse experiences (average ratings of two clinical experts) and psychometric scores with the results of ANOVA and Duncan Multiple Range comparisons are presented in TABLE 1 for individuals with CAPS $\geq$ 45 and a posterior probability > 1/2 (High CAPS-High Responder), CAPS <45 and a posterior probability >1/2 (Low CAPS-High Responder), and CAPS <45 and a posterior probability $\leq$1/2 (Low CAPS-Low Responder). There was no group for CAPS $\geq$ 45 and a posterior probability $\leq$1/2 because only one individual fell into this category. It is important to note from TABLE 1 that the Low CAPS-High Responder group did not report higher levels of symptoms than did the Low CAPS-Low Responder group. The level of trait anxiety was the only psychometric measure that produced a significant difference between these two groups, and this was in the paradoxical direction of being lower for the responders. These psychometric results suggest that the heightened physiologic reactivity in that asymptomatic group cannot be explained by the presence of partial or subthreshold PTSD. Rather, heightened physiologic reactivity appears to persist for many individuals, primarily those who once had PTSD, even though current PTSD symptoms may be low.

CONCLUDING PERSPECTIVE

The results obtained from psychophysiologic assessment of adult women sexually abused during childhood provide compelling support for incorporating a measure of symptom severity in the diagnostic evaluation of PTSD. Instruments such as the CAPS may be optimal for this purpose because they provide a composite score based on the severities of all PTSD symptoms. As noted, 15 of 16 women sexually abused during childhood with total CAPS scores $\geq$45 also showed heightened physiologic reactivity during imagery of their traumatic experiences. Given that only 66% of individuals (19 of 29) with SCID-based diagnosis of PTSD were physiologically responsive, it appears that the disorder tends to be overdiagnosed when classification is based solely on whether or not the DSM criteria are met.

It is important to recognize that the CAPS cutoff score found to be optimal for the present sample may not be applicable to other childhood sexual assault samples or other trauma populations. Herein may lie an important application of psychophysiologic assessment to the extent that it can provide an accurate assessment of emotional reexperiencing of the traumatic event.

Some evidence indicates that individuals with PTSD are not very successful in altering their physiologic responses when instructed to do so.[22,23] Thus, the presence or absence of heightened psychophysiologic reactivity to trauma-related cues may be especially helpful in aiding diagnostic determinations when there is reason to believe that self-reported symptoms may not accurately reflect underlying symptoms. However, at best, physiologic reactivity provides one estimate of an individual's current emotional state. Factors that weaken or alter the relations between trauma-related cues, emotion, and physiologic response will make test results more difficult to interpret.

In addition to the finding that women sexually abused during childhood with moderate to severe PTSD (CAPS Total score ≥ 45) almost unanimously show heightened physiologic reactivity, a substantial number of individuals with lifetime but not current PTSD (42% for SCID-based or 41% for CAPS <45 based current PTSD diagnosis) also show heightened physiologic reactivity when exposed to reminders of the traumatic event. This is consistent with results from the multisite study[6] indicating that approximately 50% of Vietnam combat veterans with lifetime PTSD remain physiologically responsive. These findings are important because they indicate that physiologic reactivity can remain high even though an individual does not meet DSM criteria for current PTSD. Furthermore, the childhood sexual abuse data suggest that the heightened reactivity observed in some individuals with lifetime PTSD is not the result of having subthreshold or "partial" PTSD. The low CAPS-High Responder subgroup consisted primarily of individuals with a DSM diagnosis of lifetime or current (based on SCID results) PTSD, and comparisons between the psychometric scores of this subgroup and those of the Low Caps-Low Responder subgroup indicated that the responsive individuals did not report significantly higher levels of current symptoms. However, it is possible that the high responder subgroup was underreporting the severity of their symptoms.

Conditioning theory has been used to explain the acquisition of strong emotional responses to cues associated with a traumatic event and the subsequent manifestation of heightened physiologic reactivity on reexposure to trauma-related stimuli.[24-26] In particular, the acquisition of conditioned fear responses seems likely, given that the response to a traumatic event is presumed to involve "intense fear, helplessness, or horror."[1] In a review of the early research literature on childhood sexual abuse, the most commonly reported finding on the initial (within 2 years) emotional effect of childhood sexual abuse was that of fear.[27] This fear could support the development of PTSD and conditioned emotional responses to cues associated with experiences of sexual abuse. Within this framework, the persistence of heightened physiologic responsivity to trauma-related cues when other PTSD symptoms have abated, as in some individuals with lifetime PTSD, could be conceptualized as a failure to extin-

TABLE 1. Group Means, Standard Deviations, and Results of ANOVA and Duncan Multiple Range Comparisons for Event Ratings and Psychometric Measures for High vs Low CAPS Total Score and Physiologic Responders vs Nonresponders

| | Current CAPS and Physiologic Responder Status | | | | | | ANOVA | | | Group Differences |
| | CAPS ≥ 45 Responder Group 1 (n = 15) | | CAPS < 45 Responder Group 2 (n = 14) | | CAPS < 45 Nonresponder Group 3 (n = 30) | | | | | |
	M	(SD)	M	(SD)	M	(SD)	F	df	p	
Event ratings										
Sexual abuse (averaged)										
Expert severity scores	8.7	(1.4)	8.4	(1.6)	8.3	(1.4)	<1	(2,56)	ns	
Impact of Event Scale	34.6	(17.6)	25.6	(18.3)	20.0	(20.6)	2.8	(2,55)	.07	1>3
Psychometrics										
Clinician Administered PTSD Scale										
Current total score	70.1	(14.9)	20.9	(11.7)	18.4	(14.6)	73.4	(2,56)	<.001	1>2,3
Lifetime total score	86.9	(18.9)	63.4	(28.5)	51.8	(31.9)	7.6	(2,56)	.001	1>2,3
Mississippi Scale—										
Civilian Version	120.0	(16.3)	81.1	(18.8)	86.6	(23.7)	15.2	(2,54)	<.001	1>2,3
Keane Scale (MMPI)	27.9	(9.6)	8.4	(6.1)	13.3	(10.3)	16.8	(2,52)	<.001	1>2,3
Beck Depression Inventory	26.5	(10.7)	7.4	(6.9)	6.3	(6.8)	28.7	(2,47)	<.001	1>2,3
Symptom Checklist 90	1.4	(0.5)	0.4	(0.3)	0.7	(0.6)	14.4	(2,49)	<.001	1>2,3
Dissociative Experiences Scale	19.8	(12.2)	8.3	(5.5)	10.7	(11.3)	4.9	(2,55)	.01	1>2,3
State-Trait Anxiety Inventory										
State	50.3	(12.5)	33.7	(9.9)	35.1	(9.8)	12.3	(2,56)	<.001	1>2,3
Trait	57.3	(11.8)	30.4	(7.7)	37.8	(11.4)	25.3	(2,55)	<.001	1>3>2

MMPI (T-scores)

	Mean	(SD)	Mean	(SD)	Mean	(SD)	F	(df)	p	
L	47.6	(5.5)	54.9	(7.5)	51.3	(7.8)	3.4	(2,52)	.04	2>1
F	74.3	(15.7)	57.6	(6.7)	61.7	(9.6)	4.9	(2,52)	.01	1>2,3
K	47.8	(6.8)	56.3	(9.3)	54.4	(8.9)	3.7	(2,52)	.03	1<2,3
F-K (raw scores)	1.0	(9.0)	-7.9	(8.2)	-6.6	(8.2)	4.7	(2,52)	.01	1>2,3
Hypochondriasis (1)	71.2	(15.4)	57.6	(10.9)	60.0	(9.2)	5.7	(2,52)	.006	1>2,3
Depression (2)	83.1	(13.0)	56.4	(9.3)	58.9	(11.1)	25.2	(2,52)	<.001	1>2,3
Hysteria (3)	72.0	(10.1)	59.8	(9.1)	61.1	(7.2)	9.0	(2,52)	<.001	1>2,3
Psychopathic deviate (4)	80.2	(12.7)	63.2	(9.3)	69.4	(10.0)	9.0	(2,52)	<.001	1>2,3
Masculinity-femininity (5)	45.5	(7.8)	52.6	(9.5)	52.1	(9.2)	2.8	(2,52)	.07	1<2,3
Paranoia (6)	68.4	(12.6)	59.3	(7.6)	63.4	(9.7)	2.8	(2,52)	.07	1>2
Psychasthenia (7)	76.0	(13.6)	53.6	(8.5)	57.3	(12.2)	14.8	(2,52)	<.001	1>2,3
Schizophrenia (8)	83.9	(18.7)	58.1	(9.6)	63.1	(14.3)	12.5	(2,52)	<.001	1>2,3
Hypomania (9)	54.8	(9.6)	55.1	(11.4)	54.3	(10.8)	<1	(2,52)	ns	
Social introversion (0)	72.6	(9.6)	52.4	(10.3)	55.9	(10.1)	16.3	(2,52)	<.001	1>2,3

guish the conditioned emotional response associated with the original traumatic event. However, extinction of the conditioned response does not appear to be a requisite for clinical improvement, at least for some individuals. This has important implications for the conceptualization and treatment of PTSD.

It has been noted[28] that findings of heightened physiologic responses and the specificity of these responses to trauma-related cues in individuals with PTSD are similar to findings from studies of specific phobia. Individuals with specific phobia demonstrate larger HR and SC responses during imagery of their phobic objects than do individuals with less specific fears and anxiety.[29,30] In fact, the potential for overlap between PTSD and phobias that have a traumatic origin, such as fear of driving that results from a severe collision, may lead to difficulty in establishing a differential diagnosis.[31] Unlike PTSD, which has multiple symptoms in addition to physiologic reactivity, a specific phobia typically involves avoidance of the phobic object and little else in the way of substantive psychopathology. The heightened physiologic responsivity seen in some individuals with lifetime, but not current, PTSD and the relative absence of other PTSD-related symptoms gives the appearance of a phobia-like disorder. Emotional distress is experienced when the individual is directly confronted with reminders of the traumatic event, but the individual is otherwise symptom free or relatively so. This suggests that using methods aimed at directly reducing emotional reactivity to memories or reminders of the traumatic event (e.g., exposure therapies) may be unnecessary in some individuals, given that symptom improvement appears possible even though physiologic responsivity remains elevated. For some individuals, successful coping with the emotional residue of a traumatic experience may involve learning to accept and adapt to their emotional responsivity to reminders of the trauma.

The presence of heightened physiologic reactivity in individuals with lifetime PTSD indicates that it is possible to be emotionally reactive to trauma-related cues and not have a diagnosis of current PTSD. But is it possible to have current PTSD and not show heightened reactivity? Previous psychophysiologic results suggest that the answer to this question is yes, given that approximately one third of individuals with a diagnosis of current PTSD are not physiologically responsive in the laboratory. However, these studies did not incorporate an estimate of symptom frequency and intensity into their diagnoses of PTSD and probably included some individuals in the PTSD category who had relatively mild symptoms. The present findings suggest that when the current PTSD group includes only those individuals with moderate to severe symptoms (CAPS $\geqq 45$), nearly all individuals show heightened physiologic reactivity. Diagnostic accuracy may be improved by incorporating a symptom severity floor into the determination, a minimal value below which the diagnosis of PTSD would not be assigned.

REFERENCES

1. AMERICAN PSYCHIATRIC ASSOCIATION. 1994. Diagnostic and Statistical Manual of Mental Disorders, 4th Ed. American Psychiatric Association. Washington, DC.
2. AMERICAN PSYCHIATRIC ASSOCIATION. 1987. Diagnostic and Statistical Manual of Mental Disorders, 3rd Ed., Revised. American Psychiatric Association. Washington, DC.

3. McFall, M. E., M. M. Murburg, D. K. Roszell & R. C. Veith. 1989. Psychophysiologic and neuroendocrine findings in posttraumatic stress disorder: A review of theory and research. J. Anxiety Disorders **3:** 243–257.
4. Shalev, A. Y. & Y. Rogel-Fuchs. 1993. Psychophysiology of the posttraumatic stress disorder: From sulfur fumes to behavioral genetics. Psychosom. Med. **55:** 413–423.
5. Orr, S. P. & D. G. Kaloupek. 1997. Psychophysiological assessment of PTSD. *In* Assessing Psychological Trauma and PTSD: A Handbook for Practitioners. J. Wilson & T. Keane, Eds.: 69–97. Guilford Publications. New York, NY.
6. Keane, T. M., L. C. Kolb, D. G. Kaloupek, S. P. Orr, R. G. Thomas, F. Hsieh & P. Lavori. 1997. Utility of psychophysiological measurement in the diagnosis of posttraumatic stress disorder: Results of a Department of Veterans Affairs Cooperative Study. Submitted.
7. Blanchard, E. B., E. J. Hickling, A. E. Taylor, W. R. Loos & R. J. Gerardi. 1994. The psychophysiology of motor vehicle accident related posttraumatic stress disorder. Behav. Ther. **25:** 453–467.
8. Blanchard, E. B., E. J. Hickling, T. C. Buckley, A. E. Taylor, A. Vollmer & W. R. Loos. 1996. The psychophysiology of motor vehicle accident related posttraumatic stress disorder: Replication and extension. J. Consult. Clin. Psychol. **64:** 742–751.
9. Shalev, A. Y., S. P. Orr & R. K. Pitman. 1993. Psychophysiologic assessment of traumatic imagery in Israeli civilian post-traumatic stress disorder patients. Am. J. Psychiatry **150:** 620–624.
10. Orr, S. P., R. K. Pitman, N. B. Lasko & L. R. Herz. 1993. Psychophysiologic assessment of posttraumatic stress disorder imagery in World War II and Korean Combat Veterans. J. Abnorm. Psychol. **102:** 152–159.
11. Pitman, R. K., S. P. Orr, D. F. Forgue, B. Altman, J. B. de Jong & L. R. Herz. 1990. Psychophysiologic responses to combat imagery of Vietnam veterans with posttraumatic stress disorder versus other anxiety disorders. J. Abnorm. Psychol. **99:** 49–54.
12. Pitman, R. K., S. P. Orr, D. F. Forgue, J. B. de Jong & J. M. Claiborn. 1987. Psychophysiologic assessment of posttraumatic stress disorder imagery in Vietnam combat veterans. Arch. Gen. Psychiatry **44:** 970–975.
13. Blanchard, E. B., L. C. Kolb, R. J. Gerardi, P. Ryan & T. P. Pallmeyer. 1986. Cardiac response to relevant stimuli as an adjunctive tool for diagnosing post-traumatic stress disorder in Vietnam veterans. Behav. Ther. **17:** 592–606.
14. Blanchard, E. B., L. C. Kolb, A. E. Taylor & D. A. Wittrock. 1989. Cardiac response to relevant stimuli as an adjunct in diagnosing post-traumatic stress disorder: Replication and extension. Behav. Ther. **20:** 535–543.
15. Davis, J. M., H. E. Adams, M. Uddo, J. J. Vasterling & P. B. Sutker. 1996. Physiological arousal and attention in veterans with posttraumatic stress disorder. J. Psychopathol. Behav. Assess. **18:** 1–20.
16. Boudewyns, P. A. & L. Hyer. 1990. Physiological response to combat memories and preliminary treatment outcome in Vietnam veteran PTSD patients with direct therapeutic exposure. Behav. Ther. **21:** 63–87.
17. Keane, T. M. & D. G. Kaloupek. 1982. Imaginal flooding in the treatment of a posttraumatic stress disorder. J. Consult. Clin. Psychol. **50:** 138–140.
18. Shalev, A. Y., S. P. Orr & R. K. Pitman. 1992. Psychophysiologic response during script-driven imagery as an outcome measure in posttraumatic stress disorder. J. Clin. Psychiatry **53:** 324–326.
19. Orr, S. P., N. B. Lasko, L. J. Metzger, N. Berry, C. Ahern & R. K. Pitman. 1997. Psychophysiologic assessment of post-traumatic stress disorder imagery in adult females who were sexually abused during childhood. Submitted.
20. Spitzer, R. L., J. B. W. Williams, M. Gibbon & M. B. First. 1990. Structured Clinical Interview for DSM-III-R—Non-Patient Edition (SCID-NP, Version 1.0). American Psychiatric Press. Washington, DC.

21. BLAKE D. D., F. W. WEATHERS, L. M. NAGY, D. G. KALOUPEK, G. KLAUMINZER & T. M. KEANE. 1990. Clinician rating scale for assessing current and lifetime PTSD: The CAPS-1. Behav. Therapist **13:** 187-188.
22. GERARDI, R. J., E. B. BLANCHARD & L. C. KOLB. 1989. Ability of Vietnam veterans to dissimulate a psychophysiological assessment for post-traumatic stress disorder. Behav. Ther. **20:** 229-243.
23. ORR, S. P. & R. K. PITMAN. 1993. Psychophysiologic assessment of attempts to simulate posttraumatic stress disorder. Biol. Psychiatry **33:** 127-129.
24. KEANE, T. M., J. A. FAIRBANK, J. M. CADDELL, R. T. ZIMERING & M. E. BENDER. 1985. A behavioral approach to assessing and treating post-traumatic stress disorder. *In* Trauma and Its Wake, the Study and Treatment of Post-traumatic Stress Disorder. C. R. Figley, Ed.: 257-294. Brunner/Mazel. New York, NY.
25. KOLB, L. C. & L. R. MULTALIPASSI. 1982. The conditioned emotional response: A subclass of the chronic and delayed post-traumatic stress disorder. Psychiatric Ann. **12:** 979-987.
26. PITMAN, R. K. 1988. Post-traumatic stress disorder, conditioning, and network theory. Psychiatric Ann. **18:** 182-189.
27. BROWNE, A. & D. FINKELHOR. 1986. Impact of child sexual abuse: A review of the research. Psychol. Bull. **99:** 66-77.
28. ORR, S. P. 1994. An overview of psychophysiological studies of PTSD. PTSD Res. Q. **5:** 1-7.
29. COOK, E. W., III, B. G. MELAMED, B. N. CUTHBERT, D. W. MCNEIL & J. LANG. 1988. Emotional imagery and the differential diagnosis of anxiety. J. Consult. Clin. Psychol. **56:** 734-740.
30. MCNEIL, D. W., S. R. VRANA, B. G. MELAMED, B. N. CUTHBERT & P. J. LANG. 1993. Emotional imagery in simple and social phobia: Fear versus anxiety. J. Abnorm. Psychol. **102:** 212-225.
31. MCNALLY, R. J. & P. A. SAIGH. 1993. On the distinction between traumatic simple phobia and posttraumatic stress disorder. *In* Posttraumatic Stress Disorder: DSM-IV and Beyond. J. T. Davidson & E. B. Foa, Eds.: 207-212. American Psychiatric Press. Washington, DC.

Noradrenergic Alterations in Posttraumatic Stress Disorder

STEVEN M. SOUTHWICK, C. A. MORGAN, III,
A. DOUGLAS BREMNER, CHRISTIAN G. GRILLON,
JOHN H. KRYSTAL, LINDA M. NAGY, AND
DENNIS S. CHARNEY

Department of Psychiatry
Yale University
VA Connecticut
950 Campbell Ave.
West Haven, Connecticut 06515

Since World War I, numerous clinicians and researchers have described signs and symptoms of sympathetic nervous system dysregulation in combat veterans who suffer from what is currently termed posttraumatic stress disorder (PTSD). These veterans return from war in a hyperaroused, vigilant, and at times agitated state that may persist or even worsen over time. To describe this chronic war-related physiologic hyperarousal, Kardiner and Spiegel[1] coined the term physioneurosis in the 1940s. They believed that physioneurosis differed from other neuroses in its profound underlying physiologic basis. Similarly, Grinker and Spiegel[2] believed that veterans with physioneurosis suffered from chronic stimulation of the sympathetic nervous system that made them appear as if they had received an injection of adrenaline.

Formal research into the nature of war-related neurobiologic alterations in sympathetic nervous system activity began as early as 1918 when Meakins and Wilson[3] exposed shell-shocked veterans to the sounds of gunfire and the smell of sulfuric fumes. Compared to healthy controls, shell-shocked veterans showed significantly greater increases in heart rate. Also in 1918, among combat veterans with shell shock, Fraser and Wilson[4] reported exaggerated increases in subjective anxiety, heart rate, and blood pressure after administration of epinephrine (EPI). Since then, a host of well-designed psychophysiologic studies have demonstrated increased physiologic reactivity to reminders of past traumas in individuals with PTSD compared to controls.[5-17]

Intrigued by the aforementioned psychophysiologic studies, a growing number of researchers have begun to investigate possible hormone and neurotransmitter alterations in individuals with PTSD. To date, alterations have been reported in a number of neurobiologic systems including catecholamine,[18] opiate,[18] and thyroid[19] systems as well as in the HPA axis.[20] That alterations have been found in multiple systems is not surprising, because numerous neurobiologic axes become activated when an organism is threatened. It has been hypothesized that parallel activation of multiple brain regions and neurotransmitter systems is critical for survival during situations of danger.[21] How these activated systems interact with one another to effect behavior is not well understood.

In the present report we focus on the noradrenergic system as it relates to PTSD. Following a brief discussion of preclinical studies on stress and norepinephrine, this chapter summarizes the current clinical literature on PTSD and norepinephrine, with particular emphasis on a series of studies investigating the effects of yohimbine hydrochloride on behavior, physiology, and biochemistry in traumatized combat veterans. Yohimbine is an alpha$_2$-adrenergic receptor antagonist that causes a robust increase in the release of norepinephrine. It has been used as a probe of the noradrenergic system in numerous psychiatric disorders.

PRECLINICAL RESEARCH

Acute stress and fear increase central and peripheral norepinephrine (NE) through effects on synthesis, release, and catabolism.[22] Stress-induced regional increases in NE turnover have been recorded in the locus coeruleus (LC), cerebral cortex, and limbic regions (hypothalamus, amygdala, and hippocampus).[23-25] The LC is particularly relevant to catecholamine systems, because it contains most of the brain's noradrenergic cell bodies. It has been proposed that the LC, in conjunction with the nucleus paragigantocellularis (PGI), may serve as the brain's central alerting or vigilance system.[26] Features that make the LC ideal for such a role include its widespread terminal fields, extensive feedback loops, and its tendency to fire synchronously between cells. With such a broad efferent network, the LC could mediate a wide range of skeletal motor, cardiovascular, neuroendocrine, and cognitive responses appropriate to situations of anxiety and fear.[22] Theoretically it might play a role in mediating traumatic levels of arousal, selectively attending to meaningful environmental stimuli, and responding to such stimuli.

Activation of the LC by direct electrical stimulation[27] or by pharmacologic agents,[27,28] such as yohimbine or piperoxane, elicits fear behaviors in primates. In contrast, fear behaviors are reduced by pharmacologic agents that decrease LC function such as opiates, benzodiazepines, and clonidine, an alpha$_2$-adrenergic receptor agonist.[27,29] Furthermore, bilateral lesions of the LC in the monkey decrease fear-related behaviors in response to threatening situations and in social group situations.[27] Finally, it was shown that stressful or fear-inducing stimuli can activate the LC. In a study of freely moving cats, confrontation with a nonthreatening novel stimulus, such as a mouse, did not cause a specific increase in LC firing, whereas confrontation with a threatening stimulus, such as a dog or an aggressive cat, caused a marked increase in firing.[30-33] These increases in LC firing were accompanied by sympathetic activation. It has been suggested that central LC activity is coordinated with the peripheral sympathetic nervous system through the PGI which has connections to both areas.[26]

Norepinephrine appears to play an important role in vigilance, selective attention, orienting behaviors, and cardiovascular responses to threatening or dangerous situations.[26] It has been shown to selectively enhance responses to strong afferent or sensory input relative to basal activity in the same neurons. The selective enhancement results in what has been termed an increase in "signal-to-noise ratio" with an increase in neuronal responsivity to relevant stimuli (signal) and a decrease in responsivity to background neuronal activity (noise). Several studies have provided evidence for a dose response relationship between norepinephrine and neuronal activity with high level of NE resulting in decreased neuronal activity and low levels of NE in increased activity.[34,35] It has further been proposed that marked increases in NE tend to interrupt vegetative behaviors such as sleeping, grooming, and eating while stimulating behaviors related to orienting and vigilance.[26]

Norepinephrine, particularly in the amygdala, also appears to play an important role in learning and memory. Intra-amygdala infusion of NE immediately after training for an inhibitory avoidance task enhances retention.[36] Naloxone, which increases release of NE through opiate receptor blockade, also facilitates retention.[37,38] On the other hand, both NE-and naloxone-induced memory enhancement are blocked by posttrial intra-amygdala infusion of beta-adrenergic antagonists.[36,39,40] The memory-enhancing effects of norepinephrine appear to be dose dependent.[36]

In addition to its role in encoding memory, NE can facilitate retrieval of memory for stress-related learning tasks. Sara and Devauges[41] argued that the effectiveness of these treatments often depends on an intact central noradrenergic system. The facilitating effects of NE on memory retrieval have received strong support from studies of the alpha$_2$-adrenergic antagonists yohimbine[42] and idazoxan. It has been argued that both external and internal cues (e.g., similar or matching neuroendocrine states) appear capable of enhancing retrieval.

CLINICAL NEUROBIOLOGIC RESEARCH

Since 1980, numerous psychophysiological studies have documented heightened sympathetic nervous system arousal in combat veterans with PTSD.[5-17] When exposed to visual or auditory reminders of combat, veterans with PTSD tend to have greater increases in blood pressure and heart rate than combat veterans with anxiety disorders other than PTSD or normal controls. Although some studies reported increases in baseline cardiovascular parameters, others found increases only in response to trauma-related stimuli. It has been suggested that basal differences in autonomic nervous system arousal may best be understood as state-related elevations secondary to anticipatory distress (i.e., the stress of the experiment).[43] On the other hand, elevations in response to trauma-related stimuli appear to reflect a consistent feature of severely traumatized veterans with PTSD. Exaggerated increases in heart rate and blood pressure to trauma-specific stimuli also have been reported in a variety of noncombat traumatized populations.[43]

Investigations of neuroendocrine and peripheral catecholamine receptor systems also provide evidence for a dysregulation of sympathetic nervous system activity in PTSD. Kosten *et al.*[44] found that 24-hour urinary NE excretion was higher in combat veterans with PTSD than in patients with schizophrenia or major depression. Furthermore, throughout hospitalization, NE excretion in the PTSD group remained markedly elevated in comparison to that of controls. This finding was replicated in one study of war veterans[45] but not in another.[46] Davidson and Baum[47] measured urinary catecholamine levels in a community sample of individuals living within 5 miles of the Three Mile Island nuclear power station 5 years after the accident. Higher urinary NE levels were detected in residents living closer to Three Mile Island than in those living 80 miles away, implying higher "stress levels" in individuals with greater exposure to the accident based on proximity. Similarly, in a 24-hour urine catecholamine study comparing sexually abused girls to demographically matched controls, DeBellis *et al.*[48] found significantly greater amounts of homovanillic acid and trends towards greater excretion of urinary vanillylmandelic acid metanephrine, and total catecholamines (epinephrine, norepinephrine, and dopamine) among the abused subjects. Thus, most 24-hour urine catecholamine studies in combat veterans, adult civilian trauma victims, and traumatized children indicate chronic elevation of catecholamine excretion. Twenty-four-hour urine studies contrast with most studies measuring resting baseline plasma NE in which subjects with PTSD generally have not differed from normal controls.[18]

Several receptor binding studies provide further evidence for dysregulation of catecholamine systems in PTSD. Among combat veterans with PTSD[49] and among traumatized children,[50] Perry *et al.* found an abnormally low number of total alpha$_2$-adrenergic receptor binding sites per platelet. Decreased platelet alpha$_2$ adrenergic receptor number also was reported in congestive heart failure[51] and borderline personality disorder.[52] It has been suggested that decreased receptor number reflects an adaptation to elevation of circulating catecholamines.[53] Furthermore, Lerer *et al.* reported lower basal cyclic AMP[54] and lower basal adenylate cyclase levels[55] among combat veterans with PTSD than among healthy controls.

A variety of challenge strategies also have been used to characterize catecholamine activity in PTSD. Using an *in vivo* preparation, Perry[50] exposed intact platelets to high concentrations of epinephrine. Platelets of patients with PTSD showed an abnormal and extensive loss of receptor protein from platelet membranes. These findings were viewed as consistent with an overtaxed and easily "fatigued" receptor-effector system that was sensitive to downregulation. In a separate series of studies, Lerer *et al.*[54,55] found lower responsiveness to isoproteronol and forskolin in lymphocyte preparations and lower responsiveness to forskolin stimulation in platelet membranes of PTSD patients than in controls.

Some challenge studies have used nontrauma-related stressors to provoke catecholamine systems. To investigate the effects of physical stress on plasma catecholamines, Hamner *et al.*[56] measured plasma catecholamine responses to rigorous exercise on a treadmill. Compared to 8 normal controls, 12 combat veterans with PTSD did not differ significantly in heart rate or maximal blood pressure response to exercise, pre- and posttest NE levels, or percentage increase in mean plasma NE. PTSD patients did, however, have a significantly greater increase in plasma 3-methoxy-4 hydroxyphenylglycol (MHPG) than did controls, suggesting increased sensitivity to noradrenergic activation in the PTSD group. On the other hand, McFall *et al.*[57] found no differences between combat veterans with PTSD and controls in heart rate, blood pressure, NE, or epinephrine responses to a film of an automobile accident that was unrelated to specific traumas experienced by subjects in the study.

Challenges with trauma-related stressors, such as the sights, sounds, and smells of personally experienced traumas, have consistently caused greater increases in cardiac indices among patients with PTSD than among controls. Catecholamine responses to personally relevant trauma stimuli also have been measured in two separate studies. Among combat veterans with PTSD compared to healthy controls, McFall *et al.*[57] reported higher levels and a parallel rise in plasma EPI during and after a combat film. Similarly, Blanchard *et al.*[58] found significantly greater increases in heart rate and plasma NE after exposure to auditory stimuli reminiscent of combat in combat veterans with PTSD than in combat veterans without PTSD.

Neuroendocrine challenge strategies also have been used to probe catecholamine systems in patients with PTSD. Noradrenergic systems specifically were studied using desipramine, clonidine, and yohimbine as challenge agents. In a study of eight traumatized women, Dinan *et al.*[59] reported no differences between traumatized subjects and controls in desipramine-stimulated growth hormone levels. The desipramine growth hormone challenge has been used to assess postsynaptic alpha$_2$-adrenergic receptor function. On the other hand, a blunted growth hormone response to intravenous clonidine in a car accident victim with PTSD was reported by Hansenne *et al.*[60] The growth hormone response to clonidine generally is thought to represent an index of noradrenergic function. Blunting suggested possible downregulation of noradrenergic receptors and heightened noradrenergic sensitivity. Finally, responses to yohimbine are reviewed below.

Yohimbine vs Placebo Challenge

To more directly probe both peripheral and central noradrenergic reactivity, yohimbine was administered to 20 combat veterans with PTSD and 18 healthy controls.[61] As noted earlier, yohimbine is an alpha$_2$-adrenergic receptor antagonist that activates noradrenergic neurons by blocking the alpha$_2$-adrenergic autoreceptor. Although yohimbine affects multiple neurotransmitter systems, its primary action is on the noradrenergic system.[62,63] Yohimbine has been shown in preclinical studies to readily cross the blood-brain barrier. Support for the use of yohimbine as a probe of central noradrenergic function in humans comes from a study of healthy controls in which yohimbine administration resulted in increased levels of cerebrospinal fluid NE.[64] Plasma MHPG is believed to represent a combination of MHPG that has crossed the blood-brain barrier from the brain and MHPG that is derived from NE that has been released from peripheral sympathetic neurons.[65]

Patients with PTSD and healthy controls received either yohimbine hydrocloride (0.4 mg/kg) or saline solution on two separate test days in double-blind fashion and in randomized balanced order. Seventy percent of the patient group experienced yohimbine-induced panic attacks and 40% had yohimbine-induced flashbacks. In contrast, no yohimbine-induced panic attacks or flashbacks were noted in the healthy controls. The subgroup of patients with yohimbine-induced panic attacks also had significantly greater increases in heart rate, sitting systolic blood pressure, and plasma MHPG than did controls. In addition to greater increases in anxiety as measured by the Panic Attack Symptom Scale, patients with PTSD experienced significant increases in the core symptoms of PTSD as reflected by a PTSD symptom scale. Specific PTSD symptoms that were affected included intrusive thoughts, flashbacks, feeling emotionally numb, and difficulty concentrating.

Yohimbine has been administered to many different psychiatric patient groups. It has not produced marked increases in anxiety among patients with schizophrenia, major depression, obsessive compulsive disorder, or generalized anxiety disorder.[66–69] However, in patients with panic disorder yohimbine also caused potentiated behavioral (anxiety symptoms), cardiovascular and biochemical responses that are similar to those seen in the PTSD group.[70-72] These similar responses suggest that PTSD and panic disorder share a common neurobiologic abnormality that is related to altered sensitivity of the noradrenergic system. Of note, because PTSD patients both with and without comorbid panic disorder experienced yohimbine-induced panic attacks, the diagnosis of panic disorder alone could not explain the study findings.[61]

Unlike patients with panic disorder (and no PTSD), many PTSD patients in this study reported intrusive traumatic thoughts and flashbacks in response to yohimbine. For example, shortly after yohimbine infusion one patient experienced intense fear, anxiety, tremulousness, diaphoresis, and memories of combat. A second patient had a flashback in which he saw, heard, and smelled the crashing of a helicopter. In many cases the intrusive thoughts were described as extremely clear and vivid as if the events recalled had happened "just the other day."

Yohimbine vs Placebo Challenge: Acoustic Startle

Exaggerated startle is a clinical physiological symptom of PTSD. It is thought to represent an objective index of central nervous system dysregulation in some traumatized individuals. In humans it typically is measured by recording the electrocardiogram of facial muscles (the amplitude of eyeblink) in response to loud acoustic stimuli.

Both preclinical and clinical studies suggest that the acoustic startle reflex may represent a good model for studying the neurochemical foundations of anxiety and fear.[73] In preclinical studies, unconditioned and conditioned fear increases the amplitude of the startle reflex. For example, if elicited in the presence of a stimulus previously paired with an aversive stimulus (such as footshock), the magnitude of the acoustic startle is increased.[74,75] Similarly, in humans, the eyeblind component of the startle reflex is potentiated by aversive imagery connoting fear, anxiety, or anger compared to imagery associated with pleasant emotions.[76] Furthermore, Grillon et al.[77] have shown that the anticipation of shock potentiates the startle reflex in healthy subjects.

Numerous investigators have shown that fear-potentiated startle in rats is generally reduced by drugs that decrease fear and anxiety in humans. For example, clonidine, morphine, and diazepam each block fear-potentiated startle in rats.[78,79] On the other hand, the amplitude of fear-potentiated startle is increased by yohimbine and piperoxane, both of which are anxiogenic in humans, especially those who have panic disorder or PTSD.[78,79] Yohimbine and piperoxane are both alpha$_2$-adrenergic receptor antagonists that activate noradrenergic neurons.

From the foregoing preclinical and clinical observations, Morgan et al. predicted that yohimbine would increase acoustic startle in normal subjects[81] and in combat veterans with PTSD.[73] Furthermore, it was predicted that subjects with PTSD, experiencing an augmented catecholaminergic response to yohimbine, would have a greater potentiation of startle than would healthy controls. Thus, yohimbine was used as a biological probe to study the effects of catecholamines on acoustic startle.

In one study,[81] yohimbine (0.4 mg/kg) or placebo was administered on two separate test days to seven healthy subjects in randomized double-blind placebo-controlled fashion. Compared to placebo, yohimbine caused significant augmentation in startle amplitude at 96, 102, 108, and 114 dB but not at 90 dB. On the yohimbine day, significant correlations were observed between startle at 102 dB and peak anxiety as well as plasma MHPG. Additionally, peak anxiety was significantly correlated with peak plasma MHPG.[73]

In a second study using a similar design, yohimbine was administered to 18 combat veterans with PTSD and to 11 age-matched combat controls (subjects who were in combat but did not develop PTSD). Yohimbine significantly increased startle amplitude at 90, 96, 102, 108, and 114 dB compared to placebo in the PTSD group but not in the group of combat controls. Taken together, these studies demonstrate that yohimbine has an excitatory effect on the magnitude of the acoustic startle response in humans, suggesting that the startle reflex is, at least in part, mediated by noradrenergic systems. Furthermore, data suggest that the exaggerated startle observed in veterans with PTSD may well be related to a hypersensitivity of noradrenergic systems in this patient population.

Yohimbine vs Placebo Challenge: PET

To more directly study CNS noradrenergic systems in combat veterans with PTSD, Bremner *et al.*[82] administered a single bolus of [F-18]2-fluoro-2-deoxyglucose to 10 combat veterans with PTSD and 10 healthy age-matched controls. This was immediately followed by either iv yohimbine (0.4 mg/kg) or placebo infusion. All subjects received both yohimbine and placebo on two separate test days under double-blind conditions and in randomized balanced order. After completion of the yohimbine or placebo infusion, subjects underwent PET scanning for 60 minutes. To determine brain metabolic activity a PET image was reconstructed 30-50 minutes after infusion.

Preclinical pharmacological and blood flow studies suggest a dose-response relation for the effects of NE on neuronal activity, brain metabolism, and blood flow with low levels of NE causing no effect or an increase in activity and high levels causing a decrease or inhibition of activity.[34,35,83,84] For example, large doses of yohimbine cause a decrease in blood flow and metabolism in brain areas that receive noradrenergic innervation including the frontal, parietal, temporal, postcentral, and occipital cortex.[83,84] Based on the foregoing preclinical studies and on the earlier reviewed evidence for increased responsivity of noradrenergic systems in patients with PTSD, it was hypothesized that yohimbine administration would result in a relative decrease in brain metabolism in neocortical areas and caudate among combat veterans with PTSD controls.

Six of the ten patients with PTSD had a yohimbine-induced panic attack and three of ten a flashback. None of the control subjects had either a panic attack or a flashback. These behavioral responses were similar to those observed in the aforementioned yohimbine PTSD studies. The metabolic response to yohimbine significantly differed between patients and controls. As a group, the healthy controls showed a tendency towards increased metabolism in neocortical brain regions including prefrontal, temporal, parietal, and orbitofrontal cortices. In contrast, the patient group showed a tendency towards decreased metabolism in these same brain regions.

The results were consistent with the notion that PTSD patients as a group released more NE than did control subjects because of their greater sensitivity to yohimbine.

This increase in NE resulted in a relative decrease in brain metabolism. It was speculated that the degree of decrease in metabolism may be related to the degree of yohimbine-induced anxiety/panic symptoms and PTSD-specific symptoms including impairment of attention and vigilance. On the other hand, it is possible that high levels of NE cause a net decrease in neuronal activity with an increase in signal-to-noise ratio that has the functional effect of potentiating recognition of relevant stimuli while dampening or suppressing background neuronal activity or "noise" with the result of increasing chronic hyperarousal and vigilance in individuals with PTSD.

Yohimbine vs mCPP vs Placebo Challenge

To test the specificity of the yohimbine response in combat veterans with PTSD and to evaluate potential serotonergic contributions to trauma-related symptoms, 26 patients and 14 healthy controls each received an intravenous infusion of yohimbine hydrochloride (0.4 mg/kg), m-chlorophenylpiperazine (mCPP) (1.0 mg/kg), or saline solution on three separate test days in a randomized balanced order and in double-blind fashion.[85] In this study, yohimbine was used as a probe of noradrenergic activity and mCPP as a probe of serotonergic activity. MCPP interacts with numerous 5HT receptor subtypes and the 5HT transporter. It acts as an antagonist at the 5HT-3 receptor,[86,87] as a partial agonist at the 5HT-1 receptor,[88-90] and as a partial agonist or antagonist at the 5HT-2 receptor.[91-93] MCPP has relatively low affinity for alpha$_1$, alpha$_2$, dopamine 1, and dopamine 2 receptors.[94,95] Serotonergic function in a number of neuropsychiatric disorders including depression, schizophrenia, obsessive compulsive disorder, panic disorder, and alcoholism has been investigated using mCPP.

As in the aforedescribed yohimbine/placebo study,[61] subjects were rated at regular intervals before and after infusion of yohimbine, mCPP, and placebo for anxiety and panic symptoms as well as PTSD-specific symptoms including intrusive memories and flashbacks. Heart rate, blood pressure, and plasma MHPG also were measured at multiple time points. Eleven of 26 patients (42%) and 1 of 14 healthy controls (7%) had a panic attack in response to yohimbine. Eight patients (31%) and no controls had a panic attack after mCPP infusion. Three patients had a panic attack in response to both active compounds. None of the patients or controls had a panic attack on their placebo day. Flashbacks occurred in eight patients after yohimbine, seven patients after mCPP, and two patients after placebo. Four subjects had flashbacks on both yohimbine and mCPP test days. No flashbacks occurred in any of the control subjects during the three test days.

Compared to controls the subgroup of patients with yohimbine-induced panic attacks had significantly greater increases in anxiety as measured by the Panic Attack Symptom Scale (PASS) and in PTSD-specific symptoms as measured by a PTSD symptom scale. No significant differences were noted in heart rate or blood pressure. Similarly, in a second subgroup of patients with mCPP-induced panic attacks, the patient group had significantly greater increases in anxiety, panic, PTSD symptoms, and diastolic blood pressure than did controls. Relative to placebo, four PTSD-specific symptoms increased significantly in response to either mCPP or yohimbine in the group of 26 PTSD patients. After adjustments for multiple statistical comparisons, the correlation between peak change over time for yohimbine and mCPP was significant only for the symptom of feeling distant from others. Furthermore, none of the 11 anxiety symptoms that increased significantly after either yohimbine or mCPP had peak changes after mCPP that significantly correlated with peak changes after yohimbine, suggesting that these agents have distinct effects on both PTSD-specific symptoms and anxiety symptoms in combat veterans with PTSD.

This study provides preliminary evidence for the presence of two neurobiologic subgroups of patients with PTSD. One subgroup appears to have increased reactivity of the noradrenergic system, whereas the other has increased reactivity of the serotonergic system. The fact that there was little correlation between the behavioral responses to yohimbine and mCPP in individual patients with PTSD further supports the possibility of neurobiolobical subtypes. It is not clear if these findings have clinical relevance. It might be predicted that PTSD patients with hypersensitivity to yohimbine would respond to pharmacologic agents that reduce noradrenergic function, whereas patients with hypersensitivity to mCPP would preferentially respond to agents with primary actions on the serotonin system.

Yohimbine vs Placebo: Family Study

The findings of the foregoing yohimbine studies suggest that PTSD and panic disorder share a common sensitivity of the noradrenergic system. Yohimbine causes exaggerated behavioral and biochemical responses in both panic disorder and PTSD but not in schizophrenia, major depressive disorder, generalized anxiety disorder, or obsessive compulsive disorder.[61] Furthermore, yohimbine rarely causes panic attacks in healthy controls.

It is possible that similar responses to yohimbine in patients with PTSD and panic disorder are caused by a shared genetically transmitted abnormality of the noradrenergic system. Preclinical and clinical studies have shown that various aspects of noradrenergic function and sensitivity may be genetically determined.[96–101] Support for the notion that PTSD and panic disorder share a common genetically transmitted noradrenergic abnormality comes from the finding that both panic disorder and PTSD appear to have a significant genetic component[102–106] and that both disorders are characterized by abnormalities of the noradrenergic system.[61,70–72]

It is also possible that the origin of yohimbine hyperresponsivity in PTSD differs from its origin in panic disorder. For example, yohimbine hyperresponsivity may be familial in patients with panic disorder, whereas it primarily is due to a unique environment, most likely the trauma itself, in patients with PTSD. A large body of preclinical data has shown that repeated stressors can cause increases in tyrosine-hydroxylase, dopamine beta-hydroxylase activity, and synaptic levels of NE metabolites.[107–109] Thus, it appears that repeated stress can cause a compensatory increase in NE synthesis, so that reexposure to limited stress results in a degree of NE release that is more appropriate for a much greater degree of stress. In addition, uncontrollable stress can cause a chronic increase in responsivity of locus coeruleus neurons to excitatory stimulation by the alpha$_2$-adrenergic antagonists yohimbine and idazoxane.

To determine if yohimbine-induced panic attacks in patients with PTSD were due to familially transmitted vulnerability for panic attacks, 24 combat veterans who participated in two yohimbine infusion studies also were interviewed about axis 1 diagnoses in themselves and in each of their first-degree relatives.[110] All probands met SCID DSM-111R criteria for PTSD. There were two comparison groups of male subjects who had participated in a separate family history study. One group was comprised of 26 healthy controls and the other of 18 subjects who met diagnostic criteria for panic disorder but not PTSD. All subjects were interviewed using the Family Health History Inventory-modified from the Family History-RDC instrument to include DSM-111R diagnostic criteria.

Fifteen PTSD subjects (62%) experienced a panic attack in response to yohimbine. The rate of panic disorder in 85 first-degree relatives of these 15 subjects was 2.4%. In 63 first-degree relatives of the nine PTSD subjects who did not experience a yohimbine-induced panic attack there was a 3.2% rate of panic disorder. The rates of panic disorder in first-degree relatives of healthy probands and panic disorder probands were 0.0% and 15.9%, respectively. Thus, the rate of panic disorder in first-degree relatives of PTSD patients with and without yohimbine-induced panic attacks was similar. Furthermore, these rates were not substantially different from the rate observed in the healthy control group. In contrast, and consistent with other published studies, the rate of panic disorder in relatives of the panic disorder probands was higher than that in healthy controls.

In addition, in a group of 34 combat veterans with PTSD (that included the foregoing 24 subjects who participated in one of two yohimbine studies), 17 (50%) met DSM-III-R criteria for comorbid panic disorder. In contrast, less than 3% of first-degree relatives met criteria for panic disorder. Thus, this study suggests that panic disorder was no more frequent in the family members of these PTSD patients than in the general population in which prevalence is estimated to range between 1% and 5%.

Data from the foregoing family history study do not support the hypothesis that a family history of panic disorder in patients with PTSD is a predisposing vulnerability for the development of panic attacks when exposed to yohimbine. They also fail to support the notion that similar responses to yohimbine in patients with PTSD and panic disorder are caused by a shared genetically transmitted abnormality of the noradrenergic system. Rather, it may be that the panic symptoms seen in patients with PTSD primarily result from nongenetic factors such as traumatic exposure, whereas these same symptoms have a greater genetic or familial origin in panic disorder patients.

DISCUSSION

The studies reviewed in this report provide strong evidence for noradrenergic dysregulation in a subgroup of individuals with chronic PTSD. Alterations in noradrenergic function are most evident during states of "stress" and not during baseline or resting conditions. Thus, consistent elevations of baseline heart rate, blood pressure, plasma epinephrine, NE, and MHPG have not been reported in this population. On the other hand, during investigations involving neuroendocrine and psychological challenges, heart rate and blood pressure as well as plasma epinephrine, NE, and MHPG have all been reported as elevated in subjects with PTSD compared to controls.[61,111]

Exaggerated responsivity of noradrenergic systems in response to stressful stimuli is consistent with a behavioral sensitization model of PTSD. In this model, biochemical, physiological, and behavioral responses to stressors increase over time.[112] Preclinical studies have described an increase in dopamine beta-hydroxylase activity, tyrosine hydroxylase, and synaptic levels of NE in repeatedly shocked animals.[107–109] These animals also appear to have increased fear-related behaviors over time.

It has been speculated that increased responsivity of noradrenergic systems contributes to a number of arousal symptoms in PTSD, including hypervigilance, exaggerated startle, and insomnia.[18,26] Norepinephrine's proposed role in hypervigilance, exaggerated startle, and insomnia is supported by preclinical studies in which NE was related to fear, selective attention, and mode-switching or orienting behaviors such as interruption of sleep and grooming.[26] Support from clinical studies has come from neuroendocrine, psychophysiological, and brain-imaging studies. For example, baseline nocturnal urinary MHPG was negatively correlated with total sleep time, and yohimbine was shown to cause an exaggerated increase in acoustic startle[73] and a decease in brain metabolism among combat veterans with PTSD compared to controls.[82]

Norepinephrine also has been implicated in the reexperiencing symptoms of PTSD. Preclinical studies repeatedly demonstrated a central role for NE in encoding memory and possibly in retrieving memory for aversive events. Among humans with PTSD a significant positive relation was reported between 24-hour urine NE levels and intrusive traumatic memories, and yohimbine was shown to induce both intrusive memories and flashbacks. Although the mechanism by which yohimbine stimulates intrusive memories and flashbacks is not understood, it is possible that by increasing NE in specific brain regions, yohimbine recreates a neurobiologic state that existed at the time of memory encoding. It is well known that memory retrieval can be facilitated by reexposure to the external context or environment in which the original learning took place. Similarly, it has been shown that recreating the internal context at the time of encoding also can be memory enhancing. For example, administration of hormones that are released during stress such as ACTH,[113] glucose,[114] and epinephrine facilitate memory retrieval for aversive events. These effects may depend on intact noradrenergic neurons. In the studies just reviewed, it is possible that the administration of yohimbine to combat veterans with PTSD resulted in increased NE release, thereby producing an internal hypercatecholaminergic state that was present at the time the traumatic memories were encoded. Accompanying subjective experiences might include fear, anxiety, and heightened arousal.

It is also possible that trauma-related external cues present during the testing procedure accounted for enhanced memory retrieval. This is unlikely, however, because the testing took place in a relatively sterile laboratory and because the same external cues were present on both active and placebo test days. Although traumatic memories were frequently elicited on active test days, they were rarely reported on placebo days.

A third possibility involves the recreation of a physiologic state present at the time of traumatic memory encoding. In a subgroup of combat veterans with PTSD, yohimbine caused diaphoresis, tremulousness, and increased blood pressure and heart rate, physiologic responses commonly observed during highly stressful experiences. The role of yohimbine-induced peripheral effects on memory retrieval is not clear.

Coadministration of yohimbine and a peripheral adrenergic blocker might help to differentiate peripheral and central effects.

The data presented in this chapter may well have treatment implications. For example, it might be predicted that symptoms of PTSD would respond to pharmacologic agents that specifically affect catecholamines. Two such agents that reduce catecholamine activity through differing mechanisms of action are clonidine and propranolol. Clonidine is an alpha$_2$-adrenergic receptor agonist and propranolol a postsynaptic beta-adrenergic blocker. Indeed, preliminary reports suggest that both agents have promise as treatments for a host of PTSD symptoms.[115]

In this report we focused on alterations in the noradrenergic system in individuals with PTSD. As noted earlier, evidence is clear in preclinical and clinical studies that other neurotransmitter systems are also affected by traumatic stress. In fact, from a neurobiologic perspective PTSD may best be understood as a multisystem disorder. It is hoped and anticipated that with better understanding of the underlying pathophysiology of PTSD more effective treatments can be developed for this often devastating disorder.

REFERENCES

1. KARDINER, A. & H. SPIEGEL. 1947. The Traumatic Neuroses of War. Paul Hoeber. New York.
2. GRINKER, R. R. & J. P. SPIEGEL. 1945. Men Under Stress. Blakiston. Philadelphia, PA.
3. MEAKINS, J. C. & R. M. WILSON. 1918. The effect of certain sensory stimulation on the respiratory rate in cases of so-called "irritable heart." Heart 7: 17-22.
4. FRASER, F. & E. M. WILSON. 1918. The sympathetic nervous system and the "irritable heart of soldiers." Br. Med. J. 2: 27-29.
5. DOBBS, D. & W. P. WILSON. 1960. Observations on the persistence of neurosis. Dis. Nerv. Syst. 21: 40-46.
6. BRENDE, J. O. 1982. Electrodermal responses in post-traumatic syndromes. J. Nerv. Ment. Dis. 170: 352-361.
7. BLANCHARD, E. B. et al. 1986. A psychophysiological study of post traumatic stress disorders in Vietnam veterans. Behav. Res. Ther. 24: 645-652.
8. BLANCHARD, E. B. et al. 1991. Changes in plasma norepinephrine to combat-related stimuli among Vietnam veterans with posttraumatic stress disorder. J. Nerv. Ment. Dis. 179: 371-373.
9. MALLOY, P. F. et al. 1983. Validation of a multimethod assessment of posttraumatic stress disorder in Vietnam veterans. J. Consult. Clin. Psychol. 51: 488-494.
10. PALLMEYER, T. P. et al. 1986. The psychophysiology of combat-induced posttraumatic stress disorder in Vietnam veterans. Behav. Res. Ther. 24: 645-652.
11. PITMAN, R. K. et al. 1987. Psychophysiologic assessment of posttraumatic stress disorder imagery in Vietnam combat veterans. Arch. Gen. Psychiatry. 44: 970-975.
12. PITMAN, R. K. 1989. Posttraumatic stress disorder, hormone, and memory (editorial). Biol. Psychiatry 26: 221-223.
13. ORR, S. P. 1990. Psychophysiologic studies of post traumatic stress disorder. In Biological Assessment and Treatment of Post Traumatic Stress Disorder. E. L. Giller, Ed.: 135-160. American Psychiatric Press. Washington, DC.
14. ORR, S. P. 1993. Psychophysiological assessment of posttraumatic stress disorder imagery in World War II and Korean combat veterans. J. Abnorm. Psychol. 102: 152-159.
15. SHALEV, A. Y. 1993. Psychophysiologic assessment of traumatic imagery in Israeli civilian patients with posttraumatic stress disorders. Am. J. Psychiatry 150: 620-624.

16. PITMAN, R. K. *et al.* 1990. Psychophysiologic responses to combat imagery of Vietnam veterans with posttraumatic stress disorder versus other anxiety disorders. J. Abnorm. Psychol. **99:** 49-54.

17. BLANCHARD, E. B. *et al.* 1991. The psychophysiology of motor vehicle accident related post-traumatic stress disorder. Biofeedback Self-Regul. **16:** 116.

18. SOUTHWICK, S. M. *et al.* 1995. Clinical studies of neurotransmitter alterations in post-traumatic stress disorder. *In* Neurobiological and Clinical Consequences of Stress: From Normal Adaptation to PTSD. M. J. Friedman, D. S. Charney & A. Y. Deutch, Eds.: 335-349. Lippincott-Raven Publishers. Philadelphia, PA.

19. MASON, J. W. *et al.* 1995. Some approaches to the study of the clinical implications of thyroid alterations in post-traumatic stress disorder. *In* Neurobiological and Clinical Consequences of Stress: From Normal Adaptation to PTSD. M. J. Friedman, D. S. Charney & A. Y. Deutch, Eds.: 367-379. Lippincott-Raven Publishers. Philadelphia, PA.

20. YEHUDA, R. *et al.* 1995. Hypothalamic-pituitary-adrenal functioning in post-traumatic stress disorder: Expanding the concept of the stress response spectrum. *In* Neurobiological and Clinical Consequences of Stress: From Normal Adaptation to PTSD. M. J. Friedman, D. S. Charney & A. Y. Deutch, Eds.: 351-365. Lippincott-Raven Publishers. Philadelphia, PA.

21. CHARNEY, D. S. *et al.* 1993. Psychobiologic mechanisms of posttraumatic stress disorder. Arch. Gen. Psychiatry **50:** 294-305.

22. ZIGMOND, M. J. *et al.* 1995. Neurochemical studies of central noradrenergic responses to acute and chronic stress: Implications for normal and abnormal behavior. *In* Neurobiological and Clinical Consequences of Stress: From Normal Adaptation to PTSD. M. J. Friedman, D. S. Charney & A. Y. Deutch, Eds.: 45-60. Lippincott-Raven Publishers. Philadelphia, PA.

23. IDA, Y. *et al.* 1985. Attenuating effect of diazepam on stress-induced increases in noradrenaline turnover in specific brain regions of rats: Antagonism by Ro15-1788. Life Sci. **37:** 2491-2498.

24. TANAKA, M. *et al.* 1986. Involvement of brain noradrenaline and opioid peptides in emotional changes induced by stress in rats. *In* Emotions: Neural and Chemical Control. Y. Oomura, Ed.: 417. Scientific Societies Press. Tokyo, Japan.

25. TSUDA, A. & M. TANAKA. 1985. Differential changes in noradrenaline turnover in specific regions of rat brain produced by controllable and uncontrollable shocks. Behav. Neurosci. **99:** 802-817.

26. ASTON-JONES, G. 1994. Locus coeruleus, stress, and post traumatic stress disorder: Neurobiological and clinical parallels. *In* Catecholamine Function in Post Traumatic Stress Disorder, Emerging Concepts. M. Murburg, Ed.: 17-62. American Psychiatric Press. Washington, DC.

27. REDMOND, D. E., JR. 1987. Studies of the nucleus locus coeruleus in monkeys and hypotheses for neuropsychopharmacology. *In* Psychopharmacology: The Third Generation of Progress. H. Y. Meltzer, Ed.: 967-975. Raven Press. New York.

28. REDMOND, D. E. & Y. H. HUANG. 1979. New evidence for a locus coeruleus norepinephrine connection with anxiety. Life Sci. **25:** 2149-2162.

29. CHARNEY, D. S. *et al.* 1990. Noradrenergic dysregulation in panic disorder. *In* Neurobiology of Panic Disorders. J. C. Ballenger, Ed.: 91-105. Alan R. Liss. New York.

30. ABERCROMBIE, E. D. & B. L. JACOBS. 1987. Single-unit response of noradrenergic neurons in the locus coeruleus of freely moving cats. I. Acutely presented stressful and nonstressful stimuli. J. Neurosci. **7:** 2837-2843.

31. ABERCROMBIE, E. D. & B. L. JACOBS. 1987. Single-unit response of noradrenergic neurons in the locus coeruleus of freely moving cats. II. Adaptation to chronically presented stressful stimuli. J. Neurosci. **7:** 2844-2848.

32. RASMUSSEN, K. *et al.* 1986. Single unit activity of locus coeruleus neurons in the freely moving cat. I. During naturalistic behaviors and in response to simple and complex stimuli. Brain Res. **371:** 324-334.

33. LEVINE, E. S. *et al.* 1990. Activity of cat locus coeruleus noradrenergic neurons during the defense reaction. Brain Res. **531:** 189-195.

34. MCCULLOCH, J. & A. M. HARPER. 1979. Factors influencing the response of the cerebral circulation to phenylethylamine. Neurology **29:** 201-207.

35. RAICHLE, M. E. *et al.* 1975. Central noradrenergic regulation of cerebral blood flow and vascular permeability. Proc. Natl. Acad. Sci. **72:** 3726-3730.

36. LIANG, K. C. *et al.* 1990. Modulating effects of posttraining epinephrine on memory: Involvement of the amygdala noradrenergic system. Brain Res. **368:** 125-133.

37. GALLAGHER, M. & B. S. KAPP. 1973. Manipulation of opiate activity in the amygdala alters memory processes. Life Sci. **23:** 1973-1978.

38. GALLAGHER, M. *et al.* 1981. Aneuropharmacology of amygdaloid systems which contribute to learning and memory. *In* The Amygdaloid Complex. Y. Ben-Ari, Ed. Elsevier/North Holland. Amsterdam.

39. MCGAUGH, J. L. *et al.* 1988. Memory-enhancing effects of posttraining naloxone: Involvement of β-noradrenergic influence in the amygdaloid complex. Brain Res. **446:** 37-49.

40. INTROINI-COLLISON, I. B. *et al.* 1989. Memory-enhancement with intra-amygdala posttraining naloxone is blocked by concurrent administration of propranolol. Brain Res. **476:** 94-101.

41. SARA, S. J. & V. DEVAUGES. 1989. Idazoxan, an α-2 antagonist, facilitates memory retrieval in the rat. Behav. Neural Biol. **51:** 401-411.

42. SARA, S. J. 1985. The locus-coeruleus and cognitive function: Attempts to relate noradrenergic enhancement of signal/noise in the brain. Physiol. Psychol. **13:** 151-162.

43. PRINS, A. *et al.* 1995. Psychophysiological evidence for autonomic arousal and startle in traumatized adult populations. *In* Neurobiological and Clinical Consequences of Stress: From Normal Adaptation to PTSD. M. J. Friedman, D. S. Charney & A. Y. Deutch, Eds.: 291-314. Lippincott-Raven Publishers. Philadelphia, PA.

44. KOSTEN, T. R. *et al.* 1987. Sustained urinary norepinephrine and epinephrine elevation in post-traumatic stress disorder. Psychoneuroendocrinology **12:** 13-20.

45. YEHUDA, R. *et al.* 1992. Urinary catecholamine excretion and severity of PTSD symptoms in Vietnam combat veterans. J. Nerv. Ment. Dis. **180:** 321-325.

46. PITMAN, R. & S. ORR. 1990. Twenty-four hour urinary cortisol and catecholamine excretion in combat-related post-traumatic stress disorder. Biol. Psychiatry **27:** 245-247.

47. DAVIDSON, L. M. & A. BAUM. 1986. Chronic stress and posttraumatic stress disorder. J. Consult. Clin. Psychol. **54:** 303-308.

48. DEBELLIS, M. D. *et al.* 1994. Urinary catecholamine excretion in sexually abused girls. J. Am. Acad. Child Adolesc. Psychiatry **33:** 320-327.

49. PERRY, B. D. *et al.* 1987. Altered platelet alpha$_2$ adrenergic binding sites in post-traumatic stress disorder. Am. J. Psychiatry **144:** 1511-1512.

50. PERRY, B. D. Neurobiological sequelae of childhood trauma: PTSD in children. *In* Catecholamine Function in Post-Traumatic Stress Disorder: Emerging Concepts. M. Murburg, Ed.: 131-158. APA Press. Washington, DC.

51. WEISS, R. T. *et al.* 1983. Platelet alpha 2 adrenoceptors in chronic congestive heart failure. Am. J. Cardiol. **52:** 101-105.

52. SOUTHWICK, S. M. *et al.* 1990. Altered platelet alpha$_2$-adrenergic binding sites in borderline personality disorder. Am. J. Psychiatry **147:** 1014-1017.

53. PERRY, B. D. *et al.* 1990. Adrenergic receptor regulation in post-traumatic stress disorder. *In* Biological Assessment and Treatment of Post-Traumatic Stress Disorder. E. L. Giller, Ed.: 87-114. APA Press. Washington, DC.

54. LERER, B. *et al.* 1987. Cyclic AMP signal transduction in post-traumatic stress disorder. Am. J. Psychiatry **144:** 1324-1327.

55. LERER, B. *et al.* 1990. Platelet adenylate-cyclase and phospholipase C activity in posttraumatic stress disorder. Biol. Psychiatry **27:** 735-744.
56. HAMMER, M. B. *et al.* 1990. Plasma dopamine and prolactin levels in PTSD. Biol. Psychiatry **27:** 72A.
57. McFALL, M. *et al.* 1990. Autonomic response to stress in Vietnam combat veterans with post-traumatic stress disorder. Biol. Psychiatry **27:** 1165-1175.
58. BLANCHARD, E. B. *et al.* 1991. Changes in plasma norepinephrine to combat-related stimuli among Vietnam veterans with post traumatic stress disorder. J. Nerv. Ment. Dis. **179:** 371-373.
59. DINAN, T. G. *et al.* 1990. A pilot study of neuroendocrine test battery in post traumatic stress. Biol. Psychiatry **28:** 665-672.
60. HANSENNE M. *et al.* 1991. The clonidine test in post traumatic stress disorder. Am. J. Psychiatry **148:** 810-811.
61. SOUTHWICK, S. M. *et al.* 1993. Abnormal noradrenergic function in posttraumatic stress disorder. Arch. Gen. Psychiatry **50:** 266-274.
62. SCATTON, B. *et al.* 1980. Antidopamine properties of yohimbine. J. Pharmacol. Exp. Ther. **215:** 494-499.
63. WINTER, J. C. & R. A. RABIN. 1992. Yohimbine as a serotonergic agent: Evidence for receptor binding and drug discrimination. J. Pharmacol. Exp. Ther. **263:** 682-689.
64. PESKIND, E. R. *et al.* 1989. Yohimbine increases cerebrospinal fluid and plasma norepinephrine but not arginine vasopressin in humans. Neuroendocrinology **50:** 286-291.
65. CHARNEY, D. S. *et al.* 1987. Neurobiological mechanisms of panic anxiety: Biochemical and behavioral correlates of yohimbine-induced panic attacks. Am. J. Psychiatry **144:** 1030-1036.
66. GLAZER, W. M. *et al.* 1987. Noradrenergic function in schizophrenia. Arch. Gen. Psychiatry **44:** 898-904.
67. HENINGER, G. R. *et al.* 1988. Alpha$_2$-adrenergic receptor sensitivity in depression: The plasma MHPG, behavioral, and cardiovascular responses to yohimbine. Arch. Gen. Psychiatry **45:** 718-726.
68. CHARNEY, D. S. *et al.* 1989. Noradrenergic function in generalized anxiety disorder: Effects of yohimbine in healthy subjects and patients with generalized anxiety disorder. Psychol. Res. **27:** 173-182.
69. RASMUSSEN, S. A. *et al.* 1987. Effects of yohimbine in obsessive-compulsive disorder. Psychopharmacology (Berl.). **93:** 308-313.
70. CHARNEY, D. S. *et al.* 1984. Noradrenergic function in panic anxiety: Effects of yohimbine in healthy subjects and patients with agoraphobia and panic disorder. Arch. Gen. Psychiatry **41:** 751-763.
71. CHARNEY, D. S. *et al.* 1987. Neurobiological mechanisms of panic anxiety: Biochemical and behavioral correlates of yohimbine-induced panic attacks. Am. J. Psychiatry **144:** 1030-1036.
72. GURGUIS, G. N. M. & T. W. UHDE. 1990. Plasma 3-methoxy-4-hydroxyphenylethylene glycol (MHPG) and growth hormone responses to yohimbine in panic disorder patients and normal controls. Psychoneuroendocrinology **15:** 217-224.
73. MORGAN, C. A. *et al.* 1995. Yohimbine facilitated acoustic startle in combat veterans with post-traumatic stress disorder. **117:** 466-471.
74. BROWN, J. S. *et al.* 1951. Conditioned fear as revealed by magnitude of startle response to an auditory stimulus. J. Exp. Psychol. **43:** 317-328.
75. DAVIS, M. & B. ASTRACHAN. 1978. Conditioned fear and startle magnitude: Effects of different footshock or backshock intensities. J. Exp. Psychol. [Anim. Behav. Proc]. **4:** 95-103.
76. COOK, E. W. *et al.* 1991. Emotional dysfunction and affective modulation of startle. J. Abnorm. Psychol. **100:** 5-13.
77. GRILLON, C. *et al.* 1992. Fear potentiated startle in humans: Effects of anticipatory anxiety on the acoustic blink reflex. Psychophysiology. In press.

78. DAVIS, M. *et al.* 1979. Noradrenergic agonists and antagonists: Effects on conditioned fear as measured by the potentiated startle paradigm. Psychopharmacology **65:** 111-118.

79. DAVIS, M. 1979. Diazepam and flurazepm: Effects on conditioned fear as measured by the potentiated startle paradigm Psychopharmacology **62:** 1-7.

80. KEHNE, J. H. & M. DAVIS. 1985. Central noradrenergic involvement in yohimbine excitation of acoustic startle: Effects of DSP4 and 6-OHDA. Brain Res. **330:** 32-41.

81. MORGAN C. A. *et al.* 1993. Yohimbine facilitated acoustic startle reflex in humans. Psychopharmacology **110:** 342-346.

82. BREMNER, J. D. *et al.* 1997. PET measurement of cerebral metabolic correlates of yohimbine administration in combat related Posttraumatic Stress Disorder. Arch. Gen. Psychiatry **54:** 246-254.

83. SAVAKI, H. E. *et al.* 1982. The central noradrenergic system in the rat: Metabolic mapping with alpha-adrenergic blocking agents. Brain Res. **234:** 65-79.

84. INOUE, M. & M. McHUGH. 1991. Pappius: The effect of alpha-adrenergic receptor blockers prazosin and yohimbine on cerebral metabolism and biogenic amine content of traumatized brain. J. Cereb. Blood Flow Metab. **11:** 242-252.

85. SOUTHWICK, S. M. *et al.* 1997. Noradrenergic and serotonergic function in Posttraumatic Stress Disorder. Arch. Gen. Psychiatry. In press.

86. IRELAND, S. J. & M. B. TYERS. 1987. Pharmacological characterization of 5-hydroxytryptamine-induced depolarization of the rabbit isolated vagus nerve. Br. J. Pharmacol. **90:** 229.

87. ROBERTSON, D. W. *et al.* 1991. MCPP but not TFMPP is an antagonist at cardiac 5-HT3 receptors. Life Sci. **50:** 599-605.

88. SCHOEFFTER, P. & D. HOYER. 1989. Interaction of arylpiperazines with 5-HT_{1A}, 5-HT_{1B}, 5-HT_{1C} and 5-HT_{1D} receptors: Do discriminatory 5-HT_{1B} receptor ligands exist? Arch. Pharmacol. **339:** 675-683.

89. SHEN, Y. *et al.* 1993. Molecular cloning and expression of a 5-hydroxytryptamine: receptor sybtype. J. Biol. Chem. **268:** 18200-18204.

90. SHELDON, P. W. & G. K. AGHAJANIAN. 1991. Excitatory responses to serotonin (5-HT) in neurons of the rat piriform cortex: Evidence for mediation by 5-HT_{1C} receptors in pyramidal cells and 5-HT_2 receptors in interneurons. Synapse **9:** 208-218.

91. CONN, P. J. & E. SANDERS-BUSH. 1987. Relative efficacies of piperazines at the phosphoinositide hydrolysis-linked serotonergic (5-HT_2 and 5-HT_{1C}) receptors. J. Pharmacol. Exp. Ther. **2142:** 552-557.

92. SHELDON, P. W. & G. K. AGHAJANIAN. Serotonin (5-HT) induces IPSP's in pyramidal layer cells of rat piriform cortex: Evidence for the involvement of a 5-HT_2 activated interneuron. Brain Res. **506:** 62-69.

93. CARVER, J. G. *et al.* 1993. The effects of 5-HT and m-chlorphenylpiperazine (m-CPP) on the efflux of [3-H]-5-HT from human perfused platelets. Br. J. Clin. Pharmacol. **35:** 473-478.

94. HAMIK, A. & S. J. PEROUTKA. 1989. 1-(m-chlorophenypiperazine interactions with neurotransmitter receptors in the human brain. Biol. Psychiatry **25:** 569-575.

95. HOYER, D. 1988. Functional correlates of serotonin 5-HT_1 recognition sites. J. Recept. Res. **8:** 59-81.

96. ANISMAN, H. *et al.* 1979. Escape performance after inescapable shock in selectively bred lines of mice: Response maintenance and catecholamine activity. J. Comp. Physiol. Psychiatry **93:** 229-241.

97. BERGER, B. *et al.* 1979. Genetically determined differences in noradrenergic input to the brain cortex: A histochemical and biochemical study in two inbred strains of mice. Neuroscience **4:** 877-888.

98. ENGBERG, G. *et al.* 1987. Locus coeruleus neurons show reduced alpha_2 receptor responsiveness and decreased basal activity in spontaneously hypertensive rats. J. Neural Transm. **69:** 71-83.

99. GAXIOLA, B. *et al.* 1984. Epinephrine-induced platelet aggregation. A twin study. Clin. Genet. **26:** 543–548.

100. PROPPING, P. & W. FRIEDL. 1983. Genetic control of adrenergic receptors on human platelets. A twin study. Human Genet. **64:** 105–109.

101. WIELAND, S. *et al.* 1986. Stock differences in the susceptibility of rats to learned helplessness training. Life Sci. **39:** 937–944.

102. KENDLER, D. S. *et al.* 1993. Panic disorder in women: A population-based twin study. Psychol. Med. **23:** 397–406.

103. NOYES, R. *et al.* 1986. Relationship between panic disorder and agoraphobia: A family study. Arch. Gen. Psychiatry **43:** 227–232.

104. MARTIN, N. G. *et al.* 1988. Anxiety disorders an neuroticism: Are there genetic factors to panic? Acta Psychiatr. Scand. **77:** 698–706.

105. DAVIDSON, J. *et al.* Familial psychiatric illness in chronic Posttraumatic Stress Disorder. Compr. Psychiatry **30:** 339–345.

106. BRESLAU, N. *et al.* 1991. Traumatic events and posttraumatic stress disorder in an urban population of young adults. Arch. Gen. Psychiatry **48:** 216–222.

107. IRWIN J. *et al.* 1986. Sensitization of norepinephrine activity following acute and chronic foot-shock. Brain Res. **379:** 98–103.

108. KARMARCY, N. R. *et al.* 1984. Footshock treatment activates catecholamine synthesis in slices of mouse brain region. Brain Res. **290:** 311–319.

109. MELIA, K. R. *et al.* 1991. Regulation of tyrosine hydroxylase (TH) in the locus coeruleus (LC) by corticotropin-releasing factor (CRF): Relation to stress and depression. Neurosci. Abstr. **16:** 444.

110. NAGY *et al.* Genetic epidemiology of panic attacks and noradrenergic response in posttraumatic stress disorder: A family history study. J. Traumatic Stress. In press.

111. MURBURG, M. M. 1994. Catecholamine Function in Posttraumtic Stress Disorder: Emerging Concepts. American Psychiatric Press. Washington, DC.

112. POST, R. M. 1992. Transduction of psychosocial stress into the neurobiology of recurrent affect disorder. Am. J. Psychiatry **149:** 999–1010.

113. MACTUTUS, C. F. *et al.* 1980. Extending the ACTH-induced memory reactivation in amnestic paradigm. Physiol. Behav. **24:** 541–546.

114. STONE, W. S. *et al.* 1990. Amphetamine, epinephrine and glucose enhancement of memory retrieval. Psychobiology **18:** 227–230.

115. KOLB, L. C. *et al.* 1984. Propranolol and clonidine in the treatment of the chronic posttraumatic stress disorders of war. *In* Posttraumatic Stress Disorder: Psychological and Biological Sequelae. B. A. van der Kolk, ed. American Psychiatric Press. Washington, DC.

Psychobiology of Sleep Disturbances in Posttraumatic Stress Disorder

THOMAS A. MELLMAN [a]

Department of Psychiatry
University of Miami School of Medicine
and
Miami Veterans Administration Medical Center
Miami, Florida 33125

Sleep disturbances are prominent features of posttraumatic stress disorder (PTSD) and are included in both the reexperiencing and heightened arousal symptom clusters in the DSM-IV. Nightmares have been referred to as a "hallmark" of PTSD[1] and are characterized to initially replicate traumatic events and feature threatening themes over time.[2] Heightened arousal symptoms related to sleep are referred to as "difficulties initiating and maintaining sleep" in the DSM-IV. Survey studies of chronic PTSD suggest that in addition to insomnia, heightened arousal symptoms manifested during sleep include body movement and awakenings with psychic and somatic anxiety symptoms that are not necessarily associated with dreaming.[3-5]

Thus, two general dimensions of sleep disturbances exist in PTSD, one pertaining to arousal regulation and the other to the expression of memories in dreams. Arousal regulation and memory processing are also fundamental to features of the disorder that manifest during wake states. Sleep can be advantageous in investigating core phenomena of psychiatric disorders in that there is less direct influence of environmental stimuli. In addition, sleep is comprised of discreet psychophysiological states that have well characterized neurobiological regulation. Given that sleep has vital restorative functions, the sleep disruption that is frequent in PTSD likely contributes to the disorder's pathogenesis and maintenance. This formulation suggests value in the development of treatments targeting sleep disturbance.

Polysomnography records electroencephalographic and other physiologic data across the sleep period, generating objective measures of sleep initiation, maintenance, architecture (distribution of sleep stages), and rapid eye movement sleep (REM) activity. Rapid eye movement sleep is the stage most specifically associated with dreaming.[6,7] In the remainder of this chapter, available phenomenological and polysomnographic findings regarding arousal patterns, dreaming, and REM physiology are reviewed. Implications for pathogenesis are discussed and preliminary observations relevant to treatment are presented.

SLEEP DISTURBANCE AND AROUSAL REGULATION IN PTSD

As previously noted, the insomnia complaints referred to in the DSM-IV and the symptomatic awakenings and body movement during sleep are common symptom

---

[a] Address for correspondence: 1201 N.W. 16th Street (116A), Miami, FL 22125.

complaints among combat veterans with PTSD[3,4] and survivors of the Nazi Holocaust.[5] Impairment of sleep maintenance with PTSD is supported by several preliminary polysomnographic studies of Israeli combat veterans with PTSD in which reduced sleep efficiency (percentage of time in bed spent sleeping) related to awakenings and movement time was reported.[8–10] Polysomnographic findings from our laboratory tend to be consistent with the subjective symptom profile of combat-related PTSD. In comparing 25 combat veterans with PTSD and controls, we also found decreased sleep efficiency and increased wake time after sleep onset, as well as more frequent micro-awakenings and gross body movement and limb movements during sleep in the PTSD group. Two recorded awakenings with anxiety featured sudden increases in autonomic activity. We have concluded from the aforementioned findings that sleep in chronic PTSD can be disrupted by intrusions of more highly aroused states and behaviors (e.g., awakening and body movement).[3] We did not find differences in sleep efficiency in a group of more acutely affected subjects with PTSD related to a natural disaster compared to that in controls. Measures of increased arousal and entries into light sleep stages, however, also implicate impairment in sustaining diminished levels of arousal in this population.[11]

Not all polysomnographic studies of PTSD support there being disturbances in maintaining sleep. In a study of 12 American combat veterans, Ross et al.[12] did not find differences in sleep efficiency or awakenings between patients and controls. An Israeli group also reported the absence of differences in sleep maintenance measures between PTSD subjects and controls. These investigators tested responses to auditory stimuli during non-REM sleep. Surprisingly, patients had increased thresholds to arousal. Reasons for this paradoxical finding, interpreted as a deepening of sleep, are unclear. The authors speculate that this phenomenon may represent a compensatory "blocking mechanism" to minimize the disruption of sleep from internal or external stimuli.[13]

IMPLICATIONS FOR PATHOGENESIS

Since subjective findings and many objective studies support disrupted sleep with PTSD, we and others postulated that chronic, partial sleep deprivation influences the development and maintenance of the disorder. Experimental evidence indicates that humans are affected by cumulative sleep loss and interruption. Increased subjective and objectively measured sleepiness was demonstrated after two consecutive nights of restricting sleep to 5 hours.[14] Induced arousals to subthreshold stimuli also affect waking performance in a dose-dependent fashion.[15] Forty-eight-hour continuous sleep deprivation in normal volunteers resulted in increased ratings of fatigue, confusion, and tension/anxiety,[16] all of which are common symptoms of PTSD patients. Panic disorder, which has phenomenological overlap with PTSD,[17] is exacerbated by sleep deprivation.[18] Finally, in an epidemiological study, insomnia was associated with increased risk for the subsequent onset of mood and anxiety disorders,[19] which represent common PTSD comorbidities.[20]

DREAMING AND RAPID EYE MOVEMENT IN PTSD

There have been many anecdotal references to dreams that occur repetitively and replicate traumatic events in chronic, combat-related PTSD. Findings from surveys and interview assessments of combat veterans support the occurrence of this phenomenon and its specificity to PTSD.[2,3] In a population that we studied 6-8 months into the wake of a natural disaster, references to the traumatic event were infrequent in diary-based dream reports. The hurricane references that did occur, however, were only in subjects who had met criteria for PTSD.[21] These observations also support replication of trauma in dreams as being specific to PTSD. We postulate that the relative infrequence of disaster references may be related to the method of assessment as well as lesser severity and impairment in the study subjects relative to clinical combat veteran populations.

The specificity of repetitive, replicative nightmares in PTSD led Ross et al.[1] to invoke a role for abnormal REM mechanisms in the disorder. The most extensive and affectively laden dreaming is associated with REM.[6,7] REM occurs at regular intervals during the sleep cycle and features cerebral activation coexisting with suppression of peripheral muscle tone. Normally, REM periods progress in length and intensity as the night progresses and become associated with more elaborate dream content.[22] In fact, nightmares in PTSD have been linked to REM and non-REM sleep.[23] In all but one study of polysomnographic recordings of awakenings precipitated by nightmares in PTSD subjects, however, episodes were preceded by REM.[2,3,12,23]

Consistent polysomnographic findings of REM in PTSD have been elusive. Reduced latency to REM (i.e., the time from the onset of sleep to the beginning of the first REM period) has been considered an important biological marker of depression,[24] which frequently overlaps PTSD.[20] Mean REM latency has not typically distinguished PTSD patients from controls. We and others commented on wide ranges of REM latency values in PTSD samples.[11,12,25] In an unpublished comparison of polysomnographic measures in PTSD and depressed patients and in controls from our laboratory, the highest and lowest values for REM latency were in the PTSD group. One explanation for a wide range of REM latency findings within and across PTSD studies could be the coexistence of pressure for REM to occur, with heightened arousal at night (as evidenced by our finding of nondiminished noradrenergic production[26]), inhibiting the onset of REM.

Several preliminary studies found reduced amounts of REM sleep with PTSD,[8-10] but this finding has also not been consistently replicated.[3,12] Both our laboratory[26] and that of Ross et al.[12] reported comparable increases in the frequency of eye movements during REM with chronic, combat-related PTSD, which has not been contradicted by other reports. In our recent study the increase in REM density was comparable to that of a comparison group with primary depression; however, the absolute amount of REM sleep was significantly lower in the PTSD group than in the depressed group.

We recently conducted multiple sleep latency tests in combat veterans with PTSD. Among 8 of 11 subjects who slept during nap opportunities, five demonstrated "sleep onset REM periods." REM activity occurred across nap opportunities and in association with high and low REM activity during the preceding night. This finding suggests that "pressure" for REM can be abnormally increased during the day in some patients with chronic PTSD. Increased REM density may also be indicative of elevated pressure for REM, in that recovery sleep following experimental REM deprivation features increased REM density.[27]

IMPLICATIONS FOR PATHOGENESIS

Pressure for REM to occur, like sleep itself, increases when either is prevented or interrupted.[27] The naps with sleep onset REM periods and increased REM density at night could therefore be interpreted as expressions of an unmet need for REM. It is possible that interruption during nighttime sleep can interfere with REM processes. Ross et al.[26] found increased phasic muscle intrusion during REM with chronic PTSD, and we reported a trend for symptomatic awakenings to arise from REM.[3]

Another reason for increased REM density and the early daytime REM onsets may be the potentially adaptive association between REM activity and states of emotional distress. Increased REM density was associated with nonpathological adaptations to bereavement.[29] Short REM latencies in a nondepressed adolescent comparison group were predicted by recent negative life events.[30] The possibility that REM has an adaptive role towards integrating traumatic memories was raised by Greenberg[25] and colleagues who observed early REM onsets in a subset of recently returned combat veterans that were associated with increased "defensive strain" during psychotherapy sessions.

Empirical support for a positive role for REM in adaptation to distressing life events was provided by the work of Cartwright and colleagues[31] who found that shorter REM latencies predicted recovery from depression in recently divorced subjects. Short REM latency was also associated with a higher dream-like quality of reports following awakenings from initial REM periods.[32] Thus, the apparent positive role for REM in emotional adaptation may in part be a function of dreaming. The mechanism by which REM and dreaming can be adaptive was postulated to be related to connections that are facilitated between current issues and affectively related memory networks.[22] Such a process would seem similar to the type of emotional processing postulated to be vital to the therapeutic benefit of psychological exposure, in which the affective and cognitive valence of distressing memories are increased and modified.[33] An additional similarity of REM phenomena to a psychotherapeutic condition is the possibility for experiencing threat in a state of physical relaxation. That characteristics of memory networks can be altered in relation to REM is supported by the evidence linking REM and information processing.[34,35]

Evidence from animal studies[36] and preliminary evidence from humans[37] indicate that periods of active learning are followed by increases in REM activity. Animal studies further indicate that the acquisition of recently learned tasks is interfered with by deprivation of critical REM periods.[34]

The available evidence suggests that the role of REM in learning depends on the nature of the learning task. Recall for complex stories, in contrast to word lists, is reported to be affected by REM loss.[35] There is also evidence that recall for types of words is differentially affected by the intervening sleep state, with the recall of words associated with personal discomfort being more specifically linked to REM.[38] Thus, a relation of REM and the processing of memories related to emotions was supported. The work of Smith and colleagues has dissected relationships of sleep states and learning via experiments utilizing selective REM deprivation versus non-REM sleep interruption. These investigators found the posttraining improvement in tests that involved verbal and visual procedural learning to be disrupted by REM deprivation. Such specificity was not found for declarative learning tasks classified as involving explicit memory.[34]

It remains speculative that learning processes linked to REM are related to emotional adaptation. It seems likely, nonetheless, that the occurrence of learning consolidation during REM indicates a capacity for emotional processing via modification of memory networks. However, dreaming in PTSD patients appears to incorporate a restricted network of memories compared to the more diffuse elements of normal dreams. Thus, dream mentation may reenforce trauma-related behavioral responses to concurrent stressors and preoccupations that manifest in chronic PTSD. To evaluate this hypothesis, we recently developed a method for rating the degree to which dreams in combat veterans replicate traumatic events without distortion or incorporation of contemporaneous references. Preliminary findings support a relationship of such tendencies in dream reports to overall PTSD severity and functional impairment.

TREATMENT IMPLICATIONS

A consistent finding in the literature is that approximately a fourth to a third of those exposed to the severe end of threatening trauma develop PTSD.[20] A critical issue for secondary prevention is to determine who among those exposed are at greatest risk. Many risk factors were recently elaborated in the literature. In our study following Hurricane Andrew, the group with PTSD and related morbidity endorsed greater degrees of sleep disturbance than did the group not manifesting PTSD. The group positive for morbidity also was found to endorse greater degrees of sleep disturbance before the hurricane, even though they had been screened to have not had active psychiatric disorders during the preceding 6 months.[11] We preliminarily replicated the association with pre-event sleep disturbance in a study of acute PTSD symptoms following severe accidental injury. Thus, sleep disturbance may be a practical target, that is straightforward to assess, for screening populations at risk for PTSD.

Fragmentation of sleep related to repetitive arousal may be an important target symptom for treatment. Although no study has demonstrated robust pharmacological impact on PTSD, amitriptyline was found to have a modest therapeutic impact in combat veterans with chronic PTSD.[39] Although amitriptyline, like other antidepressants, suppresses REM, it is often selected in clinical practice because it facilitates sleep initiation and maintenance.

We have been interested in determining if consolidating sleep by diminishing arousability is a useful strategy for intervention during acute trauma responses. This rationale led to an open evaluation of a brief application of hypnotic medication in four acutely traumatized subjects. All four subjects reported increased consolidated sleep times and reduced PTSD symptom severity 1 week after discontinuing medication compared to the baseline period. Thus, evaluation of acute intervention for sleep disruption following trauma merits more extensive and controlled evaluation.

If REM can facilitate emotional adaptation and if the interpretation of recent polysomnographic findings as suggesting a functional REM deficit is correct, then there are implications for treatment. Phenomenological overlap and comorbidity of PTSD with mood and anxiety disorders suggest a potential benefit of antidepressant medications for PTSD symptoms. A review of the available data on monoamine oxidase inhibitors and tricyclic antidepressants concluded that the therapeutic effects are only modest.[40] The property of these medications for suppressing REM sleep is a limitation for treating PTSD. This consideration led to our interest in piloting the use of the recently approved antidepressant nefazodone in PTSD. Nefazodone's pharmacological effects are thought to be primarily serotonergic, yet unlike other serotonergic antidepressants, nefazodone does not suppress, and in some subjects enhances, REM.[41] The three subjects with PTSD whose sleep we recorded at baseline and during nefazodone treatment had similar amounts of REM sleep, and consistent with findings from depression studies,[41] had less frequent awakenings and movement arousals during treatment. Dream reports were not increased during an open label trial, and five subjects recorded dream reports on a sleep/dream diary form at baseline and during treatment. Although some of the dreams reported during nefazodone treatment continued to have disturbing qualities, all five pairs of dream reports were rated as less replicative of "a traumatic experience." These observations are preliminary; however, they challenge the assumption of REM suppression as the means of ameliorating PTSD nightmares.

Behavioral therapies involving exposure appear to have the best documented efficacy for PTSD.[42] Sleep-related symptoms in the disorder are relevant targets for behavioral intervention. Treatments designed for insomnia symptoms often focus on conditioned apprehension towards initiating sleep. In PTSD, conditioned apprehension may be related to both traumatic experiences and recurrent distressing nightmares. Chronic nightmare sufferers have benefited from exposure techniques that focus on nightmare content.[43] There is a preliminary positive report of one such technique, nightmare rehearsal, in PTSD patients.[44]

SUMMARY

Sleep disturbances are prominent complaints of PTSD patients. Some, but not all, of the polysomnographic studies support the occurrence of sleep disruption. The main dimensions of sleep disturbance in the disorder relate to arousal regulation and REM-related functions of dreaming and memory processing. Both of these issues are relevant to the pathogenesis of PTSD and manifestations of the disorder during wake states. Studies elucidating the effects of treatment on sleep parameters are an important direction for future research.

ACKNOWLEDGMENTS

The author would like to acknowledge the contributions of recent collaborators in this research including Bruce Nolan, MD, Daniella David, MD, Anna Fins, PhD, Karen Esposito, MD, PhD, Amparo Benitez, DO, Joanne Hebding, R.PSG.T., and Lydia Barza.

REFERENCES

1. Ross, R. J., W. A. Ball, K. A. Sullivan & S. N. Caroff. 1989. Sleep disturbances as the hallmark of posttraumatic stress disorder. Am. J. Psychiatry **146:** 6977-6970.

2. VAN DER KOLK, B., R. BLITZ, W. A. BURR, S. SHERRY & E. HARTMANN. 1984. Nightmares and trauma: A comparison of nightmares after combat with lifelong nightmares in veterans. Am. J. Psychiatry **141:** 187-190.

3. MELLMAN, T. A., R. KULICK-BELL, L. E. ASHLOCK & B. NOLAN. 1995. Sleep events in combat-related post-traumatic stress disorder. Am. J. Psychiatry **152:** 110-115.

4. INMAN, D. J., S. M. SILVER & K. DOGHRAMJI. 1990. Sleep disturbance in post-traumatic stress disorder: A comparison with non-PTSD insomnia. J. Traumatic Stress **3:** 429-437.

5. ROSEN, J., C. F. REYNOLDS, A. L. YEAER, P. R. HOUCK & L. F. HURWITZ. 1990. Sleep disturbances in survivors of the Nazi holocaust. Am. J. Psychiatry **148:** 62-66.

6. DEMENT, W. & N. KLEITMAN. 1957. The relation of eye movements during sleep to dream activity: An objective method for the study of dreaming. J. Exp. Psychol. **53:** 339-346.

7. FOULKES, W. D. 1962. Dream reports from different stages of sleep. J. Abnorm. Soc. Psychol. **65:** 14-25.

8. LAVIE, P., A. HEFEZ, G. HALPERIN & D. ENOCH. 1979. Long-term effects of traumatic war-related events on sleep. Am. J. Psychiatry **136:** 175-178.

9. HEFEZ, A., L. METZ & P. LAVIE. 1987. Long-term effects of extreme situational stress on sleep and dreaming. Am. J. Psychiatry **144:** 344-347.

10. GLAUBMAN, H., M. MIKULINCER, A. PORAT, O. WASSERMAN & M. BIRGER. 1990. Sleep of chronic posttraumatic patients. J. Traumatic Stress **3:** 255-263.

11. MELLMAN, T. A., D. DAVID, R. KULICK-BELL, J. HEBDING & B. NOLAN. 1995. Sleep disturbance and its relationship to psychiatric morbidity following hurricane Andrew. Am. J. Psychiatry **152:** 1659-1663.

12. ROSS, R. J., W. A. BALL, D. F. DINGES, N. B. KRIBBS, A. R. MORRISON, S. M. SILVER & F. D. MULVANEY. 1994. Rapid eye movement sleep disturbance in posttraumatic stress disorder. Biol. Psychiatry **35:** 195-202.

13. DAGAN, Y., P. LAVIE & A. BLEICH. 1991. Elevated awakening thresholds in sleep stage 3-4 in war-related post-traumatic stress disorder. Biol. Psychiatry **30:** 618-622.

14. CARSKADON, M. A. & W. C. DEMENT. 1981. Cumulative effects of sleep restriction on daytime sleepiness. Psychophysiology **18:** 107-113.

15. MAGEE, J., J. HARSH & P. BADIA. 1987. Effects of experimentally-induced sleep fragmentation on sleep and sleepiness. Psychophysiology **24:** 528-534.

16. NEWHOUSE, P. A., G. BELENKY, M. THOMAS, D. THORNE, H. C. SING & J. FERTIG. 1989. The effects of d-Amphetamine on arousal, cognition, and mood after prolonged total sleep deprivation. Neuropsychopharmacology **2:** 153-164.

17. MELLMAN, T. A. & G. C. DAVIS. 1985. Combat-related flashbacks in postraumatic stress disorder: Phenomenology and similarity to panic attacks. J. Clin. Psychiatry **46:** 379-382.

18. ROY-BYRNE, P. P., T. W. UHDE & R. M. POST. 1986. Effects of one night's sleep deprivation on mood and behavior on patients with panic disorder. Arch. Gen. Psychiatry **43:** 895-899.

19. FORD, D. E. & D. B. KAMEROW. 1989. Epidemiologic study of sleep disturbances and psychiatric disorders: An opportunity for prevention? JAMA **262:** 1479-1484.

20. KESSLER, R. C., A. SONNEGA, E. BROMET, M. HUGHES & C. B. NELSON. 1995. Posttraumatic stress disorder in the National Comorbidity Survey. Arch. Gen. Psychiatry **52:** 1048-1060.

21. DAVID, D. & T. A. MELLMAN. 1995. Dreams following Hurricane Andrew. American Psychiatric Association 148th Annual Meeting. NR69

22. CARTWRIGHT, R. D. 1994. Dreams and their meaning. *In* Principles and Practice of Sleep Medicine, 2nd Ed. M. Krieger *et al.,* Eds. W.B. Saunders Co. Philadelphia.

23. KRAMER, M., L. S. SCHOEN & L. KINNEY. 1984. The dream experience in dream disturbed Vietnam veterans. *In* Post-traumatic Stress Disorders: Psychological and Biological Sequelae. B. van der Kolk, Ed. American Psychiatric Press. Washington, DC.

24. KUPFER, D. J. 1976. REM latency—A psychobiological marker for primary depressive disease. Biol. Psychiatry **11:** 159-174.

25. GREENBERG, R. 1967. Dream interruption insomnia. J. Nerv. Ment. Dis. **144:** 18-21.
26. MELLMAN, T. A., A. KUMAR, R. L. KULICK-BELL, M. KUMAR & B. NOLAN. 1995. Nocturnal/ daytime urine noradrenergic measures and sleep in combat-related PTSD. Biol. Psychiatry **38:** 174-179.
27. REYNOLDS, C. F., D. J. BUYSSE, D. J. KUPFER, C. C. HOCH, P. R. HOUCH, J. MATZZIE & C. J. GEORGE. 1990. Rapid eye movement sleep deprivation as probe in elderly subjects. Arch. Gen. Psychiatry **47:** 1128-1136.
28. ROSS, R. J., W. A. BALL, D. F. DINGES, N. B. KRIBBS, A. R. MORRISON, S. M. SILVER & F. D. MULVANEY. 1994. Motor dysfunction during sleep in posttraumatic stress disorder. Sleep **17:** 723-732.
29. REYNOLDS, C. F., C. C. HOCH, D. J. BUYSSE, P. R. HOUCH, M. SCHLERNITZAUER, R. E. PASTERNACK, E. FRANK, S. MAZUMDAR & D. J. KUPFER. 1993. Sleep after spousal bereavement: A study of recovery from stress. Biol. Psychiatry **34:** 791-797.
30. WILLIAMSON, D. E., R. E. DAHL, B. BIRMAHER, R. R. GOETZ, B. NELSON & N. D. RYAN. 1995. Stressful life events and EEG sleep in depressed and normal control adolescents. Biol. Psychiatry **37:** 859-865.
31. CARTWRIGHT, R. D., H. KRAVITZ, C. I. EASTMAN & E. WOOD. 1991. REM Latency and the recovery from depression: Getting over divorce. Am. J. Psychiatry **148:** 1530-1535.
32. CARTWRIGHT, R. D. & S. R. LLOYD. 1993. Early REM sleep: A compensatory change in depression? Psychiatry Res. **51:** 245-252.
33. FOA, E. B., B. O. ROTHBAUM, D. S. RIGGS & T. B. MURDOCK. 1991. Treatment of posttraumatic stress disorder in rape victims: A comparison between cognitive-behavioral procedures and counseling. J. Consult. Clin. Psychol. **59:** 715-723.
34. SMITH, C. 1995. Sleep states and memory processes. Behav. Brain Res. **69:** 137-145.
35. TILLEY, A. J. & J. A. C. EMPSON. 1978. REM sleep and memory consolidation. Biol. Psychol. **6:** 293-300.
36. SMITH, C. & L. LAPP. 1986. Prolonged increase in both PS and number of REMS following a shuttle avoidance task. Physiol. Behav. **36:** 1053-1057.
37. SMITH, C. & L. LAPP. 1991. Increases in number of REMs and REM density in humans following an intensive learning period. Sleep **14:** 325-330.
38. CARTWRIGHT, R. D., S. LLOYD, E. BUTTERS, L. WEINER, L. MCCARTHY & J. HANCOCK. 1975. Effects of REM time on what is recalled. Psychophysiology **12:** 561-568.
39. DAVIDSON, J., H. KUDLER, R. SMITH *et al.* 1990. Treatment of post-traumatic stress disorder with amitryptyline and placebo. Arch. Gen. Psychiatry **47:** 259-266.
40. SOUTHWICK, S. M., R. YEHUDA, E. L. GILLER & D. S. CHARNEY. 1994. Use of tricyclics and monoamine oxidase inhibitors in the treatment of PTSD: A quantitative review. *In* Catecholamine Function in Posttraumatic Stress Disorder: Emerging Concepts. American Psychiatric Press. Washington, DC.
41. ARMITAGE, R., A. J. RUSH, M. TRIVEDI, J. CAIN & H. P. ROFFWARG. 1994. The effects of nefazodone on sleep architecture in depression. Neuropsychopharmacology **10:** 123-127.
42. SOLOMON, S. D., E. T. GERRITY & A. M. MUFF. 1992. Efficacy of treatments of posttraumatic stress disorder. JAMA **268:** 633-638.
43. KELLNER, R., J. NEIDHARDT, B. KRAKOW & D. PATHAK. 1992. Changes in chronic nightmares after one session of desensitization or rehearsal instructions. Am. J. Psychiatry **149:** 659-663.
44. THOMPSON, K., M. HAMILTON & J. WEST. 1995. Group treatment for nightmares in veterans with combat-related PTSD. NCP Clin. Q. Fall: 13-17.

Psychobiological Effects of Sexual Abuse

A Longitudinal Study

FRANK W. PUTNAM [a,c] AND
PENELOPE K. TRICKETT [b]

[a]*Unit on Developmental Traumatology*
Behavioral Endocrinology Branch
National Institute of Mental Health
Bethesda, Maryland 20892-2668

[b]*Department of Psychology*
University of Southern California
Los Angeles, California

Child maltreatment is common in the United States and probably in most countries. US Government statistics for 1994 (most recent data available) report over 1 million substantiated cases, an increase of 27% over 1990.[1] Official 1994 incidence rates by maltreatment type are: neglect, 8/1,000 children; physical abuse, 2/1,000; sexual abuse, 2/1,000; and emotional abuse/medical neglect, 1/1,000. General population surveys, which include many cases not reported to authorities, suggest annual rates as high as 19/1,000 children for physical abuse and 11/1,000 for sexual abuse.[2] In their national survey of 2,000 children aged 10–16 years, Finkelhor and Dziuba-Leatherman[2] found that only one in four incidents of victimization were reported to authorities.

Research links multiple psychiatric symptoms and disorders to histories of maltreatment. Psychiatric outcomes vary to some degree according to the type of maltreatment. However, many victims experience multiple forms of maltreatment and/or exhibit combinations of symptoms and disorders. Indeed, the heterogeneity and overlap of maltreatment outcomes have confounded attempts to identify abuse-specific responses for clinical and forensic purposes.

Recent studies indicate that child maltreatment alters biological systems. Although preliminary, these studies find an array of stress-related biological systems significantly affected by maltreatment and related family environment factors including hypothalamic-pituitary-adrenal axis dysregulation; increased catecholamines; altered growth and physical development; immune dysfunction; and decreased hippocampal volume.

The discovery of biological dysfunctions associated with traumatic experiences is changing the direction of research on maltreatment-related psychopathology. Prior to these discoveries, research largely focused on possible psychological mechanisms.

[c]Address for correspondence: Frank W. Putnam, MD, Bldg 15K, UDT, NIMH, 9000 Rockville Pike, Bethesda, MD 20892-2668 (tel: (301) 496-4431; fax: (301) 402-1218; e-mail: PUT@CU. NIH.GOV).

Investigators are now better able to factor in relevant biological systems and to draw upon a range of animal experimental models for hypotheses. In addition, powerful new biotechnologies are being applied to these questions.

Recent associations between maltreatment experiences and biological effects promise to inform basic questions. How are behavioral and cognitive symptoms related to biological dysfunctions? How similar are the biological effects of maltreatment with those of other traumatic stressors, such as combat, accidents, and disasters? How reversible are biological effects? Do different types of maltreatment, such as sexual and physical abuse, have differential effects on a given biological system? Can biological abnormalities be used as forensic evidence? Can biological measures predict diagnosis and treatment response or suggest new forms of treatment? Do trauma-associated biological alterations produce a different "type" of individual? (For examples, see discussions in refs. 3 and 4.)

THE ROLE OF DEVELOPMENT

Greater understanding of the relationships between childhood maltreatment outcomes and underlying biological mechanisms requires taking into account the role of child development in the evolution of psychopathology. Maltreatment, especially neglect, often begins at an early age and frequently spans a sizable portion of childhood. From animal and primate studies, we know that this developmental period is crucial to the maturation of neuroendocrine systems. During certain "critical periods," small or transient environmental insults may have disproportionate effects on the subsequent function of biological systems. We know little about such windows of vulnerability in humans, but research suggests that they do exist and perhaps account for some of the apparent heterogeneity in maltreatment outcomes.

The addition of developmental inputs to the outcome equation provides an opportunity to integrate several largely independent domains of knowledge about the effects of maltreatment. To tease out mechanistic interrelationships, however, investigators must trace simultaneous psychological, social, and biological developmental trajectories over time. This is a formidable task. New forms of assessment (e.g., salivary hormone levels and computer-administered testing) are easing the difficulty and intrusiveness associated with collecting biological and psychological data from children.[5] However, young children remain difficult to study, and many measures of psychopathology are not valid below the age of 8 years. Thorny ethical considerations further complicate this work.[6]

PSYCHOBIOLOGICAL EFFECTS OF SEXUAL ABUSE

The longitudinal study, "The Psychobiological Effects of Sexual Abuse," is one of the first to prospectively trace the course of psychological, social, cognitive, and biological factors thought to be important contributors to maltreatment outcome. Prior research has significantly associated a range of psychiatric symptoms and disorders with sexual abuse. These include: depression, suicidality, self-mutilation, somatization, sexual behavior problems, dissociative identity disorder, borderline personality disorder, substance abuse (in women), and posttraumatic stress disorder (PTSD).[7,8] Many investigators suggest that this diversity is more apparent than real and that a set of basic developmental disruptions link ostensible clinical differences.[9,10]

Conceptualizing childhood sexual abuse as a model of chronic, developmentally embedded trauma, we are interested in understanding the interaction of developmental, psychological, biological, and social factors on long-term outcomes (both positive and negative) in abused girls.[11] To highlight developmental contributions, we initially focused on the critical pubertal transition period. Occurring over a 3- to 4-year span, puberty is associated with a host of psychological and social changes including attainment of a new image of self, establishment of intimate relationships with the opposite sex, and beginning the process of independence from the family of origin. It is also a period in which many forms of psychopathology are first manifest, particularly for females. Current and planned assessments also cover the important transition from adolescence into young adulthood.

Subjects

The subjects are 164 girls together with a nonabusing caretaker, usually their mother. Sexually abused girls ($n = 77$) were referred by Washington, DC area child protective service agencies. Although many received outside treatment at some point, they are not a clinically selected sample. Inclusion in the study was based on meeting sexual abuse criteria and the active participation of a primary caretaker.[12] Comparison girls ($n = 72$) were recruited through newspaper ads and notices in social service agencies. As a group, controls were matched on age, race, socioeconomic status, and family constellation. To avoid attracting comparison families covertly interested in sexual abuse, the purpose of the study was disguised under the title, "Normal female growth and development." Debriefing occurred during the first informed consent process.

Descriptions of the sample vary slightly across published reports because of exclusion of subjects based on missing data for relevant measures. In addition to the sexually abused and comparison girls, a third comparison group, "General Maltreatment" ($n = 15$), was created for comparison girls discovered to have been maltreated in some fashion and includes a few sexually abused girls who were subsequently found not to satisfy our inclusion criteria.

TABLE 1 describes the characteristics of the sexual abuse experiences in our sample. They come from inner-city, suburban, and semi-rural neighborhoods. About 40% are minority (35% African-American and 5% Hispanic or Asian), and most come from low to middle class families (mean Hollingshead score 35.4 ± 16.6). The average age at entry into the study was 11 ± 3 years.

Design

The study employs a cross-sequential design.[13] The sample initially spanned ages 6-15 years to facilitate cross-sectional analyses centered around the transition through puberty. Children were grouped in 2-year age cohorts and are followed forward in time with periodic evaluations. Subject recruitment began in December 1987 and

TABLE 1. Sexual Abuse Characteristics ($n = 77$)

Variable	Mean/Percent	SD
Abuse count (number of types of abuse)	2.81	1.35
Age of onset (yr)	7.90	3.34
Duration (mo)	26.23	29.58
Perpetrator		
Biological father	23.4%	
Father figure	58.4%	
Other	18.2%	
Physical violence	51.9%	
Multiple perpetrators	41.6%	

continued until June 1992. To date, most children have been evaluated three or four times. Evaluation timepoints 1, 2, and 3 (designated T1, T2, and T3, respectively) occurred approximately 1 year apart. Time 4 (T4) evaluation is currently underway. Multiple timepoints permit plotting of individual and group developmental trajectories. Specific age effects can be examined with pooled cohort data, for example, analyses of children aged 8–9 years may include those children aged 8–9 on entry together with children who became 8–9 at some point during the study.

Measures

Many measures are required to trace the developmental pathways of the psychological, biological, and social constructs being followed. To improve construct validity, assessments must cross social contexts (e.g., home, school, and peers) to evaluate a child's performance in different settings. Furthermore, a variety of response formats are required to capture self-appraisals, the assessments of others working with the child, and the child's performance on standardized tests. Measures must assess normal processes, such as internalization of locus of control or development of self-esteem, as well as psychopathological outcomes.

The study includes: child self-reports, parent, teacher, and therapist reports, as well as researcher-administered interviews and tests. It also includes a set of standardized social interactions (mother/child, research assistant/child) which are videotaped and later scored by coders blinded to group status and research hypotheses. For example, in the "Strange Man" segment during the T1 evaluation, girls were scored on 90 nonverbal behaviors exhibited during an 8-minute standardized interaction with a male research assistant, whom they had not previously met.[14]

Biological measures were selected to: (1) investigate similarities between maltreatment effects and other traumatic stressors; (2) examine hypothesized hormone-behavior relationships; (3) measure physical and physiological development; and (4) investigate responses to stressor challenges Hypothalamic-pituitary-adrenal (HPA) axis measures include plasma cortisol, morning resting, and stressed salivary cortisols in all subjects. Twenty-four-hour urinary free cortisols and ACTH responses to a corticotropin releasing hormone (CRH) infusion test were obtained in a subset of subjects. Serial salivary-cortisols spanning a computer-administered mental rotation task investigate HPA response to a neutral (nontraumatic) stressor.

Hypothalamic-pituitary-gonadal axis hormones include: follicle stimulating hormone, luteinizing hormone, estrogen, estradiol, and progesterone. Plasma levels of the androgens testosterone, delta-4 androstenedione, and dehydroepiandrosterone (DHEA) were collected for correlation with aggressive, suicidal, somatic, and hypersexual behaviors. Thyroid studies, 24-hour urinary catecholamine levels, and antinuclear antibodies were also obtained for subjects participating in the CRH infusion protocol.

To assess physiological reactivity and autonomic regulation, continuous heart rate and vagal tone data are collected across neutral (mental rotation) and traumatic (a comprehensive trauma interview) stressors. Videotaped facial expression (coded by the Ekman system[15]) will be compared with simultaneous physiological data to examine congruence/dissociation of affective and psychophysiological responses to traumatic reminders. Sitting and standing heart rate and blood pressure are also obtained. Restlessness and motor activity are measured by a wrist actometer. Physical growth and development are measured by height, weight, and Tanner staging of secondary sex characteristics. A subset of the sample is being recruited for magnetic resonance imaging (MRI) of hippocampal volume to investigate possible trauma-associated degeneration.

Mothers participate in the study through extensive interviews and self-report measures covering family history, family environment, and child-rearing attitudes and practices. A developmental history is obtained from the mother at T1 and is updated at each timepoint. Mothers also complete measures assessing their own history and current functioning. A substantial percentage (54%) of the mothers of abused girls were themselves sexually abused.[16] However, 17% of the mothers of comparison girls were also sexually abused. As part of our investigation of the transgenerational aspects of familial sexual abuse, mothers complete questionnaires about their family of origin.

RESULTS

Results published to date primarily involve cross-sectional (T1) data. Reports including longitudinal (T1-T3) data are in press and others are in preparation.

HPA Axis Dysregulation

The HPA axis is a major stress response system.[17] Recent studies report abnormalities in combat-related PTSD.[3] Using an indwelling intravenous catheter, we collected plasma cortisol samples at 0, 20, and 40 minutes. Analyzing T1 and partial T2 data, we found evidence of higher morning and lower afternoon plasma cortisol levels in abused girls than in controls.[18] A comparison of the 0-40-minute curve showed that abused girls had significantly higher time-integrated cortisol levels and displayed a different profile with a steeper slope in response to the stress of placing the iv. At 40 minutes, mean plasma cortisol for the controls was below the 0-minute time point, whereas for the abused girls it was significantly above the 0-minute baseline. This suggests significant dysregulation of the HPA axis to minor stressors in the abused girls.

HPA axis regulation was further characterized in a self-selected subset of abused and control subjects.[19] Plasma ACTH and total and free plasma cortisol responses to ovine CRH (oCRH) were measured in 13 sexually abused and 13 comparison girls. Twenty-four-hour urinary free cortisol was also collected. The abused girls showed significantly lower basal and net oCRH-stimulated ACTH levels and significantly reduced total ACTH responses. Their total, free basal, and oCRH-stimulated plasma cortisol and 24-hour urinary free cortisol levels did not differ from those of controls.

These data (together with reports by other investigators) indicate that sexual abuse (and likely other forms of maltreatment) is associated with dysregulatory responses of the HPA axis. These data are consistent with the hypothesis that prior stress (probably associated with sexual abuse and related family dynamics) produced hypersecretion of CRH which induced an adaptive downregulation of CRH receptors in the anterior pituitary. Similar HPA axis adaptations have been reported in animal models. These finding differ somewhat from those reported for combat-related PTSD. (It should be noted that only one of the girls participating in the CRH study met DSM-IIIR criteria for PTSD.) Our findings, however, are compatible with the larger point made by Yehuda and McFarlane,[3] that trauma-associated biological responses involve changes in the regulatory dynamics of neuroendocrine pathways.

Catecholamine Levels

Catecholamines (norepinephrine, epinephrine, and dopamine) have long been implicated in stress and trauma responses. Elevated levels of 24-hour urinary catecholamines have been found in combat veterans. Yehuda et al.[20] found that dopamine levels were significantly correlated with intrusive flashbacks, avoidance, and hyperarousal symptoms in Vietnam veterans. In subjects participating in the CRH infusion study, we found elevated 24-hour urinary catecholamines in the sexually abused girls compared with the controls. When corrected for height (the strongest developmental covariate), only homovanillic acid levels were significantly different; however, there were trends for total catecholamine synthesis, metananephrine, and vanillylmandelic acid. These findings suggest that maltreatment effects on sympathetic nervous system activity are similar to those of traumatic stressors such as combat; for examples, see ref. 21.

Immune Function

Animal studies show that a variety of stressors can alter immune function.[17] These effects may be mediated through the HPA axis and/or sympathetic nervous system, both of which suppress immune function in response to acute stress. The thymus is a key component of the immune system and is believed to play an important role in preventing the formation of antibodies against the self (autoantibodies). Early studies by Selye[22] showed that restrained rats have thymic involution and lymphopenia. Autopsy study of abused and neglected Japanese children found a significant decrease in thymus weight compared to that of comparison children who were victims of accidents or homicides, but did not have histories of abuse.[23] Severity and length of abuse were correlated with the degree of thymic involution.

Antinuclear antibody is a general term for autoantibodies against cell nuclear proteins. Although low titers of autoantibodies occur in most individuals, the presence of high antinuclear antibody levels is thought to reflect failure of the immune system to suppress autoreactive lymphocytes. We found a twofold higher incidence of plasma antinuclear antibodies in abused subjects than in control subjects participating in the CRH infusion protocol.[24] This difference was not statistically significant, in part because of the racial imbalance of this self-selected sample. (African-American females have significantly increased autoimmune phenomena compared with Caucasian females.[25]) Comparisons with a white adult female sample revealed significant differences among abused girls but not controls.[24]

Although preliminary, these data are congruent with animal and human studies indicating that stress-induced immune system alterations can occur. Depression (which is significantly associated with maltreatment in our sample and in many studies) has also been implicated in increased autoimmune antibody titers. Preliminary analyses of mother-reported rates of colds, flu, and other minor illnesses suggest disproportionate levels in abused girls. School absences are also much higher among abused girls, although the reasons for such absences cannot be determined from school records.[26] It is possible that abuse-related immune dysfunction increases susceptibility to infectious and autoimmune diseases.

Hormone/Behavior Correlations

Preliminary analyses of relationships between hormones and behaviors associated with maltreatment, such as aggression, somatization, depression, and dissociation, find complex relationships that sometimes differ for controls and abused girls. For example, somatization as measured by the Child Behavioral Checklist (CBCL) is significantly positively correlated ($r = 0.27$, $p < 0.05$) with delta-4 androstenedione in controls and equally significantly negatively correlated ($r = -0.27$, $p < 0.05$) in abused girls.[27] Child Depression Inventory scores show a similar pattern of opposite correlations.

Pathological Dissociation

Recent interest in pathological dissociation as a response to trauma has spurred over a hundred studies involving an array of traumatic stressors. Reviews and meta-analyses of these data find strong linkages between dissociative symptoms and traumatic exposures.[28,29] We are following the developmental trajectories of dissociative symptoms and behaviors in our sample. Compared with our controls, sexually abused girls have significantly elevated dissociation scores at T1, T2, and T3.[30,31]

Dissociation scores are strongly correlated with general measures of psychopathology such as the CBCL. Analysis of teacher evaluations found that dissociative and hyperactive behaviors were the best predictors of poor academic and social performance.[26] Scores on the Child Dissociative Checklist (CDC) are also the single best predictor of inappropriate sexualized behaviors at T1, T2, and T3.

Dissociation scores, however, are not significantly correlated with hypnotizability.[31] Neither (unlike dissociation) is hypnotizability correlated with measures of trauma severity. These findings support recent studies showing little or no relation between standardized measures of dissociativity and hypnotizability or between hypnotizability and trauma.[29] It is clear that pathological dissociation and hypnotizability, which are often conceptualized as psychobiologically one and the same, are different processes.[29]

Characteristics of Sexual Trauma and Predictions of Outcomes

Reviews of sexual abuse studies note the heterogeneity of outcomes, the enormous variance within a sample with respect to any given outcome, and the fact that even common outcomes, such as depression, are typically present in a minority of subjects in a given sample.[12] We explored the interrelationships among abuse variables including: (1) severity of the abusive act (e.g., penetration vs fondling); (2) duration and/or frequency; (3) use of force and/or violence; (4) relationship to the perpetrator; and (5) age of onset of the abuse.[12] We find these variables to be highly intercorrelated. For example, in our sample, the younger the child at abuse onset, (1) the more severe the abuse in terms of the number of types of abuse, (2) the longer the duration, and (3) the more likely the perpetrator is to be the biological father.

The results of these analyses are too involved to be detailed here (see ref. 12), but they suggest several cautions. First, significant differences appear between biological fathers and other father figures (e.g., stepfathers and mothers' live-in boyfriends). In our sample, sexual abuse by a biological father is a predictor of sexual acting out, aggressive delinquent behavior, the presence of a disruptive behavior disorder diagnosis, and other externalizing psychopathology. These relationships do not hold for nonbiological father figures despite similarities in other abuse variables. Second, the high intercorrelations among traditional abuse severity variables indicate that analyses of severity-outcome relationships must partial out intercorrelations and use multivariate statistical methods. It is possible that similar confounds, as yet not identified, exist for other traumatic stressors.

DISCUSSION

Preliminary biological findings have important implications for understanding the outcomes associated with child maltreatment. They indicate that major stress response systems such as the HPA axis, sympathetic nervous system, and immune system may be significantly altered by maltreatment and related family environmental experiences. Abnormalities of the HPA axis can have significant affective, cognitive, and behavioral effects, as demonstrated by disorders such as Addison's disease and Cushing's syndrome as well as by administration of exogenous cortisol. The HPA axis is capable of powerful immunosuppressive effects. Increased catecholamine levels have been implicated in PTSD symptoms. They may also contribute to the high levels of restlessness and motor activity in maltreated children noted by many investigators. Trauma/stress-induced decreases in immune competence could have ripple effects throughout the life span if they increase susceptibility to infectious diseases. If such effects increase risk for autoimmune disorders, they could be devastating.

Dissociation proves to be a robust correlate of many forms of psychopathology in both sexually abused and comparison girls across development. It appears to be a fundamental form of psychopathology analogous to depression or anxiety. We are currently investigating the relationship of pathological dissociation to traumatic, familial, social, academic, and biological variables. Of particular interest is the contribution of dissociation to the psychobiological regulation of responses to traumatic stressors.

Preliminary results suggest that abused and comparison girls differ in: (1) levels of stress-related hormones and neurotransmitters; (2) regulatory dynamics of neuroendocrine systems; (3) neuroendocrine responses to stressors; and (4) patterns of correlations between some hormones and behaviors. These findings must be replicated and extended in other studies, but they suggest that biological alterations are an important characteristic of responses to maltreatment. Biological alterations likely interact with development to influence the type and expression of pathological symptoms and behaviors in child and adult victims of maltreatment.

REFERENCES

1. U.S. DEPARTMENT OF HEALTH AND HUMAN SERVICES. 1996. Child maltreatment 1994: Reports from the States to the National Center on Child Abuse and Neglect. U.S. Government Printing Office. Washington, DC.
2. FINKELHOR, D. & J. DZIUBA-LEATHERMAN. 1994. Children as victims of violence: A national survey. Pediatrics **94:** 413-420.
3. YEHUDA, R. & A. C. MCFARLANE. 1995. Conflict between current knowledge about posttraumatic stress disorder and its original conceptual basis. Am. J. Psychiatry **152:** 1705-1713.
4. WALLER, N. G., F. W. PUTNAM & E. B. CARLSON. 1996. Types of dissociation and dissociative types. Psychol. Methods. **1:** 300-321.
5. PUTNAM, F. 1996. Special methods for trauma research with children. *In* Trauma Research Methodology. E. Carlson, Eds.: 153-173. Sidran Press. Lutherville, MD.
6. PUTNAM, F., M. LISS & J. LANDSVERK. 1996. Ethical issues in maltreatment research with children and adolescents. *In* Ethical Issues in Mental Health Research with Children and Adolescents. K. Hoagwood, P. Jensen & C. Fisher, Eds.: 113-132. Erlbaum. Mahwah, NJ.
7. TRICKETT, P. & C. MCBRIDE-CHANG. 1995. The developmental impact of different forms of child abuse and neglect. Dev. Rev. **15:** 311-337.
8. PUTNAM, F. 1997. Child and Adolescent Dissociative Disorders: A Developmental Perspective. Guilford. New York. In press.
9. COLE, P. M. & F. W. PUTNAM. 1992. The effect of incest on self and social functioning: A developmental psychopathological perspective. J. Consult. Clin. Psychol. **60:** 174-184.
10. VAN DER KOLK, B., D. PELCOVITZ, S. ROTH, F. MANDEL, A. MCFARLANE & J. HERMAN. 1996. Dissociation, somatization, and affect regulation: The complexity of adaptation to trauma. Am. J. Psychiatry **153** (Festschrift Suppl.): 83-93.
11. TRICKETT, P. K. & F. W. PUTNAM. 1993. Impact of child sexual abuse on females: Towards a developmental, psychobiological integration. Psychol. Sci. **4:** 81-87.
12. TRICKETT, P., A. REIFFMAN, L. HOROWITZ, & F. PUTNAM. 1997. Characteristics of sexual abuse trauma and the prediction of developmental outcomes. *In* Rochester Symposium

on Developmental Psychopathology, Vol 8. D. Cicchetti & S. Toth, Eds. University of Rochester Press. Rochester, NY. In press.

13. WOHLWILL, J. 1973. The Study of Behavioral Development. Academic Press. New York.

14. MAUSERT-MOONEY, R., P. TRICKETT & F. PUTNAM. 1993. Appeal and vulnerability patterns in girl victims of incest. Paper presented at the Annual Meeting of the American Psychological Association. Toronto.

15. EKMAN, P. 1972. Emotion in the Human Face: Guidelines for Research and an Integration of Findings. Pergamon. Press. New York.

16. EVERETT, B., K. COOPER, P. TRICKETT & F. PUTNAM. 1996. Mothers and daughters and child sexual abuse: Legacies of loss, trauma and abuse. Paper presented at the XIVth Biennial Conference of the International Society for the Study of Behavioral Development. Quebec City.

17. DE BELLIS, M. D. & F. W. PUTNAM. 1994. The psychobiology of childhood maltreatment. Child Adolesc. Psychiatric Clin. N. Am. 3: 1-16.

18. PUTNAM, F., P. TRICKETT, K. HELMERS, L. DORN & B. EVERETT. 1991. Cortisol abnormalities in sexually abused girls. Poster presented at the Annual Meeting of the American Psychiatric Association. Washington, DC.

19. DE BELLIS, M. D., G. P. CHROUSOS, L. D. DORN, L. BURKE, K. HELMERS, M. A. KLING, P. K. TRICKETT & F. W. PUTNAM. 1994. Hypothalamic-pituitary-adrenal axis dysregulation in sexually abused girls. J. Clin. Endocrinol. Metab. 78: 249-255.

20. YEHUDA, R., S. SOUTHWICK, E. L. GILLER, X. MA & J. W. MASON. 1992. Urinary catecholamine excretion and severity of PTSD symptoms in Vietnam combat veterans. J. Nerv. Mental Dis. 180: 321-325.

21. CHARNEY, D. S., A. Y. DEUTCH, J. H. KRYSTAL, S. M. SOUTHWICH & M. DAVIS. 1993. Psychobiological mechanisms of posttraumatic stress disorder. Arch. Gen. Psychiatry 50: 294-305.

22. SELYE, H. 1936. A syndrome produced by diverse noxious agents. Nature 138: 32-36.

23. FUKUNAGA, T., Y. MIZOI, A. YAMASHITA, M. YAMADA, Y. YAMAMOTO, Y. TATSUNO & K. NISHI. 1992. Thymus of abused/neglected children. Forensic Sci. Int. 53: 69-79.

24. DE BELLIS, M., L. BURKE, P. TRICKETT & F. PUTNAM. 1996. Antinuclear antibodies and thyroid function in sexually abused girls. J. Traumatic Stress 9: 369-378.

25. STEINBERG, A. 1992. Systemic lupus erythematosus. In Cecil Textbook of Medicine. J. Wyngaarden, L. Smith & J. Bennett, Eds.: 1522-1527. W. B. Saunders. Philadelphia.

26. TRICKETT, P., C. MCBRIDE-CHANG & F. PUTNAM. 1994. The classroom performance and behavior of sexually abused females. Dev. Psychopathol. 6: 183-194.

27. TRICKETT, P., E. SUSMAN & F. PUTNAM. 1994. Hormones and behavior in sexually abused girl victims of incest. Paper presented at the Annual Meeting of the American Psychological Association. Washington, DC.

28. VAN IJZENDOORN, M. & C. SCHUENGEL. 1996. The measurement of dissociation in normal and clinical populations: Meta-analytic validation of the Dissociative Experiences Scale (DES). Clin. Psychol. Rev. 16: 365-382.

29. PUTNAM, F. W. & E. B. CARLSON. 1997. Dissociation, hypnosis and trauma: Myths, metaphors and mechanisms. In Dissociation, Memory and Trauma. D. Bremner & C. Marmar, Eds. American Psychiatric Press. Washington, DC. In press.

30. PUTNAM, F. W., K. HELMERS & P. K. TRICKETT. 1993. Development, reliability and validity of a child dissociation scale. Child Abuse & Neglect 17: 731-741.

31. PUTNAM, F. W., K. HELMERS, L. A. HOROWITZ & P. K. TRICKETT. 1994. Hypnotizability and dissociativity in sexually abused girls. Child Abuse & Neglect 19: 645-655.

Preliminary Evidence for Abnormal Cortical Development in Physically and Sexually Abused Children Using EEG Coherence and MRI[a]

MARTIN H. TEICHER, YUTAKA ITO,[b]
CAROL A. GLOD, SUSAN L. ANDERSEN,
NATALIE DUMONT, AND ERIKA ACKERMAN

Department of Psychiatry
Harvard Medical School
and
Developmental Biopsychiatry Research Program
McLean Hospital
Belmont, Massachusetts 02178

Physical or sexual abuse during childhood has been associated with the development of an array of psychiatric disorders including multiple personality disorder,[1] borderline personality disorder,[2,3] and refractory psychosis.[4] Childhood physical abuse may also sensitize patients to the later development of posttraumatic stress disorder (PTSD).[5] We postulated that early deprivation or abuse could result in neurobiological abnormalities responsible for subsequent psychiatric disorders.[6] Green *et al.*[7] found that soft neurological signs and nonspecific EEG abnormalities were more common in abused children. Green[8] proposed that this was an additional source of trauma amplifying the impact of the abusive environment. Davies[9] reported that 17 of 22 sampled survivors of childhood incest had abnormal EEGs, and 36% had clinical seizures. He postulated that this handicap was a risk factor for being sexually abused and exploited by family members. Recently, we hypothesized that early childhood abuse or trauma could affect the development of the cerebral cortex and limbic system.[6,10–14]

VULNERABLE NEUROBIOLOGICAL TARGETS

The brain is a plastic organ whose final form and function are guided by genes but sculpted by early experience. Although early stress and trauma could conceivably have an impact on all known aspects of postnatal brain development, we postulated that some brain regions and functions may be particularly vulnerable.[14] These targets include the hippocampus, amygdala, prefrontal cortex, and corpus callosum.

[a]The research reported in this review is supported by National Institute of Mental Health grant MH-53636 (to M.H.T.) and NARSAD Young Investigator Award (to C.A.G.).

[b]Present address: Department of Psychiatry, Teikyo University, Tokyo, Japan.

160

Hippocampus

The hippocampus plays a critical role in memory storage and retrieval,[15] and may be a primary locus for the generation of dissociative states.[16] The hippocampus and parahippocampal gyrus may play a dominant role in the pathophysiology of generalized anxiety and panic disorder.[17] Furthermore, the septal area and hippocampus are crucial components of the behavioral inhibitory system, whose degree of inhibitory influence is modulated by serotonergic inputs.[18] Thus, the hippocampal area may subserve anxiogenic, dissociative, amnestic, and disinhibitory sequelae of trauma. The hippocampus is a likely target for the effects of early stress as neurogenesis continues into postnatal life, and the cellular organization of the hippocampus can be markedly affected by levels of corticosteroids, which can exert both reversible and irreversible effects on hippocampal pyramidal cells.[19]

Amygdala

The interconnecting amygdaloid nuclei have been strongly implicated in the control of aggressive, oral, and sexual behavior.[15] Amygdaloid nuclei are also critically involved in the formation of emotional memory and in stress-induced memory enhancement.[20] The amygdaloid nuclei are some of the most sensitive brain structures to the development of kindling, in which repeated intermittent stimulation produces greater and greater alterations in neuronal excitability that may eventually result in seizures.[21,22] van der Kolk and Greenberg[23] have proposed that repeated traumatization, particularly child abuse, may lead to limbic kindling and to the emergence of inappropriate aggression and sexual activity.

Prefrontal Cortex

The prefrontal cortex is critical for the temporal organization of behavior and integrates motor activity and speech with recent sensory information.[24] By the nature of its connections it is ideally suited to subserve "executive" cognitive functions and to control elements of attention and reward.[25] Recent studies indicate that the prefrontal cortex serves as working memory, holding relevant information "on-line" and updating past and current information on a moment-to-moment basis.[26] The prefrontal cortex appears to be crucial for detecting changes in the external environment and for discriminating between internally and externally derived models of the world.[27] Damage to the prefrontal cortex, particularly irritative lesions, can produce marked changes in personality with emergence of impulsive behavior, "emotional incontinence," poor self-control, impaired attention, deficient capacity to monitor reality, and dulled awareness of the consequences of one's actions.[15,27]

The prefrontal cortex has the most delayed ontogeny of any brain region. Major projections to the prefrontal cortex scarcely begin to myelinate until adolescence, and development continues well into the third decade.[28-31] Dopamine and other monoamine projections to the prefrontal cortex are specifically activated by stress.[32-34] Thus, it is conceivable that stress activates the developing prefrontal cortex and alters its development. We have theorized that stress may produce precocial maturation of the prefrontal cortex, leading to signs of early maturation ("parentified child"), but it may arrest the development of this region, preventing it from reaching full adult capacity.[14]

Corpus Callosum and Hemispheric Integration/Dominance

Evidence suggests that the degree and direction of brain laterality are controlled by genetic, hormonal, and experiential factors.[35-38] Denenberg[36] has shown in animals that early experience exerts significant effects on the structure of the corpus callosum. Interestingly, these effects are gender specific. Cynader *et al.*[39] have also shown in kittens that the normal bidirectional flow of information from the right and left hemispheres through the corpus callosum can be affected by early experience. In extreme circumstances the corpus callosum can be so affected that communication becomes entirely unidirectional. In such a situation a portion of one hemisphere becomes capable of transmitting information to the corresponding region of the other hemisphere and can affect its activity. However, this portion of the receiving hemisphere is unable to exert any influence on the transmitting hemisphere. This could lead to an extreme instance of hemispheric dominance. Human research suggests that lateralized differences in frontal cortical activity may be established very early in life and play a decisive role in temperamental reactions.[40] It is conceivable that early stress, through effects on the corpus callosum and cortex, could influence the degree of hemispheric integration or produce patterns of anomalous dominance. This, in turn, could lead to various forms of psychopathology.[12]

CLINICAL STUDIES

Early Abuse and Ratings of Limbic Dysfunction in Adulthood

To explore the potential relationship between early abuse and limbic system dysfunction, we devised a self-report questionnaire, the Limbic System Checklist-33 (LSCL-33; 10), to evaluate the frequency with which patients experienced 33 symptoms often encountered as ictal temporal lobe epilepsy (TLE) phenomena, based on the work of the Spiers *et al.*[41] These items consisted of paroxysmal somatic disturbances, brief hallucinatory events, visual phenomena, automatism, and dissociative experiences. From the items a total score was derived, as well as subscale scores for somatic, sensory, behavioral, and mnemonic disturbances. Psychometric evaluation indicated that LSCL-33 scores had high test-retest reliability ($r = 0.92$; $n = 16$). Scores were low in normal controls (<10) and elevated in patients with documented TLE (>23). LSCL-33 scores correlated well with the Dissociative Experience Scale[42] ($r = 0.81$, $n = 16$) and the somatization ($r = 0.65$) and psychoticism ($r = 0.57$) subscales of the Hopkins Symptom Checklist-90.[43]

To evaluate the association between early abuse and limbic system dysfunction, we studied 253 adults presenting for outpatient psychiatric assessment (mean age 34 years, 58% female). The Life Experience Questionnaire (LEQ[44]) was used to ascertain abuse history, which had a prominent effect on total LSCL-33 scores (p < 0.0001). Subjects who report no abuse ($n = 109$) had mean LSCL-33 scores of 13.6 ($\pm$ 11.3).

Total LSCL-33 scores were 38% greater in patients with physical abuse, but not sexual abuse ($p < 0.01$, $n = 77$), and were 49% greater in patients with sexual abuse, but not physical abuse ($p < 0.02$, $n = 26$). Patients who acknowledged both physical and sexual abuse ($n = 41$) had scores 113% greater than that of patients denying abuse ($p < 0.0001$). LSCL-33 scores from both males and females were affected by abuse in the same manner.

As expected, abuse before the age of 18 had a greater impact than did abuse after age 18. Patients who were sexually (but not physically) abused before age 18 had scores that were 66% higher than those of patients who were never abused ($p < 0.003$). In contrast, patients who were sexually (but not physically) abused after age 18 had scores that were no different from those of nonabused patients. Similarly, subjects who were physically abused (but not sexually) before age 18 had scores that were 52% higher than those of nonabused patients ($p < 0.004$), whereas patients physically abused after age 18, with no history of sexual abuse, had scores that were not significantly greater than those of nonabused patients. Although age of first abuse was a significant factor for those patients subjected to either physical *or* sexual abuse, patients with physical *and* sexual abuse were strongly affected regardless of age of first abuse. Compared to nonabused patients, subjects with combined physical and sexual abuse prior to age 18 had scores that were 147% greater ($p < 0.0001$), whereas patients abused both physically and sexually for the first time after age 18 had scores 127% greater ($p < 0.0002$).

These findings are consistent with our hypothesis that early childhood abuse may lead to limbic system dysfunction. However, several limitations are present. First, the LSCL-33 is a new instrument, and further analysis of the validity and reliability of this scale is necessary. Confirmation of limbic system dysfunction through more direct assessment of brain function or anatomy is crucial. Second, abuse history was derived entirely from self-report with no attempt to provide any degree of independent confirmation. The second study was designed to remedy these deficiencies.

Association between Early Abuse and EEG Abnormalities in Childhood

The aim of this study was to ascertain if early abuse was associated with direct evidence of neurobiological abnormalities. A chart review was conducted to blindly examine the association between different types of abuse and quantifiable abnormalities on imaging, EEG, and neuropsychological testing.[11] Medical records of 115 consecutive admissions to a child and adolescent psychiatric hospital were reviewed. Eleven cases were eliminated because of possible preexisting neurological abnormalities. The remaining 104 patients were on average 13 years old. Sixty percent were adolescents (13 years or older) and 51% were male.

Neurological assessments were divided into four categories: imaging studies (CT or MRI scans), electrophysiological studies (EEG or BEAM), neurological examination, and neuropsychological testing. Each category was rated as normal or abnormal. Overall, 98% of the neurological assessment categories were scored identically by the two assigned clinician raters. Discrepancies were satisfactorily resolved by a blind third clinician rater, who agreed with one of the two discrepant scores. Four groups were established on the basis of abuse ratings. Subjects in the nonabused group had no evidence of abuse in any of the four categories ($n = 27$). Patients in the psychological abuse group had experienced psychological abuse or neglect, but had not been physically or sexually abused ($n = 22$). Patients in the overall physical/sexual abuse group had experienced probable or definite physical or sexual abuse ($n = 55$). Patients in the severe physical/sexual abuse subgroup had a documented history of severe physical or sexual abuse ($n = 38$).

No differences were noted between abused and nonabused patients in the prevalence of abnormal neurological examinations or abnormal neuropsychological tests. Abnormal EEG studies were found in 26.9% of the nonabused patients, but in 54.4% of the patients with a history of early trauma ($p = 0.021$). Abnormal EEG studies were observed in 42.9% of the patients with psychological abuse, 59.6% of the total sample with physical/sexual abuse ($p = 0.014$), and 71.9% of the subsample with serious physical/sexual abuse ($p = 0.0013$). Most abnormal EEG results occurred in frontotemporal or anterior regions. In the nonabused group, 19.2% of the patients had abnormalities within this area. In contrast, 47.1% of abused patients had EEG abnormalities in this region ($p = 0.018$). Abused and nonabused patients differed most clearly in the prevalence of left-sided frontotemporal abnormalities ($p = 0.036$). They did not differ in the prevalence of either right-sided abnormalities ($p > 0.8$) or abnormalities that were seen bilaterally or were not specifically localized ($p > 0.5$). Neuropsychological test results were reviewed for evidence of right-left hemispheric asymmetries (i.e., substantially better visual-spatial ability than verbal performance). Overall, in the nonabused group, left-hemisphere deficits were 2.25-fold more prevalent than right-hemisphere deficits. In the total abuse group, left-sided deficits were 6.67-fold more prevalent than right, and left hemisphere deficits were eightfold more prevalent than right-sided deficits in patients with a history of psychological abuse. Therefore, abuse appears to be associated with an increased prevalence of left-sided EEG abnormalities and an increased prevalence of right-left hemispheric asymmetries.

Right-Left Evoked Response Asymmetry during Recall of Unpleasant Early Memories in Psychologically Traumatized Subjects

Probe auditory evoked potentials (AEPs) represent a cost-effective means of studying functional hemispheric activity. Schiffer *et al.*[13] used probe attenuation as a measure of hemispheric activity to further study the effects of early trauma on cerebral laterality. We specifically sought to assess whether early traumatic experience affected the degree of right-sided activation during recall of a painful childhood memory. To evaluate this hypothesis, hemispheric brain activity was measured in adult subjects under two conditions: first, during recall of a neutral memory, and then during recall of an unpleasant affectively laden early experience. Probe AEPs were used as an index of hemispheric activity. Subjects were exposed to repeated auditory clicks, while measuring the amplitude of the average evoked potential EEG response. While exposed to the clicks, the subjects were asked to engage in a mental activity. Theoretically, if one hemisphere is more actively involved in a competing mental activity than the other hemisphere, then AEPs recorded over the more distracted hemisphere should be weaker.[45-47]

Twelve unmedicated right-handed adult volunteers who had a history of psychological abuse were recruited and compared to 12 similar normal controls. No participants had an active DSM-IIIR Axis I or II disorder. Electrodes were applied at C3 and C4 and referenced to linked ear electrodes. The subjects fixed and maintained gaze on a mark in front of them throughout each recording period and were closely watched for eye movements. They were first asked to remember and reflect on a recent ordinary work or school situation. They were asked to raise their right hand at the wrist at the start and to lower it when they were actively remembering the situation. Recording of AEPs commenced when they lowered their hands (binaural 86-dB clicks at 3 Hz × 250 ms; 300–600 epochs). If it appeared that a readable evoked potential response had not been obtained, the recording was repeated. Following the recording, the subject was given several queries taken from the Profile of Mood States (POMS) scale to monitor their level of tension, anger, sadness, hopelessness, nervousness, panic, and guilt. A psychiatrist then engaged the subject in an empathic psychiatric interview lasting about 15 minutes in which he endeavored to have the subject share, with emotion, a painful childhood memory. When the psychiatrist felt that the subject was affectively reexperiencing the memory, the subject was asked to try to continue to maintain memory and mood, but without speech or motion, so that evoked potentials could be measured. Following the recording, the abbreviated POMS scale was again used to measure emotional state. The unpleasant memory task was always presented after the neutral memory task because of concern that the lingering effects of the unpleasant memories would interfere with the neutral task. The averaged AEP response from each condition was blindly read by an experienced research electroencephalographer to obtain N1 and P2 peaks.

For each task an asymmetry index, $100 \times (C3 - C4)/(C3 + C4)$, was calculated from measurements of the N-P amplitudes at C3 (left auditory cortex) and C4 (right auditory cortex). These leads were used to reduce contaminating effects of volume conduction. Of the 24 subjects studied, four had to be eliminated because at least one of their tracings did not show clearly defined peaks. The final subject pool consisted of 10 subjects (32.9 yr; M5/F5) who had experienced significant childhood trauma and 10 subjects (33.0 yr; M4/F6) without childhood trauma. No significant difference was noted between the POMS scores of the two groups during the neutral memories. Subjects in both groups had higher mean abbreviated POMS scores following the unpleasant memory than following the neutral memory. A few significant differences between groups in POMS subscales were noted following the unpleasant memory. The most significant difference between groups was for changes in the degree of hopelessness.

Significant changes were noted in the asymmetry index as a consequence of the neutral vs unpleasant memory condition ($F[1,18] = 8.61$, $p = 0.009$), and there was a significant memory condition by group interaction ($F[1,18] = 6.32$, $p = 0.02$). The victim group displayed significant left dominant asymmetry during the neutral memory (asymmetry index = -15.9; $p < 0.02$) and relative right dominance during the unpleasant memory (asymmetry index = $+12.2$; $p < 0.10$). Overall, these subjects displayed a highly significant shift in their asymmetry index between memory conditions ($p = 0.007$). On the other hand, the control group did not display a significant asymmetry during either the neutral task (asymmetry index = -2.1; ns) or the unpleasant memory task (asymmetry index = $+0.1$; ns). Neither was there a significant shift in asymmetry index between the two tasks ($p = 0.746$). Analysis of covariance was used as a partial means of testing whether group differences between controls and victims in the degree of asymmetry shift were a consequence of group differences in the degree of emotional response to the memories. Statistically significant group differences in the degree of shift persisted even when change in emotional responses were used as covariates. Hence, differences between groups in the degree of asymmetry shift did not appear to be a direct consequence of differences in expressed emotional response. These findings suggest the intriguing possibility that the two hemispheres may function more autonomously in patients with a history of childhood abuse.

Early Abuse and Development of Cortical EEG Coherence in Children

The goal of this study was to ascertain if early childhood trauma was associated with alterations in the pattern or degree of cortical development. EEG coherence is a sophisticated quantitative technique that can provide important information about brain development. Briefly, EEG coherence assesses the degree of synchrony between two EEG leads across a portion of the bandwidth. EEG coherence is determined by two primary compartments.[48,49] The first compartment represents the short axonal connections of neighboring pyramidal cells, whereas the second compartment represents long axonal propagation via intracortical association pathways. These two compartments exert opposite effects on coherence. Local cortical connections process and alter the signal, so coherence decreases with cortical differentiation. In contrast, long axon pathways propagate the signal without distortion. Thus, coherence increases with myelination and development of association pathways.

Many studies have shown that coherence measures can provide useful information about brain development. EEG coherence has been fruitfully applied to the study of normal development, mental retardation, and learning disorders.[50,51] Coherence measures have also been reported to be particularly useful, and more powerful than spectral EEG measures, in discerning differences between controls and patients with schizophrenia.[52–57] EEG coherence measures appear well suited for detecting the relatively subtle structural brain abnormalities that presumably occur in schizophrenia, and coherence is less susceptible to medication effects than is spectral EEG.[52,53] EEG coherence changes throughout childhood and adolescence, in concert with Piaget's stages of intellectual development.[50] Thus, EEG coherence is a suitable technique to test the hypothesis that early childhood abuse affects cortical maturation and laterality.

Fifteen child or adolescent inpatients (mean age 10.7 ± 2.5 yr, M : F = 7 : 8, 10 medicated) with a history of intense physical or sexual abuse, confirmed by the Department of Social Services, were recruited. The controls were 15 healthy volunteers (10.1 ± 3.1 yr, M : F = 6 : 9), assessed by clinical interview and the Child Behavior Checklist.[58,59] All subjects were between 6 and 15 years of age, were right handed, and had no history of neurological disorders or abnormal intelligence. No subject had a learning disorder diagnosis. Diagnostic data were derived from discharge diagnosis (DSM-IIIR) and structured clinical interviews.

EEG measures (QSI-9000; Ontario, Canada) were obtained from 19 gold electrodes of the International 10-20 System[60] referenced to linked ear lobes. Eye movements were detected using a bipolar vertical electrooculogram lead. A single forehead electrode served as ground. Electrode resistances were below 5 K ohms. Typical amplification was 80 or 40 K, with bandpass filters set at 0.5-30 Hz. Sampling time was 9.77 ms. Subjects were instructed to minimize movement and to be alert during the tests. At least 8 minutes of eyes-closed resting EEG were recorded. Results were carefully examined to eliminate epochs with eye movement or muscle artifact. About 40 seconds (16 epochs) of artifact free recording were selected for analysis.

Intrahemispheric coherence measures were computed for the alpha (8-13.6 Hz) frequency band according to Thatcher *et al.*[48] Measures of EEG coherence between all combinations of the eight lateralized leads per hemisphere (28 measurements) were averaged to provide a composite hemisphere measure. These measures were log transformed (log(X/(100-X))) to obtain gaussian distributions for statistical analysis.[48,61] Lateralized differences were assessed by calculating a laterality index on the nontransformed composite data. The laterality index was defined as 100 × (Left − Right)/Averaged(Left + Right).

To minimize the number of statistical comparisons, data were aggregated into composite measures, and only discrete prespecified hypothesis were tested. Three primary questions were addressed. First, was there any evidence for asymmetric cortical development? This was tested by ascertaining whether there was a difference between abused patients and controls in the average level of right vs left hemisphere alpha coherence. If this were true, then the next justifiable question would be whether these asymmetries could be localized to particular regions. The method of Besthorn *et al.*[62] was used to calculate average short-distance coherence for each lead. The third question, given evidence for an overall asymmetry in EEG coherence, was whether the asymmetry was a consequence of abnormalities in myelination or cortical differentiation. This was assessed by calculating the rate of decay of alpha EEG coherence over intraelectrode unit distance. Thatcher *et al.*[48] proposed that the rate of decline in coherence over distance reflected the ratio of short axon fibers to long axon fibers and that a rapid rate of decline was associated with a greater degree of cortical differentiation. To calculate the rate of decay, all common reference intrahemispheric coherence measures were grouped into three levels of distance on the basis of intraelectrode unit distance within the 10-20 system grid. Rate of decay was calculated for each subject using a power decay function ($y = Ax^{-b}$), where b is the decay slope.

The first question was whether significant differences existed in composite left hemisphere versus right hemisphere coherence. A significant interaction emerged between hemisphere and group ($F[1,27] = 7.76$, $p < 0.01$), which was influenced by age ($F[1,27] = 8.39$, $p = 0.007$), but not gender. Abused children had greater average left hemisphere coherence than did normal children ($F[1,27] = 8.56$, $p = 0.007$), but a comparable degree of right hemisphere coherence ($F[1,27] = 0.11$, $p > 0.7$). In controls, the average age-covaried, within-subject laterality index was −3.21%, indicating a nonsignificantly lower level of left vs right hemisphere coherence. In contrast, abused children had an average laterality index of +7.21%, indicating significantly greater left vs right coherence ($p < 0.02$). The prominent difference between groups in the degree and direction of the laterality index is indicative of a reversed cerebral asymmetry ($F[1,27] = 7.41$, $p = 0.01$). Within the abused group, medication use appeared to have a prominent effect on the degree of asymmetry ($F[1,12] = 11.47$, $p = 0.005$). Unmedicated abused patients had a much greater (and more abnormal) laterality index than did abused patients receiving pharmacotherapy (unmedicated: +17.7%; medicated: +1.4%).

No apparent relationship was noted between degree of asymmetry and diagnosis. Abused children meeting DSM-IIIR criteria for major depression ($n = 6$) had about the same laterality index as did abused children who did not meet criteria (+6.0 vs +7.3; $F[1,13] = 0.04$, ns). There were also no asymmetry differences between abused children who did ($n = 6$) or did not meet criteria for PTSD (+9.2 vs +5.2; $F[1,13] = 0.53$, ns) or who met ($n = 7$) or did not meet criteria for conduct or oppositional defiant disorder (+10.2 vs +3.9; $F[1,13] = 1.12$, $p > 0.3$). The association between abuse and EEG coherence also emerged in a subgroup of seven children subjected only to sexual abuse without concomitant physical abuse. Age-covaried laterality index was +10.9 in the abused and −3.6 in controls ($F[1,19] = 12.48$, $p = 0.002$). This lends support to the notion that the coherence abnormalities are not a consequence of direct physical injury.

Neighboring electrode pairs were averaged to ascertain the most significant regions of common reference alpha hemispheric asymmetry. In abused subjects, significant left > right asymmetries (based on log transformed values) were observed in central (C3-C4; $p < 0.05$), posterior temporal (T5-T6; $p < 0.02$), and parietal regions (P3-P4; $p < .001$). No significant regional asymmetry was found in normals. Abused subjects differed from normal subjects in degree of asymmetry in central (C3-C4; $p = 0.02$), temporal (T3-T4; $p < 0.10$; T5-T6; $p < 0.03$), and parietal regions (P3-P4; $p < 0.055$).

Common reference alpha EEG coherence decayed markedly over distance, and the rate of decay was well fit by a power function. In normal controls, coherence decayed at a numerically more rapid rate in the left hemisphere (composite group slope = −1.213) than in the right hemisphere (group slope = −1.088), which is consistent with anatomical studies that indicate greater fissuring and higher cell density in the left hemisphere of normal subjects. In contrast, pediatric patients with a history of severe abuse had a lower rate of decay in the left hemisphere than the right hemisphere (composite group slop = −0.922 vs −0.970; Group X hemisphere interaction $F[1,27] = 4.53$, $p < 0.05$). Overall, normal controls had, on average, a 16.3% *greater* rate of coherence decay (age corrected) in their left vs right hemisphere, whereas abused subjects had a 6.8% *lower* rate of coherence decay in their left vs right hemisphere ($F[1,27] = 4.59$, $p < 0.04$). These findings suggest that coherence differences between abused children and controls are a result of diminished left hemisphere differentiation in the abused group. Differences between abused patients and controls were robust, topographically widespread, and more statistically significant than were coherence abnormalities previously reported in schizophrenic subjects.[52-57] Overall, this study represents one of the first experimental attempts to test the hypothesis that early childhood abuse may have a significant impact on cortical development. The present findings of reversed hemispheric asymmetry and greater left hemisphere coherence in abused subjects support this hypothesis.

Corpus Callosum Morphology of Abused or Neglected Children

The corpus callosum is the major myelinated fiber tract in the brain that connects the right and the left hemispheres. We hypothesized that the functional differences in the lateralization of EEG coherence and evoked potentials observed in children and adults who suffered early abuse may be associated with attenuated maturation of the corpus callosum. To test this hypothesis, medical records of 115 consecutive pediatric patients admitted to McLean Hospital were reviewed. Patients were eliminated for possible preexisting neurological abnormalities unrelated to abuse, including loss of consciousness and neurological complications. All subjects had normal intelligence except one who was evaluated as learning disordered and another patient with borderline mentality. MRI records were available on 51 subjects from this group. Mean age was 12.9 ± 2.9 years, and 52% were male. Records were blindly reviewed by two independent raters using all clinical information and Department of Social Service investigative reports to ascertain if the children had a history of physical abuse, sexual abuse, psychological abuse (witnessing domestic violence, verbal abuse), or neglect. Physical, sexual, and psychological abuse was scored as 0, 1, or 2 to indicate that there was no abuse, abuse of modest severity, or documented and severe abuse. Neglect was scored as present or absent.

Magnetic resonance images consisted of T1 weighted scans obtained from a GE 1.5 Tesla Signa magnet. Archived films were scanned into a computer workstation with OPTIMAS and subsequently analyzed with IMAGE (National Institutes of Health, v 1.55). All anatomical measurements of the corpus callosum were obtained from the midsagittal image. An automated algorithm was used to divide the corpus callosum into seven regions as defined by Witelson.[63] To control for differences in corpus callosum size due to age or gender,[64] regional volume was corrected for total brain volume. Statistical differences between groups were calculated using multivariate analysis of covariance (MANCOVA), with age as a covariate. MRI measurements were performed by independent researchers blind to all clinical variables.

Data were analyzed to determine if there was a relationship between relative regional corpus callosum size and history of physical, sexual, psychological abuse or neglect and whether these effects differed by gender. Both physical abuse and neglect produced strong effects on regional corpus callosum size that varied by gender (physical abuse: $F[12,78] = 3.35$, $p < 0.0006$; neglect: $F[6,41] = 3.30$, $p < 0.01$). Neither sexual abuse nor psychological abuse was associated with alterations in regional corpus callosum size (sexual abuse $F[12,78] = 0.49$, $p > 0.9$; psychological abuse $F[12,78] = 1.19$, $p > 0.3$). Physical abuse was associated with the most prominent gender-specific alterations in region 4 of the corpus callosum ($F[2,44] = 6.08$, $p = 0.005$), which largely interconnects right and left motor cortex. Physically abused males had a 25.5% reduction in the relative volume of this region ($p < 0.03$). In contrast, physically abused females had a nonsignificant 17.4% increase in volume ($p = 0.16$). Neglect exerted gender-specific statistical effects on regions 3 ($F[1,46] = 4.20$, $p < 0.05$), 4($F[1,46] = 8.63$, $p = 0.005$), and 6 ($F[1,46] = 14.35$, $p = 0.0004$). These regions interconnect premotor, motor, and superior temporal/posterior parietal regions, respectively.[63] As with physical abuse, neglect was associated with gender-dichotomous effects. Neglected males had a 24.8% reduction in region 3 ($F[1,23] = 12.21$, $p < 0.002$), and a 25.6% reduction in region 4 ($F[1,23] = 10.26$, $p = 0.003$). Neglected females had an 89.0% increase in region 1 ($F[1,22] = 8.85$, $p = 0.007$) and a 51.6% increase in region 6 ($F[1,22] = 11.18$, $p = 0.003$). It should be born in mind that abnormally large regions of the corpus callosum can also reflect pathology.

Bulges may be caused by failure of fibers to cross the callosum, remaining instead within the body, analogous to formation of Probst body in callosal agenesis (P. Henninger, personal communication, 1996). Whereas physical abuse and neglect were associated with prominent alterations in corpus callosum anatomy, no differences were noted in total brain size as a consequence of the abuse condition.

Physical abuse and neglect were associated with alterations in the regional anatomy of the corpus callosum that varied by gender. Physical abuse or neglect in males was associated with decreased size of the rostral body and anterior midbody of the corpus callosum. Neglect in females was associated with increased size of the rostrum and isthmus of the corpus callosum. Three questions need to be addressed. First, why were physical abuse and neglect rather than sexual or psychological abuse associated with alterations in the corpus callosum? Second, how come physical abuse and neglect were associated with very different alterations in males and females? Third, what are the possible neuropsychiatric implications of these observations.

One possible reason that physical abuse and neglect may be associated with greater effects is that these forms of abuse may be more likely to occur at very early ages including infancy. Also, neglect differs from other forms of abuse, as it basically involves a lack of appropriate stimulation or interaction. Animal studies indicate that early postnatal brain development may be more affected by the presence or absence of stimulation than by the specific nature of the stimulation. Prominent gender differences in the relation between corpus callosum anatomy and early experience are hard to explain, but are consistent with previous findings. Denenberg[36] found that early experience exerted sex-dependent effects on brain laterality of rats. The regions of the corpus callosum associated with physical abuse or neglect in males are involved in the interconnection of premotor and motor cortex. Giedd et al.[65] found a decrease in region 3 in boys with attention deficit/hyperactivity disorder (ADHD) that was inversely correlated with the degree of hyperactivity/impulsivity. Thus, there is some overlap in MRI findings between childhood abuse and ADHD in males. Glod and Teicher[66] recently showed that children with early abuse and PTSD were more active than normal children, but were less hyperactive than children with classic ADHD. We proposed that childhood trauma may produce a phenocopy of ADHD.[66] Neglect in females was associated with major alterations in regions 1 and 6 that interconnect aspects of the prefrontal cortex and superior temporal cortex. These alterations may bear on the laterality of mood and emotional expression. Studies are in progress to ascertain the association between regional callosal size and measures of laterality in males and females with childhood abuse.

CAVEATS AND CAUTIONS

Although the studies we conducted are consistent with our primary hypothesis, the findings are correlational in nature and cannot prove the hypothesis. Alternative explanations can also be entertained. For instance, it is possible that the observed abnormalities were not a consequence of abuse, but a risk factor for being abused. While this is plausible, it seems unlikely that most abused individuals acted in a certain manner (because of the neurobiological abnormalities) to invite their own abuse. A more complex alternative is that these abnormalities were inherited and were associated with increased risk of abusive behavior on the part of parents or relatives. Designing ethical studies to tease apart these hypotheses will be challenging. However, animal research provides some support for the primary hypothesis by showing that early experience can exert marked effects on hemispheric laterality.[36]

The most interesting findings to emerge from this program of research are the consistent evidence that early abuse appears to be associated with left hemisphere abnormalities and a reversed left/right hemisphere asymmetry. Our findings are also very consistent with those of Stein *et al.* (this volume) who found that the left but not the right hippocampus was smaller in women with a history of childhood sexual abuse than in normal controls. From these observations we can hypothesize that early abuse exerts a more deleterious effect on left cortical and hippocampal development and may impede hemispheric integration and establishment of normal left cortical dominance.[13] Muller[38] theorized that borderline personality disorder may be the result of deficient hemispheric integration. Other theorists have speculated that a dissociation of hemispheric function may be present in alexithymia[67] and PTSD.[68,69]

Research on hemispheric function strongly suggests that the right hemisphere plays a pivotal role in the perception and expression of emotion[70] particularly negative emotions.[71–74] Deficient right and left hemisphere integration could result in the misperception of affect and foster a situation in which the right and left cerebral cortex may act in an uncooperative manner, giving rise to intrapsychic conflict and splitting.[37,38]

If it is true that early abuse affects brain development, why should the left hemisphere be more vulnerable than the right? There are a number of possibilities. The most trivial explanation is that left-sided abnormalities are secondary to physical injury resulting from head trauma. Right-handed adults may be more likely to strike a child on the left side of the head, although anecdotal information suggests that physically abused children are often struck from behind as well. None of the subjects in the EEG coherence study was known to have sustained traumatic head injury, but we cannot be certain that they did not experience lesser injury. Coherence abnormalities were also present in patients subject only to sexual abuse, making this hypothesis less likely. The second explanation may be sampling bias. It is conceivable that early abuse could affect the development of either hemisphere; however, individuals presenting with psychiatric disturbances may be those with the most pronounced left hemisphere pathology. The third hypothesis is that early stress may activate neurotransmitter systems that are asymmetrically distributed, such as norepinephrine,[75] serotonin,[76,77] or dopamine.[78] Aside from their transmitter functions, these monoamines strongly influence several facets of brain development.[79–83] Thus, overactivating these systems may produce lateralized developmental effects. The fourth hypothesis is that abnormalities in left hemisphere development stem from concomitant verbal abuse, which conceivably could suppress the development of left hemisphere linguistic centers. The fifth hypothesis is that the more rapidly developing hemisphere would be more vulnerable to the consequences of stress. During the first few months the right hemisphere develops more rapidly than the left with more advanced dendritic outgrowth in Broca's area and motor cortex.[84] However, by 5-6 months of age dendritic growth in the left hemisphere surpasses that in the right and continues at a rapid pace for the next few years. Between 3 and 6 years of age the right hemisphere begins to accelerate in its development, although the left hemisphere remains more highly differentiated. Hence, abuse from 6 months until 3-6 years of age may have the greatest differential effect on the left hemisphere. Further research will be required to verify these observations and test these hypotheses.

REFERENCES

1. SACHS, R., J. GOODWIN & B. BRAUN. 1986. The role of childhood abuse in the development of multiple personality. *In* Multiple Personality and Dissociation. B. Braun & R. Kluft, Eds. Guilford. New York, NY.
2. STONE, M. H. 1981. Borderline syndromes: A consideration of subtypes and an overview, directions for research. Psychiatr. Clin. N. Am. **4:** 3-13.
3. HERMAN, J. L., J. C. PERRY & B. A. VAN DER KOLK. 1989. Childhood trauma in borderline personality disorder. Am. J. Psychiatry **146:** 490-495.
4. BECK, J. C. & B. VAN DER KOLK. 1987. Reports of childhood incest and current behavior of chronically hospitalized psychotic women. Am. J. Psychiatry **144:** 1474-1476.
5. BREMNER, J. D. *et al.* 1993. Childhood physical abuse and combat-related posttraumatic stress disorder in Vietnam veterans. Am. J. Psychiatry **150:** 235-239.
6. TEICHER, M. H. 1989. Psychological factors in neurological development. *In* Neurobiological Development. Nestlé Nutrition Workshop, Vol 12. P. Evrard & A. Minkowski, Eds.: 243-258. Raven Press. New York, NY.
7. GREEN, A. *et al.* 1981. Neurological impairment in maltreated children. Child Abuse Neglect **5:** 129-134.
8. GREEN, A. H. 1983. Dimensions of psychological trauma in abused children. J. Am. Assoc. Child Psychiatry **22:** 231-237.
9. DAVIES, R. K. 1979. Incest: Some neuropsychiatric findings. Int. J. Psychiatry Med. **9:** 117-121.
10. TEICHER, M. H. *et al.* 1993. Early childhood abuse and limbic system ratings in adult psychiatric outpatients. J. Neuropsychiatry Clin. Neurosci. **5:** 301-306.
11. ITO, Y. *et al.* 1993. Increased prevalence of electrophysiological abnormalities in children with psychological, physical, and sexual abuse. J. Neuropsychiatry Clin. Neurosci. **5:** 401-408.
12. TEICHER, M. H. *et al.* 1994. Early abuse, limbic system dysfunction, and borderline personality disorder. *In* Biological and Neurobehavioral Studies of Borderline Personality Disorder. K. Silk, Ed. : 177-207. American Psychiatric Association Press. Washington, DC.
13. SCHIFFER, F., M. H. TEICHER & A. C. PAPANICOLAOU. 1995. Evoked potential evidence for right brain activity during recall of traumatic memories. J. Neuropsychiatry Clin. Neurosci. **7:** 169-175.
14. TEICHER, M. H. *et al.* 1996. Neurophysiological mechanisms of stress response in children. *In* Severe Stress and Mental Disturbances in Children. C. Pfeffer, Ed.: 59-84. American Psychiatric Association Press. Washington, DC.
15. PINCHUS, J. H. & G. J. TUCKER. 1978. Behavioral Neurology: 58-79. Oxford. New York, NY.
16. MESULAM, M.-M. 1981. Dissociative states with abnormal temporal lobe EEG: Multiple personality and the illusion of possession. Arch. Neurol. **38:** 176-181.
17. TEICHER, M. H. 1988. Biology of anxiety. Med. Clin. N. Amer. **72:** 791-814.
18. DEPUE, R. A. & M. R. SPOONT. 1986. Conceptualizing a serotonin trait: A behavioral dimension of constraint. Ann. N.Y. Acad. Sci. **487:** 47-62.
19. SAPOLSKY R. M. *et al.* 1990. Hippocampal damage associated with prolonged glucocorticoid exposure in primates. J. Neurosci. **10:** 2897-2902.
20. McGAUGH, J. L. *et al.* 1990. Involvement of the amygdaloid complex in neuromodulatory influences on memory storage. Neurosci. Biobehav. Rev. **14:** 425-431.

21. GODDARD, C. V., D. C. McINTRYE & C. K. LEECH. 1969. A permanent change in brain functioning resulting from daily electrical stimulation. Exp. Neurol. **25:** 295-330.

22. POST, R. M., D. R. RUBINOW & J. C. BALLENGER. 1984. Conditioning, sensitization and kindling: Implications for the course of affective illness. *In* Neurobiology of Mood Disorders. R. M. Post & J. C. Ballenger, Eds.: 432-466. Williams & Wilkins. Baltimore, MD.

23. VAN DER KOLK, B. & M. S. GREENBERG. 1987. The psychobiology of the trauma response: Hyperarousal, constriction, and addiction to traumatic reexposure. *In* Psychological Trauma. B. van der Kolk, Ed.: 63-87. American Psychiatric Press. Washington, DC.

24. FUSTER, J. M. 1991. The prefrontal cortex and its relation to behavior. Prog. Brain Res. **87:** 201-211.

25. WEINBERGER, D. R. 1987. Implications of normal brain development for the pathogenesis of schizophrenia. Arch. Gen. Psychiatry **44:** 660-669.

26. GOLDMAN-RAKIC, P. S. 1994. Working memory dysfunction in schizophrenia. J. Neuropsychiatry Clin. Neurosci. **6:** 348-357.

27. KNIGHT, R. T., M. F. GRABOWECKY & D. SCABINI. 1995. Role of human prefrontal cortex in attention control. Adv. Neurol. **66:** 21-34.

28. GOLDMAN, P. S. 1971. Functional development of the prefrontal cortex in early life and the problem of neuronal plasticity. Exp. Neurol. **32:** 366-387.

29. ALEXANDER, G. E. & P. S. GOLDMAN. 1978. Functional development of the dorsolateral prefrontal cortex: An analysis utilizing reversible cryogenic depression. Brain Res. **143:** 233-249.

30. FUSTER, J. M. 1980. The Prefrontal Cortex: Anatomy, Physiology, and Neuropsychology of the Frontal Lobe. Raven Press. New York, NY.

31. WEINBERGER, D. R. 1987. Implications of normal brain development for the pathogenesis of schizophrenia. Arch. Gen. Psychiatry **44:** 660-669.

32. REINHARD, J. F. JR., M. J. BANNON & R. H. ROTH. 1982. Acceleration by stress of dopamine synthesis and metabolism in prefrontal cortex: Antagonism by diazepam. Naunyn-Schmiedeberg's Arch. Pharmacol. **318:** 374-377.

33. KNORR, A. M., A. Y. DEUTCH & R. H. ROTH. 1989. The anxiogenic β-carboline FG-7142 increases *in vivo* and *in vitro* tyrosine hydroxylation in the prefrontal cortex. Brain Res. **495:** 335-361.

34. DEUTCH, A. Y. & R. H. ROTH. 1990. The determinants of stress induced activation of the prefrontal cortical dopamine system. Progr. Brain Res. **85:** 367-403.

35. GALIN, D. 1977. Lateral specialization and psychiatric issues: Speculations on development and the evolution of consciousness. Ann. N.Y. Acad. Sci. **299:** 397-411.

36. DENENBERG, V. H. 1983. Lateralization of function in rats. Am. J. Physiol. **245:** R505-R509.

37. JOSEPH, R. 1988. The right cerebral hemisphere: Emotion, music, visual-spatial skills, body-image, dreams, and awareness. J. Clin. Psychol. **44:** 630-673.

38. MULLER, R. J. 1992. Is there a neural basis for borderline splitting? Compr. Psychiatry **33:** 92-104.

39. CYNADER, M., F. LEPORE & J. P. GUILLEMOT. 1981. Inter-hemispheric competition during postnatal development. Nature **290:** 139-140.

40. FOX, N. A. & R. J. DAVIDSON. 1986. Taste-elicited changes in facial signs of emotion and the asymmetry of brain electrical activity in human newborns. Neuropsychologia **24:** 417-422.

41. SPIERS, P. A. *et al.* 1985. Temporolimbic epilepsy and behavior. *In* Principles of Behavioral Neurology. M.-M. Mesulam, Ed.: 289-326. F. A. Davis. Philidelphia, PA.

42. BERNSTEIN, E. M. & F. W. PUTNAM. 1986. Development, reliability and validity of a dissociation scale. J. Nerv. Ment. Dis. **174:** 727-735.

43. DEROGATIS, L. R. *et al.* 1974. The Hopkins symptoms checklist (HSCL): A self-report symptom inventory. Behav. Sci. **19:** 1-15.

44. BRYER, J. B. *et al.* 1987. Childhood sexual and physical abuse as factors in adult psychiatric illness. Am. J. Psychiatry **144:** 1426–1430.

45. PAPANICOLAOU, A. C. & J. JOHNSTONE. 1984. Probe evoked potentials: Theory, method and applications. Int. J. Neurosci. **24:** 107–131.

46. PAPANICOLAOU, A. C. *et al.* 1983. Evoked potential indices of selective hemispheric engagement in affective and phonetic tasks. Neuropsychologia **21:** 401–405.

47. PAPANICOLAOU, A. C. *et al.* 1983. Cerebral activation patterns in an arithmetic and a visuospatial processing task. Int. J. Neurosci. **20:** 289–294.

48. THATCHER, R. W., P. J. KRAUSE & M. HRYBYK. 1986. Cortico-cortical associations and EEG coherence: A two compartment model. Electroenceph. Clin. Neurophysiol. **64:** 123–143.

49. THATCHER, R. W. 1992. Cyclic cortical reorganization during early childhood. Brain Cogn. **20:** 24–50.

50. THATCHER, R. W., R. A. WALKER & S. GIUDICE. 1987. Human cerebral hemispheric development at different rates and ages. Science **236:** 1110–1113.

51. MAROSI, E. *et al.* 1992. Maturation of the coherence of EEG activity in normal and learning-disabled children. Electroenceph. Clin. Neurophysiol. **83:** 350–357.

52. FORD, M. R., J. W. GOETHE & D. K. DEKKER. 1986. EEG coherence and power in the discrimination of psychiatric disorders and medication effects. Biol. Psychiatry **21:** 1175–1188.

53. MERRIN, E. L., T. C. FLOYD & G. FEIN. 1989. EEG coherence in unmedicated schizophrenic patients. Biol. Psychiatry **25:** 60–66.

54. HOFFMAN, R. E. *et al.* 1991. EEG coherence of prefrontal areas in normal and schizophrenic males during perceptual activation. J. Neuropsychiatry Clin. Neurosci. **3:** 169–175.

55. MICHELOGIANNIS, S., N. PARITSIS & P. TRIKAS. 1991. EEG coherence during hemispheric activation in schizophrenics. Eur. Arch. Psychiatry Clin. Neurosci. **241:** 31–34.

56. MORRISON-STEWART, S. L. *et al.* 1991. Coherence on electroencephalography and aberrant functional organisation of the brain in schizophrenic patients during activation tasks. Br. J. Psychiatry **159:** 636–644.

57. NAGASE, Y. *et al.* 1992. EEG coherence in unmedicated schizophrenic patients: Topographical study of predominantly never medicated cases. Biol. Psychiatry **32:** 1028–1034.

58. ACHENBACH, T. M. 1978. The child behavior profile I. Boys ages 6 through 11. J. Consult. Clin. Psychol. **46:** 478–488.

59. ACHENBACH, T. M., & C. S. EDELBROCK. 1979. The child behavior profile II. Boys aged 12 to 16 and girls aged 6 to 11 and 12 to 16. J. Consult. Clin. Psychol. **47:** 223–233.

60. JASPER, H. H. 1958. Report of the Committee on Methods of Clinical Examination in Electroencephalography. Electroencephalogr. Clin. Neurophysiol. **10:** 370–375.

61. OKEN, B. S. & K. H. CHIAPPA. 1988. Short-term variability in EEG frequency analysis. Electroencephalogr. Clin. Neurophysiol. **69:** 191–198.

62. BESTHORN, C. *et al.* 1994. EEG coherence in Alzheimer disease. Electroencephalogr. Clin. Neurophysiol. **90:** 242–245.

63. WITELSON, S. F. 1989. Hand and sex differences in the isthmus and genu of the human corpus callosum. Brain **112:** 799–735.

64. GIEDD, J. N. *et al.* 1996. A quantitative MRI study of the corpus callosum in children and adolescents. Dev. Brain Res. **91:** 274–280.

65. GIEDD, J. N. *et al.* 1994. Quantitative morphology of the corpus callosum in attention deficit hyperactivity disorder. Am. J. Psychiatry **151:** 665–669.

66. GLOD, C. A. & M. H. TEICHER. 1996. Relationship between early abuse, posttraumatic stress disorder, and activity levels in prepubertal children. J. Am. Acad. Child Adolesc. Psychiatry **34:** 1384–1393.

67. TENHOUTEN, W. D. *et al.* 1987. Alexithymia and the split brain. V. EEG alpha-band interhemispheric coherence analysis. Psychother. Psychosom. **47:** 1–10.

68. HENRY, J. P. *et al.* 1992. Shared neuroendocrine patterns of post-traumatic stress disorder and alexithymia. Psychosom. Med. **54:** 407–415.

69. ZEITLIN, S. B. *et al.* 1989. Interhemispheric transfer deficit and alexithymia. Am. J. Psychiatry **146:** 1434-1439.
70. ROSS, E. D. 1980. The aprosodias: Functional-anatomic organization of the affective components of language in the right hemisphere. Arch. Neurol. **38:** 561-569.
71. HIRSCHMAN, R. S. & M. A. SAFER. 1982. Hemispheric differences in perceiving positive and negative emotions. Cortex **18:** 569-580.
72. SILBERMAN, E. K. & H. WEINGARTNER. 1986. Hemispheric lateralization of functions related to emotion. Brain Cogn. **5:** 322-353.
73. BOROD, J. C. 1992. Interhemispheric and intrahemispheric control of emotion: A focus on unilateral brain damage. J. Consult. Clin. Psychol. **60:** 339-348.
74. TOMARKEN, A. J. *et al.* 1992. Individual differences in anterior brain asymmetry and fundamental dimensions of emotion. J. Pers. Soc. Psychol. **64:** 676-687.
75. OKE, A. 1979. Lateralization of norepinephrine in human thalamus. Science **200:** 1411-1413.
76. ARATO, M. *et al.* 1991. Serotonergic interhemispheric asymmetry: Neurochemical and pharmaco-EEG evidence. Prog. Neuro-Psychopharm. Biol. Psychiatry **15:** 759-764.
77. ARATO, M. *et al.* 1991. Serotonergic interhemispheric asymmetry: Gender differences in the orbital cortex. Acta Psychiatr. Scand. **84:** 110-111.
78. FLOR-HENRY, P. 1984. Hemispheric laterality and disorders of affect. *In* Neurobiology of Mood Disorders. R. M. Post & J. C. Ballenger, Eds.: 467-480. Williams & Wilkins. Baltimore, MD.
79. NELSON, S. B., M. A. SCHWARTZ & J. D. DANIELS. 1985. Clonidine and cortical plasticity: Possible evidence for noradrenergic involvement. Brain Res. **355:** 39-50.
80. SOTO-MOYANO, R. *et al.* 1991. Yohimbine early in life alters functional properties of interhemispheric connections of rat visual cortex. Brain Res. Bull. **26:** 259-263.
81. AZMITIA, E. C. & P. M. WHITAKER-AZMITIA. 1991. Awakening the sleeping giant: Anatomy and plasticity of the brain serotonergic system. J. Clin. Psychiatry **52** (Suppl): 4-16.
82. TODD, R. D. 1992. Neural development is regulated by classical neuro-transmitters: dopamine D2 receptor stimulation enhances neurite outgrowth. Biol. Psychiatry **31:** 794-807.
83. GELBARD, H. A. 1990. Dopamine D1 receptor development depends of endogenous dopamine. Dev. Brain Res. **56:** 137-140.
84. GALABURDA, A. M. 1984. Anatomical asymmetries in the human brain. *In* Biological Foundations of Cerebral Dominance. N. Geschwind & A. M. Galaburda, Eds. Harvard University Press. Cambridge, MA.

Issues in the Developmental Neurobiology of Traumatic Stress

ROBERT S. PYNOOS, ALAN M. STEINBERG,
EDWARD M. ORNITZ, AND ARMEN K. GOENJIAN

Trauma Psychiatry Program
Department of Psychiatry and Biobehavioral Sciences
and
Brain Research Institute
UCLA School of Medicine
300 Medical Plaza
Los Angeles, California 90024

A NEURODEVELOPMENTAL PERSPECTIVE

Over the last decade, significant advances have been made in characterizing the neurobiology of traumatic stress reactions among adults. Increasing evidence for a similar phenomenology of posttraumatic stress disorder (PTSD) symptoms in adults and school-age children and adolescents[1-3] provides a compelling rationale for the possibility of common neurobiological alterations. If present, such alterations in children and adolescents would be of special concern in view of the potential adverse impact on a wide range of developmental processes.

We recently presented a developmental psychopathology model of traumatic stress in childhood.[4] Such a model emphasizes the complex interrelationship of trauma and developmental progression and the essential linkage between disrupted and normal development. Analogously, investigation of the neurobiology of PTSD among children and adolescents will need to be embedded in a neurodevelopmental framework. This paper provides an overview of selected areas of neurodevelopment and recent findings relevant to this research enterprise.

A key feature of our developmental model of childhood traumatic stress is the prominent role assigned to the trauma-related formation of expectations, as these are expressed in the thought, emotion, behavior, and biology of the developing child. Such traumatic expectations dramatically alter the sense of safety and security of the environment and interpersonal life and the child's sense of personal integrity. Ultimately, a comprehensive neurodevelopmental approach to traumatic stress among children and adolescents will place such investigation within the broader context of the child's evolving capacity for appraising, processing, and responding to danger, trauma, and posttrauma reminders.

OVERVIEW OF DEVELOPMENTAL NEUROBIOLOGY

Investigation of the developmental neurobiology of PTSD requires detailed attention to complex issues in three broad areas. These areas, as proposed by Ornitz,[5] include: (1) maturation of specific brain structures through progressive incremental changes or growth spurts at particular ages, including periods of cortical growth and reorganization; (2) functional physiological correlates, including attention to parallel development among independent subsystems; and (3) associated capacities for cognition and emotional regulation and behavioral responses.

In terms of the maturation of specific brain structures, evidence indicates four periods of major structural change in brain development corresponding with early childhood (15 months to 4 years), late childhood (6-10 years), puberty, and mid-adolescence.[5] These stages in brain growth and cortical reorganization overlap developmental advances in cognitive and emotional function. They also appear to correspond to a progression in children's ability to estimate external danger and to consider preventive and protective intervention by themselves or others.[6]

Based on different sets of experimental evidence, investigators have proposed different ways in which structural brain maturation and childhood traumatic experiences interact. For example, Nadel[7] discussed the importance of differential rates of maturation of the amygdala, hippocampus, and prefrontal regions in terms of relative changes in posttrauma symptoms from alarm reactions, panic, and phobia to posttraumatic stress symptoms from infancy through childhood. He and Jacobs highlighted the role of the hippocampus, its postnatal development, and its progressive and critical function in providing spatial context to danger experiences within a multiple memory system framework.[8,9]

Perry and colleagues[10] proposed that childhood trauma, by differentially affecting maturation of subsystems of the brain, sets their relative contribution to future appraisal of danger and response to traumatic reminders. They argue, for example, that early childhood trauma can alter limbic, mid-brain, and brain stem structures through "use-dependent" modifications secondary to prolonged alarm reactions. They also discuss how cortical development can be retarded by early deprivation and neglect or promoted by an enriched environment, thereby affecting the important adaptive role of cortical modulation of limbic, mid-brain, and brain stem responses to danger and fear. Finally, they express concern over potential long-term adverse developmental effects of combined decreased cortical modulation and increased limbic, mid-brain, and brain stem reactivity on cognition, impulse control, aggressivity, and emotional regulation.

We have described how trauma-induced changes in neuromodulation and physiological reactivity may constitute biological analogs of traumatic expectations.[11] These include CNS response to trauma-related cues and increased focused attention on external stimuli to detect danger and make appropriate defensive responses.[12] Similar to responses to novel stimuli found among inhibited children,[13] these changes may initiate "anticipatory bias," a "state of preparedness" for extreme negative emotions, and "anxiety of premonitions." These traumatic expectations may be associated with recurrent bouts of fear, thrill seeking, or aggression, which seriously affect a child's emerging self-concept, including self-attributions of cowardliness, courage, and fearlessness.[4] Rieder and Cicchetti[14] cogently argued that these changes may have a deleterious effect on general information processing.

Teicher and his colleagues[15] discussed the need to consider the structural impact of early childhood trauma in light of developing hemispheric lateralization in brain organization. Such considerations may prove important to the interpretation of findings of structural deficits among adults with PTSD who may have suffered early childhood trauma.[16,17] In addition, Teicher proposed that early trauma may accelerate neurodevel-

opment in specific brain regions, with subsequent arrest in those regions at a subopti-
mal level.[18] In fact, Bremner *et al.*[18a] recently showed that adults with PTSD who
had experienced childhood abuse had significantly reduced left hippocampal volume
relative to matched controls. Conversely, Ornitz and Pynoos[19] proposed that traumatic
experiences during unstable periods of neurodevelopmental consolidation can induce
regression to an earlier stage of neural structure and function. They emphasize the
potential differential effect of childhood trauma during periods of relative plasticity
or consolidation of neurophysiological pathways.

In terms of the second area, functional physiological correlates, several studies
have indicated changes in hormonal and physiological function associated with child
and adolescent trauma. Putnam and colleagues[20,21] discussed the implications of neurohormonal alterations secondary to childhood sexual abuse occurring during critical
periods in the maturation of hormonal and neuroendocrine systems. Because the
prevalence of certain patterns of sexual abuse varies with age and gender, they argue
for a longitudinal model that recognizes the interaction between the type, frequency,
and duration of trauma and neurodevelopmental stage. The outcome may have secondary developmental consequences, such as precocious sexual development, which
often carry additional developmental risks.

Perry and colleagues[22–24] demonstrated sustained changes in autonomic function
at baseline, downregulation of platelet alpha$_2$-adrenergic receptors, and bidirectional
patterns of reactivity to traumatic reminders among severely traumatized children with
PTSD. These findings suggest underlying alterations in neurohormonal modulation.
Goenjian and colleagues[25] documented chronic PTSD-related alterations in HPA axis
function among adolescents with chronic PTSD similar to those reported among
adults, indicating that common neuroendocrine alterations may occur across age
groups. Ornitz and Pynoos[19] reported alterations in modulation of the acoustic startle
reflex among children exposed to catastrophic violence, indicating the effects of
traumatic exposure on the function of maturing inhibitory startle modulation pathways.
The details of the latter two studies are summarized in the following sections.

HPA AXIS ALTERATIONS AMONG ADOLESCENTS 5 YEARS
AFTER THE 1988 EARTHQUAKE IN ARMENIA

The 1988 catastrophic earthquake in Armenia was one of the most devastating
natural disasters of the 20th century. Spitak, the city closest to the epicenter, was
virtually destroyed with enormous rates of injury and mortality. At the time of the
earthquake, children from this city had been in schools that totally collapsed, with
over half the student body killed. Surviving children had experienced extreme threat
to life, witnessed horrifying deaths, heard agonizing screams from those buried in
the rubble, and suffered extensive loss of family members. Gumri, a city 20 miles
from the epicenter, sustained relatively less damage and loss of life. The children in
Spitak suffered prolonged severe post-earthquake adversities and chronic exposure
to traumatic reminders, including the sights of earthquake debris and unrepaired,
heavily damaged buildings.

As part of our longitudinal studies of children and adolescents from this region,[3,26]
basal cortisol, basal 3-methoxy-4-hydroxyphenylglycol (MHPG) levels, and dexa-

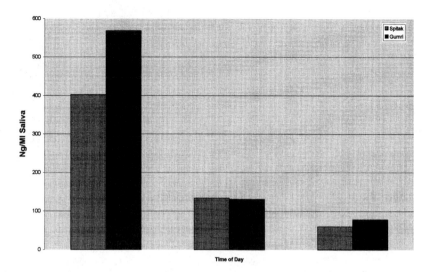

FIGURE 1. Basal salivary cortisol levels among adolescents in Armenia 5 1/2 years after the 1988 earthquake ($n = 37$) on Day 1 at 8:00 AM, 4:00 PM, and 11:00 PM.

methasone suppression of cortisol were measured among 37 mid-adolescents who, as pre-adolescents, were exposed to earthquake-related trauma in these two cities.[25] Five years after the earthquake, baseline saliva samples were obtained on Day 1 at 8:00 AM, 4:00 PM, and 11:00 PM, after which 0.5 mg of dexamethasone was administered. Saliva samples were again obtained at 8:00 AM and 4:00 PM on Day 2.

Findings indicate that the more symptomatic adolescents living in Spitak had: (1) significantly more severe PTSD symptoms; (2) lower 8:00 AM Day 1 basal cortisol levels (FIG. 1); (3) a more rapid decline in MHPG levels over Day 1; and (4) greater 4:00 PM Day 2 suppression of cortisol (FIG. 2). Severity of category B (Intrusion) symptoms was negatively correlated with 8 AM day 1 basal cortisol levels and positively correlated with percentage of suppression by dexamethasone. This latter finding suggests that persistent intrusive symptoms may constitute continued episodes of distress and evoke repeated stress responses which, over time, alter HPA axis function.

This biological profile (i.e., low basal cortisol and hypersuppression by dexamethasone) is the same as that reported among adults with chronic PTSD.[27] Consistent with the adult literature,[28] adolescents in this study who reported comorbid depression with PTSD had this "PTSD" profile rather than that characteristic of primary depression. The debate over underlying pathophysiological mechanisms and potential long-term consequences takes on added meaning when one considers that among these subjects such alterations occurred during formative developmental transitions from late childhood through puberty to mid-adolescence. In addition, these chronic alterations may condition a pattern of biological stress response to future traumatic or stressful life events. Recent evidence from one adult study indicated that an earlier history of trauma is associated with an attenuated acute cortisol response to a subsequent traumatic experience in adulthood.[29]

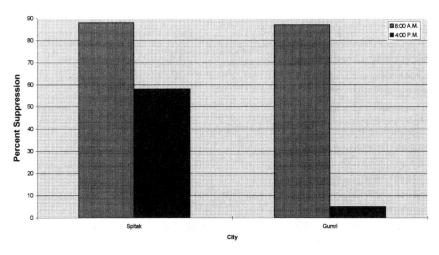

FIGURE 2. Percentage of suppression after dexamethasone among adolescents in Armenia 5 1/2 years after the 1988 earthquake ($n = 37$) on Day 2 at 8:00 AM and 4:00 PM.

MODULATION OF STARTLE IN PTSD

The startle response is a defensive mechanism found in all mammalian species including man.[30] The direct startle pathway in the brain stem is modified by extrinsic mechanisms, two of which are of particular importance to PTSD. In the rat, fear-potentiated startle is the enhancement of the startle response by association with cues that have previously been associated with painful stimuli. In the human, fear potentiation of startle occurs under conditions of threat of painful stimuli, e.g., shock anticipation in the laboratory.[30a] Pre-pulse modulation of startle response is the inhibition of enhancement of the startle response induced by nonstartling stimuli occurring less than 300 ms or more than 1400 ms, respectively, before the starting stimulus.[5,19] Fear potentiation of startle has been noted in adults with PTSD,[31] but it has yet to be studied in children or adolescents with PTSD. Prepulse modulation of startle was studied in adults and children with PTSD.[19] FIGURE 3 depicts the current state of knowledge about brain regions and pathways that modulate fear potentiation and prepulse inhibition of acoustic startle.

Startle modulation in children is different from that in adults in some respects and similar in others. The most striking developmental effect involves prepulse modulation of startle. There is a robust developmental effect on both inhibitory and facilitatory prepulse modulation of startle, with pre-school children failing to show prepulse-induced startle inhibition, while showing exaggerated prepulse-induced startle facilitation. TABLE 1 illustrates the normal developmental course of acquisition of startle inhibition. This developmental effect has been attributed to neuronal pathways extrinsic to the direct startle pathway, as described in FIGURE 3. FIGURE 3 suggests that PPI of startle is mediated by prefrontal and limbic-cortico-striatal-pallidal-brainstem pathways, while fear-potentiated startle is mediated by an independent pathway involving perirhinal-amygdala and striatal pathways to the direct startle pathway in the pons. However, a very recent study[31a] suggests that amygdala mechanisms may also influence PPI through pathways yet to be precisely defined.

Ornitz and Pynoos[19] reported disturbances in inhibitory startle modulation among school-aged children exposed to catastrophic violence. In this study, acoustic startle responses were measured among six children with PTSD who had been in a direct extreme life-threatening situation from a sniper who shot at their school playground with a semiautomatic weapon. From 17-21 months after this traumatic event, their responses were compared to those of six age-matched controls. Acoustic startle responses were recorded as eye blink reflexes. Startle responses were modulated by nonstartling acoustic prestimulation (warning stimuli) to study inhibition and facilitation of the startle reaction.

The findings indicated that the children with PTSD exhibited a significantly reduced level of age-related normal prepulse inhibition (PPI) of startle response, suggesting chronic alteration in PPI modulatory circuitry (FIG. 4, top panel). Additionally, another schoolage child with PTSD was evaluated 3 months after witnessing his father's murder, again by fire from an assailant's semiautomatic rifle. He was restudied on three occasions over the following 2 years. This boy initially exhibited a significant exaggerated startle, with loss of prepulse inhibitory modulation. His initial profile resembled that of a 4-5 year-old child, with evidence of facilitation to a sustained prepulse stimulus (800 ms) as well as a lack of inhibition after short prepulse warning intervals (FIG. 4, bottom panel). The serial evaluations indicated a 2-year lag before achieving an age-appropriate pattern of startle modulation.

Such an extended neurophysiological recovery represents a significant time span over a schoolage child's course of development. The loss of inhibitory control over the startle reflex may interfere with the acquisition of latency skills, such as increased control over activity level and the capacity for reflection, academic learning, and focused attention. In this regard, we found a strong association between the degree of exposure and the presence of new-onset attention deficit disorder symptoms among exposed children 1 year after the school playground sniper attack.[36] Putnam[37] also reported on attention deficit disorder symptoms among prepubertal victims of sexual abuse.

DEVELOPMENTAL CONSIDERATIONS IN FUTURE STUDIES OF TRAUMA-RELATED EFFECTS ON CHILDREN'S INFORMATION PROCESSING

There is increasing interest in studying the effects of trauma on physiological mechanisms that contribute to information processing, such as endogenous event-related potentials. Several researchers[38-40] have presented preliminary evidence for an attenuated P300 among adult patients with PTSD. Disruption of noradrenergic innervation of cortical and limbic structures involved in the generation of P300 by locus coeruleus results in the attenuation of P300 responses recorded at the surface of the monkey cortex.[42a] Future studies among children and adolescents should take into account the developmental course of neurophysiological indicators of information processing and, in a similar manner to the startle, document specific vulnerabilities

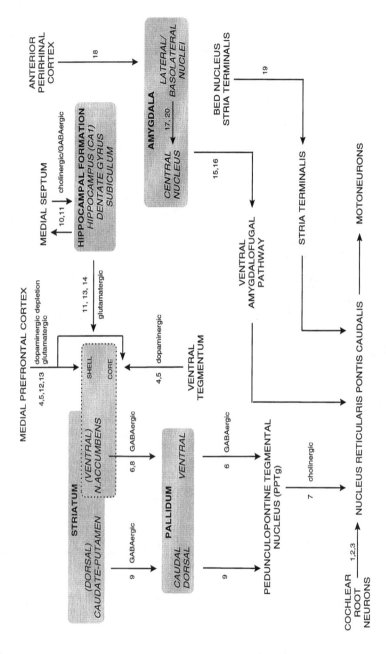

FIGURE 3. (*See legend on facing page.*)

FIGURE 3. Diagram of brain centers and pathways involved in modulating prepulse inhibition (PPI) and fear potentiation of acoustic startle. Numbers indicate references (listed below) that provide evidence to support the diagrammed pathways. For the auditory startle response, the direct startle pathway originates in the cochlear root neurons, passes through the nucleus reticularis pontis caudalis (nRPC), and terminates in motor neurons.[1-3] PPI is mediated by an inhibitory cholinergic projection from the pedunculopontine tegmental nucleus (PPTg) impinging on the nRCP.[7] Fear potentiation is mediated by pathways from both the amygdala and the bed nucleus of the stria terminalis impinging on the nRCP. The acquisition of fear to explicit cues involves the transmission of information from the lateral/basolateral nuclei to the central nucleus of the amygdala,[17,20] whereas recent studies suggest that acquisition of fear to contextual cues depends on both the central nucleus of the amygdala[15,16] and the bed nucleus of the stria terminalis.[19] The effectiveness of the amygdala in mediating fear-potentiated startle depends on the transmission of information on the conditioned stimulus (explicit cue) from the anterior perirhinal cortex.[18] In contrast, PPI is modulated primarily by the striatum, particularly the nucleus accumbens, via GABAergic striatopallidal pathways impinging on the PPTg.[6,8,9] Nucleus accumbens' influence over PPI is, in turn, modulated by inputs from the ventral tegmentum,[4,5] medial prefrontal cortex,[12,13] and the septohippocampal system.[11,13,14]

Overactivity of the mesolimbic dopamine system, involving D_2 receptors in the nucleus accumbens, reduces PPI. Such activation results from interaction between ascending dopaminergic input originating in the ventral tegmentum and activation of glutamate receptors in the nucleus accumbens core, and the resulting disruption of PPI can be opposed by the D_2 antagonist haloperidol. In contrast, disruption of PPI in the nucleus accumbens shell cannot be reversed by D_2 receptor blockage.[5] These complex regional effects of dopamine-glutamate interactions within the nucleus accumbens are in turn modulated by descending dopaminergic and glutamatergic influence from more rostral structures. Medial prefrontal cortical amelioration of mesolimbic dopaminergic activity in the nucleus accumbens protects PPI. Depletion of medial prefrontal cortex dopamine reduces PPI.[12] Hence, the action of the medial prefrontal dopaminergic system on PPI opposes that of dopaminergic mechanisms within the nucleus accumbens; dopamine in the medial prefrontal cortex exerts inhibitory control over striatal dopaminergic systems. Also, cell damage in both the medial prefrontal cortex and the hippocampus increases sensitivity to disruption of PPI by dopaminergic receptor activation in the nucleus accumbens.[13,14] However, activation of the septohippocampal system by cholinergic and GABAergic transmission originating in the medial septum also results in impairment of PPI. This source of PPI disruption may involve glutamate receptors in the nucleus accumbens without interacting with dopaminergic mechanisms.[10,11]

REFERENCES FOR FIGURE 3

1. LEE, Y., D. E. LOPEZ, E. G. MELONI, & M. DAVIS. 1996. A primary acoustic startle pathway: Obligatory role of cochlear root neurons and the nucleus reticularis pontis caudalis. J. Neurosci. **16:** 3775–3789.

2. LINGENHÖHL, K. & E. FRIAUF. 1994. Giant neurons in the rat reticular formation: A sensorimotor interface in the elementary acoustic startle circuit? J. Neurosci. **14:** 1176–1194.

3. YEOMANS, J. S. & P. W. FRANKLAND. 1996. The acoustic startle reflex: Neurons and connections. Brain Res. Rev. **21:** 301–314.

4. WAN, F. J., M. A. GEYER & N. R. SWERDLOW. 1995. Presynaptic dopamine-glutamate interactions in the nucleus accumbens regulate sensorimotor gating. Psychopharmacology **120:** 433–441.

5. WAN, F. J. & N. R. SWERDLOW. 1996. Sensorimotor gating in rats is regulated by different dopamine-glutamate interactions in the nucleus accumbens core and shell subregions. Brain Res. **722:** 168–176.

6. SWERDLOW, N. R. & M. A. GEYER. 1993. Prepulse inhibition of acoustic startle in rats after lesions of the pedunculopontine tegmental nucleus. Behav. Neurosci. **107:** 104–117.

(*Figure 3 legend continued*)

7. Koch, M., M. Kungel & H. Herbert. 1993. Cholinergic neurons in the pedunculopontine tegmental nucleus are involved in the mediation of prepulse inhibition of the acoustic startle response in the rat. Exp. Brain Res. **97:** 71–82.

8. Kodsi, M. H. & N. R. Swerdlow. 1995. Ventral pallidal GABA-A receptors regulate prepulse inhibition of acoustic startle. Brain Res. **684:** 26–35.

9. Kodsi, M. H. & N. R. Swerdlow. 1995. Prepulse inhibition in the rat is regulated by ventral and caudodorsal striato-pallidal circuitry. Behav. Neurosci. **109:** 912–928.

10. Caine, S. B., M. A. Geyer & N. R. Swerdlow. 1992. Hippocampal modulation of acoustic startle and prepulse inhibition in the rat. Pharmacol. Biochem. and Behav. **43:** 1201–1208.

11. Koch, M. 1996. The septohippocampal system is involved in prepulse inhibition of the acoustic startle response in rats. Behav. Neurosci. **110:** 468–477.

12. Bubser, M. & M. Koch. 1994. Prepulse inhibition of the acoustic startle response of rats in reduced by 6-hydroxydopamine lesions of the medial prefrontal cortex. Psychopharmacology **113:** 487–492.

13. Swerdlow, N. R., B. K. Lipska, D. R. Weinberger, D. L. Braff, G. E. Jaskiw & M. A. Geyer. 1995. Increased sensitivity to the sensorimotor gating-disruptive effects of apomorphine after lesions of medial prefrontal cortex or ventral hippocampus in adult rats. Psychopharmacology **122:** 27–34.

14. Lipska, B. K., N. R. Swerdlow, M. A. Geyer, G. E. Jaskiw, D. L. Braff & D. R. Weinberger. 1995. Neonatal excitotoxic hippocampal damage in rats causes post-pubertal changes in prepulse inhibition of startle and its disruption by apomorphine. Psychopharmacology **122:** 35–43.

15. Rosen, J. B., M. Hitchcock, C. B. Sananes, M. J. D. Miserendino & M. Davis. 1991. A direct projection from the central nucleus of the amygdala to the acoustic startle pathway: Anterograde and retrograde tracing studies. Behav. Neurosci. **105:** 817–825.

16. Hitchcock, J. M. & M. Davis. 1991. Efferent pathway of the amygdala involved in conditioned fear as measured with the fear-potentiated startle paradigm. Behav. Neurosci. **105:** 826–842.

17. Campeau, S. & M. Davis. 1995. Involvement of subcortical and cortical afferents to the lateral nucleus of the amygdala in fear conditioning measured with fear-potentiated startle in rats trained concurrently with auditory and visual conditioned stimuli. J. Neurosci. **15:** 2312–2327.

18. Rosen, J. B., J. M. Hitchcock, M. J. D. Miserendino, W. A. Falls, S. Campeau & M. Davis. 1992. Lesions of the perirhinal cortex but not of the frontal, medial prefrontal, visual, or insular cortex block fear-potentiated startle using a visual conditioned stimulus. J. Neurosci. **12:** 4624–4633.

19. Davis, M., J. C. Gewirtz, K. A. McNish & M. Kim. 1995. The roles of the amygdala and bed nucleus of the stria terminalis (BNST) in the acquisition of fear potentiated startle using both explicit and contextual cues. Neurosci. Abstr. 479.22.

20. Sananes, C. B. & M. Davis. 1992. *N*-Methyl-D-aspartate lesions of the lateral and basolateral nuclei of the amygdala block fear-potentiated startle and shock sensitization of startle. Behav. Neurosci. **106:** 72–80.

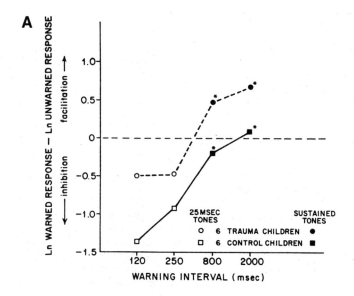

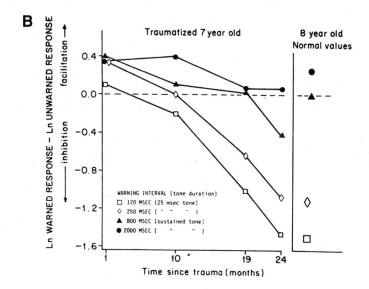

FIGURE 4. (A) Prepulse modulation of startle amplitude in PTSD and normal children. **(B)** Prepulse modulation of startle amplitude in a school-age boy with PTSD over a 2-year period.

TABLE 1. Normal Developmental Course of Startle Inhibition[32-35]

1. Prior to about 4 years of age, inhibitory startle modulation is weak or absent, whereas facilitatory startle modulation to sustained prestimulation is strong in early infancy.
2. Both inhibitory and facilitatory startle modulation show, respectively, peak losses in startle inhibition and peak gains in startle facilitation at about 4.5 years of age.
3. Progressive increase in inhibition and decrease in facilitation follow until, by 8 years of age, mature values are obtained.

TABLE 2. Development of Endogenous Event-Related Potentials, Indices of the Maturation of Information Processing[5,41,42]

1. The N200 wave (early stimulus classification as novel/deviant versus background or expected) is large and long in latency between 4 and 7 months of age, after which there is progressive reduction in amplitude and latency throughout childhood and adolescence.
2. The P300 wave (categorization and discrimination), which is not present in infancy, has been demonstrated at 3 years of age. Its amplitude increases to maximum values between 3.7 and 6 years of age, decreasing to adult values between 10 and 13 years of age.
3. The developmental peak in P300 amplitude in response to target stimuli at 4.5 years of age coincides with the developmental peak of loss of inhibitory startle modulation and the associated peak increment of facilitatory startle modulation.
4. The latency of P300 follows a different pattern from that of amplitude. It decreases exponentially between 5 and 14 years of age.

at critical periods of neuroplasticity and consolidation. TABLE 2 provides an overview of the development of the N200 and P300.

A marker of information processing such as the P300 may be relevant to clinically observable differences among children and adolescents (as well as adults) in the ability to make timely cognitive discriminations among traumatic reminders and their reference to specific traumatic moments. Such discriminatory capacity is an important component in the recovery process,[4] even in terms of the return to more homeostatic levels of autonomic arousal after reminders and the risk of transition from phasic to tonic neurophysiological arousal.[43] Similar developmental considerations are germane to the study of other trauma-induced attentional disturbances as well as sleep disorders.

BEHAVIORAL ANIMAL MODEL OF PTSD

Returning to the third main area of developmental neurobiology, the behavioral consequences of neuroanatomical and neurophysiological alterations, we recently described a behavioral animal model of PTSD.[44] The model featured repeated exposures to a situational reminder of a prior brief electric shock and included assessment of two behavioral parameters, exploratory behavior in a neutral environment and in a fear-provoking environment and the magnitude of the startle reflex to acoustic stimuli. This model differs from a fear-enhanced startle paradigm, in which a link

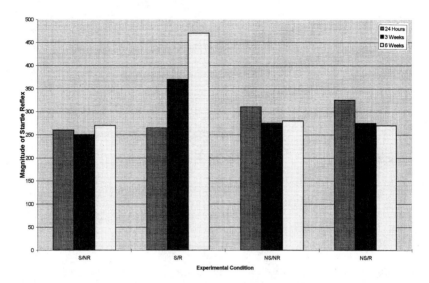

FIGURE 5. Magnitude of acoustic startle reflex at 24 hours, 3 weeks, and 6 weeks ($n = 120$). S/NR, shock with no reminders; S/R, shock with reminders; NS/NR, no shock with no reminders; NS/R, no shock with reminders.

between a conditioned stimulus and an unconditioned stimulus is established through classic conditioning. By contrast, in this paradigm, the animal is reexposed to situational reminders without any external reinforcement and without desensitization.

Subjects for this study included 150 male C57bl/6 mice. Animals were housed five per cage. Cages were randomly assigned to one of four groups: Shock/With Situational Reminders; Shock/Without Situational Reminders; No Shock/With Situational Reminders; and No Shock/Without Situational Reminders. Animals from each group were tested at each of three time points: 24 hours, 3 weeks, and 6 weeks. To avoid bias introduced by previous testing, animals were tested only once at either of the three test intervals. Therefore, this study employed three cohorts of experimental animals for each of the experimental groups. FIGURES 5 and 6 present the findings on acoustic startle and behavior in a fear-provoking environment.

The findings indicated an initial, but unsustained, increase in locomotor activity in a neutral environment due to traumatic stress. Exposure to situational reminders was associated with a progressive increase over time in the magnitude of the startle reflex (FIG. 5) and persistent bidirectional abnormal behavioral patterns in a fear-provoking environment (FIG. 6). Exposure to situational reminders also produced an increase in fighting, with eruption of catastrophic violence after 6 weeks of 1-minute per week exposure to the situational reminder. This animal model appears to produce behavioral changes analogous to those in patients with PTSD.

Exaggerated startle reactions predicted increased overall severity and chronicity of posttraumatic stress reactions in adults[45] and children.[3,46] This animal model specifically suggests a central role of situational reminders in the exacerbation of startle reactivity. Our study after the 1988 Armenian earthquake suggested that chronic

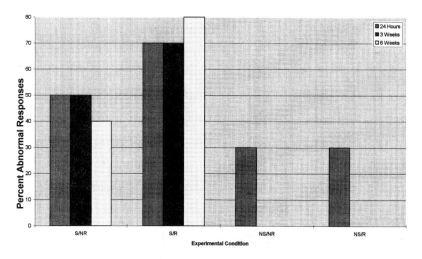

FIGURE 6. Percentage of animals exhibiting abnormal responses on the elevated plus maze ($n = 80$). S/NR, shock with no reminders; S/R, shock with reminders; NS/NR, no shock with no reminders; NS/R, no shock with reminders.

exposures to situational reminders, in the form of damaged buildings and sites where injury or death occurred, contributed to long-term symptoms of heightened arousal.[3,26]

The finding of such a powerful effect of reexposure to nonconditioned traumatic reminders in our animal model has important implications for future studies of neurobiological and behavioral correlates of PTSD. First, there is an urgent need to incorporate appropriate assessment of the type, frequency, and response to traumatic reminders. To date, there have been no systematic investigations of the natural course of situational reminders in the study of PTSD, and studies have not typically considered differences in the rates of exposure to reminders among subjects.

We presented elsewhere a preliminary typology of traumatic reminders derived from our clinical descriptive research with children and adolescents.[47] We also suggested that what may constitute situational reminders to children and adolescents varies with developmental stage as well as experience. Attention to the presence of a traumatic reminder in the child's daily environment may be critical to understanding the clinical course and providing effective intervention.

Our findings after the 1994 Northridge earthquake in Los Angeles documented that the overall severity of posttraumatic stress reactions at 5 months was strongly related to the degree of initial exposure, frequency of exposure to traumatic reminders, and current level of physiological reactivity to reminders.[48] After the earthquake, one schoolage child had a persistent sleep disturbance despite several months of psychotherapy. On closer scrutiny, the clinician learned that the child went to bed each night staring at a prominent crack in the wall. Even a temporary solution, with the boy covering the crack with a handpainted paper mural, helped to restore his ability to sleep, while a more permanent repair was scheduled.

In terms of the emerging personality of the child, we reviewed evidence for the effects of traumatic experiences on a number of personality parameters, including the dimension of fearfulness, courage, and fearlessness.[4] The bidirectional changes in behavior in a fear-provoking environment produced in the animal model has several developmental implications. Future studies in children and adolescents should examine for bimodal distributions of, or oscillations in, fear-related behaviors. Any such bimodal distribution would then need to be examined for the interplay of genetic predisposition and prior experience.

Investigation of trauma-induced exaggeration or discontinuity in preexisting temperamental characteristics will require a neurodevelopmental interactive model. For example, Kagan[13] described a group of preschool children who were unusually inhibited in reactivity to, or avoidant of, novel situations. In the transition from preschool to school age, resolution of this inhibited pattern of response occurred in many of these children. What would happen if such a child in transition experienced a traumatic event? It might reverse this developmental progression, resulting in an exaggeration of this preexisting trait, with an accelerated consolidation into the emerging personality of the child. Of note, Kagan[13] proposed that this pattern of inhibition is related to genetic factors that govern fear responses mediated by the central nucleus of the amygdala, the brain region also associated with fear-enhanced startle.[49,50]

The most unexpected and disturbing finding of our animal study was the emergence of catastrophic cohort aggression among group-housed mice exposed to weekly situational reminders. This finding points to the importance of investigating traumatic reminder-related dysregulation of aggression in children and adolescents. Studies need to account for the developmental progression in the use of hostile versus instrumental aggression.[51] They also need to examine cohort phenomena when studying irritability, hostile aggression, and propensity to retaliatory violence.

Using this animal paradigm, we are currently using autoradiographic imaging to investigate the underlying function of brain structures in response to situational reminders. We are also examining factors that may contribute to cohort aggressive behavior, including changes in latency to aggressive action. Latency to aggression may be an important parameter for understanding maturation in the use of hostile versus instrumental aggression in children and adolescents.

AN EVOLUTIONARY BIOLOGY PERSPECTIVE

We would propose that understanding of the neurobiology of danger, trauma, and PTSD requires an expanded evolutionary perspective beyond the traditional fight/flight paradigm, one that includes the human's capacity for considering protective intervention. Such evolving capacity should be studied over the course of ontogenesis as it correlates with neurodevelopment. As an example, we[4] described a relationship between the neurophysiological maturation of prepulse inhibition of startle and the evolving content of children's intervention fantasies in response to a direct life threat or witnessing life threat or injury. The lack of inhibitory modulation of the startle in early childhood promotes avoidant, escape, or search behavior, and corresponds to a developmental stage characterized by conscious thoughts of turning away from danger and seeking out external protection and intervention. Acquisition of inhibitory modulation of the startle, which occurs at approximately 8 years of age, corresponds to a developmental stage in which children actively begin to entertain conscious thoughts and fantasies of personally addressing, disarming, or directly harming the source of danger. Children begin to construct intervention fantasies that anticipate dangerous situations to prevent or avert danger. By early adolescence, when inhibitory modulation of the startle reflex is consolidated, thoughts or fantasies of intervention are typically accompanied by decisions about whether to intervene directly.

In addition, a comprehensive neurodevelopmental approach places posttraumatic stress reactions in an evolutionary biology framework. A sociobiological perspective raises the question of the utility to the individual, as well as consequent utility to the group, of such intense, complex, and often enduring biological, mental, behavioral, and cultural responses associated with traumatic stress.[52] For example, PTSD reactions among children and adolescents may serve to: (1) increase proximity to attachment figures in the presence of danger and readiness for protective action of self and other, and (2) accelerate strivings for self-efficacy in the presence of danger when protective intervention of attachment figures is absent or fails. In addition, recurrent or chronic posttraumatic distress, while a significant source of suffering for the individual, may serve to mobilize sustained intervention on behalf of the family, group, or community to promote prevention or protective action. Traumatic events in childhood can initiate life-long preoccupation with intervention fantasies that remain relatively fixed or evolve with maturity and experience. These intervention preoccupations may themselves strongly influence future career choices, preferences for geographical residence, and parenting behavior, which have cross-generational ramifications.[11]

REFERENCES

1. PYNOOS, R. S., C. FREDERICK, K. NADER, W. ARROYO, A. M. STEINBERG, S. ETH, F. NUNEZ & L. A. FAIRBANKS. 1987. Life threat and posttraumatic stress in school-age children. Arch. Gen. Psychiatry **44:** 1057-1063.
2. NADER, K., R. S. PYNOOS, L. A. FAIRBANKS & C. FREDERICK. 1990. Children's PTSD reactions one year after a sniper attack at their school. Am. J. Psychiatry **147:** 1526-1530.
3. PYNOOS, R. S., A. K. GOENJIAN, M. TASHJIAN, M. KARAKASHIAN, R. MANJIKIAN, R. G. MANOUKIAN, A. M. STEINBERG & L. A. FAIRBANKS. 1993. Posttraumatic stress reactions in children after the 1988 Armenian earthquake. Br. J. Psychiatry **163:** 239-247.
4. PYNOOS, R. S., A. M. STEINBERG & R. WRAITH. 1995. A developmental model of childhood traumatic stress. *In* Manual of Developmental Psychopathology. D. Cicchetti & D. J. Cohen, Eds.: 72-93. John Wiley & Sons. New York.
5. ORNITZ, E. M. 1996. Developmental aspects of neurophysiology. *In* Child and Adolescent Psychiatry: A Comprehensive Textbook, 2nd Ed. E. Lewis, Ed.: 39-51. Williams & Wilkins. Baltimore, MD.
6. PYNOOS, R. S., A. M. STEINBERG & L. ARONSON. 1997. Traumatic experiences: The early organization of memory in school-age children and adolescents. *In* Trauma and Memory: Clinical and Legal Controversies. P. Appelbaum, P. M. Elin & L. Uyehara, Eds.: 272-288. Oxford University Press. New York.
7. NADEL, L. 1994. Hippocampus: Effects of alterations in timing of development. *In* Developmental Time and Timing. G. Turkewitz & D. A. Devenny, Eds.: 233-252. Lawrence Erlbaum Associates, Inc. Hillside, NJ.
8. JACOBS, W. T., L NADEL & V. C. HAYDEN. 1992. Anxiety disorders. *In* Cognitive Science and Clinical Disorders. D. J. Stein & J. E. Young, Eds.: 211-233. Academic Press, Inc. San Diego, CA.
9. NADEL, L. 1992. Multiple memory systems. What and why. J. Cognit. Sci. **4:** 179-188.

10. PERRY, B. D., R. A. POLLARD, T. L. BLAKLEY, W. L. BAKER & D. VIGILANTE. 1995. Childhood trauma, the neurobiology of adaptation and use-dependent development of the brain: How "states" become "traits." Infant Ment. Health J. **16:** 271-291.

11. PYNOOS, R. S. 1996. The repercussion of traumatic expectations within and across generations. 6th International Psychoanalytic Association Conference, London, March.

12. KRYSTAL, J. H., T. KOSTEN, B. D. PERRY, S. SOUTHWICK, J. MASON & E. L. GILLER. 1989. Neurobiological aspects of post-traumatic stress disorder: Review of clinical and preclinical studies. Behav. Ther. **20:** 177-193.

13. KAGAN, J. 1991. A conceptual analysis of the affects. J. Am. Psychoanal. Assoc. **39:** 109-130.

14. REIDER, C. & D. CICCHETTI. 1989. Organizational perspective on cognitive control functioning and cognitive-affective balance in maltreated children. Dev. Psychol. **25:** 382-393.

15. TEICHER, M. H., C. A. GLOD, J. SURREY & C. SWEET, JR. 1993. Early childhood abuse and limbic system ratings in adult psychiatric outpatients. J. Neuropsychiatry Clin. Neurosci. **5:** 301-306.

16. BREMNER, J. D., S. M. SOUTHWICK, D. R. JOHNSON, R. YEHUDA & D. S. CHARNEY. 1993. Childhood physical abuse and combat-related posttraumatic stress disorder in Vietnam veterans. Am. J. Psychiatry **150:** 235-239.

17. BREMNER, J. D., P. RANDALL, T. M. SCOTT, R. A. BRONEN, J. P. SEIBYL, S. M. SOUTHWICK, R. C. DELANEY, G. MCCARTHY, D. S. CHARNEY & R. B. INNIS. 1995. MRI-based measurement of hippocampal volume in patients with combat-related posttraumatic stress disorder. Am. J. Psychiatry **152:** 973-981.

18. TEICHER M. H. Ann. N.Y. Acad. Sci. (This volume).

18a. BREMNER, J. D., P. RANDALL, E. VERMETTEN, L. STAIB, R. A. BRONEN, C. MAZURE, S. CAPELLI, G. MCCARTHY, R. B. INNIS & D. S. CHARNEY. 1997. Magnetic resonance imaging-based measurement of hippocampal volume in posttraumatic stress disorder related to childhood physical and sexual abuse. A preliminary report. Biol. Psychiatry **41:** 23-32.

19. ORNITZ, E. M. & R. S. PYNOOS. 1989. Startle modulation in children with posttraumatic stress disorder. Am. J. Psychiatry **146:** 866-870.

20. PUTNAM, F. W. & P. K. TRICKETT. 1993. Child sexual abuse: A model of chronic trauma. Psychiatry **56:** 82-95.

21. DE BELLIS, M. D., G. P. CHROUSOS, L. D. DORN, L. BURKE, K. HELMERS, M. A. KLING, P. K. TRICKETT & F. W. PUTNAM. 1994. Hypothalamic-pituitary-adrenal axis dysregulation in sexually abused girls. J. Clin. Endocrinol. Metab. **78:** 249-255.

22. PERRY, D. B., S. M. SOUTHWICK & E. L. GILLER. 1990. Adrenergic receptors in post-traumatic stress disorder. *In* E. L. Giller, Ed.: 89-114. Biological Assessment and Treatment of Post-Traumatic Stress Disorder. American Psychiatric Press, Washington, DC.

23. PERRY, D. B. 1994. Neurobiological sequelae of childhood trauma: Post-traumatic stress disorders in children. *In* M. Murberg, Ed.: 253-276. Catecholamines in Post-Traumatic Stress Disorder: Emerging Concepts. American Psychiatric Press. Washington, DC.

24. PERRY, B. D., R. A. POLLARD, W. L. BAKER, C. STURGES, D. VIGILANTE & T. L. BLAKLEY. 1995. Continuous heart rate monitoring in maltreated children (Abstr.). Annual meeting of the American Academy of Child and Adolescent Psychiatry. New Research.

25. GOENJIAN, A. K., R. YEHUDA, R. S. PYNOOS, A. M. STEINBERG, M. TASHJIAN, R. K. YANG, L. M. NAJARIAN & L. A. FAIRBANKS. 1996. Basal cortisol and dexamethasone suppression of cortisol and MHPG among adolescents after the 1988 earthquake in Armenia. Am. J. Psychiatry **153:** 929-934.

26. GOENJIAN, A. K., R. S. PYNOOS, A. M. STEINBERG, L. M. NAJARIAN, J. R. ASARNOW, I. KARAYAN, M. GHURABI & L. A. FAIRBANKS. 1995. Psychiatric co-morbidity in children after the 1988 earthquake in Armenia. J. Am. Acad. Child Adoles. Psychiatry **34:** 1174-1184.

27. YEHUDA, R., E. L. GILLER, S. M. SOUTHWICK, M. T. LOWY & J. W. MASON. 1991. Hypothalamic-pituitary-adrenal dysfunction in posttraumatic stress disorder. Biol. Psychiatry 30: 1031-1048.

28. YEHUDA, R., S. M. SOUTHWICK, G. NUSSBAUM, V. WAHBY, E. L. GILLER & J. W. MASON. 1990. Low urinary cortisol secretion in patients with post-traumatic stress disorder. J. Nerv. Ment. Dis. 178: 366-369.

29. RESNICK, H. S., R. YEHUDA, R. K. PITMAN & D. W. FOY. 1995. Effect of previous trauma on acute plasma cortisol level following rape. Am. J. Psychiatry 152: 1675-1677.

30. DAVIS, M. 1992. The role of the amygdala in conditioned fear. In Amygdala: Neurobiology Aspects of Emotion, Memory and Mental Dysfunction. Aggleton, Ed.: 255-306. Wiley-Liss. New York.

30a. GRILLON, C., C. A. MORGAN, S. M. SOUTHWICK, M. DAVIS & D. S. CHARNEY. 1996. Baseline startle amplitude and prepulse inhibition in Vietnam veterans with posttraumatic stress disorder. Psychiatry Res. 64: 169-178.

31. MORGAN, C. A., C. GRILLON, S. M. SOUTHWICK, M. DAVIS & D. S. CHARNEY. 1995. Fear-potentiated startle in posttraumatic stress disorder. Biol. Psychiatry 38: 378-385.

31a. WAN, F. J. & N. R. SWERDLOW. 1997. The basolateral amygdala regulates sensorimotor gating of acoustic startle in the rat. Neuroscience 76: 715-724.

32. GRAHAM, F. K., B. D. STROCK & B. L. ZEIGLER. 1981. Excitatory and Inhibitory influences on reflex responsiveness. In Minnesota Symposium on Child Psychology. Vol. 14. W. A. Collins, Ed.: 1-38. Lawrence Erlbaum Associates. Hillsdale, NJ.

33. ORNITZ, E. M., D. GUTHRIE, A. R. KAPLAN & S. J. LANE. 1986. Maturation of startle modulation. Psychophysiology 23: 624-634.

34. ORNITZ, E. M., D. GUTHRIE, S. J. LANE & T. SUGIYAMA. 1990. Maturation of startle facilitation by sustained prestimulation. Psychopsysiology 27: 298-308.

35. ORNITZ, E. M., D. GUTHRIE, M. SADEGHPOUR & T. SUGIYAMA. 1991. Maturation of prestimulation-induced startle modulation in girls. Psychophysiology 28: 11-20.

36. PYNOOS, R. S. & K. NADER. 1986. Childhood exposure to mass violence: Psychological first aid and approaches to treatment. NIMH Center for Mental Health Studies of Emergencies: Long term effects of mass violence. Rockville, MD.

37. PUTNAM, F. W. 1993. Dissociative disorders in children: Behavioral profiles and problems. Child Abuse and Neglect 17: 39-45.

38. MCFARLANE, A. C., D. L. WEBER & C. R. CLARK. 1993. Abnormal stimulus processing in posttraumatic stress disorder. Biol. Psychiatry 34: 311-320.

39. CHARLES, G., M. HANSENNE, M. ANSSEAU, R. MACHOWSKI, M. SCHITTECATTE & J. WILMOTTE. 1995. P300 in posttraumatic stress disorder. Biol. Psychiatry 32: 72-74.

40. METZGER, L. J., S. P. ORR, N. B. LASKO, N. J. BERRY & R. K. PITMAN. 1996. Evidence for diminished P3 amplitudes in PTSD. Paper presented 12th Annual Meeting of the International Society for Traumatic Stress Studies. San Francisco, CA.

41. COURCHESNE, E. 1978. Neurophysiological correlates of cognitive development: Changes in long-latency event-related potentials form childhood to adulthood. Electroencephal. Clin. Neurophysiol. 45: 468-482.

42. COURCHESNE, E. 1983. Cognitive components of the event-related brain potential: Changes associated with development. In Tutorials in ERP Research: Endogenous Components. A. W. K. Gaillard & W. Ritter, Eds.: 329-344. North-Holland, Amsterdam.

42a. PINEDA, J. A., S. L. FOOTE & H. J. NEVILLE. 1989. Effects of locus coeruleus on auditory long-latency, event-related potentials in monkey. J. Neurosci. 9: 81-93.

43. PITMAN, R. K. 1988. Post-traumatic stress disorder, conditioning, and network theory. Psychiatric Ann. 18: 182-189.

44. PYNOOS, R. S., R. F. RITZMANN, A. M. STEINBERG, A. K. GOENJIAN & I. PRISECARU. 1996. A behavioral animal model of PTSD featuring repeated exposures to situational reminders. Biol. Psychiatry 39: 129-134.

45. WEISAETH, L. 1989. A study of behavioral responses to an industrial disaster. Acta Psychiatrica Scand. Suppl. 355 80: 13-24.

46. Yule, W. & R. M. Williams. 1990. Post-traumatic stress reactions in children. J. Traumatic Stress **3:** 279-295.

47. Pynoos, R. S., K. Nader & J. March. 1991. Childhood post-traumatic stress disorder. *In* The Textbook of Child and Adolescent Psychiatry. J. Weiner, Ed.: 955-984. American Psychiatric Press. Washington, DC.

48. Wang, A., R. S. Pynoos, Q. James & M. Wong. 1994. Los Angeles earthquake, 1994: School district reduction of trauma effects. Symposium. American Academy of Child and Adolescent Psychiatry Annual Meeting. New York.

49. Davis, M. 1992. The role of the amygdala in conditioned fear. *In* The Amygdala. J. P. Affleton, Ed. Wiley-Liss. New York.

50. LeDeux, J. E., J. Iwata, P. Cicchetti & D. J. Reis. 1986. Different projections of the central amygdaloid nucleus mediate autonomic and behavioral correlates of conditioned fear. J. Neurosci. **8:** 2517-2529.

51. Atkins, M., D. Stoff, M. L. Osborne & K. Brown. 1993. Distinguishing instrumental and hostile aggression: Does it make a difference? J. Abnorm. Child Psychol. **21:** 355-365.

52. Nesse, R. M. 1991. What good is feeling bad? The evolutionary benefits of psychic pain. The Sciences **31:** 30-37.

The Role of Early Adverse Life Events in the Etiology of Depression and Posttraumatic Stress Disorder

Focus on Corticotropin-Releasing Factor[a]

CHRISTINE HEIM, MICHAEL J. OWENS,
PAUL M. PLOTSKY, AND CHARLES B. NEMEROFF [b]

Laboratory of Neuropsychopharmacology
Department of Psychiatry and Behavioral Sciences
Emory University School of Medicine
Atlanta, Georgia 30322

The remarkable progress in neurobiological research techniques has now been applied to investigate the pathogenesis of psychiatric disorders. A large body of literature has confirmed an important biological basis for a majority of severe psychiatric disorders, such as affective and anxiety disorders, including posttraumatic stress disorder (PTSD).[1] At the beginning of this century, Sigmund Freud's psychoanalytical theory was the major etiological approach for the explanation of psychopathology. According to this theory, conflicts in early life constitute a causal factor for the development of psychological disorders.[2]

In addition to convincing evidence for a genetic contribution in the development of mood and anxiety disorders,[3–5] evidence for a preeminent role of psychosocial stressors in the pathogenesis of these disorders has also been obtained. For example, episodes of major depression are often preceded by stressful life events[6] or are mutually related to episodes of stress.[7] In a study of identical twins by Kendler *et al.*,[8] lifetime stressors, including childhood abuse and neglect as well as stressful life events in adulthood, were identified as predictors of major depression. In the case of PTSD, a stressful life event outside the range of usual human experiences is required for a diagnosis of the disorder according to DSM-IV criteria.[9] The inclusion of a stressful event as an etiological factor in the DSM-IV differentiates PTSD from other psychiatric disorders. However, less than one quarter of traumatized individuals subsequently develop syndromal PTSD, suggesting that the disorder does not merely represent a normative reaction to extreme stress.[10] Increasing evidence indicates that the occurrence and persistence of PTSD in response to trauma depends on many factors including other stressful life events[11–13] as well as minor psychosocial stressors and daily stressors[14] before or after the onset of the traumatic event. Furthermore, recent studies suggest a strong relation between early adverse life events, that is,

[a]This research was supported by National Institutes of Health grant MH-42088.

[b]Address for correspondence: Charles B. Nemeroff, MD, PhD, Department of Psychiatry and Behavioral Sciences, Emory University School of Medicine, WMB, Suite 4000, 1639 Pierce Drive, Atlanta, GA 30322 (tel: (404) 727-8382; fax: (404) 727-3233; e-mail: cnemero@emory.edu).

childhood physical abuse[15,16] and negative parenting behavior,[17] and the development of PTSD in response to combat exposure.

Given these observations, it is plausible that alterations in stress-responsive neurobiological systems might be the link between stressful experiences and the development of psychopathology in the genetically vulnerable individual. Since the seminal studies of Selye,[18] the stress response has been associated with activation of the hypothalamic-pituitary-adrenal (HPA) axis, which is regulated by corticotropin-releasing factor (CRF). There are several reasons why CRF has been considered the major neurohumoral candidate in mediating stress experiences and subsequent pathology: (1) Because of its widespread distribution throughout the central nervous system (CNS) and its known effects when administered centrally, CRF is assumed to be the major regulator of not only the neuroendocrine, but also the behavioral, immune, and autonomic stress responses; (2) central administration of synthetic CRF to laboratory animals produces many signs and symptoms reminiscent of stress, depression, and anxiety; (3) increasing evidence is consistent with an enhanced CNS CRF activation in depression and PTSD; and (4) in laboratory animals, exposure to stress induces changes in the CRF system and, moreover, long-term alterations in CRF neurons are observed in adult animals after exposure to stress in early life. In the following pages, studies of the effects of early adverse life events on CRF neurons and the relationship of these findings to mood and anxiety disorders are reviewed.

THE MAJOR REGULATOR OF THE STRESS RESPONSE: CRF

As early as 1948, Harris suggested that the release of pituitary hormones was controlled by the hypothalamus. In the 1950s, Safran and Schally[19] and Guillemin and Rosenberg[20] independently described the existence of a factor in hypothalamic extracts capable of stimulating the secretion of adrenocorticotropin (ACTH) from anterior pituitary cells. Due to extensive methodological difficulties, the 41 amino acid sequence of CRF was isolated and characterized after a delay of more than 25 years by Vale and colleagues[21] in 1981. Immunohistochemical and radioimmunoassay mapping studies revealed a widespread distribution of CRF-containing neurons in the CNS, including not only the hypothalamus, but also the cerebral cortex, the limbic system, and brain stem areas. An equally widespread distribution of CRF mRNA and two CRF receptor subtypes throughout the brain has also been demonstrated using *in situ* hybridization and Northern blot analysis as well as autoradiographic and biochemical methods. The widespread distribution of CRF, CRF mRNA, and CRF receptors in the CNS points to the multipotential role of this peptide as a neuroendocrine regulator and neurotransmitter. The presence of CRF in limbic and cortical brain regions further supports its importance in mediating the stress response. The occurrence of CRF in brain stem regions that also contain catecholaminergic and serotonergic neurons points to a role for CRF in modulating monoaminergic neurotransmitter systems and autonomic stress responses. (See ref. 22 for review.)

EFFECTS OF CENTRAL CRF ADMINISTRATION

Central administration of CRF to laboratory animals produces many physiological and behavioral changes that parallel many signs of stress in animals and symptoms of depression and anxiety in humans, including increases in heart rate and mean arterial pressure, bidirectional changes of gastrointestinal function, suppression of exploratory behavior, induction of grooming behavior, increases in locomotor activity, reduction of feeding behavior and food intake as well as disruption of reproductive behavior. Furthermore, centrally administered CRF potentiates acoustic startle responses, facilitates fear conditioning, enhances shock-induced freezing and fighting behavior, and produces long-lasting behavioral sensitization to the effects of psychostimulants. (See refs. 22–24 for review.)

Many of the anxiogenic effects of CRF have been postulated to be mediated by activation of the central noradrenergic system. To localize the site of action of CRF in the brain, we used microinjection techniques to directly administer CRF into distinct brain regions. Microinjection of CRF into the locus coeruleus, a major site of CNS noradrenergic cell bodies, resulted in a pronounced decrease in exploratory behavior in a novel environment in rats.[25] In another study, an increase in fearful behavior was apparent in rats exposed to a conflict test after microinjection of CRF into the locus coeruleus or into the nearby parabrachial nucleus.[26] Physiologically, microinjection of CRF into the locus coeruleus was reported to increase neuronal firing rates[27] as well as tyroxine hydroxylase activity[28] and to induce the release of excitatory amino acids.[29] However, discordant results have also been obtained.[30,31] Due to its modulatory effect on the locus coeruleus, CRF might be involved in the regulation of arousal and vigilance.[23]

Consistent with the neuroanatomical links between the locus coeruleus and the amygdala, microinjection of CRF into the locus coeruleus increases concentrations of norepinephrine metabolites in the amygdala.[25] Microinjection of CRF directly into the amygdaloid nuclei produces fear-related behavior, characterized by facilitation of conditioned avoidance and decreased exploratory behavior.[32] Conversely, microinjection of the antagonist α-helical CRF$_{9-41}$ into the amygdala attenuates shock-induced freezing.[33] Lesioning of the amygdaloid complex completely blocks CRF-induced potentiation of startle responses, indicating a role of the amygdala in encoding emotional memories.[34]

It therefore would appear that increased activity of the CNS CRF neuronal system could plausibly account for many symptoms of major depression, such as sleep disruption, alterations in arousal, and loss of appetite and libido. Furthermore, numerous symptoms of PTSD, including hypervigilance, increased autonomic reactivity in response to stress, avoidance behavior, and potentiated startle responses, might be due to an increased activity of brain CRF systems. Moreover, a comparable dysregulation of stress-responsive neuronal systems might cause the remarkable symptom overlap and the frequent comorbidity between major depressive disorder and PTSD.

NEUROENDOCRINE ALTERATIONS IN DEPRESSION AND PTSD

The consistent finding of HPA hyperactivity in major depression characterized by hypercortisolemia, a decreased number of glucocorticoid receptors in lymphocytes, and resistance of cortisol to suppression by dexamethasone supports the hypothesis of an increased hypothalamic CRF release in this disorder. (See ref. 35 for review.)

In response to exogenous CRF administration, patients with major depression exhibit a blunting of the ACTH response with a normal cortisol response,[36,37] suggesting a downregulation of adenohypophyseal CRF receptors as a consequence of hypothalamic CRF hypersecretion and/or an increased feedback action of circulating cortisol on the pituitary corticotrophs. The former hypothesis is substantially supported by a series of findings in depressed patients and suicide victims. We have observed an increased concentration of CRF-like immunoreactivity in lumbar cerebrospinal fluid (CSF) of drug-free depressed patients compared to patients with other psychiatric disorders and healthy controls,[38] a finding that was replicated in several separate studies.[39] Increased CRF concentrations were also measured in cisternal CSF collected postmortem from suicide victims.[40] In two reports, Raadsheer *et al.*[41,42] demonstrated marked increases in CRF and CRF mRNA expression in postmortem tissue of depressed patients compared to controls. Interestingly, we observed a decrease of CSF CRF concentrations in depressed patients 24 hours after a regimen of electroconvulsive therapy, suggesting that CRF hyperactivity is a state, rather than a trait, marker of major depression.[43] Antidepressants, including desipramine, fluoxetine, and venlafaxine, have all been reported to reduce CSF CRF concentrations.[39,44] CSF measures reflect extrahypothalamic, nonhypophyseal CRF activity; however, these measures do not allow for the identification of specific CRF neuronal circuits that contribute to the observed increases in CSF CRF concentrations. Postmortem studies in suicide victims revealed a decreased density of CRF receptors in the frontal cortex of suicide victims, most of whom probably suffered from major depression.[45] Finally, our results from structural imaging studies demonstrating increased pituitary volumes and adrenal hypertrophy in patients with major depression support the hypothesis of increased hypothalamic CRF secretion in this disorder.[46]

Because PTSD is a consequence of exposure to extreme stress and it often is comorbid with major depression, the HPA axis has been scrutinized in PTSD. In initial studies, Vietnam war veterans with PTSD demonstrated decreased rather than increased 24-hour urinary cortisol secretion compared to depressed patients and healthy controls.[47,48] Subsequently, Yehuda and her colleagues[49] identified low urinary cortisol levels, "supersuppression" of cortisol to a low dose of dexamethasone, and an increased number of glucocorticoid receptors in lymphocytes as specific neuroendocrine correlates of PTSD. This pattern is clearly in contradistinction to neuroendocrine alterations in major depression. (See ref. 49 for review.) In chronobiological studies, an increased ratio between nadir and peak cortisol levels during the diurnal cycle has been observed in PTSD patients.[50] Based on these findings, taken together with clinical observations of increased HPA responses to emotional stress, Yehuda *et al.*[51] suggested that PTSD is characterized by a hyperdynamic, hyperregulated HPA axis which allows a maximal stress response that is effectively controlled by negative feedback inhibition. In a recent study, an increased feedback action of circulating cortisol on the HPA axis in PTSD was confirmed by the observation of exaggerated ACTH responses to "pharmacological adrenalectomy" induced by metyrapone.[52] The latter result also showed pronounced central CRF activity in patients with PTSD despite apparent hypocortisolism. A blunted ACTH and a normal cortisol response to CRF challenge have consistently been reported in Vietnam war veterans with PTSD[53] and sexually abused girls.[54] Interpretation of these results is somewhat difficult, as many subjects studied by Smith *et al.*[53] suffered from comorbid major depression, and the sexually abused girls studied by de Bellis *et al.*[54] mainly suffered from dysthymia, while PTSD was not diagnosed at all. However, in contrast to depression, the blunted ACTH responses occurred in the presence of normal basal cortisol levels, excluding the possibility of increased feedback action by elevated baseline cortisol levels. In contrast to the results of de Bellis *et al.,*[54] Kaufman and colleagues observed exaggerated ACTH responses and normal cortisol responses in sexually abused girls with major depression who were at greater risk for PTSD and under chronic psychosocial stress (personal communication), suggesting that early trauma results in both sensitization of the pituitary and adrenocortical hyporesponsiveness. Decreased adrenocortical responsivity in the CRF stimulation test was also observed in women with chronic pelvic pain, many of whom were sexually abused and had PTSD (Heim, Ehlert, Hanker & Hellhammer, in preparation). Thus, results in the CRF stimulation test are inconsistent and do not allow a definite conclusion with respect to central CRF activity in PTSD. The recently observed elevation of CSF CRF levels in Vietnam war veterans with PTSD, however, supports the assumption of a central CRF hyperactivity in PTSD.[55] In the same study, decreased CSF somatostatin concentrations were observed in PTSD patients. Consistent with the assumption of a stimulatory effect of CRF on the noradrenergic system, evidence for increased noradrenergic activity in PTSD was reported.[56,57] Interestingly, patients with PTSD demonstrate symptomatic increases and exacerbations of flashbacks in response to central noradrenergic stimulation by the selective α_2-receptor antagonist yohimbine.[58]

CRF AND EXPERIMENTAL STRESS

As just indicated, there is considerable evidence that CRF is the major physiological regulator of mammalian endocrine, behavioral, immune, and autonomic stress responses. In recent studies, responses of the central CRF system to the induction of experimental stress were investigated in animal models, including paradigms of acute and chronic stress in adult animals as well as exposure to stress in neonatal animals.

Acute Stress

It has long been known that acute stress exposure results in activation of the HPA axis.[8] In an early study, we observed a 52% reduction of CRF-like immunoreactivity in the median eminence of rats following exposure to acute cold stress, which presumably reflects the release of the peptide into the portal circulation.[59] Consistent with the observation of a pronounced induction of stress-like behavior by microinjection of CRF into the locus coeruleus (*vide supra*), a twofold increase in CRF concentration after acute stress was observed in this brain area. Furthermore, de Goeij *et al.*[60] reported a decrease in CRF as well as arginine vasopressin (AVP) immunoreactivity in the external zone of the median eminence in response to acute immobilization stress. Whitnall[61] identified a selected depletion of CRF neurons that coexpress AVP after acute stress, whereas there was no effect on the AVP-deficient CRF cell population. Interestingly, an increased AVP content in the median eminence accompanied by exaggerated ACTH, but reduced adrenal reponses to novelty stress, as well as an increased number of hippocampal corticosteroid receptors were observed in rats 28 days after exposure to a single footshock session,[62] a result with particular relevance to the pathophysiology of PTSD.

Acute hypersecretion of CRF could plausibly induce a desensitization or downregulation of CRF receptors in the brain or anterior pituitary. However, Hauger *et al.*[63,64] failed to demonstrate any changes in central or pituitary CRF binding sites after acute immobilization stress.

Chronic Stress

More relevant to the understanding of the pathophysiology of mood and anxiety disorders is the consideration of effects of chronic stress on neuroendocrine regulation. Exposure of animals to repeated stress usually results in increased basal adrenocortical activity and desensitization of pituitary and adrenal responses to the repeated stressor. (See ref. 49 for review.) Such habituation is stressor specific and depends on factors such as intensity and predictability.[65,66] Attenuation of pituitary-adrenal hormone secretion is also evident after continuous stress or prolonged pharmacological stimulation.[67] In humans and primates, reduced basal adrenocortical activity has been observed under several conditions of chronic stress.[68–71] Possible mechanisms include downregulation of pituitary CRF receptors due to CRF hypersecretion, increased feedback action due to stress-induced corticosterone release, or stress-induced demand for release overcoming the capacity for synthesis. The two latter mechanisms are unlikely because adaptation has also been observed in adrenalectomized animals[67] and because animals show substantial HPA responses to a superimposed novel stressor.[72] Rather, CNS mechanisms are likely to be involved.

Using an unpredictable stress protocol over a 2-week period, we observed a marked increase of CRF immunoreactivity in the locus coeruleus and a decrease of CRF concentration in the median eminence.[59] In another study, a 50% decrease of CRF content in the paraventricular nucleus (PVN) was observed in rats after chronic electroconvulsive shock treatment/stress.[73]

After 7 days of intermittent footshock, Imaki *et al.*[74] measured twofold increases in CRF mRNA expression in the hypothalamus using Northern blot analysis and in the PVN using *in situ* hybridization. Recently, Herman *et al.*[75] reported a 61% increase of CRF mRNA and a 16% increase of AVP mRNA in the PVN of rats exposed to a variable stressor paradigm over 30 days. The increase in transcription activity presumably occurs in reaction to the decline of CRF peptide content in the PVN. These findings contrast the results of de Goeij *et al.*,[60] suggesting a principal role for AVP in maintaining the sustained HPA activation during chronic stress.

CRF receptor density was shown to be altered in response to changes in CRF availability. Hauger *et al.*[63] observed a time-dependent reduction of pituitary CRF binding during 48 hours of continuous restraint stress, which was correlated to the decrease of CRF immunoreactivity in the median eminence. In a more recent study, the same group reported a downregulation of pituitary CRF receptors after 4 and 10 days of intermittent immobilization.[64] In both studies, exaggerated responses to a superimposed stressor were observed despite CRF receptor downregulation, indicative of the importance of other ACTH secretagogues or adrenal sensitivity. Hauger and colleagues[63] failed to reveal any CRF receptor changes in the CNS. In contrast, Anderson *et al.*[76] measured a decrease of CRF binding in the frontal cortex after 3 days and in the hypothalamus after 14 days of intermittent footshocks. Furthermore, widespread changes in the number of CRF binding sites were observed in tree shrews exposed to natural psychosocial stress.[77] In the pituitary level and the hippocampus, chronic psychosocial stress produced a significant reduction of CRF receptor number; increased binding was observed in the frontal cortex, amygdala, and other cortical areas.

In summary, chronic stress in adult animals results in changes in CNS CRF neurons and receptors in various brain regions, some of which are involved in neuroendocrine and behavioral regulation. These changes are concordant with the findings of increased CSF CRF concentrations in depressed patients and in patients with PTSD. The CRF hyperactivity goes along with adaptive changes in CRF mRNA and CRF receptors in the CNS and anterior pituitary. Downregulation of pituitary binding sites parallels findings of blunted responsiveness to CRF in major depression. In PTSD, results from the CRF challenge test are less conclusive. Comparable to findings in suicide victims, Anderson *et al.*[76] report a downregulation of CRF receptors in the frontal cortex of chronically stressed animals; however, Fuchs and Flügge[77] observed an opposite effect in tree shrews.

Early Life Stress

More than three decades ago, the pioneering work of Levine[78] and Denenberg[79] and their colleagues showed that exposure of infant animals to mild stress permanently reduces adrenocortical responses to subsequent stressors in adult life. In recent studies, Meaney and his colleagues further evaluated HPA alterations in rats exposed to handling in the first 2 weeks of life. (see ref. 80 for a review.) Handled rats demonstrated significantly lower ACTH and corticosterone secretion in response to a variety of stressors as well as a faster return of corticosterone to baseline levels after cessation of the handling as compared to nonhandled rats.[81] Administration of dexamethasone or corticosterone in various doses suppressed stress-induced HPA activation to a greater extent in handled rats than in nonhandled rats, suggesting an enhanced feedback sensitivity of the HPA axis. Consistent with this assumption, binding studies revealed a specific upregulation of glucocorticoid receptor number, and *in situ* hybridization studies indicated an increased glucocorticoid receptor mRNA expression in hippocampal tissue from neonatally handled rats.[81-84] Experimental manipulation of feedback effects showed that the feedback exerted by basal corticosterone levels, which is increased due to upregulation of glucocorticoid receptors, is critical to the induction of stress hyporesponsiveness.[85] Increased suppression of the axis is also reflected within the CNS. Median eminence concentrations of CRF and AVP as well as hypothalamic CRF mRNA levels are significantly decreased in handled rats.[85,86] These findings are thought to reflect a reduction in the readily releasable pool of these peptides, as handled rats, for example, show a lower CRF release from the median eminence in response to restraint stress.[86]

It should be noted, however, that in most animal paradigms of experimental stress, the procedure of handling represents the normal condition for ''control''

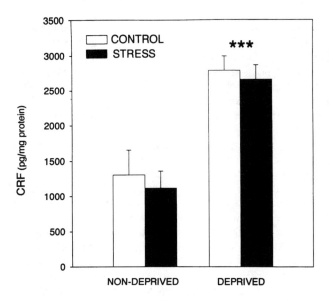

FIGURE 1. Immunoreactive CRF (means ± SEM) in the median eminence in four experimental groups: non-deprived/control ($n = 10$); non-deprived/stress ($N = 11$); deprived/control ($n = 15$); deprived/stress ($n = 15$). ***$p > 0.0001$ versus all non-deprived rats. (Reprinted, with permission, from Ladd *et al.*[87])

laboratory animals, whereas nonhandling might be considered as stressful in terms of deprivation of expected handling/activity. Thus, the foregoing results might rather reflect increased HPA activation and decreased feedback sensitivity in nonhandled rats compared to normally reared control animals. Consistent with this perspective are findings from studies showing that deprivation of the infant animal from maternal care for prolonged periods results in virtually opposite long-term neuroendocrine alterations as neonatal handling stress. Plotsky and Meaney[86] observed significantly increased ACTH and corticosterone responses to restraint or novelty stress in rats that were exposed to daily maternal separation for 3 hours in the first 2 weeks of life. In response to dexamethasone, maternally deprived rats showed an escape from suppression, reflecting a decreased feedback sensitivity of the HPA axis. The concentration of immunoreactive CRF in the median eminence and of CRF mRNA expression in the PVN is increased. In a recent study by our group,[87] rats that were deprived for 6 hours per day from day 10 until weaning (day 21) exhibited a significant increase in basal plasma ACTH concentrations. Consistent with the results of Plotsky and Meaney,[86] the ACTH response to a mild footshock was significantly higher in deprived rats than in the nondeprived controls. However, no differences were noted in either basal or stress-induced corticosterone levels. These results impressively parallel findings in a subgroup of sexually abused girls (Kaufman *et al.*, personal communication, *vide supra*). Again, maternally deprived rats exhibited markedly increased CRF concentrations in the median eminence (FIG. 1); moreover, pituitary CRF binding sites were decreased, indicative of CRF hypersecretion. In this study,

CRF concentrations were also measured in other brain regions. Increased concentrations of immunoreactive CRF were observed in the parabrachial nucleus, which adjoins the locus coeruleus and is a site of anxiogenic actions of CRF.[26] In subsequent studies, maternal deprivation produced a persistent, long-lasting increase in CRF mRNA expression in the PVN, amygdala, and bed nucleus as well as hyperresponsiveness of the HPA axis to acute stress. These effects are reversed by treatment with the clinically effective selective serotonin reuptake inhibitor paroxetine (Plotsky *et al.*, in preparation).

To some extent, maternal separation is an exception compared to milder stressors, regarding the acute stress response of the infant rat. From days 4 to 14, many species exhibit a stress hyporesponsive phase, which is characterized by subnormal or unmeasurable HPA responses to certain stressors. However, infant rats can mount a pronounced endocrine response when exposed to maternal separation. Thus, we observed significant rises in plasma corticosterone levels both in 10-day-old and in 18-day-old rats subjected to maternal deprivation.[88] Further measures showed that this stress-induced HPA activation was mediated by release of hypothalamic CRF. In the 10-day-old rat pups, CRF concentrations in the median eminence were reduced after 24 hours of maternal separation most likely because of secretion of CRF into the portal blood. This finding is consistent with findings on acute stress responses in adult rats (*vide supra*). In 18-day-old rats, no significant changes in median eminence CRF concentrations were observed. Together with the observation of a 50% reduction of pituitary CRF receptors, a sustained synthesis and release of CRF in the maternally deprived 18-day-old rats can be assumed. We also observed decreased pituitary CRF binding sites after maternal deprivation in 12-day-old rats.[89] Surprisingly, 24-hour maternal deprivation increased CRF receptors in various brain regions, including the frontal cortex, hypothalamus, hippocampus, amygdala, and cerebellum. Thus, target neurons of CRF might be sensitized by maternal deprivation. Compatible with the concept of sensitization, these rats exhibited an enhanced endocrine responsiveness to acute heterologous stressors. The findings show that maternal separation acutely affects the central CRF system, inducing a state of sensitization early in life.

In the presence of variation of results according to the intensitiy of early life stressors as well as profound species differences, it is still unclear how these findings can be generalized to humans. Thus, in a recent study, we attempted to design a paradigm that adequately parallels stress experiences in early human life.[90] Nonhuman primates (*Macaca radiata*) were assigned to differential rearing conditions over 12 weeks, in which the mothers and their 3- to 6-month-old infants were confronted with different foraging demands. Mothers with constantly low foraging demands could easily reach food without any effort, whereas mothers with constantly high foraging demands had to work for their food. In the variable foraging demand group, mothers were exposed to unpredictable conditions with respect to food access, perhaps resulting in a diminished perception of "security" in the infants with respect to maternal attachment. After the experimental period, primates were subjected to normal colony conditions until young adulthood (2–4 years). These young adult bonnet macaques, which were reared while their mothers were under the variable foraging demand condition, exhibited significantly elevated CSF CRF concentrations compared to primates reared by mothers under either consistently low or consistently high foraging demands (Fig. 2). CSF CRF concentrations did not correlate with CSF

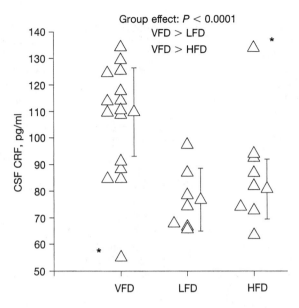

FIGURE 2. CSF CRF concentrations in grown bonnet macaques whose mothers were exposed to low, high, and variable foraging demands during infancy. Pooled data are expressed as means ± SD (*-not used for the determination of mean group concentrations). (Reprinted, with permission, from Coplan *et al.*[90])

cortisol concentrations. Indeed, CSF cortisol was actually lower in animals exposed to the variable foraging demand. Moreover, CSF somatostatin concentrations were also reduced (unpublished observations). The dissociation between increased central CRF activity and adrenal hypoactivity and the reduction in CSF somatostatin levels exactly parallel the results obtained in patients with PTSD (*vide supra*). In this regard, it is interesting that adult bonnet macaques exposed to adverse rearing conditions in the same paradigm demonstrate stable traits of anxiety.[91] In response to central noradrenergic stimulation by administration of the selective α_2-adrenoceptor antagonist yohimbine, a behavioral hyperresponsiveness was observed characterized by a higher number of anxiety-related behavioral changes.[92]

In summary, considerable evidence indicates that early life stress affects the central CRF system, resulting in long-term alterations in the stress-responsive neuroendocrine system. Untoward early life events induce a persistent increase in CRF neuronal activity, paralleling findings of elevated CSF CRF concentrations in depression and PTSD. CRF hypersecretion seems to be accompanied by sensitization of the stress response despite CRF receptor downregulation at the adenohypophysis. This finding exactly parallels the concept of sensitization of the HPA axis in PTSD, which allows the organism to maximally respond to stress.[52] Also like PTSD, early life stress is associated with behavioral sensitization to noradrenegic stimulation. The observation of adrenocortical hyporesponsiveness in maternally deprived animals parallels findings in sexually abused girls and women with chronic pelvic pain at high risk of

PTSD and might contribute to the development of hypocortisolism. Comparable to neuroendocrine alterations in PTSD, early handling stress induces an up-regulation of glucocorticoid receptors; however unlike PTSD, early handling is associated with decreased instead of increased CRF activity and blunted stress responses. Additionally, as noted earlier, interpretation of the results from this paradigm depends on which condition is considered stressful. Thus, the observation of sensitization of the pituitary and adrenocortical hyporesponsiveness to stress together with upregulation of gluco-corticoid receptors 2 weeks after a single footshock session in adult rats (*vide supra*) might be considered a more valid model of PTSD.

CONCLUSION

According to the stress diathesis model, stress, particularly early in life, can contribute to the development of psychopathology in the genetically vulnerable individual. It has been shown that major depression and PTSD are closely linked to stressful experiences, including early life stress. Accordingly, accumulated evidence suggests that both disorders are characterized by hyperactivity of one or more populations of CRF-containing neurons which mediate endocrine, behavioral, immune, and autonomic stress responses. Similar hyperactivity of CNS CRF neurons is observed in animals subjected to experimental chronic stress. Moreover, long-lasting alterations of the central CRF system occur in animals exposed to severe stress in early life. Thus, early stressful experiences in humans might render the individual vulnerable to the effects of stress, resulting in an increased risk for developing psychopathology by actions on CRF neurons and/or receptors. Clearly, more data are needed to elucidate the mechanisms of this sensitization. The overall goal of biological research in psychiatry is to find new ways of prevention, detection, and treatment of psychopathology. Because dysregulation of the central CRF system may be the common feature of major depression and PTSD, both disorders arguably being related to early life stress, the preventive and therapeutic benefit of selective CRF-receptor antagonists should be explored. Based on the findings that early stress produces persistent alterations in the CNS, it is plausible that psychotherapy or pharmacological intervention early in life may prevent the neurobiological consequences of early life stress. The findings of persistent effects of early life stress on CRF neurons and receptors represent one potential neurobiological substrate for the traditional psychoanalytical view. Future studies should clearly evaluate reactions to early life stress and its link to stress responsiveness in later life. The question of why some individuals tend to react with depression and hypercortisolism and other individuals develop PTSD and hypocortisolism in response to stress, with both syndromes associated with increased CNS CRF secretion, requires further scrutiny.

REFERENCES

1. Schatzberg, A. F. & C. B. Nemeroff. 1995. The Textbook of Psychopharmacology. American Psychiatric Press. Washington, DC.
2. Freud, S. 1966. The Standard Edition of the Complete Psychological Works of Sigmund Freud. Vol. 1. Hogarth. London.

3. NATHAN, K. I., D. L. MUSSELMAN, A. F. SCHATZBERG & C. B. NEMEROFF. 1995. Biology of mood disorders. *In* Textbook of Psychopharmacology. A. F. Schatzberg & C. B. Nemeroff, Eds.: 439-478. American Psychiatric Press. Washington, DC.
4. STEIN, M. B. & T. W. UHDE. 1995. Biology of anxiety disorders. *In* Textbook of Psychopharmacology. A. F. Schatzberg & C. B. Nemeroff, Eds.: 501-522. American Psychiatric Press. Washington, DC.
5. TRUE, W. R., J. RICE, S. A. EISEN, A. C. HEATH, J. GOLDBERG, M. J. LYONS & J. NOWAK. 1993. Arch. Gen. Psychiatry **50:** 257-264.
6. DUNNER, D., V. PATRICK & R. R. FIEVE. 1979. Am. J. Psychiatry **136:** 508-511.
7. HAMMEN, C., J. DAVILA, G. BROWN, A. ELLICOTT & M. GITLIN. 1992. J. Abnorm. Psychol. **101:** 45-52.
8. KENDLER, K. S., R. C. KESSLER, M. C. NEALE, A. C. HEATH & L. J. EAVES. 1993. Am. J. Psychiatry **150:** 1139-1148.
9. AMERICAN PSYCHIATRIC ASSOCIATION. 1995. Diagnostic and Statistical Manual of Mental Disorders, Fourth Edition. American Psychiatric Association. Washington, DC.
10. YEHUDA, R. & A. C. MCFARLANE. 1995. Am. J. Psychiatry **152:** 1705-1713.
11. RUCH, L. O., S. M. CHANDLER & R. A. HARTER. 1980. J. Health Soc. Behav. **21:** 248-260.
12. MCFARLANE, A. C. 1988. J. Nerv. Ment. Dis. **174:** 4-14.
13. YEHUDA, R., B. KAHANA, J. SCHMEIDLER, S. M. SOUTHWICK, S. WILSON & E. L. GILLER. 1995. Am. J. Psychiatry **152:** 1815-1818.
14. GREEN, B. L. & M. A. BERLIN. 1987. J. Clin. Psychol. **43:** 643-649.
15. BREMNER, J. D., S. M. SOUTHWICK, D. R. JOHNSON, R. YEHUDA & D. S. CHARNEY. 1993. Am. J. Psychiatry **150:** 235-239.
16. ZAIDI, L. Y. & D. W. FOY. 1994. J. Traumatic Stress **7:** 33-42.
17. MCCRANIE, E. W., L. A. HYER, P. A. BOUDEWYNS & M. G. WOODS. 1992. J. Nerv. Ment. Dis. **180:** 431-438.
18. SELYE, H. 1936. Nature **138:** 32-36.
19. SAFFRAN, M. & A. V. SCHALLY. 1955. Can. J. Biochem. Physiol. **33:** 408-415.
20. GUILLEMIN, R. & B. ROSENBERG. 1955. Endocrinology **57:** 599-607.
21. VALE, W., J. SPIESS, C. RIVIER & J. RIVIER. 1981. Science **213:** 1394-1397.
22. OWENS, M. J. & C. B. NEMEROFF. 1991. Pharmacol. Rev. **43:** 425-473.
23. DUNN, A. J. & C. W. BERRIDGE. 1990. Brain Res. Rev. **15:** 71-100.
24. KOOB, G. F., S. C. HEINRICHS, F. MENZAGHI, E. M. PICH & K. T. BRITTON. 1994. Sem. Neurosci. **6:** 221-229.
25. BUTLER, P. D., J. M. WEISS, J. C. STOUT & C. B. NEMEROFF. 1990. J. Neurosci. **10:** 176-183.
26. WEISS, J. M., J. STOUT, M. AARON, M. J. OWENS & C. B. NEMEROFF. 1994. Brain Res. Bull. **35:** 561-572.
27. VALENTINO, R. J., S. L. FOOTE & G. ASTON-JONES. 1983. Brain Res. **270:** 363-367.
28. MELIA, K. R. & R. S. DUMAN. 1991. Proc. Natl. Acad. Sci. USA **88:** 8382-8386.
29. SINGEWALD, N., G. Y. ZHOU, F. CHEN & A. PHILIPPU. 1996. Neurosci. Letts. **204:** 45-48.
30. LANDRY, J. C., Z. N. STOWE, M. J. OWENS, P. M. PLOTSKY & C. B. NEMEROFF. 1994. Soc. Neurosci. Abstr. **20:** 553. 2.
31. BORSODY, M. K. & J. M. WEISS. 1996. Brain Res. **7:** 149-168.
32. LIANG, K. C. & E. H. Y. LEE. 1988. Psychopharmacology **96:** 232-236.
33. SWIERGIEL, A. H., L. K. TAKAHASHI & N. H. KALIN. 1993. Brain Res. **623:** 229-234.
34. HITCHCOCK, J. & M. DAVIS. 1986. Behav. Neurosci. **100:** 11-22.
35. ROTHSCHILD, A. J. 1993. Psychiatric Ann. **23:** 662-670.
36. GOLD, P. W., G. CHROUSOS, C. KELLNER, R. POST, A. ROY, P. AUGERINOS, H. SCHULTE, E. OLDFIELD & D. L. LORIAUX. 1984. Am. J. Psychiatry **141:** 619-627.
37. HOLSBOER, F., A. GERKEN, G. K. STALLA & O. A. MUELLER. 1985. Biol. Psychiatry **20:** 276-286.
38. NEMEROFF, C. B., E. WIDERLOV, G. BISSETTE, H. WALLEUS, L. KARLSSON, K. EKLUND, C. D. KILTS, P. T. LOOSEN & W. VALE. 1984. Science **226:** 1342-1344.

39. OWENS, M. J., P. M. PLOTSKY & C. B. NEMEROFF. 1996. Peptides and affective disorders. *In* S. J. Watson, Ed.: 259-293. Biology of Schizophrenia and Affective Disorders. American Psychiatric Press. Washington, DC.
40. ARATO, M., C. M. BANKI, G. BISSETTE & C. B. NEMEROFF. Biol. Psychiatry 25: 355-359.
41. RAADSHEER, F. C., W. J. HOOGENDIJK, F. C. STAM, F. J. TILDERS & D. F. SWAAB. 1994. Neuroendocrinology 60: 436-444.
42. RAADSHEER, F. C., J. J. VAN HEERIKHUIZE, P. J. LUCASSEN, W. J. HOOGENDIJK, F. J. TILDERS & D. F. SWAAB. 1995. Am. J. Psychiatry 152: 1372-1376.
43. NEMEROFF, C. B., G. BISSETTE, H. AKIL & M. FINK. 1991. Br. J. Psychiatry 158: 59-63.
44. KALIN, N. H. 1996. Animal Models of Depression and Anxiety: Utility in New Drug Development. ISPNE XXVIIth Congress Abstracts: 52.
45. NEMEROFF, C. B., M. J. OWENS, G. BISSETTE, A. C. ANDORN & M. STANLEY. 1988. Arch. Gen. Psychiatry 45: 577-579.
46. KRISHNAN, K. R. R. 1993. Psychiatric Ann. 23: 671-675.
47. MASON, J. W., E. L. GILLER, T. R. KOSTEN, R. B. OSTROFF & L. PODD. 1986. J. Nerv. Ment. Dis. 174: 145-159.
48. YEHUDA, R., S. M. SOUTHWICK, G. NUSSBAUM, V. WAHBY, E. L. GILLER & J. W. MASON. 1990. J. Nerv. Ment. Dis. 178: 366-369.
49. YEHUDA, R., E. L. GILLER, S. M. SOUTHWICK, M. T. LOWY & J. W. MASON. 1991. Biol. Psychiatry 30: 1031-1048.
50. YEHUDA, R., M. H. TEICHER, R. A. LEVENGOOD, R. L. TRESTMAN & L. J. SIEVER. 1994. Ann. N.Y. Acad. Sci. 746: 378-380.
51. YEHUDA, R., E. L. GILLER, R. A. LEVENGOOD, S. M. SOUTHWICK & L. J. SIEVER. 1995. Hypothalamic-pituitary-adrenal functioning in posttraumatic stress disorder. *In* Neurobiological and Clinical Consequences of Stress. M. J. Friedman, D. S. Charney & A. Y. Deutch, Eds.: 351-366. Lippincott-Raven. Philadelphia, PA.
52. YEHUDA, R., R. A. LEVENGOOD, J. SCHMEIDLER, S. WILSON, L. S. GUO & D. GERBER. 1996. Psychoneuroendocrinology 21: 1-16.
53. SMITH, M. A., J. DAVIDSON, J. C. RITCHIE, H. KUDLER, S. LIPPER, P. CHAPPELL & C. B. NEMEROFF. 1989. Biol. Psychiatry 26: 349-355.
54. DEBELLIS, M. D., G. P. CHROUSOS, L. D. DORN, L. BURKE, K. HELMERS, M. A. KLING, P. K. TRICKETT & F. W. PUTNAM. 1994. J. Clin. Endocrinol. Metab. 78: 249-255.
55. BREMNER, J. D., J. LICINO, A. DARNELL, J. H. KRYSTAL, M. J. OWENS, S. M. SOUTHWICK, C. B. NEMEROFF & D. S. CHARNEY. Am. J. Psychiatry. In press.
56. KOSTEN, T. R., J. W. MASON, E. L. GILLER & L. HARKNESS. 1987. Psychoneuroendocrinology 12: 13-20.
57. PERRY, B. D., S. M. SOUTHWICK & E. L. GILLER. 1987. Am. J. Psychiatry 144: 1511-1512.
58. SOUTHWICK, S. M., J. H. KRYSTAL, D. R. JOHNSON, L. M. NAGY, A. NICOLAU, G. R. HENINGER & D. S. CHARNEY. 1993. Arch. Gen. Psychiatry 50: 266-274.
59. CHAPPELL, P. B., M. A. SMITH, C. D. KILTS, G. BISSETTE, J. C. RITCHIE, C. ANDERSON & C. B. NEMEROFF. 1986. J. Neurosci. 6: 2908-2914.
60. DE GOEIJ, D. C., R. KVETNANSKY, M. H. WHITNALL, D. JEZOVA, F. BERKENBOSCH & F. J. H. TILDERS. 1991. Neuroendocrinology 53: 150-159.
61. WHITNALL, M. H. 1989. Neuroendocrinology 50: 702-707.
62. VAN DIJKEN, H. H., D. C. DE GOEIJ, W. SUTANTO, J. MOS, E. R. DE KLOET & F. J. H. TILDERS. 1993. Neuroendocrinology 58: 57-64.
63. HAUGER, R. L., M. A. MILLAN, M. LORANG, J. P. HARWOOD & G. AGUILERA. 1988. Endocrinology 123: 396-405.
64. HAUGER, R. L., M. LORANG, M. IRWIN & G. AGUILERA. 1990. Brain Res. 532: 34-40.
65. PITMAN, D. L., J. E. OTTENWELLER & B. H. NATELSON. 1988. Physiol. Behav. 43: 47-55.
66. BASSETT, J. R. & K. D. CAIRNCROSS. 1973. Physiol. Behav. 10: 901-907.
67. RIVIER, C. & W. VALE. 1987. Endocrinology 121: 1320-1328.
68. FRIEDMAN, S. B., J. W. MASON & D. A. HANBURG. 1963. Psychosom. Med. 25: 364-376.
69. BOURNE, P. G., R. M. ROSE & J. W. MASON. 1968. Arch. Gen. Psychiatry 19: 135-140.

70. CAPLAN, R. D., S. COBB & J. R. FRENCH. 1979. J. Psychosom. Res. **23:** 181-192.
71. MASON, J. W., J. V. BRADY & G. A. TOLLIVER. 1968. Psychosom. Med. **30:** 608-630.
72. ARMARIO, A., J. HIDALGO & M. GIRALT. 1988. Neuroendocrinology **47:** 263-267.
73. HERMAN, J. P., M. K. H. SCHÄFER, C. D. SLADEK, R. DAY, E. A. YOUNG, H. AKIL & S. J. WATSON. 1989. Brain Res. **501:** 235-246.
74. IMAKI, T., J. L. NAHAN, C. RIVIER, P. E. SAWCHENKO & W. VALE. 1991. J. Neurosci. **11:** 585-599.
75. HERMAN, J. P., D. ADAMS & C. PREWITT. 1995. Neuroendocrinology **61:** 180-190.
76. ANDERSON, S. M., G. J. KANT & E. B. DE SOUZA. 1993. Pharmacol. Biochem. Behav. **44:** 755-761.
77. FUCHS, E. & G. FLÜGGE. 1995. Psychoneuroendocrinology **20:** 33-51.
78. LEVINE, S. 1957. Science **126:** 405-406.
79. DENENBERG, V. H. 1964. Psychol. Rev. **71:** 335-351.
80. MEANEY, M. J., B. TANNENBAUM, D. FRANCIS, S. BHATNAGAR, N. SHANKS, V. VIAU, D. O'DONNELL & P. M. PLOTSKY. 1994. Sem. Neurosci. **6:** 247-259.
81. MEANEY, M. J., D. H. AITKEN, V. VIAU, S. SHARMA & A. SARIEAU. 1989. Neuroendocrinology **50:** 597-604.
82. MEANEY, M. J. & D. H. AITKEN. 1985. Dev. Brain Res. **22:** 301-304.
83. MEANEY, M. J., D. H. AITKEN, S. R. BODNOFF, L.-J. INY, J. E. TATAREWICZ & R. M. SAPOLSKY. 1985. Behav. Neurosci. **99:** 765-770.
84. O'DONNELL, D., S. LAROCQUE, J. R. SECKL & M. J. MEANEY. 1994. Mol. Brain Res. **26:** 242-248.
85. VIAU, V., S. SHARMA, P. M. PLOTSKY & M. J. MEANEY. 1993. J. Neurosci. **13:** 1097-1105.
86. PLOTSKY, P. M. & M. J. MEANEY. 1993. Mol. Brain Res. **18:** 195-200.
87. LADD, C. O., M. J. OWENS & C. B. NEMEROFF. 1996. Endocrinology **137:** 1212-1218.
88. PIHOKER, C., M. J. OWENS, C. M. KUHN, S. M. SCHANBERG & C. B. NEMEROFF. 1993. Psychoneuroendocrinology **18:** 485-493.
89. NEMEROFF, C. B., M. J. OWENS, S. J. PLOTT & S. LEVINE. 1993. Soc. Neurosci. Abstr. **19:** 1.
90. COPLAN, J. D., M. W. ANDREWS, L. A. ROSENBLUM, M. J. OWENS, S. FRIEDMAN, J. M. GORMAN & C. B. NEMEROFF. 1996. Neurobiology **93:** 1619-1623.
91. ROSENBLUM, L. A. & G. S. PAULLY. 1984. Child Dev. **55:** 305-314.
92. ROSENBLUM, L. A., J. D. COPLAN, S. FRIEDMAN, J. M. GORMAN & M. W. ANDREWS. 1994. Biol. Psychiatry **35:** 221-227.

Performance of PTSD Patients on Standard Tests of Memory

Implications for Trauma[a]

J. WOLFE [b,c,d] AND L. K. SCHLESINGER [b,d]

[b]*Women's Health Sciences Division*
National Center for PTSD and

[c]*Tufts University School of Medicine*
Boston, Massachusetts 02130

Use of neuropsychological tests in posttraumatic stress disorder (PTSD) began approximately 10 years ago with the growing interest in reported concentration and memory problems in trauma survivors. Clinicians in particular were familiar with patients' descriptions of difficulties attending to and recalling basic factual data while concomitantly reporting distressing, intermittently recurrent intrusive memories of traumas. This seeming dichotomy in performance could be roughly characterized in two ways: (1) a nonspecific concentration or memory deficit in this disorder, and (2) the tendency to selectively attend to or encode cues related to traumatic experiences. These two approaches had differing implications: a focus on memory problems in general could suggest a more basic cognitive disturbance previously described in other anxiety and depressive disorders, with limited specificity for PTSD, or an alteration in learning or processing capabilities that might be distinctive for trauma syndromes.[1,2]

This paper provides an overview of the topic of memory performance in PTSD, beginning with common etiological frameworks that have been employed to examine this issue. Next, extant use of neuropsychological tests, including standard and empirical measures, are reviewed followed by a summation of performance findings to date. The article concludes by reviewing the concordance between current models of memory disturbances and cognitive changes in PTSD and proposes a series of issues that need to be addressed in future research on this topic.

CONCEPTUAL MODELS

Basic Memory Models

The application of general theories of memory to purported learning deficits in PTSD is relatively broad at this time. Some models have suggested that recall and learning could be adversely affected by factors ranging from fluctuations in general

[a]This research was supported by a Department of Veterans Affairs Medical Research Service Award to J.W.

[d]Address for correspondence: DVA Medical Center (116B-3), 150 S. Huntington Ave., Boston, MA 02130.

attention or concentration to decreased motivation or affective condition of the respondent (e.g., depression).[3] These observations reflect mechanisms that have relevance for understanding the cognitive deficits found in other major psychiatric disorders (e.g., major depression and panic disorder). These models generally predict that memory problems in affective or anxiety disorders stem from processing deficits that are based in affective and sensory dysregulation.[4] Still, although PTSD shares certain phenomenological characteristics with these disorders (e.g., agitation and depressed mood), currently few, if any, empirical data exist to confirm any commonality in either core memory disturbances or underlying functional mechanisms.

More detailed probes into memory changes in PTSD have speculated that alterations in certain brain neurotransmitter systems (e.g., catecholamines) are likely to have an impact on memory and recall. Preclinical and clinical research in fact substantiate that noradrenaline and, recently, serotonin, are linked to basic changes in attention and concentration (e.g., disruptions in selective attention).[5] Furthermore, psychobiological research in PTSD confirms that central noradrenaline functions are abnormal in PTSD,[6] and preclinical research demonstrates that noradrenergic neurons in the thalamus and amygdala are selectively activated by stress. Since fear conditioning, a basic component of PTSD, is mediated through sensory pathways in subcortical brain systems that project to the thalamus and amygdala, it is not surprising that PTSD patients might evidence disruptions in cognitive processing, at least under conditions of high arousal or fear.[7] Thus, memory changes in this disorder could stem from the involvement of complex neural mechanisms and brain chemicals implicated in the response (or adaptation) to intense fear.[8]

Support for neurotransmitter relevance in cognition in PTSD is also found in the growing number of studies which show that PTSD is associated with significantly slowed reaction times on tasks involving the detection of target stimuli,[5] a finding that has been supported for both neutral[5] as well threat-based stimuli.[9-11] One possible explanation for these findings is that sustained or selective attentional disturbances affect the rate and depth of subsequent processing, rendering individuals vulnerable to interference, complex processing demands, and inefficient encoding. In this scenario, neurochemical dysregulation in PTSD is linked to memory problems largely through disturbances in attentional systems, the normal foundation for preserved recall.

Evidence of decreased hippocampal volume in some PTSD patients has recently suggested that actual neuroanatomic changes in the brain, possibly at the limbic or paralimbic level, might be linked to the development of cognitive changes.[12] Research by a number of investigators[13] has emphasized the importance of subcortical structures, such as the hippocampus, for certain components of memory (e.g., the explicit memory processing needed for memory consolidation). Accordingly, the permanency of memory traces could be impacted by structural changes in these brain regions. Still, despite preliminary data, empirical evidence that ties subtle neuroanatomical alterations to measurable cognitive change remains limited at this time[14] as does the specificity of such a finding for PTSD.[15]

Network Memory Models

In contrast to general models of memory, information-processing network models propose that memory changes or deficits in PTSD depend on the existence of closely interlinked, semantic networks whose associational nodules are laid down during trauma.[16,17] These trauma-specific associations often generalize to other stimuli through secondary and higher order conditioning and are subsequently activated during the intense reexperiencing phenomena and phasic arousal found in PTSD. Recently, Metcalfe and Jacobs[18] suggested certain neuroanatomic correlates for network memory models in PTSD. Specifically, the hippocampus is seen as related to a "cool-cognition" dimension, while the amygdala is associated with a "hot-emotion" function. On the basis of this differentiation, the two brain structures are separately implicated in PTSD: traumatization, for example, substantially impacts the "cool" system by disabling certain of its functional cognitive capabilities, while the "hot" system associated with the amygdala becomes hyperresponsive. In actual neurologic disease, hippocampal disturbances would likely result in cognitive deficits in spatial perception, spatial memory, and episodic memory, while overall cognitive skills remain intact. In PTSD, where involvement of this brain region is likely to be more diffuse or nonspecific, cognitive abilities could remain intact, but fear-provoking stimuli would be liable to encoding in the absence of an adequate temporospatial context. Accordingly, many trauma memories could not be reliably retrieved from episodic memory. In contrast to the preceding, activation of the amygdala and associated structures could contribute to the phasic appearance of intense, intrusive thoughts and trauma memory fragments.

Overall, models like these help to emphasize the critical role played by stimuli with affective connotations, suggesting that PTSD is not necessarily linked to any clearcut storage or retrieval deficit per se but, rather, to disruptions at the intial encoding level, at least for certain types of information. Furthermore, these models offer some of the first evidence for bidirectionality in memory performance in PTSD; that is, under certain conditions, memory abilities could actually be enhanced, while under others, they are diminished.

Resource Allocation Models

Resource allocation models are similar to network models in that they propose the effects of an interlinked series of cognitive mechanisms in PTSD. Similar to cognitive and memory models for clinical depression, resource allocation theories suggest that the selective deployment of attentional skills to certain stimuli leads to their heightened accessibility. Under particular conditions, however (e.g., those involving competing task demands or complex, multilevel processing), the performance by a PTSD patient suffers appreciably because of the competition among fixed allocation resources. In this scenario, the level or complexity of a task could produce interference or disruption in required inhibition by drawing focused attention elsewhere. Consequently, the rapidity or accuracy of recall is likely to be seriously compromised. Research by McNally and colleagues[19] is particularly informative in this area. These investigators conducted experimental cognitive studies in PTSD and found growing evidence that certain characteristics of this disorder substantially disrupt correlates of normal information processing. As a result, some PTSD patients demonstrate measurable disturbances in normal attention and attendant recall when fear-based or trauma stimuli are used. Furthermore, the data suggest that cognitive patterns in PTSD are notable for a pronounced bias towards high threat stimuli. Additional studies are required to determine whether baseline attention and memory are intact during more complex tasks in the context of these demonstrated aberrations at higher levels.

ASSESSMENT PARADIGMS

To assess memory in PTSD, clinicians and researchers have selected from a range of extant neuropsychological tests, with a primary interest on recall and effects of interference. Tests of recognition memory have generated somewhat greater interest, probably because of their less challenging nature in a population not known to have discrete brain lesions. Standard memory tests (e.g., Wechsler Memory Scale[20] and its revised version [WMS(-R)][21]) have been used to assess immediate and delayed verbal and nonverbal visual memory,[22] while more complex tasks (e.g., California Verbal Learning Test [CVLT][23] and Selective Reminding Test [SRT][24,25]) are employed when the study of memory correlates (e.g., retention capacity, efficiency, and interference effects) are of interest.

To date, studies using tests such as the WMS(-R) have yielded, at best, equivocal evidence for memory impairment in PTSD.[26] Overall, these and other data[27] suggest that most PTSD patients are not likely to have appreciable memory deficits *in the absence of* histories of diagnosed neurologic disease, head injury with loss of consciousness, or notable developmental (learning) disabilities, all factors that could impact memory performance independently. Because of high rates of these problems, the association of any defects in learning and memory in these patients cannot always be readily or definitively linked to PTSD, particularly without the use of more sophisticated tests known to dissociate among various etiologies.[28] In addition, tests such as the WMS(-R) are likely to lack sufficient difficulty for use with some PTSD patients who perform at a test's upper limits because of their higher functional status. Accordingly, such tests will fail to detect all but the most serious memory problems. In contrast, tests such as the CVLT, which are more challenging and contain measures of disparate memory abilities (e.g., retention over trials, primacy and recency, and effects of interference) are potentially more useful in PTSD.[29]

Still, without the testing of other higher cortical functions, it is difficult to assess if memory functions alone are affected in PTSD or if the performance of these patients reflects more generally disrupted cognitive abilities (e.g., frontally mediated processing inefficiencies). It is noteworthy that within some PTSD populations (e.g., combat veterans), high proportions of participants are likely to have learning disabilities or other developmental problems in their backgrounds[3,28,30] Such data raise speculation about whether earlier, predisposing characteristics constitute a vulnerability in this disorder for either the development of PTSD following trauma exposure or the manifestation of deficits in proximal domains (i.e., memory) when tested as adults.[31] As such, neuropsychologists and others might be well advised to assess a broader range of functions (including sequencing and organizational skills) which typically underlie the performance of memory tasks when evaluating PTSD in certain populations.[32] This approach would place memory assessment within a larger context and could help address whether memory systems per se are disrupted by this disorder or whether alterations represent more basic, structural, or systemic anomalies.

Generally, more definitive memory changes are found when experimental neuro-psychological tests are employed with PTSD patients.[33,34] These tasks are typically more challenging in their attentional, memorial, and processing requirements; further-more, their design permits the breaking apart of various memory components, enabling improved content analysis. To date, research findings have provided data in two important domains: (1) the nature of selective processing and retention in PTSD, and (2) the capacity for general recall under varying demand conditions.

Current findings suggest that individuals with PTSD in fact demonstrate changes in the processing of emotionally salient material[35] as well as in attention. These data confirm an enhanced attentional bias for trauma salient or trauma congruent stimuli. When complex processing tasks are employed, these alterations are likely to be seen in conjunction with markedly increased response latencies, suggesting the reallocation of attentional resources (as evidenced on Stroop tasks when emotionally laden words are employed[10,15,36]) and a pronounced susceptibility to trauma congruent interference. Whether these deficits will be confirmed on tasks involving nontraumatic stimuli is unclear at this time. However, it is essential that research be structured so that effects of stimulus content can be dissembled from basic processing and memorial requirements if correlates of memory in PTSD are to be elucidated.[37,38]

CURRENT EMPIRICAL FINDINGS

To summarize, findings of cognitive deficits in PTSD can be classified broadly in two categories: (1) those providing evidence for equivocal or no deficits across a range of functions (e.g., attention, verbal fluency, and visual tracking) and (2) those supporting memory deficits in verbal or visuospatial domains. A brief review of empirical research in each is provided.

Yehuda et al.[29] administered standard neuropsychological tests to individuals with and without PTSD and found that PTSD patients generally performed within normal limits on a variety of attention, immediate memory, and cumulative learning tasks. However, when tasks involved interference conditions, the performance of PTSD patients, specifically their capacity for retention, diminished. This finding preliminar-ily strengthens the argument that memory defects in PTSD may reflect underlying attentional disturbances. Evidence of other subtle cognitive changes comes from research involving the use of standard and experimental neuropsychological para-digms. Uddo et al.[39] examined the performance of male veterans with PTSD and found learning inefficiencies marked by decrements in cumulative learning across trials, a pattern not observed in individuals without this disorder. In addition, the performance of PTSD patients was characterized by more perseverative errors, prob-lems in fluency and tracking, and sensitivity to proactive interference. Together, these deficits suggest the possibility of changes in brain mechanisms that support more complex and efficient learning.

Other evidence for minor cognitive and memory alterations comes from experi-ments on autobiographical memory in PTSD.[19,40] McNally et al.[19,40] found that PTSD patients tended to overgeneralize on tasks involving personal recall, suggesting limita-tions in their ability to distinguish effectively among various salient cues. Similarly, Schwarz et al.[41] demonstrated that individuals exposed to trauma were susceptible to altering their retrospective reports of events, regardless of age. These changes included distortions in proximity to the event as well as in event sequencing. Furthermore, greater perceptual memory changes were associated with increasing levels of PTSD symptoms. However, these performance patterns were also associated with symptoms of anxiety and depression; hence, the specificity of this finding for PTSD is unclear.

Use of experimental laboratory tests of cognition offer a better opportunity to disentangle the components of memory performance in PTSD. To date, changes in recall have been found using both explicit (with conscious awareness) and implicit (without conscious awareness) memory paradigms. Because prior research on these memory systems suggests that they are distinct from each other, such findings might imply that memory problems in PTSD are diffuse or nonspecific, rather than selective.[42] However, closer examination of research findings shows that certain characteristics of memory tasks may play a role.

In terms of actual recall capabilities, data from explicit memory studies remain equivocal. Although Yehuda et al.[29] found that explicit memory in PTSD was intact, other studies have found evidence of impairment.[13] According to resource allocation models, one possible explanation is that explicit memory performance in PTSD is impacted by the diminution of attentional resources during processing conducted under conscious control. This theory, espoused by Siegel,[13] suggests that the emotional reactivity caused during trauma leads to cognitive disruption by dividing attentional resources and disturbing focal attention and effortful learning. Furthermore, only explicit memory is affected because material processed under less than full conscious awareness (i.e., implicit memory) is afforded greater scrutiny, especially when the content is emotionally salient. This model is predicated on the assumption that only conscious, effortful learning is disrupted within an integrated memory system.

Other data, which are not inherently contradictory, suggest that implicit memory remains intact or is potentially enhanced in PTSD. Using resource allocation or memory network models, this performance pattern could stem from an intensified focus on material that has prime informational importance, that is, data relating to conditions of threat or intense fear. Some research studies have hypothesized that this process is analogous to PTSD's reexperiencing symptom cluster, that is, behavioral manifestations of efforts to reintegrate unabsorbed cognitive and affective elements associated with the trauma.[43] In fact, several studies show that implicit memory performance in PTSD is likely either to (1) exceed that of normal control subjects or (2) be enhanced relative to PTSD patients' explicit memory abilities.[33,44] Importantly, these findings are most robust when threat consonant stimuli are employed, again suggesting the importance of conditioned associations. Together with evidence from autobiographical tasks, implicit memory data appear to confirm that the observed memory and learning alterations in PTSD stem more from affectively based effects of stimulus content rather than disruptions in basic memory systems per se.

Despite the early stage of neuroscientific research in PTSD, data identifying more selective memory problems offer some evidence for linkages between the pathophysiology of this disorder and memory. Sutker et al.[45] examined a pair of monozygotic adult twins and found that only the twin with PTSD showed deficits on tasks of nonverbal memory. New studies using brain imaging also offer preliminary evidence concerning brain change in PTSD and its relevance for cognitive status.

Bremner *et al.*[12] studied male Vietnam combat veterans with PTSD and found evidence for significant reduction in right hippocampal density (8%) compared to that of participants without this disorder. Furthermore, volumetric decrease was associated with concurrent deficits in *verbal,* short-term memory as measured by the WMS. Measures of other brain regions (e.g., temporal lobes) in these patients did not show similar decreases, suggesting the possibility that the hippocampus could play a distinctive role in the mediation of traumatic stress and its associated features.

Although these results are compelling, findings from other neuroanatomically based studies in PTSD suggest greater discretion. Stein[14] studied female survivors of childhood sexual abuse with and without PTSD and observed diminished right hippocampal density in abuse survivors as a group, irrespective of PTSD status. Thus, severe trauma exposure, rather than the ensuing PTSD, might be a determining factor. Furthermore, this study failed to demonstrate the presence of notable memory deficits in women either with or without PTSD, suggesting that hippocampal density was not directly implicated in the genesis of memory changes. Still, these studies reflect the complexity of content and methodological issues that will need to be addressed, including gender, age, intensity of trauma exposure, and symptom duration.

Data from studies in the neurosciences offer other evidence for contexts in which more localized memory deficits might occur in PTSD. Basic neurological research in patients undergoing temporal lobectomy, for example, has demonstrated the strong relationship between these brain regions and preserved functions of verbal and visual memory, substantiating the normal neural substrates for these functions.[46–49] Furthermore, Trenerry *et al.*[50] recently showed that destruction (i.e., removal) of portions of certain underlying subcortical areas (e.g., right hippocampus) produces similarly noteworthy declines in visual memory. However, most PTSD patients are not thought to have discrete brain lesions. Accordingly, evidence for the link between known structural damage and particular cognitive skills is far more substantial than that proposed for most psychiatric conditions.

CONCLUSION

Growing research suggests that certain cognitive alterations occur in PTSD. These changes are generally characterized by a preferential bias or increased attention associated with the presentation of threat-related stimuli, despite processing latencies. Accordingly, PTSD patients may evidence seemingly enhanced learning and retention of some trauma stimuli. In other instances, deficits in explicit recall are documented, but these are not uniformly observed. Importantly, the conditions under which explicit memory deficits occur are not well understood and are likely to reflect diverse factors such as baseline cognitive abilities, history of learning disabilities, and contributions of mood states.

Results of both enhanced and decreased memory functioning in PTSD raise the possibility of a bidirectional memory model. Such a model is consonant with the phenomenology of PTSD which reflects alternating elements of phasic sensitization/hyperreactivity and avoidance/numbing. As brain and behavioral mechanisms of PTSD are better understood, complex interactions between intrinsic cortical and external or contextual factors should help to elucidate the conditions under which various cognitive mechanisms operate. Still, certain methodological issues warrant mention. First, future research should address the specificity of any observed memory changes for this disorder. To date, studies have relied nearly exclusively on contrasts between PTSD and well-adjusted samples, precluding critical diagnostic comparisons. Subsequent studies will need to employ a range of appropriate, matched psychiatric comparison groups to demonstrate the ways in which deficits are specific to PTSD and not generic to psychiatric disturbance overall[51] or subsets of anxiety and affective disorders in particular. Relatedly, study designs should more carefully assess extant comorbidities in PTSD patients and control groups, especially given the high rates of comorbid disorders in PTSD and the demonstrated impact of such disorders (e.g., major depression) on memory performance.

Second, improved assessment of baseline cognitive abilities in respondents is strongly recommended. This should be conducted across the range of cortical functions, so that evaluation of learning and memory skills can be considered in the appropriate context and at various levels of difficulty. Special attention should be paid to the possibility of early developmental anomalies or learning disabilities given the growing interest in family genetics and inborn vulnerabilities for conditions such as PTSD.[31,52] Third, the performance of PTSD patients on neuropsychological measures to date indicates that more sophisticated tests of memory and attention are needed. Currently, interpretation of some study results is constrained by potential ceiling effects of certain tests, limiting the ability to detect subtle performance alterations. Also, both standard and experimental neuropsychological tests should be employed that permit closer examination of critical components of learning and memory, for example, response latencies, sequential processing, span of apprehension, and susceptibility to various forms of interference. Finally, we encourage the development of prospective studies in trauma-exposed young individuals with and without the PTSD diagnosis, as this research offers the opportunity to examine contributions of age, developmental status, plasticity, and adaptational mechanisms to cognitive performance across the spectrum of stress responses.

SUMMARY

Mental health professionals have employed a variety of clinical and experimental neuropsychological tests for exploring purported memory alterations in PTSD. Protocols range from standard tests of immediate and delayed learning, recall, and recognition to elaborate paradigms using experimental stimuli for assessment of information-processing skills. Whereas the former have typically focused on general learning and memory capabilities, experimental paradigms have examined the role of trauma-related cues and their impact on remembering. Findings to date suggest that memory abilities in PTSD patients range from intact to mildly impaired on general tests of verbal or visual memory. At the same time, memory tests involving trauma-specific stimuli point to alterations in cognitive information processing, specifically, an attentional bias manifested by changes in speed, accuracy, and depth of processing. The role of a semantic information network involving enhanced specificity for trauma cues is discussed along with possible implications for brain structures and theories of PTSD.

REFERENCES

1. KUYKEN, W. & C. R. BREWIN. 1994. Intrusive memories of childhood abuse during depressive episodes. Behav. Res. Ther. **32:** 525-528.
2. FOA, E. B., G. STEKETEE & B. O. ROTHBAUM. 1989. Behavioral/cognitive conceptualizations of post-traumatic stress disorder. Behav. Ther. **20:** 155-176.
3. WOLFE, J. & D. S. CHARNEY. 1991. Use of neuropsychological assessment in posttraumatic stress disorder. Psychol. Assess. **3:** 573-580.
4. KING, D. A., E. D. CAINE & C. COX. 1993. Influence of depression and age on selected cognitive functions. Clin. Neuropsychologist **7:** 443-453.
5. MCFARLANE, A. C., D. L. WEBER & C. R. CLARK. 1993. Abnormal stimulus processing in posttraumatic stress disorder. Biol. Psychiatry **34:** 311-320.
6. SOUTHWICK, S. M., J. H. KRYSTAL, C. A. MORGAN, D. JOHNSON, L. M. NAGY, A. NICOLAOU, G. R. HENINGER & D. S. CHARNEY. 1993. Abnormal noradrenergic function in posttraumatic stress disorder. Arch. Gen. Psychiatry **50:** 266-274.
7. TEICHER, M. H., C. A. GLOD, J. SURREY & C. SWETT. 1993. Early childhood abuse and limbic system ratings in adult psychiatric outpatients. J. Neuropsychiatry Clin. Neurosci. **5:** 301-306.
8. CHARNEY, D. S., A. Y. DEUTCH, J. H. KRYSTAL, S. M. SOUTHWICK & M. DAVIS. 1993. Psychobiological mechanisms of posttraumatic stress disorder. Arch. Gen. Psychiatry **50:** 294-305.
9. MCNALLY, R. J., D. L. LUEDKE, J. K. BESYNER, R. A. PETERSON, K. BOHM & O. J. LIPS. 1987. Sensitivity to stress relevant stimuli in posttraumatic stress disorder. J. Anxiety Disord. **1:** 105-116.
10. FOA, E. B., U. FESKE, T. B. MURDOCK, M. J. KOZAC & P. R. MCCARTHY. 1991. Processing of threat related information in rape victims. J. Abnorm. Psychol. **100:** 156-162.
11. MCNALLY, R. J., S. P. KASPI, B. C. RIEMANN & S. B. ZEITLIN. 1990. Selective processing of threat cues in posttraumatic stress disorder. J. Abnorm. Psychol. **99:** 398-402.
12. BREMNER, J. D., P. RANDALL, T. M. SCOTT, R. A. BRONEN, J. P. SEIBYL, S. M. SOUTHWICK, R. C. DELANEY, G. MCCARTHY, D. S. CHARNEY & R. B. INNIS. 1995. MRI-based measurement of hippocampal volume in patients with combat-related posttraumatic stress disorder. Am. J. Psychiatry **152:** 971-981.
13. SIEGEL, D. J. 1995. Memory, trauma, and psychotherapy: A cognitive science review. J. Psychother. Pract. Res. **4:** 93-122.
14. STEIN, M. B. 1997. Structural brain changes in PTSD: Does trauma alter neuroanatomy? Ann. N.Y. Acad. Sci., this volume.
15. BRYANT, R. A. & A. G. HARVEY. 1995. Processing threatening information in posttraumatic stress disorder. J. Abnorm. Psychol. **104:** 537-541.
16. CHEMTOB, C. M., H. L. ROITBLAT, R. S. HAMADA, J. G. CARLSON & C. T. TWENTYMAN. 1988. A cognitive action theory of Post-Traumatic Stress Disorder. J. Anxiety Disord. **2:** 253-275.
17. PITMAN, R. K. 1988. Post-traumatic stress disorder, conditioning, and network theory. Psychiatr. Ann. **18:** 182-189.
18. METCALFE, J. & W. J. JACOBS. 1996. A "hot-system/cool system" view of memory under stress. PTSD Res. Q. **7:** 1-3.
19. MCNALLY, R. J., N. B. LASKO, M. L. MACKLIN & R. K. PITMAN. 1995. Autobiographical memory disturbance in combat-related posttraumatic stress disorder. Behav. Res. Ther. **33:** 619-630.
20. WECHSLER, D. 1974. Wechsler Memory Scale Manual. The Psychological Corporation. San Antonio, TX.
21. WECHSLER, D. 1987. Wechsler Memory Scale-Revised Manual. The Psychological Corporation. San Antonio, TX.
22. BREMNER, J. D., T. M. SCOTT, R. C. DELANEY, S. M. SOUTHWICK, J. W. MASON, D. R. JOHNSON, R. B. INNIS, G. MCCARTHY & D. S. CHARNEY. 1993. Deficits in short-term memory in posttraumatic stress disorder. Am. J. Psychiatry **150:** 1015-1019.

23. Delis, D. C., J. H. Kramer, E. Kaplan & B. A. Ober. 1987. California Verbal Learning Test: Adult Version. The Psychological Corporation. San Antonio, TX.

24. Buschke, H. & P. A. Fuld. 1974. Evaluating storage, retention, and retrieval in disordered memory and learning. Neurology **24:** 1019-1025.

25. Hannay, H. J. & H. S. Levin. 1985. Selective Reminding Test: An examination of the equivalence of four forms. J. Clin. Exp. Neuropsychol. **7:** 251-263.

26. Levy, C. L. 1988. Agent orange exposure and posttraumatic stress disorder. J. Nerv. Ment. Dis. **176:** 242-245.

27. Speed, N., B. Engdahl, J. Schwartz & R. Eberly. 1989. Posttraumatic stress disorder as a consequence of the POW experience. J. Nerv. Ment. Dis. **177:** 147-153.

28. Centers for Disease Control. 1988. Health status of Vietnam veterans. J.A.M.A. **259:** 2701-2724.

29. Yehuda, R., R. S. E. Keefe, P. D. Harvey, R. A. Levengood, D. K. Gerber, J. Geni & L. J. Siever. 1995. Learning and memory in combat veterans with posttraumatic stress disorder. Am. J. Psychiatry **152:** 137-139.

30. McCranie, E. W., L. A. Hyer, P. A. Boudewyns & M. G. Woods. 1992. Negative parenting behavior, combat exposure, and PTSD symptom severity: Test of a person-event interaction model. J. Nerv. Ment. Dis. **180:** 431-438.

31. True, W. R., J. Rice, S. A. Eisen, A. C. Heath, J. Goldberg, M. J. Lyons & J. Nowak. 1993. A twin study of genetic and environmental contributions to liability for posttraumatic stress symptoms. Arch. Gen. Psychiatry **50:** 257-264.

32. Kaplan, E. 1990. The process approach to neuropsychological assessment of psychiatric patients. J. Neuropsychiatry Clin. Neurosci. **2:** 72-87.

33. Wolfe, J., P. C. Ouimette, K. R. Chrestman, D. Kaloupek & S. G. Joaquim. 1997. Implicit and explicit memory for military words in female veterans, Red Cross, and USO volunteers of the Vietnam era. Submitted.

34. Kaszniak, A. W., P. D. Nussbaum, M. R. Berren & J. Santiago. 1988. Amnesia as a consequence of male rape: A case report. J. Abnorm. Psychol. **97:** 100-104.

35. Thrasher, S. M., T. Dalgleish & W. Yule. 1994. Information processing in post-traumatic stress disorder. Behav. Res. Ther. **32:** 247-254.

36. Cassiday, K. L., R. J. McNally & S. B. Zeitlin. 1992. Cognitive processing of trauma cues in rape victims with post-traumatic stress disorder. Cognit. Ther. Res. **16:** 283-295.

37. Vrana, S. R., A. Roodman & J. C. Beckham. 1995. Selective processing of trauma-relevant words in posttraumatic stress disorder. J. Anxiety Disord. **9:** 515-530.

38. Schacter, D. L. & J. F. Kihlstrom. 1989. Functional amnesia. In Handbook of Neuropsychology. F. Boller & J. Grafman, Eds. Elsevier Publications. Amsterdam.

39. Uddo, M., J. J. Vasterling, K. Brailey & P. B. Sutker. 1993. Memory and attention in combat-related post-traumatic stress disorder (PTSD). J. Psychopathol. Behav. Assess. **15:** 43-52.

40. McNally, R. J., B. T. Litz, A. Prassas, L. M. Shin & F. W. Weathers. 1994. Emotional priming of autobiographical memory in post-traumatic stress disorder. Cognition Emotion **8:** 351-367.

41. Schwarz, E. D., J. M. Kowalski & R. J. McNally. 1993. Malignant memories: Post-traumatic changes in memory in adults after a school shooting. J. Trauma Stress **6:** 545-553.

42. Schacter, D. L., C. Y. P. Chiu & K. N. Ochsner. 1993. Implicit memory: A selective review. Annu. Rev. Neurosci. **16:** 159-182.

43. Layton, B. S. & K. Wardi-Zonna. 1995. Posttraumatic stress disorder with neurogenic amnesia for the traumatic event. Clin. Neuropsychologist **9:** 2-10.

44. Zeitlin, S. B. & R. J. McNally. 1991. Implicit and explicit memory bias for threat in post-traumatic stress disorder. Behav. Res. Ther. **29:** 451-457.

45. Sutker, P. B., A. N. Allain & J. L. Johnson. 1993. Clinical assessment of long-term cognitive and emotional sequelae to World War II prisoner-of-war confinement: Comparison of pilot twins. Psychol. Assess. **5:** 3-10.

46. JONES-GOTMAN, M. 1986. Right hippocampal excision impairs learning and recall of a list of abstract designs. Neuropsychologia **24:** 659-670.
47. KATZ, A., I. A. AWAD, A. K. KONG, G. J. CHELUNE, R. I. NAUGLE, E. WYLLIE, G. BEAUCHAMP & H. LUDERS. 1989. Extent of resection in temporal lobectomy for epilepsy II: Memory changes and neurological complications. Epilepsia **30:** 763-771.
48. MEYER, V. & A. J. YATES. 1955. Intellectual changes following temporal lobectomy for psychomotor epilepsy: Preliminary communication. J. Neurol. Neurosurg. Psychiatry **18:** 44-52.
49. MILNER, B. 1968. Visual recognition and recall after right temporal-lobe excision in man. Neuropsychologia **6:** 191-209.
50. TRENNERY, M. R., C. R. JACK, JR., G. D. CASCINO, F. W. SHARBROUGH & R. J. IVNIK. 1996. Sex differences in the relationship between visual memory and MRI hippocampal volumes. Neuropsychology **10:** 343-351.
51. CHAPMAN, L. & J. CHAPMAN. 1969. Illusory correlations as an obstacle to the use of valid psychodiagnostic signs. J. Abnorm. Psychol. **74:** 271-280.
52. KING, D. W., L. A. KING, D. W. FOY & D. W. GUDANOWSKI. 1996. Prewar factors in combat-related posttraumatic stress disorder: Structural equation modeling with a national sample of female and male Vietnam veterans. J. Consult. Clin. Psychol. **64:** 520-531.

Implicit and Explicit Memory for Trauma-Related Information in PTSD[a]

RICHARD J. McNALLY [b]

Department of Psychology
Harvard University
Cambridge, Massachusetts 02138

The phenomenology of posttraumatic stress disorder (PTSD) strongly suggests that memory abnormalities underlie many symptoms. Persons with PTSD report involuntary retrieval of horrific autobiographical memories as expressed in intrusive thoughts, nightmares, and flashbacks. They may also experience memory deficits for either certain aspects of traumatic events themselves or information unrelated to trauma.

Despite the prominence of self-reported memory problems in PTSD, only recently have researchers applied the experimental paradigms of neuropsychology and cognitive psychology to elucidate these phenomena in the laboratory.[1,2] One potentially useful way of organizing memory data is to distinguish between *content-independent* and *content-dependent* abnormalities.[3] Content-independent abnormalities denote dysfunctions that occur irrespective of the meaning of the information processed. Studies on short-term memory deficits,[4] for example, exemplify this line of research. Work in this area is in the tradition of neuropsychology.

Content-dependent abnormalities denote disturbances that arise only when individuals process information that has personal emotional significance. Studies on anxiety disorders, including PTSD, have uncovered memory biases that are operative only when patients process threatening or trauma-relevant input.[3] Work in this area is in the tradition of cognitive experimental psychology and exemplifies the growing hybrid domain of cognition-emotion research.

This article reviews the research on content-dependent memory abnormalities in PTSD. Studies on explicit and implicit memory biases for trauma cues are covered. Explicit memory is expressed on tests that require conscious recollection of previous experiences (e.g., free recall). Implicit memory is revealed when these experiences affect performance on a test that does not require conscious recollection (e.g., perceptual identification).

MEMORY BIASES FOR TRAUMA-RELATED INFORMATION

Intrusive symptoms imply that information about trauma is primed and readily accessible in PTSD. If enhanced accessibility underlies these symptoms, persons with

[a] Preparation of this chapter was supported in part by National Institute of Mental Health grant 51927 awarded to the author.

[b] Address for correspondence: Department of Psychology, Harvard University, 33 Kirkland Street, Cambridge, MA 02138 (tel: (617) 495-3853; fax: (617) 495-3728; e-mail: rjm@wjh.harvard.edu).

PTSD should exhibit an explicit memory bias for material related to trauma under controlled laboratory conditions. That is, they ought to show superior recollection of words related to trauma in comparison with other words and in comparison with trauma-exposed persons without the disorder. Consistent with this hypothesis, Vrana et al.[5] reported that Vietnam combat veterans with PTSD recalled more words related to trauma than did Vietnam combat veterans without PTSD. Litz et al.,[6] on the other hand, did not find enhanced recognition memory for trauma words in veterans with combat-related PTSD relative to healthy combat veterans. This null effect may be partly attributable to their use of a recognition rather than a recall test; the former is seldom affected by emotional variables such as word valence or diagnostic status.[3]

PTSD patients describe intrusive symptoms as occurring outside their conscious control. Such phenomenologic reports imply that mechanisms underlying the activation of these symptoms may be automatic. Accordingly, researchers have used implicit memory tests to investigate whether PTSD is associated with automatic biases favoring the processing of trauma-related information. In a study of Vietnam combat veterans with and without PTSD, McNally and Amir[7] used a perceptual identification procedure to test for an implicit memory bias favoring trauma cues. Participants first saw a series of trauma words, positive words, and neutral words on a computer screen. On a subsequent perceptual identification test, they again saw these ("old") words intermixed with ("new") distractor words of the same type. Each word flashed on the screen for only 100 ms and was replaced by a visual pattern mask comprising different characters (e.g., #%$*& #) that made it difficult to perceive the word. Subjects attempted to identify these briefly presented words. The results revealed that both groups accurately identified old words more often than new words, thereby demonstrating implicit memory for the former. However, there was no evidence for enhanced perceptual identification of trauma words in the PTSD group. Because performance on perceptual identification tasks is influenced more by the physical shape of words than by their meaning, it is perhaps not surprising that PTSD patients did not exhibit an implicit memory bias for trauma cues.

To investigate implicit memory for conceptually richer materials than single words, Amir et al.[8] adapted the "white noise" paradigm of Jacoby et al.[9] In this experiment, Vietnam combat veterans with and without PTSD heard a series of prerecorded trauma sentences (e.g., "The chopper landed in hot LZ.") and neutral sentences (e.g., "The shiny apple sat on the table."). They later heard these old sentences intermixed with new trauma and neutral sentences, each accompanied by white noise of either low, medium, or high volume.

Participants were asked to judge the volume of the noise that accompanied each sentence. Implicit memory for old sentences is revealed when individuals rate the noise accompanying these sentences as less loud than that accompanying new sentences, and an implicit memory bias for material related to trauma is demonstrated when the difference between volume ratings for new minus old sentences is greater for trauma sentences than for neutral sentences. That is, previous exposure to a sentence renders it easier to hear when it subsequently recurs against a background of white noise; consequently, white noise of a certain volume does not seem as loud when it accompanies a familiar sentence than an unfamiliar one. Therefore, ratings of perceived volume serve as indices of previous exposure (i.e., memory) for the sentences they accompany. The results indicated that PTSD patients exhibited enhanced implicit memory for trauma sentences than for neutral sentences, whereas healthy combat veterans exhibited the opposite pattern. Although findings were similar across the three noise levels, the effect was statistically significant only at the loudest volume.

In summary, some data suggest that explicit memory for trauma-related material is enhanced in persons with PTSD relative to trauma-exposed persons without the disorder. There is provisional evidence of enhanced implicit memory for conceptually complex input related to trauma in PTSD as well.

DIRECTED FORGETTING AND CHILDHOOD SEXUAL ABUSE

Some experts believe that children traumatized by sexual abuse develop a dissociative encoding style that enables them to disengage attention from terrifying stimuli during abuse episodes and to redirect it elsewhere.[10,11] Presumably, attending to innocuous cues (e.g., wallpaper patterns) blunts an otherwise overwhelmingly frightening experience.[12]

McNally et al.[13] used a directed forgetting paradigm to test for a possible dissociative encoding style in women with histories of childhood sexual abuse with and without PTSD. Participants viewed a series of trauma words (e.g., *abused*), positive words (e.g., *celebrate*), and neutral words (e.g., *mailbox*) that appeared one at a time on a computer screen. Each word was immediately followed by an instruction either to remember or to forget the word. Participants later received free recall, cued recall, and recognition tests for all words irrespective of original instructions. Cognitive psychologists have shown that most individuals exhibit a "directed forgetting" effect whereby they recall words that they were instructed to remember better than words they were instructed to forget.[14] Moreover, superior recall for remember-words relative to forget-words is attributable to better initial encoding of remember-words rather than to inhibition ("repression") of forget-words.[15] Therefore, if psychiatrically impaired survivors of childhood sexual abuse are especially adept at disengaging attention from trauma cues, they ought to show memory deficits for trauma-remember words relative to positive-remember and neutral-remember words.

The results were wholly inconsistent with this dissociative encoding hypothesis. Impaired survivors did, indeed, exhibit memory deficits, but only for positive-remember and neutral-remember words, not for trauma-remember words. Furthermore, they tended to remember trauma words they were supposed to forget. Healthy survivors exhibited typical directed forgetting effects: they recalled remember-words better than forget-words regardless of word valence. There was no difference in memory performance between those who reported having recovered memories of trauma and those who had always remembered their abuse.

Taken together, these data suggest that people with PTSD readily encode and therefore recall trauma-related material and that persistent rumination about trauma may disrupt encoding for nontraumatic material. To the extent that intrusive thoughts impair concentration, it should be difficult for survivors with PTSD to encode and recall the nontrauma words they are supposed to remember. Although these findings are clearly inconsistent with the dissociative encoding hypothesis, they do not establish that impaired survivors did not dissociate during abuse episodes in childhood.

AUTOBIOGRAPHICAL MEMORY DISTURBANCE

While investigating mood and memory in depressed and suicidal patients, Williams and his colleagues[16,17] discovered that these individuals had great difficulty accessing specific personal memories in response to cue words. Unlike nondepressed individuals, these patients tended to retrieve "overgeneral" memories, especially in response to positive cues. Thus, in response to words such as *happy,* healthy control participants easily remembered specific events (e.g., "the day we left to go on holiday"), but depressed participants usually retrieved a categoric memory that did not refer to any specific episode despite instructions to retrieve a specific memory (e.g., "when I play squash").[18]

Difficulties in retrieving specific personal memories strongly predicts failure to recover from major depression.[19] This memory abnormality is also associated with poor problem-solving skills.[18] Most probably, difficulty remembering specific details regarding how one attempted to deal with problems in the past hampers one's ability to learn from experience.

Several experiments have uncovered a link between overgeneral memory and a history of trauma in general and PTSD in particular.[20-22] In the first experiment, Vietnam combat veterans with PTSD, relative to healthy combat veterans, exhibited difficulties recalling specific personal memories in response to cue words having either neutral (e.g., *appearance*), positive (e.g., *kindness*), or negative (e.g., *panic*) emotional meaning.[20] Although they had been trained to retrieve specific episodes in response to cue words, PTSD subjects reverted to an overgeneral mode of retrieval as the experiment progressed. PTSD patients who had been exposed to reminders of trauma (i.e., a combat audio-videotape) had more difficulty accessing specific memories than did those who had been exposed to an emotionally neutral videotape. This suggests that reminder-induced preoccupation with traumatic events may consume attentional resources to such an extent that PTSD patients have little remaining capacity to search memory effortfully in tasks requiring accessing of specific autobiographical episodes.

In the second experiment,[21] Vietnam combat veterans with and without PTSD attempted to retrieve specific autobiographical memories exemplifying traits denoted by negative (e.g., *guilty*) and positive (e.g., *loyal*) cue words. Healthy veterans had little problem accessing specific memories, especially in response to positive cues. In contrast, those with PTSD had difficulty accessing specific memories to both kinds of cues. These "overgeneral" memory problems were far more marked in PTSD subjects who arrived at the laboratory wearing Vietnam War regalia (e.g., POW/MIA buttons, fatigues, and a loaded gun) than in those who did not. Healthy combat veterans never wore regalia. Regalia-wearing PTSD participants disproportionately retrieved memories from the war, unlike other subjects who overwhelmingly recalled specific memories from the last few weeks. The striking self-presentational style of wearing one's military regalia in everyday life is not only emblematic of psychological fixation to a war fought more than two decades ago, but also a marker for autobiographical memory disturbance. The overgeneral memory problems evident in PTSD patients who are "still in Vietnam" may underlie their difficulties envisioning the future, as reflected in the symptom of "future foreshortening." Difficulty remembering the past may render it difficult to envision the future.

Kuyken and Brewin[22] reported further evidence linking autobiographical memory dysfunction to a history of trauma. They found that depressed women who had been sexually abused as children exhibited difficulties retrieving specific personal memories in response to cue words, whereas depressed women who had not been abused did not. These researchers, however, did not assess for PTSD.

Difficulties in retrieving specific autobiographical memories converge with findings showing diminished hippocampal volume in PTSD.[23] Individuals with compromised anatomical structures that support autobiographical memory may have especial difficulty retrieving details of their past.

SUMMARY

Experiments on content-dependent memory abnormalities in PTSD suggest several conclusions. First, PTSD patients exhibit enhanced recall of words related to trauma relative to trauma-exposed persons with the disorder. Recognition tests, however, appear insensitive to these effects.

Second, PTSD patients do not exhibit implicit memory biases for trauma cues on implicit memory tasks that are strongly influenced by perceptual (e.g., orthographic) aspects of input. They may, however, exhibit enhanced implicit memory for trauma-related material on conceptually more complex tasks.

Third, directed forgetting research suggests that adult survivors of childhood sexual abuse who have PTSD exhibit memory deficits only for neutral and positive material, not for material related to their abuse. Psychiatrically healthy survivors exhibit normal memory performance in this paradigm.

Fourth, autobiographical memory research indicates that trauma survivors, especially those with PTSD, are characterized by difficulties retrieving specific memories from their past in response to cue words. These findings are especially dramatic in Vietnam combat veterans whose self-presentational style suggests a fixation to the war and a failure of their autobiography to unfold.

REFERENCES

1. McNALLY, R. J. 1995. Cognitive processing of trauma-relevant information in PTSD. PTSD Res. Q. **6:** 1-6.
2. McNALLY, R. J. Cognitive approaches to trauma and memory. *In* Trauma and Memory. A. C. Tishelman, E. Newberger & C. Newberger, Eds. Harvard University Press. Cambridge, MA. In press.
3. McNALLY, R. J. 1996. Cognitive bias in the anxiety disorders. Nebr. Symp. Motiv. **43:** 211-250.
4. BREMNER, J. D., T. M. SCOTT, R. C. DELANEY, S. M. SOUTHWICK, J. W. MASON, D. R. JOHNSON, R. B. INNIS, G. McCARTHY & D. S. CHARNEY. 1993. Deficits in short-term memory in posttraumatic stress disorder. Am. J. Psychiatry **150:** 1015-1019.
5. LITZ, B. T., F. W. WEATHERS, V. MONACO, D. S. HERMAN, M. WULFSOHN, B. MARX & T. M. KEANE. 1996. Attention, arousal, and memory in posttraumatic stress disorder. J. Traumatic Stress **9:** 497-519.
6. VRANA, S. R., A. ROODMAN & J. C. BECKHAM. 1995. Selective processing of trauma-relevant words in posttraumatic stress disorder. J. Anxiety Dis. **9:** 515-530.

7. McNALLY, R. J. & N. AMIR. 1996. Perceptual implicit memory for trauma-related information in posttraumatic stress disorder. Cognition & Emotion **10:** 551-556.
8. AMIR, N., R. J. McNALLY & P. S. WIEGARTZ. 1996. Implicit memory bias for threat in posttraumatic stress disorder. Cog. Ther. Res. **20:** 625-635.
9. JACOBY, L. L., L. G. ALLAN, J. C. COLLINS & L. K. LARWILL. 1988. Memory influences subjective experiences: Noise judgments. J. Exp. Psychol. Learn. Mem. Cogn. **14:** 240-247.
10. GELINAS, D. J. 1983. The persisting negative effects of incest. Psychiatry **46:** 312-332.
11. TERR, L. C. 1991. Childhood traumas: An outline and overview. Am. J. Psychiatry **148:** 10-20.
12. HERMAN, J. L. & E. SCHATZOW. 1987. Recovery and verification of memories of childhood sexual trauma. Psychoanal. Psychol. **4:** 1-14.
13. McNALLY, R. J., L. J. METZGER, N. B. LASKO & R. K. PITMAN. 1997. Directed forgetting of trauma cues in adult survivors of childhood sexual abuse with and without posttraumatic stress disorder. Submitted.
14. JOHNSON, H. M. 1994. Processes of successful intentional forgetting. Psychol. Bull. **116:** 274-292.
15. BASDEN, B. H., D. R. BASDEN & G. J. GARGANO. 1993. Directed forgetting in implicit and explicit memory tests: A comparison of methods. J. Exp. Psychol. Learn. Mem. Cogn. **19:** 603-616.
16. WILLIAMS, J. M. G. & K. BROADBENT. 1986. Autobiographical memory in suicide attempters. J. Abnorm. Psychol. **95:** 144-149.
17. WILLIAMS, J. M. G. & B. H. DRITSCHEL. 1988. Emotional disturbance and the specificity of autobiographical memory. Cognition & Emotion **2:** 221-234.
18. EVANS, J., J. M. G. WILLIAMS, S. O'LOUGHLIN & K. HOWELLS. 1992. Autobiographical memory and problem-solving strategies of parasuicide patients. Psychol. Med. **22:** 399-405.
19. BRITTLEBANK, A. D., J. SCOTT, J. M. G. WILLIAMS & I. N. FERRIER. 1993. Autobiographical memory in depression: State or trait marker? Br. J. Psychiatry **162:** 118-121.
20. McNALLY, R. J., B. T. LITZ, A. PRASSAS, L. M. SHIN & F. W. WEATHERS. 1994. Emotional priming of autobiographical memory in post-traumatic stress disorder. Cognition & Emotion **8:** 351-367.
21. McNALLY, R. J., N. B. LASKO, M. L. MACKLIN & R. K. PITMAN. 1995. Autobiographical memory disturbance in combat-related posttraumatic stress disorder. Behav. Res. Ther. **33:** 619-630.
22. KUYKEN, W. & C. R. BREWIN. 1995. Autobiographical memory functioning in depression and reports of early abuse. J. Abnorm. Psychol. **104:** 585-591.
23. GURVITS, T. V., M. E. SHENTON, H. HOKAMA, H. OHTA, N. B. LASKO, M. W. GILBERTSON, S. P. ORR, R. KIKINIS, F. A. JOLESZ, R. W. McCARLEY & R. K. PITMAN. 1996. Magnetic resonance imaging study of hippocampal volume in chronic, combat-related posttraumatic stress disorder. Biol. Psychiatry **19:** 433-444.

Trauma, Dissociation, and Memory

DAVID SPIEGEL

Department of Psychiatry & Behavioral Sciences
Stanford University School of Medicine
Stanford, California 94305–5544

Dissociation is a failure to integrate aspects of identity, memory, perception, and consciousness. Individuals with dissociative disorders usually report a history of exposure to traumatic stressors. Dissociative symptoms are included in the DSM-IV definition of posttraumatic stress disorder (PTSD) and are required for a diagnosis of acute stress disorder. Several appealing models for a neural basis of dissociation have recently appeared and are reviewed.

DISSOCIATION

Dissociation is both a normal component of a normal phenomenon (hypnosis) and may occur spontaneously by itself to a degree that may reach pathological proportions.[1] To become intensely involved in a central object of consciousness, one must restrict conscious processing of perceptions, thoughts, memories, or motor activities at the periphery.[2] These experiences may range from the simple, such as a hand feeling not as much a part of the body as usual, to the complex. Even rather intense emotional states or sensory experiences may be dissociated.[3] Some may involve memory alterations, such as dissociative amnesia for a traumatic event, as well as identity and motor function, as in a fugue episode in which for a period of hours to months an individual functions as though he or she had a different name and residence. Such experiences can be both induced and reversed with the structured use of hypnosis.[4]

The dissociative disorders represent a disturbance in the integrated organization of identity, memory, perception, or consciousness.[5] Events normally experienced on a smooth continuum become isolated from the other mental processes with which they would ordinarily be contiguous. Clinically, this can result in specific deficits. When the dissociation specifically involves memory, it produces dissociative amnesia. When it involves identity, dissociative fugue or dissociative identity (formerly multiple personality) disorder occurs. Dissociation of perception yields depersonalization disorder, whereas that of consciousness results in acute stress disorder or dissociative trance disorder, which includes various trance and possession states. They are in this sense a disturbance in the organization or structure of mental contents rather than in the contents themselves. Memories in dissociative amnesia are not so much distorted as they are segregated one from another. The problem is the failure of integration rather than a reflection of the contents of the fragments.[6]

Dissociated information is temporarily and reversibly unavailable to consciousness, but it may nonetheless influence conscious (or other unconscious) experience analogous to priming.[7,8] Out of sight does not mean out of mind. A rape victim may have no conscious memory of the crime, yet become anxious when exposed to stimuli reminiscent of the event.[3]

DISSOCIATIVE AMNESIA

Dissociative effects on memory will be examined from the perspective of dissociation as a continuum from normal to pathological segregation of mental contents.[9] Memory storage processes may be particularly influenced by dissociative phenomena. The nature of memory storage and the potential for retrievability are profoundly influenced by the associative matrix in which the memories are laid down, for example, explicit versus implicit,[10] episodic versus semantic[11] or declarative versus procedural.[12] Associative networks, the co-occurrence of related activated associations, are at the heart of connectionist models of memory.[13] It therefore makes sense that mental processes that segregate one set of associations from another might well impair memory storage or retrieval.[7]

Functional disorders of memory have been traditionally conceptualized as deficits in memory retrieval.[6] Amnesia has been described as occurring when information that is potentially ''available'' is currently not ''accessible'' for recollection because of some kind of retrieval problem.[11] However, some kinds of functional memory disorders may be related to organizational and storage deficits as well.

If the state of mind at the time of trauma is altered or hypnotic-like, the way the memories are stored may be influenced by this narrowness of focus. The range of associations may be more limited, and therefore those that exist more intense. Strong affect, for example, which is usually associated with traumatic memories, may influence both storage and retrieval.[14] There is evidence that mood congruence between the state in which memories were stored and that in which they are retrieved improves recall.[15] Similarly, another form of salient state dependency involves the dissociative state itself. To the extent that individuals do enter a spontaneous dissociated state during trauma, memories may be stored in a manner that reflects this state (e.g., narrower range of associations to context). There may be fewer cross-connections to other related memories.[1,6] Furthermore, retrieval should be facilitated by being in a similar dissociated state, that is, hypnosis. Trauma can be conceptualized as a sudden discontinuity in experience. This may lead to a process of memory storage which is similarly discontinuous with the usual range of associated memories. This may explain the ''off/on'' quality of dissociative amnesia and its reversibility with techniques such as hypnosis.[16,17]

Such disorders of memory usually follow some form of acute traumatic stress and may be gradual or sudden in onset.[18–21] They are usually reversible with psychotherapeutic techniques including hypnosis, which may be used to access memory that is otherwise unavailable to consciousness. In contrast to repressed memories, dissociated ones are usually composed of discrete periods of time lost from consciousness.[17] Thus, the patient may complain of ''losing time,'' being unaware of what happened between one specific time and another. Occasionally, however, such patients may not present with such a complaint, that is, they may not be aware of or ''remember'' their failure to remember. Instead, the complaint may come from others that the patient apparently was unaware of certain events, had no memory for a given period of time, or could not recognize certain persons or usually familiar places.

> A Vietnam combat veteran described a period of complete memory loss covering several weeks which commenced immediately after he learned that a Vietnamese child he had informally 'adopted' had been killed in the Tet Offensive. Although he had 3

previous years of uninterrupted service in Vietnam, and 15 prior years of good to excellent conduct ratings in the Army, he became unable to function, and was evacuated and eventually discharged for psychiatric reasons. Initial diagnoses included antisocial personality disorder, schizophrenia, and bipolar disorder, and he spent 4 years in various Army and Veterans Administration Hospitals, becoming increasingly depressed and suicidal. Using hypnosis, he was able to recall consciously for the first time the events subsequent to the boy's death. He relived with intense affect discovering the body, commandeering an ambulance, and setting booby traps for Vietcong. He tearfully relived burying the child and began grieving the loss, with an improvement in his chronic suicidal depression.[22]

Phone calls to people identified in his recollected memories indicated that some of the events were correct but others were not. A soldier he thought had been killed during the Offensive was alive, for example.

The information kept out of consciousness nonetheless has effects on it, consistent with the suicidal depression observed in the case just described.

That such amnesia for traumatic events does occur is most convincingly demonstrated by Williams.[23,24] She obtained hospital records of 129 women indicating emergency room contact for sexual or physical abuse and interviewed them 17 years later. The results of these interviews were striking: 38% did not report the abuse that had been recorded or any sexual abuse by the same perpetrator. Indeed, 12% reported no abuse at all.[23] An additional 16% (10% of the whole sample) of the women who did remember the abuse reported that there was a period in their lives when they could not remember it.[24] In fact, if the analysis was conservatively restricted to only those with recorded medical evidence of genital trauma and whose accounts were rated as most credible (in the 1970s), 52% did not remember the sexual abuse. It should be noted that this lack of memory was not diagnosed as a dissociative disorder, but the interviews were not designed to establish the presence or absence of a psychiatric disorder.

DISSOCIATION AND TRAUMA

An important development in the modern understanding of dissociative disorders is the exploration of the link between trauma and dissociation. Trauma can be understood as the experience of being made into an object, a thing, the victim of someone else's rage, of nature's indifference. Traumatic stress is the ultimate experience of helplessness and loss of control over one's body. There is growing clinical and some empirical evidence that dissociation may occur especially as a defense during trauma, an attempt to maintain mental control just as physical control is lost.[4,18,25–31] One patient with dissociative identity disorder reported "going to a mountain meadow full of wild flowers" when she was being sexually assaulted by her drunken father. She would concentrate on how pleasant and beautiful this imaginary scene was as a way of detaching herself from the immediate experience of terror, pain, and helplessness. Such individuals often report seeking comfort from imaginary playmates or imagined protectors or absorbing themselves in the pattern of the wallpaper. Many rape victims report floating above their body, feeling sorry for the person being assaulted below them.

Fifteen studies of immediate psychological reactions within the first month follow-ing a major disaster provide evidence of a high prevalence of dissociative symptoms, and some show that such symptoms are strong predictors of the development of PTSD. These studies examined the experiences of survivors, victims, and their families, and rescue workers in a variety of disasters: the Coconut Grove fire,[32] the 1972 Buffalo Creek flood disaster caused by the collapse of a dam,[33] automobile and other accidents and serious illnesses;[34,35] correctional officers' experience as hostages in a New Mexico penitentiary;[36] the collapse of the Hyatt Regency Hotel skywalk in Kansas City;[37] a lightening strike disaster that killed one child with others present;[38] a 1984 tornado that devastated a North Carolina community;[39] an airplane crash-landing;[40] an ambush in a war zone in Namibia;[41] the 1989 Loma Prieta earthquake in the San Francisco Bay Area;[29,31] the Oakland-Berkeley firestorm;[30] witnessing an execution;[42] and shootings in a high rise office building.[30]

POSTTRAUMATIC DISSOCIATIVE SYMPTOMS

Stupor involves a dulling of the senses and decreases in behavioral responsiveness and has been described in many survivors of automobile accidents.[34] In the immediate aftermath of the Buffalo Creek disaster, survivors reported "disorganization and sluggishness in thinking and decision making."[33,p296] All of the correctional officers held hostage in the Hillman[36] study reported feeling "dazed or in a 'state of shock' " (p. 1195).

Derealization symptoms were a common response to the earthquake (e.g., 40% reported "unreal surroundings"[29]), and some survivors of the Buffalo Creek disaster reported transient hallucinations and delusions.[33] Thirty percent of the accident/illness survivors[35] reported experiences that had a dream-like quality. For example, one survivor recalled that at the time of the accident "My sight seemed filtered through a blue piece of tissue paper with spots of red and yellow".[35,p379] Derealization experi-ences were also reported by several (3 of 14) soldiers ambushed in Namibia[41] and 54% of the airline crash survivors.[40]

Depersonalization was reported by 25% of the earthquake survivors (e.g., self detaching from body"[29]). In the accident survivor study,[34] depersonalization was frequently reported. For example, one survivor reported that: "It was as though I was separate from myself and watching, like in a dream when you are watching yourself."[35,p381]

Amnesia or memory impairment was reported by 29% of the Bay Area earthquake victims[24] and by 8 of 14 soldiers directly involved in the Namibia ambush.[41] Impair-ment of memory or concentration was reported by 79% of the airplane crash-landing survivors.[40] One boy in the lightning strike disaster had total amnesia for the event.[38] Research on hostage-taking situations report studies of survivors of life-threatening events indicate that more than half have experienced feelings of unreality, automatic movements, lack of emotion, and the sense of detachment.[35,39,43] Depersonalization and hyperalertness are prominent experiences during trauma.[34,44]

Numbing, loss of interest, and an inability to feel deeply about anything were reported in about a third of the survivors of the Hyatt Regency skywalk collapse[37] and in a similar proportion of survivors of the North Sea oil rig collapse.[45] This is consistent with our studies of survivors of the Loma Prieta earthquake.[29] A quarter of a sample of normal students reported marked depersonalization during and immediately after the earthquake, and 40% described derealization, the surroundings seeming unreal or dream-like. Although the most common reported memory disturbance was intrusive recollection, 29% of the sample reported difficulties with everyday memory. One survivor of the Oakland/Berkeley firestorm who had lost his house reported a strange sense of detachment during the fire:

> It was as though I was watching myself on television. I had this image of myself talking to a policeman, asking if I could go to my home, and whether he had any information about where my son was. I thought that I seemed rather unemotional, and decided that I had better stay that way in order not to upset my wife. It felt like I was watching the experience rather than having it.

A subjective sense of numbing was suggested by the reports of 5 of 14 soldiers involved in the Namibia ambush who were reported to have experienced constricted affect.[4] Correctional officers reported than when they were kept hostage, with repeated beatings, the beating ceased to be painful.[36] For example, one hostage said: "I could see my body moving so I knew that I had been kicked . . . but I didn't feel anything" (p. 1195).

Dissociative symptoms have also been retrospectively reported to occur during combat. Bremner et al.[28] administered the Dissociative Experiences Scale (DES) to 85 Vietnam veterans, 53 with PTSD and 32 with medical problems. The DES scores of those with PTSD were twice as high as those obtained among the comparison sample. Veterans with PTSD have been found to obtain higher scores on measures of hypnotizability.[48,46]

DISSOCIATIVE SYMPTOMS AS PREDICTORS OF PTSD

Dissociative symptoms, especially numbing, have been rather strong predictors of later posttraumatic stress disorder.[30,47,48] Thus, physical trauma seems to elicit dissociation or compartmentalization of experience and may often become the matrix for later posttraumatic symptoms, such as dissociative amnesia for the traumatic episode. Indeed, more extreme dissociative disorders, such dissociative identity disorder, have been conceptualized as chronic posttraumatic stress disorders.[25,26,49] Children exposed to multiple traumas are more likely to use dissociative mechanisms which include spontaneous trance episodes.[50] Recollection of trauma tends to have an off-on quality involving either intrusion or avoidance[51] in which victims either intensively relive the trauma as though it were recurring or have difficulty remembering it.[39,52,53] Thus, physical trauma seems to elicit dissociative responses.

Acute Stress Disorder. The evidence just reviewed on the prevalence of dissociative and other symptoms in the immediate aftermath of trauma was the basis for including acute stress disorder (ASD) as a new diagnosis in the DSM-IV.[20,53] It is diagnosed when high levels of dissociative, anxiety, and other symptoms occur within 1 month of trauma and persist for at least 2 days, causing distress and dysfunction. Such individuals must have experienced or witnessed physical trauma and responded with intense fear, helplessness, or horror. This "A" criterion of the DSM-IV requirements for ASD is identical to that of PTSD. The individual must have at least three of the following five dissociative symptoms: depersonalization, derealization, amnesia, numbing, or stupor. In addition, the trauma victim must have one symptom from each of the three classic PTSD categories: intrusion of traumatic memories, including nightmares and flashbacks; avoidance; and anxiety or hyperarousal. If symptoms persist beyond 1 month, the person receives another diagnosis based on symptom patterns. Likely candidates are dissociative, anxiety, or posttraumatic stress disorders.

POSSIBLE NEURAL MECHANISMS OF DISSOCIATIVE AMNESIA

This volume is designed to address the psychobiology of PTSD, and therefore I have undertaken to review the available evidence on the neurophysiological mechanisms that may underlie the dissociative elements of posttraumatic symptoms.

Hippocampal Damage. Exciting recent findings from the PTSD group at the West Haven VA[54] demonstrate reduced right hippocampal volume in MRI studies of Vietnam veterans with PTSD as compared with those who do not have PTSD. The severity of symptoms was associated with the degree of volume reduction. This finding was recently replicated by Stein, this time with reduction of left hippocampal volume, among incest survivors (Stein *et al.*, this volume). Given the crucial role of the hippocampus in memory storage and retrieval, dysregulation of memory in PTSD, including intrusive recollection, avoidance, hyperarousal in response to trauma-related stimuli, and dissociative amnesia, could be explained through impaired hippocampal function. Reduced hippocampal volume in PTSD suggests that damage to this region, possibly through chronic dysregulation of the HPA,[55,56] could underlie dissociative amnesia, because there are cortisol receptors on hippocampal neurons.

Thalamocortical Pathways. The thalamus integrates perceptual and cognitive information and has been proposed as a site of dissociative symptoms.[57] The thalamus modulates access of perceptual information to limbic structures and the cortex. The thalamus projects to the frontal cortex, the cingulate gyrus which shifts attention, the amygdala, and the hippocampus, thereby influencing attention and access of the cortex to sensory input as well as its modulation by emotion via the locus coeruleus and limbic system. Thalamic activity is reduced in slow-wave sleep, interrupting perceptual processing, but it is phasically active during REM sleep. The connections to limbic as well as to cortical attentional and perceptual processing areas provide a plausible structure for the disruption of memory and perception by trauma-related affect.

Amygdala. Control of affective arousal mediated by the amygdala modulates memory retention. It has been known that affective arousal can increase memory storage and retrieval, especially for events central to the affectively arousing stimulus.[52] Recently a neural mechanism for this has been uncovered. McGaugh and colleagues[14] showed a film to volunteers with one of two interpretations provided, one designed to arouse affect (the film depicts a serious and permanently disabling injury) and the other not (it shows a routine trip to the hospital). Memory was better in the arousing condition, but this increase was blocked when subjects were given propranalol, a beta-adrenergic blocker. This implicates the amygdala in affective enhancement of memory and also links mechanisms that block affective arousal to inhibition of noradrenergic activity in general and amygdala function in particular. Thus, dissociative mechanisms leading to affective numbness may inhibit noradrenergic arousal and reduce activity in the amygdala, locus ceruleus, and other basal structures associated with affective arousal. This could in turn explain otherwise puzzling memory deficits for traumatic experiences.

Modulation of Cortical Perceptual Processing. ERP studies indicate that alteration of perception under hypnosis results in changes in portions of the waveform affected by inattention and meaning.[58–60] In particular, hypnotic hallucination designed to obstruct perception of visual and somatosensory stimuli results in reduction of amplitude of early (P100) and late (P300) components of the waveform. Thus, the subjectively reduced perception typical of, for example, hypnotic analgesia is accompanied by reduced ERP amplitude to perception in that modality. More recent investigation has identified both common reductions in components such as P100 which are attention related and others that are not (P200).[60] In the visual system this finding was localized to the left occipital cortex, consistent with work indicating imagery generation in that region.[61]

Similarly, hypnotic amnesia affects attentional components of the ERP and a late negative component (N400), but not late positive components, consistent with intact implicit but not explicit memory processing.[62] Recent PET studies show that response to true versus false recollections can be distinguished through activation of parietal auditory association cortex.[63] Thus, modulation of perceptual response to stimuli in the primary sensory association cortices could affect storage and retrieval of memories of these events, potentially linking dissociative responses during trauma that might modulate perceptual encoding to dissociative amnesia afterwards.

Temporal Lobes. There is classical evidence from the neurology literature of dissociative symptoms, including behavioral automatisms, amnesia, and fugue, during ictal periods of complex partial and *petit mal* seizures.[64] For example, Feindel and Penfield[65] reported that 78% of a series of 155 patients with temporal lobe epilepsy had behavioral automatisms and amnesia. Indeed, dissociated behavior and memory are the most prominent features of this form of epilepsy.[66,67]

Dissociative symptoms also emerge during interictal periods among seizure disorder patients.[67–69] However, some studies indicate less similarity between dissociative disorder and epileptic patients.[70–72] A related but different issue is the prevalence of neurological indicators of seizure disorder among DID patients. In thus review of 100 cases, Putnam *et al.*[73] found that 10% of cases had temporal lobe epilepsy, the same figure that Coons and collaborators found among their sample of 50 patients.[74] This incidence is considerably higher than the base rate for epilepsy. Among the subset of patients who underwent EEG measurements, 7 of 30 (23%) had abnormal EEGs. Devinsky *et al.*[75] studied six DID patients suspected of having seizure disorders as well. Although there were minor EEG abnormalities in three of the six patients, none was found to have epilepsy.

These studies consistently support the notion that patients with seizure disorders experience more dissociative phenomena (e.g., depersonalization, derealization) than do normal controls, although epileptics do not generally show the same frequency or symptom profile as do full-fledged dissociative disorder patients. This literature makes it clear that dissociative symptoms involving disturbances in the integration of memory, identity, and consciousness occur frequently secondary to seizure activity, both ictal and interictal.

Corpus Callosum. The capacity for relatively independent function by the two cerebral hemispheres has been well illustrated in the work of Gazzaniga,[76] Sperry,[77] Hugdahl,[78] and others. Studies of callosectomy patients have shown that there may be recognition without awareness or inability to describe an object presented to the left visual field. Clearly the corpus callosum and the commissures play a role in integrating perceptual and lexical input. One patient who had a large chromophobe adenoma removed reported that prior to the surgery he would see or think of something and would have to struggle with something that he called a "practice tape" before articulating what he had seen or thought. After the surgery, which removed a tennis-ball sized mass between his temporal lobes, he reported speaking automatically, without this delay in translating thought into words. Although this kind of dissociation of cognitive functions may seem a long way from clinical dissociation, interhemispheric interaction has long been postulated as a possible mechanism for repression.[79]

Relative disconnection of cortical information processing may activate dysphoric affect. There is evidence[80] that the amount of combat exposure is related to the intensity of posttraumatic imagery. Many victims of trauma are beset with unbidden images of the traumatic event.[51] A highway construction worker who was struck by a car traveling at 60 miles per hour said in his hospital bed, "I keep seeing that car coming at me. I realize he is ignoring the pylons—he is going to hit me." Most trauma victims experience their recollections of these events as images and sensations, not as words. This may be especially problematic, as there is evidence that dysphoria is localized to the function of the right frontal pole,[81] which is part of the hemisphere that is specialized for imagery processing.[82] Activation of the right frontal pole is associated with depressive affect, whereas activation of the left frontal pole is associated with elevation of mood. It therefore could be that the intrusion of images from a traumatic experience might be especially activating of depressive affect. Conversely, the translation of such images into lexical form, via explaining the experience to others or specifically in psychotherapy, might transfer the locus of activity to the left hemisphere, the lexical processor, thereby elevating affect as well.

MODEL OF THE NEUROPHYSIOLOGY OF POSTTRAUMATIC DISSOCIATION

The dissociative state seems to be a frequent, if not ubiquitous, response to a traumatic experience. Many rape victims report floating above their body, feeling sorry for the person being assaulted below. Given the effectiveness of hypnotic states in reducing or eliminating pain,[83–85] it would be surprising if individuals with the requisite hypnotic capacity for analgesia to serious traumatic injury did not mobilize and use that ability during traumatic experience. The evidence reviewed here indicates that distortions of time, memory, and perception, including depersonalization and derealization episodes, are common during trauma. However, this dissociative state, which may be adaptive in fending off the acute emotional impact of traumatic events and improving adaptation to traumatic stress by allowing for focus on survival and other coping strategies, may lose its adaptiveness over the ensuing period of days or weeks. McFarlane (this volume) has shown that dissociative symptoms within 24 hours of motor vehicle accidents do not predict the development of posttraumatic stress disorder, but by 10 days they do. In other words, the persistence of dissociative symptoms beyond the immediate peritraumatic period becomes a predictor of PTSD, whereas their initial occurrence does not.

The model in this chapter is that these dissociative states, which may be common and adaptive at the time of trauma, become maladaptive over time in that they allow for reactivation of traumatic memories with reduced opportunity to process and control them. Thus, the lack of control, dysphoria, and helplessness that typifies the traumatic effect is reinforced rather than modulated by repetition. Affect is either overmodulated, as in numbing, detachment, and avoidance, or undermodulated, as in flashbacks and hyperarousal responses. Traumatic memories are reactivated rather than transformed, thereby reinflicting trauma rather than working it through. This model would hold that the problem in dissociative disorders is that the systems of the brain that facilitate integration and modulation of affect and synthesis of information across sensory modalities and between images and lexical processing are reduced. Sites for this in the brain include the hippocampus, which contextualizes information, the thalamus, which links various sensory inputs to cognition, the corpus callosum, which links left and right hemisphere functioning, and frontal cortex, which re-processes information.

Rausch's recent PET work (this volume) indicates that PTSD is associated with hyperactivity of the hippocampus, amygdala, and visual association cortex (lingual and fusiform gyri) and hypoactivity in Broca's area. This suggests hyperfunction of the portions of the brain responsible for emotion, memory, and imagery, three aspects of cognition that are strongly activated in PTSD. But of equal or even greater interest is the hypoactivity of Broca's area. It suggests inhibition of lexical processing. This is consistent with Teicher's data (this volume) showing EEG abnormalities in the left but not in the right hemisphere in victims of childhood sexual abuse. The picture that potentially emerges from these data is a state of intrusive reactivation of traumatic memories with affective loading and intense imagery along with impaired ability to reprocess these memories in lexical terms. Thus, the data suggest that the dissociative phenomena, while helpful initially, may limit the brain's ability to reprocess traumatic memories. In this pathway, reactivation of the memory reelicits neuradrenergic arousal, intensifies recollection and visual imagery, and reduces the ability to talk about and presumably transform the traumatic memories. The non-PTSD pathway would involve presumably reduced intrusion through hippocampal activity, reduced limbic loading, better thalamic and corpus callosum functioning, and normal activation of Broca's area, thereby facilitating reprocessing of traumatic memories so that their activation of affect and imagery is modulated over time.

Interestingly, this process is typical of psychotherapy, in which affect, memory, and images are transformed through words. The critical variable may well be the ability to recontextualize on reexposure to stimuli reminiscent of the traumatic stressor, including traumatic memories (Foa, this volume). Hippocampal dysfunction, inferred through reduced hippocampal volume (Stein, this volume, and ref. 86), may indicate limited ability to alter context. The combination of frontal and temporal hyperactivation, possible isolation of the right hemisphere with its relative suppression of positive affect, and stimulation of affective arousal through the amygdala may provide a context for retraumatization and repetition rather than transformation of traumatic memories. Thus, the dissociative effect of circumscribing memory, identity, perception, affect, and consciousness during trauma may inhibit integration and thereby perpetuate PTSD symptoms over time.

CONCLUSION

The literature reviewed makes it clear that dissociative symptoms involving failure of integration of aspects of memory, perception, identity, and consciousness occur at higher than normal frequency in the immediate aftermath of trauma and that the prevalence of such symptoms predicts the development of later posttraumatic stress disorder. Such disturbances may be related to unusual attentional states (intensity of focus) or dissociative reactions during traumatic events. These discontinuities of mental experience are plausibly related to alterations in the activity of those portions of the brain responsible for integrating information. Clearly no definitive model of dissociative neural processes is possible at this time, but malfunction of both deep and cortical structures has been implicated. Disruptions of activity in the hippocampus, thalamus, and amygdala can reduce access to or integration of memory traces. Disruption of sensory processing in the cortex may impair storage of traumatic memories and therefore their subsequent retrieval, perhaps via heightened attentional focus involving the anterior cingulate and frontal cortex. Finally, impaired communication between cerebral hemispheres has yielded evidence of dissociative phenomena. This relative isolation of perception, affect, and memory have be perpetuated by inhibition of lexical processing centers. Dissociation has been termed "knowing without awareness." Further research on posttraumatic brain function should help to increase our awareness of the brain processes that underlie our ability to know about traumatic experiences.

REFERENCES

1. HILGARD, E. 1986. Divided Consciousness: Multiple Controls in Human Thought and Action. Wiley. New York.
2. POSNER, M. I. & S. E. PETERSEN. 1990. The attention system of the human brain. Annu. Rev. Neurosci. **13:** 25–42.
3. SPIEGEL, D. 1991. Dissociation and Trauma. American Psychiatric Press Review of Psychiatry. A. Tasman & S. M. Goldfinger, Eds. **10:** 261–275. American Psychiatric Press. Washington, DC.
4. BUTLER, L. D., R. E. F. DURAN, P. JASIUKAITIS, C. KOOPMAN & D. SPIEGEL. 1996. Hypnotizability and traumatic experience: A diathesis-stress model of dissociative symptomatology. Am. J. Psychiatry **153:** 42–63.
5. AMERICAN PSYCHIATRIC ASSOCIATION. 1994. Diagnostic and Statistical Manual of Mental Disorders. 4th Ed. (DSM-IV). American Psychiatric Press. Washington, DC.
6. EVANS, F. J. & J. F. KIHLSTROM. 1973. Posthypnotic amnesia as disrupted retrieval. J. Abnorm. Psychol. **82:** 317–323.
7. KIHLSTROM, J. F. 1987. The cognitive unconscious. Science **237:** 1445–1452.
8. SCHACTER, D. L. 1992. Understanding implicit memory. A cognitive neuroscience approach. Am. Psychol. **47:** 559–569.
9. SPIEGEL, H. & N. SHAINESS. 1963. The dissociation-association continuum. J. Nerv. Ment. Dis. **136:** 374–378.

10. SCHACTER, D. L. 1987. Implicit Memory: History and Current Status. J. Exp. Psychol. Learn. Mem. Cognit. **13:** 501-518.

11. TULVING, E. 1983. Elements of Episodic Memory. Clarendon Press. Oxford.

12. SQUIRE, L. R. 1987. Memory and Brain. Oxford University Press. New York.

13. RUMELHART, D. & J. McCLELLAND. 1986. Parallel Distributed Processing: Explorations in the Microstructure of Cognition. The MIT Press. Cambridge.

14. CAHILL, L., B. PRINS, M. WEBER & J. L. McGAUGH. 1994. Beta-adrenergic activation and memory for emotional events. Nature **371:** 702-704.

15. BOWER, G. H. 1981. Mood and Memory. Am. Psychol. **36:** 129-148.

16. SPIEGEL, H. & D. SPIEGEL. 1987. Trance and Treatment: Clinical Uses of Hypnosis. Basic Books. New York.

17. LOEWENSTEIN, R. J. 1991. Psychogenic amnesia and psychogenic fugue: A comprehensive review. *In* American Psychiatric Press Review of Psychiatry. A Tasman & S. M. Goldfinger, Eds. **10:** 189-222. American Psychiatric Press. Washington, DC.

18. SPIEGEL, D., T. HUNT *et al.* 1988. Dissociation and hypnotizability in posttraumatic stress disorder. Am. J. Psychiatry **145:** 301-305.

19. SPIEGEL, D. 1990. Hypnosis, dissociation, and trauma: Hidden and overt observers. *In* Repression and Dissociation: Implications for Personality Theory, Psychopathology, and Health. J. L. Singer, Ed.: 121-142. University of Chicago Press. Chicago.

20. SPIEGEL, D. & E. CARDENA. 1990. New uses of hypnosis in the treatment of posttraumatic stress disorder. J. Clin. Psychiatry **51:** 39-43.

21. LOEWENSTEIN, R. L. 1991. Dissociative amnesia and fugue. *In* American Psychiatric Press Review of Psychiatry. A. Tasman & S. M. Goldfinger, Eds. Vol. 10. American Psychiatric Press. Washington, DC.

22. SPIEGEL, D. 1981. Vietnam grief work using hypnosis. Am. J. Clin. Hypn. **24:** 33-40.

23. WILLIAMS, L. M. 1994. Recall of childhood trauma: A prospective study of women's memories of child sexual abuse. J. Consult. Clin. Psychol. **62:** 1167-1176.

24. WILLIAMS, L. M. 1995. Recovered memories of abuse in women with documented child victimization histories. J. Traumatic Stress **8:** 649-673.

25. SPIEGEL, D. 1984. Multiple personality as a post-traumatic stress disorder. Psychiatr. Clin. North Am. **7:** 101-110.

26. KLUFT, R. P. 1985. The natural history of multiple personality disorder. Childhood Antecedents of Multiple Personality. R. P. Kluft, Ed.: 197-238. American Psychiatric Press. Washington, DC.

27. PUTNAM, F. W. 1985. Dissociation as a response to extreme trauma. *In* Childhood Antecedents of Multiple Personality. R. P. Kluft, Ed.: 65-97. American Psychiatric Press. Washington, DC.

28. BREMNER, J. D., S. SOUTHWICK *et al.* 1992. Dissociation and posttraumatic stress disorder in Vietnam combat veterans. Am. J. Psychiatry **149:** 328-332.

29. CARDEÑA, E. & D. SPIEGEL. 1993. Dissociative reactions to the San Francisco Bay Area earthquake of 1989. Am. J. Psychiatry **150:** 474-478.

30. KOOPMAN, C., C. CLASSEN *et al.* 1994. Predictors of posttraumatic stress symptoms among survivors of the Oakland/Berkeley, Calif., firestorm. Am. J. Psychiatry. **151:** 888-894.

31. MARMAR, C. R., D. S. WEISS *et al.* 1994. Peritraumatic dissociation and posttraumatic stress in male Vietnam theater veterans. Am. J. Psychiatry **151:** 902-907.

32. LINDEMANN, E. 1944(94). Symptomatology and management of acute grief. Am. J. Psychiatry **151:** 155-160.

33. TITCHENER, J. L. & F. T. KAPP. 1976. Disaster at Buffalo Creek. Family and character change at Buffalo Creek. Am. J. Psychiatry **133:** 295-299.

34. NOYES, R., JR., P. R. HOENK *et al.* 1977. Depersonalization in accident victims and psychiatric patients. J. Nerv. Ment. Dis. **164:** 401-407.

35. NOYES, R., JR. & R. KLETTI. 1977. Depersonalization in response to life-threatening danger. Compr. Psychiatry **18:** 375-384.

36. HILLMAN, R. G. 1981. The psychopathology of being held hostage. Am. J. Psychiatry **138:** 1193-1197.
37. WILKINSON, C. B. 1983. Aftermath of a disaster: The collapse of the Hyatt Regency Hotel skywalks. Am. J. Psychiatry **140:** 1134-1139.
38. DOLLINGER, S. J. 1985. Lightning-strike disaster among children. Br. J. Med. Psychol. **58**(Pt. 4): 375-383.
39. MADAKASIRA, S. & K. F. O'BRIEN. 1987. Acute posttraumatic stress disorder in victims of a natural disaster. J. Nerv. Ment. Dis. **175:** 286-290.
40. SLOAN, P. 1988. Post-traumatic stress in survivors of an airplane crash-landing: A clinical and exploratory research intervention. J. Traumatic Stress **1:** 211-229.
41. FEINSTEIN, A. 1989. Posttraumatic stress disorder: A descriptive study supporting DSM-III-R criteria. Am. J. Psychiatry **146:** 665-666.
42. FREINKEL, A., C. KOOPMAN *et al.* 1994. Dissociative symptoms in media eyewitnesses of an execution. Am. J. Psychiatry **151:** 1335-1339.
43. SLOAN, T. B. 1988. Neurologic monitoring. Crit. Care Clin. **4:** 543-557.
44. NOYES, R. & D. SLYMAN. 1978. The subjective response to life-threatening danger. Omega **9:** 313-321.
45. HOLEN, A. 1993. The North Sea Oil Rig Disaster. Plenum. New York.
46. STUTMAN, R. K. & E. L. BLISS. 1985. Posttraumatic stress disorder, hypnotizability, and imagery. Am. J. Psychiatry **142:** 741-743.
47. MACFARLANE, A. C. 1986. Posttraumatic morbidity of a disaster. J. Nerv. Ment. Dis. **174:** 4-14.
48. SOLOMON, Z., M. MIKULINCER *et al.* 1989. Combat stress reaction: Clinical manifestations and correlates. Milit. Psychol. **1:** 35-47.
49. SPIEGEL, D. 1986. Dissociating damage. Am. J. Clin. Hypn. **29:** 123-131.
50. TERR, L. C. 1991. Childhood traumas: An outline and overview [see comments]. Am. J. Psychiatry **148:** 10-20.
51. HOROWITZ, M. 1976. Stress Response Syndromes. Aronson. New York.
52. CHRISTIANSON, S. & E. LOFTUS. 1987. Memory for traumatic events. Applied Cognit. Psychol. **1:** 225-239.
53. SPIEGEL, D. & E. CARDENA. 1991. Disintegrated experience: The dissociative disorders revisited. J. Abnorm. Psychol. **100:** 366-378.
54. BREMNER, J. D., S. M. SOUTHWICK *et al.* 1995. Etiological factors in the development of posttraumatic stress disorder. *In* Does Stress Cause Psychiatric Illness? C. M. Mazure, Ed. American Psychiatric Press. Washington, DC.
55. SAPOLSKY, R., L. KREY *et al.* 1985. Prolonged glucocorticoid exposure reduces hippocampal neuron number. Implication for aging. J. Neurosci. **5:** 1222-1227.
56. MCEWEN, B. S. 1993. Stress and the individual: Mechanisms leading to disease. Arch. Int. Med. **153:** 2093-2101.
57. KRYSTAL, J. H., A. L. BENNETT *et al.* 1995. Toward a cognitive neuroscience of dissociation and altered memory functions in post-traumatic stress disorder. *In* Neurobiological and Clinical Consequences of Stress: From Normal Adaptation to PTSD. M. J. Friedman, D. S. Charney & A. Y. Deutch, Eds.: 239-269. Lippincott-Raven. Philadelphia.
58. SPIEGEL, D., S. CUTCOMB *et al.* 1985. Hypnotic hallucination alters evoked potentials. J. Abnorm. Psychol. **94:** 249-255.
59. SPIEGEL, D., P. BIERRE *et al.* 1989. Hypnotic alteration somatosensory perception. Am. J. Psychiatry **144:** 299-302.
60. JASIUKAITIS, P., B. NOURIANI *et al.* 1996. Left hemisphere superiority for event-related potential effects of hypnotic obstruction. Neuropsychologia **34:** 661-669.
61. FARAH, M. J., L. L. WEISBERG *et al.* 1990. Brain activity underlying imagery: Event-related potentials during mental image generation. J. Cognit. Neurosci. **1:** 302-316.
62. ALLEN, J. J., W. G. IACONO *et al.* 1995. An event-related potential investigation of posthypnotic recognition amnesia. J. Abnorm. Psychol. **104:** 421-430.

63. SCHACTER, D. L., E. REIMAN, T. CURRAN, L. S. YUN, D. BANDY, K. B. McDERMOTT & H. L. ROEDIGER. 1996. Neuroanatomical correlates of veridical and illusory recognition memory: Evidence from positron emission tomography. Neuron **17:** 267-274.
64. MAYEUX, R., M. P. ALEXANDER et al. 1979. Poriomania. Neurology **29:** 1616-1619.
65. FEINDEL, W. & W. PENFIELD. 1954. Localization of discharge in temporal lobe automatism. Arch. Neurol Psychiatry **72:** 605-630.
66. BLUMER, D. & A. E. WALKER. 1969. Memory in temporal lobe epileptics. The Pathology of Memory. G. A. Tallan & N. C. Waugh, Eds.: 65-73. Academic Press. New York.
67. SCHENK, L. & D. BEAR. 1981. Multiple personality and related dissociative phenomena in patients with temporal lobe epilepsy. Am. J. Psychiatry **138:** 1311-1316.
68. MESULAM, M. M. 1981. Dissociative states with abnormal temporal lobe EEG. Arch. Neurol. **38:** 176-181.
69. BENSON, D. F., B. MILLER et al. 1986. Dual personality associated with epilepsy. Archives **43:** 471-474.
70. LOEWENSTEIN, R. J. & F. W. PUTNAM. 1988. A comparative study of dissociative symptoms in patients with complex partial seizures, multiple personality disorder and posttraumatic stress disorder. Dissociation **1:** 17-23.
71. ROSS, C. A. 1989. Multiple Personality Disorder: Diagnosis, Clinical Features and Treatment. John Wiley & Sons. New York.
72. DEVINSKY, O., F. PUTNAM et al. 1989. Dissociative states and epilepsy. Neurology **39:** 835-840.
73. PUTNAM, F. W., J. J. GUROFF et al. 1986. The clinical phenomenology of multiple personality disorder: Review of 100 recent cases. J. Clin. Psychiatry **47:** 285-293.
74. COONS, P. M., E. S. BOWMAN et al. 1988. Multiple personality disorder. A clinical investigation of 50 cases. J. Nerv. Ment. Dis. **176:** 519-527.
75. DEVINSKY, O., E. FELDMANN et al. 1989. Autoscopic phenomena with seizures. Arch. Neurol **46:** 1080-1088.
76. GAZZANIGA, M. S. 1989. Organization of the human brain. Science **245:** 947-952.
77. SPERRY, R. W. 1974. Lateral specialization in the surgically separated hemisphere. In F. O. Schmitt & F. G. Worden, Eds.: 5-19. The Neurosciences: Third Study Program. Cambridge. MIT Press.
78. HUGDAHL, K. 1995. Psychophysiology: The Mind-Body Perspective. Harvard University Press. Cambridge.
79. GALIN, D. 1977. Lateral specialization and psychiatric issues: Speculations on development and the evolution of consciousness. Ann. N.Y. Acad. Sci. **299:** 397-411.
80. MUESER, K. T. & R. W. BUTLER. 1987. Auditory hallucination in combat-related chronic posttraumatic stress disorder. Am. J. Psychiatry **144:** 299-302.
81. DAVIDSON, J. R., H. S. KUDLER et al. 1993. Predicting response to amitriptyline in posttraumatic stress disorder. Am. J. Psychiatry **150:** 1024-1029.
82. KOSSLYN, S. M. & O. KOENIG. 1992. Wet Mind: The New Cognitive Neuroscience. Free Press. New York.
83. HILGARD, E. R. & J. R. HILGARD. 1975. Hypnosis in the Relief of Pain. William Kauffman. Los Altos, CA.
84. SPIEGEL, D. & J. R. BLOOM. 1983. Group therapy and hypnosis reduce metastatic breast carcinoma pain. Psychosom. Med. **45:** 333-339.
85. LANG, E. V., J. S. JOYCE et al. 1996. Self-hypnotic relaxation during interventional radiological procedures: Effects on pain perception and intravenous drug use. Int. J. Clin. Exp. Hypnosis **44:** 106-119.
86. BREMNER, J. D., P. RANDALL et al. 1995. MRI-based measurement of hippocampal volume in patients with combat-related posttraumatic stress disorder. Am. J. Psychiatry **152:** 973-981.

The Neurobiology of Emotionally Influenced Memory

Implications for Understanding Traumatic Memory

LARRY CAHILL [a]

Center for the Neurobiology of Learning and Memory
University of California, Irvine
Irvine, California 92697-3800

The usefulness of all the passions consists in their strengthening and prolonging in the soul thoughts which are good for it to conserve. . . . And all the harm they can do consists in their strengthening and prolonging these thoughts more than is necessary.
Descartes, *The Passions of the Soul,* 1650

This chapter addresses the neurobiological basis of long-term memory formation for emotional events. The central thesis is: Storage of memory for emotionally arousing events is modulated by an endogenous neurobiological system[1] which is normally inactive in nonemotionally arousing learning situations, but which becomes active in emotionally stressful learning situations to insure that the strength of memory for an event is, in general, proportional to its importance.[2,3] Two neurobiological elements, at minimum, are considered fundamental to this system: (1) endogenous stress hormones released during emotional events (in particular, the catecholamines epinephrine and norepinephrine) and (2) the amygdaloid complex (AC).

Much of the evidence supporting this view comes from studies involving animal subjects and is reviewed in detail elsewhere[1,3] (Roozendaal *et al.,* this volume). This chapter concentrates on recent experiments that confirm in human subjects this view of the neurobiology of memory for emotional events. First, psychological evidence concerning the influence of emotion on memory in humans is briefly reviewed. Next, some experiments from animal literature on the role of stress hormones and the AC in emotional memory are described, followed by a synopsis of recent investigations into the neurobiological mechanisms of human emotional memory. Finally, potential applications of these findings to understanding and treating disorders of emotional memory are explored.

[a] Address for correspondence: Dr. Larry Cahill, CNLM, Bonney Center, University of California, Irvine, CA 92697-3800 (tel: (714)824-5250; fax: (714)824-2952; e-mail: lcahill@darwin.bio. uci.edu).

INFLUENCE OF EMOTION ON MEMORY

In his remarkably prescient discussion of the emotion-memory relationship, Stratton[4] addressed many issues still considered critical today. He noted, for example, that emotional arousal can affect memory not only for the emotional event itself, but also for experiences occurring both shortly before and shortly after the event. He noted that emotion may either enhance memory (hypermnesia) or impair memory (hypomnesia) and occasionally even create a "curious combination of both these effects."

Stratton[4] also anticipated an issue central to this chapter, namely, the modulation of memory by endogenous "drugs," that is, stress hormones, released during emotional events: "The effect of emotion [on memory] would seem to be analogous to that of certain drugs, where a certain dose excites, while a still greater dose depresses." Stratton's observations clearly anticipate the now well-established "inverted-U" relationship between dose and memory typically found with memory-enhancing drugs and hormones.

Referring to hypermnesia for events experienced during a period of emotional excitement, Stratton[4] commented that a person may recall "in almost photographic detail the total situation at the moment of shock." It is this vivid, seemingly "photographic" memory which inspired the descriptive term "flashbulb memory," originally coined by Brown and Kulik[5] and implying the existence of a biologically distinct mechanism underlying the formation of these memories. The term "flashbulb memory," which suggests that emotionally influenced memories are perfectly accurate and not subject to decay, appears to be a misnomer.[6] Perhaps as a partial consequence of this misnomer, considerable controversy has ensued about the accuracy of flashbulb memories. Neisser[7] and McCloskey et al.[8] pointed out that memories of highly emotional events are not necessarily free of errors. Consequently, they argued that such memories should not be considered a distinct category and that there is no need to posit a "separate mechanism" to account for them.

It is not necessary that emotionally influenced memories be perfect and immune to decay for their formation to be explained by the existence of a distinct biological mechanism. Furthermore, much evidence indicates that memories for highly emotional events are qualitatively different from other types of memories. They are generally both more accurate and less susceptible to decay than are memories of events that do not produce a strong emotional reaction.[6,9-14] As summarized in what follows, studies involving animal and human subjects indicate that neurobiologically distinct memory storage processes operate during and after periods of emotional excitement.

BRAIN MECHANISMS OF EMOTIONAL MEMORY: STRESS HORMONES AND THE AMYGDALOID COMPLEX

Gold and McGaugh[2] proposed that peripheral stress hormones released during and after an emotionally arousing event influence brain memory storage processes for the event. Over the last 20 years, considerable research testing this hypothesis was reported, and evidence now strongly suggests that stress hormones, in particular the catecholamines epinephrine and norepinephrine acting at β-adrenergic receptors, influence memory.[3,15] For example, injections of epinephrine immediately after a learning event influence memory for the event.[16] The effects of posttraining stress hormone injections on memory are time dependent, that is, they affect subsequent retention only when administered soon after a training experience, indicating that the hormones act on memory storage processes.[16,17] An additional feature of the action of catecholamine stress hormones on memory is that they can both enhance and impair memory under appropriate conditions. In general, low doses enhance, while higher doses impair memory.[15,16] This feature of stress hormone action on memory provides an important parallel to the effects of emotion on memory.[4]

The brain region most clearly implicated in the influence of stress hormones on memory is the AC, a group of interconnected nuclei in the medial temporal lobe. The AC has long been believed to be involved with emotional behavior[18] and with hormonal responses to stress.[19,20] Considerable evidence also indicates that the AC is involved in learning, especially during emotionally stressful situations. For example, research from several laboratories in recent years has focused on the role of the AC in pavlovian fear conditioning (LeDoux, this volume; Davis, this volume). The degree to which the AC is involved in learning appears to reflect the degree to which the training conditions induce stress hormone release.[21]

Animal subject studies indicate further that other stress hormones (such as adrenocortical hormones) influence memory processes, that individual AC nuclei serve different roles in memory, and that the AC influences memory storage in other brain regions[3,22] (Roozendaal et al., this volume). However, two "core" predictions of animal subject investigations are that enhanced memory for emotional events requires the action of catecholamine stress hormones and the AC. These predictions have now been tested in humans.

CATECHOLAMINE INVOLVEMENT IN EMOTIONALLY INFLUENCED MEMORY IN HUMANS

Recently, we studied the role of catecholamines in emotionally influenced memory in human subjects.[23] We compared the effect of blockade of β-adrenergic receptors (at which the catecholamines epinephrine and norepinephrine act) on memory for emotionally neutral and emotionally charged material. Subjects took either a placebo or the β-adrenergic blocking drug propranolol (Inderal) 1 hour prior to viewing either an emotionally neutral story or a closely matched but more emotionally arousing story. At one phase of the emotional story (referred to as "phase 2") the boy, walking with his mother to visit his father at work, is critically injured in a car crash as his mother watches. Retention of the stories was tested in a surprise memory test 1 week later. As expected, placebo subjects showed enhanced retention of the emotional story (phase 2) compared to the retention of subjects who viewed the neutral story. Propranolol administration did not effect memory for the neutral story, but impaired memory for the arousing story (FIG. 1). The results are consistent with other evidence indicating that chronic β-blocker treatment impairs the enhancing effect of physical activity on memory.[24] Taken together, these studies strongly support the view derived from animal studies[1] that enhanced memory associated with arousal in humans involves the activation of β-adrenergic receptors.

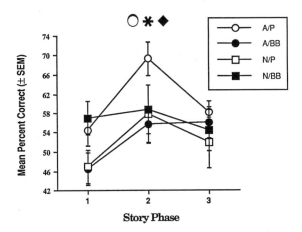

FIGURE 1. Memory test performance of subjects taking either a placebo or propranolol (Inderal) 1 hour before viewing either an emotional or a neutral story. The emotional story elements were introduced into the middle phase of the emotional story (phase 2). Enhanced memory for these elements was seen only in the placebo group. Memory in the arousal story/ placebo group for story phase 2 was significantly better than that for either phase 1 ($\bigcirc$, $p <$ 0.01) or phase 3 ($\star$, $p < 0.05$). No other group showed any significant differences in retention between any story phases. Propranolol blocked the enhancing effect of emotion on memory: $\blacklozenge$, $p < 0.02$ compared to the arousal/beta-blocker (A/BB) group score for story phase 2. A/P = arousal story/placebo. A/BB = arousal story/beta-blocker. N/P = neutral story/placebo. N/BB = neutral story/beta-blocker. (Reprinted with permission from ref. 23.)

AMYGDALOID COMPLEX INVOLVEMENT IN EMOTIONALLY INFLUENCED MEMORY IN HUMANS

At least since the famous report of Scoville and Milner[25] in which the amnesic patient H.M. was first described, a role for the AC in what is now commonly called "declarative" (or "conscious") memory in humans has been questioned. Although several patients in this study had AC damage, the authors concluded that memory loss occurred "whenever the hippocampus and hippocampal gyrus were damaged bilaterally . . . but not otherwise."[25] However, considerable evidence from animal studies implicates the AC in types of emotionally influenced memory that can be considered "declarative," such as memory for a single training event (e.g., one-trial avoidance learning; see Roozendaal *et al.*, this volume). And, as just described, evidence from animal studies indicates a role for the AC for arousing (i.e., stress hormone-activating) learning situations.[3,21]

Evidence from studies involving human subjects now indicates that the AC is selectively involved with enhanced long-term, declarative memory associated with emotionally arousing events. Evidence for the role of the human AC in declarative memory comes from two main sources: studies of AC activity using brain-imaging techniques and investigations of rare patients with brain damage centered on, or confined to, the AC.

Cahill *et al.*[26] examined long-term memory for emotional material in a patient with selective AC damage and control subjects using the same emotional story

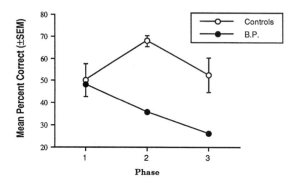

FIGURE 2. Memory test performance for controls and patient B.P. Controls show the expected increase in memory for the phase of the story in which the emotional elements were introduced (phase 2). Patient B.P., who has a selective, bilateral amygdala lesion, showed no evidence of enhanced memory for the emotional story elements. (Reprinted with permission from ref. 26.)

paradigm previously shown to be sensitive to β-adrenergic blockade.[23] As expected, control subjects' retention for the emotional story elements (phase 2) was superior to that for the relatively nonemotional elements (phase 1, FIG. 2). In contrast, patient B.P. showed no evidence of enhanced phase 2 recall despite normal phase 1 recall. This finding has been replicated and extended on a second AC-lesioned patient (Adolphs, Cahill *et al.,* in preparation), and together with findings from a third AC-lesioned patient,[27] provides strong confirmation of the view that the AC is selectively involved with long-term, emotionally influenced, conscious recall in humans.

Additional evidence for this conclusion comes from studies using positron emission tomography (PET). Cahill *et al.*[28] used the PET technique to measure regional cerebral glucose metabolism in subjects while they viewed a series of emotionally arousing (aversive) films and again while they viewed a series of similar, but relatively neutral films. Retention of the films was tested 3 weeks later. Activity of the right amygdala while watching the emotional films correlated highly (r = +0.93) with retention of those films (FIG. 3). However, activity of the right amygdala while viewing the neutral films did not correlate with recall of those films. These results confirm in healthy humans the view that the AC is selectively involved with enhanced memory associated with emotional arousal.[3,21] Another PET investigation implicated the right AC in retrieval of traumatic memories in PTSD patients.[29]

IMPLICATIONS FOR THE PREVENTION AND TREATMENT OF TRAUMATIC MEMORY

PTSD appears to be in large part a disorder of memory, particularly of conscious memory. Perhaps the most characteristic feature of PTSD is "intrusive" memories, exceptionally strong, conscious memories of traumatic events, so strong that they are easily provoked by stimuli associated with the traumatic event or simply intrude on the consciousness of the patient unbidden. Although there is considerable evidence

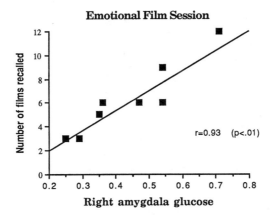

FIGURE 3. Scatterplot of right amygdaloid complex (AC) relative glucose metabolic rate versus recall of a series of relatively emotionally arousing films. The activity of the right AC while viewing the films was highly correlated with the number of films recalled. Activity of the same region while subjects viewed a series of relatively nonemotional films was not correlated with recall. (Reprinted with permission from ref. 28.)

for the existence of nonconscious forms of memory for emotional events,[30,31] understanding PTSD will likely require understanding how these exceptionally strong, conscious memories are formed and maintained.

The evidence summarized in the previous sections suggests that conscious memory for emotional events is modulated by an endogenous mechanism consisting minimally of the AC and stress hormones (especially those acting at β-adrenergic receptors). Emotional arousal may act via this mechanism to increase the strength of memory, that is, the degree to which memories are consciously accessible.[10]

The action of this memory-modulating system, whose role is adaptive within the normal range of emotional events, may also help explain disorders of memory associated with extremely emotional events. It has been suggested that PTSD patients may be caught in a positive feedback loop[32,33] in which each reexperiencing episode (intrusive memory, flashback) produces a stress hormone (especially adrenergic) response. This response then acts to strengthen the memory which produced it, thereby increasing the likelihood of reexperiencing the memory.[33]

Several prominent characteristics of PTSD fit well with this hypothesis of its pathogenesis. For example, PTSD is characterized by hypersensitivity of the sympathetic adrenomedullary system. Twenty-four-hour urinary epinephrine and norepinephrine concentrations are higher in patients with PTSD than in other diagnostic groups.[34] Noradrenergic hypersensitivity in PTSD patients was also demonstrated by Southwick and colleagues[35] who found a significantly greater adrenergic plasma response in PTSD patients than in controls when challenged with intravenous injections of yohimbine (an α_2-adrenergic antagonist). The yohimbine injections also produced panic attacks and flashbacks in a large percentage of PTSD patients, but not in control subjects.[35] Similarly, Blanchard et al.[36] reported that in comparison with control subjects, veterans with PTSD had heightened noradrenergic response to combat-related sounds. The evidence reviewed in this chapter suggests that heightened adrenergic responsiveness may strengthen and maintain memory for the traumatic event in a PTSD patient.

Another line of research further implicates the proposed memory-modulating system in the pathogenesis of PTSD. There are many indications from animal research that the modulation of memory by emotional arousal depends critically on stress hormone-related influences from the peripheral nervous system[37,38] (Roozendaal *et al.*, this volume). If the formation of PTSD involves the memory-modulating system, then anything that impairs influences between the peripheral nervous system and the brain may decrease the likelihood of developing PTSD after a traumatic event. Furthermore, the greater the disruption of peripheral influences, the smaller the likelihood of developing PTSD should be.

This prediction has recently been confirmed in a study of veterans with spinal cord injury (Radnitz *et al.*, submitted for publication). Of several trauma-related risk factors examined, the level of spinal cord injury was the most consistent predictor of PTSD diagnosis and symptom severity. Specifically, quadriplegics were significantly *less* likely than paraplegics to develop PTSD, despite enduring what could be considered the more severe injury. This somewhat counter-intuitive finding fits well, however, with the view that PTSD is a disorder of an endogenous memory-modulating system that is critically dependent on peripheral influences. Supporting this interpretation is the fact that baseline levels of norepinephrine and epinephrine are lower in quadraplegics than in healthy controls, presumably because of lost input from supraspinal centers.[39] Thus, it seems likely that the normal adrenergic response to recall of a traumatic event (and hence modulation of memory by the adrenergic response) is suppressed in quadriplegic patients.

The "positive feedback loop" hypothesis[33] suggests that β-adrenergic blocking drugs may be effective in either treating or preventing the formation of PTSD. An open-trial study of propranolol in 12 PTSD patients reported improvements in PTSD symptoms over a six-month period in most patients.[40] Unfortunately, no controlled studies of β-blocker treatment for PTSD have been reported.

If it is the case that "kindling-like," irreversible increases in nervous system excitability develop in PTSD[41] (Post, this volume), then a proactive strategy designed to prevent PTSD formation may prove more effective than attempts to treat established PTSD. For example, suppression of β-adrenergic activity either before or as quickly as possible after a traumatic event may help prevent the formation of PTSD. Appropriate β-blocker treatment as quickly as possible after a trauma, such as rape, or before an individual enters a traumatic situation, such as combat or the scene of a disaster, should, according to the views developed here, reduce the likelihood of PTSD formation. Experiments to test this possibility are underway.

SUMMARY

Substantial evidence from animal and human subject studies converges on the view that memory for emotionally arousing events is modulated by an endogenous memory-modulating system consisting, at minimum, of stress hormones and the amygdaloid complex. Within the normal range of emotions experienced, this system is viewed as an evolutionarily adaptive method of creating memory strength that is, in general, proportional to memory importance. In conditions of extreme emotional stress, the operation of this normally adaptive system may underly the formation of strong, "intrusive" memories characteristic of PTSD. An improved understanding of the neurobiology of memory modulation should lead to an improved ability to treat or prevent traumatic memories.

REFERENCES

1. McGAUGH, J. L. 1992. *In* The Handbook of Emotion and Memory: Research and Theory. S.-A. Christianson, Eds.: 245-268. Lawrence Erlbaum Assoc. Hillsdale.
2. GOLD, P. E. & J. L. McGAUGH. 1975. *In* Short-Term Memory. D. Deutsch & J. A. Deutsch, Eds.: 355-378. Academic Press, Inc. New York.
3. CAHILL, L & J. L. McGAUGH. 1996. Current Opin. Neurobiol. **6**: 237-242.
4. STRATTON, G. M. 1919. Psychol. Rev. **26**: 474-486.
5. BROWN, K. & J. KULIK. 1977. Cognition **5**: 73-99.
6. BOHANNON, J. N. & V. L. SYMONS. 1992. *In* Affect and Accuracy in Recall: The Problem of Flashbulb Memory. E. Winograd & U. Neisser, Eds. Cambridge University Press. New York.
7. NEISSER, U. 1982. *In* Memory Observed: Remembering in Natural Contexts. U. Neisser, Ed.: 43-48. Freeman. San Francisco.
8. McCLOSKEY, M., C. WIBLE & N. J. COHEN. 1988. J. Exp. Psych Gen. **117**: 336-338.
9. CONWAY, M. A., S. J. ANDERSON, S. F. LARSEN, C. M. DONNELLY, M. A. McDANIEL, A. G. R. McCLELLAND, R. E. RAWLES & R. H. LOGIE. 1994. Mem. Cognit. **22**: 326-343.
10. CAHILL, L. & J. L. McGAUGH. 1995. Consc. Cognit. **4**: 410-421.
11. BURKE, A., F. HEUER & D. REISBERG. 1992. Mem. Cognit. **20**: 277-290.
12. YUILLE, J. C. & J. L. CUTSHALL. 1986. J. Appl. Psychol. **71**: 291-301.
13. PILLEMER, D. B. 1984. Cognition **16**: 63-80.
14. CHRISTIANSON, S.-A. & E. LOFTUS. 1987. Appl. Cog. Psychol. **1**: 225-239.
15. McGAUGH, J. L. 1989. Ann. Rev. Neurosci. **12**: 255-287.
16. GOLD, P. E. & J. L. McGAUGH. 1977. *In* Neuropeptide Influences on Brain and Behavior. L. H. Miller, C. A. Sandman & A. J. Kastin, Eds.: 127-143. Raven Press. New York.
17. GOLD, P. & R. B. VAN BUSKIRK. 1975. Behav. Biol. **13**: 145-153.
18. WEISKRANTZ, L. 1956. J. Comp. Physiol. Psychol. **49**: 381-391.
19. DUNN, J. D. & J. WHITENER. 1986. Neuroendocrinology **42**: 211-217.
20. REDGATE, E. S. 1970. Endocrinology **86**: 806-811.
21. CAHILL, L. & J. L. McGAUGH. 1990. Behav. Neurosci. **104**: 532-543.
22. PACKARD, M., L. CAHILL & J. L. McGAUGH. 1994. Proc. Natl. Acad. Sci. USA **91**: 8477-8481.
23. CAHILL, L., B. PRINS, M. WEBER & J. L. McGAUGH. 1994. Nature **371**: 702-704.
24. NIELSON, K. A. & R. A. JENSEN. 1994. Behav. Neurol. Biol. **62**: 190-200.
25. SCOVILLE, B. & W. B. MILNER. 1957. J. Neurol. Neurosurg. Psychiatry **29**: 11-21.
26. CAHILL, L., R. BABINSKY, H. MARKOWITSCH & J. L. McGAUGH. 1995. Nature **377**: 295-296.
27. BABINSKY, R., P. CALABRESE, H. F. DURWEN, H. J. MARKOWITSCH, D. BRECHTELSBAUER, L. HEUSER & W. GEHLEN. 1993. Behav. Neurol. **6**: 167-170.
28. CAHILL, L., R. HAIER, J. FALLON, M. ALKIRE, C. TANG, D. KEATOR, J. WU & J. L. McGAUGH. 1996. Proc. Natl. Acad. Sci. USA **93**: 8016-8021.
29. RAUCH, S. L., B. A. VAN DER KOLK, R. E. FISLER, N. M. ALPERT, S. P. ORR, S. R. SAVAGE, A. J. FISCHMAN, M. A. JENIKE & R. K. PITMAN. Arch. Gen. Psychiatry **53**: 380-387.
30. TOBIAS, B. A., J. F. KIHLSTROM & D. L. SCHACTER. 1992. *In* The Handbook of Emotion and Memory. S. A. Christianson, Ed.: 67-92. Lawrence Erlbaum Assoc. Hillsdale.
31. LEDOUX, J. E. 1995. Ann. Rev. Psychol. **46**: 209-235.

32. EYSENCK, H. J. & M. J. KELLY. 1987. *In* Cognitive Processes and Pavlovian Conditioning in Humans. D. Graham, Ed.: 251–286. Wiley. New York.
33. PITMAN, R. K. 1989. Biol. Psychiatry **26:** 221–223.
34. YEHUDA, R., E. L. GILLER, S. M. SOUTHWICK, B. KAHANA, D. BOISONEAU, X. MA. & J. MASON. 1994. *In* Catecholamine Function in Posttraumatic Stress Disorder. M. M. Murburg, Ed.: 203–220. American Psychiatric Press. Washington.
35. SOUTHWICK, S. M., J. H. KRYSTAL, C. A. MORGAN, D. JOHNSON, L. M. NAGY, A. NICOLAOU, G. R. HENINGER & D. S. CHARNEY. 1993. Arch. Gen. Psychiatry **50:** 266–274.
36. BLANCHARD, E. B., L. C. KOLB, A. PRINS, S. GATES & G. C. McCoy. 1991. J. Nerv. Ment. Dis. **179:** 371–373.
37. PACKARD, M., C. L. WILLIAMS, L. CAHILL & J. L. McGAUGH. 1995. *In* Neurobehavioral Plasticity. N. E. Spear, L. P. Spear & M. L. Woodruff, Eds.: 149–185. Lawrence Erlbaum Associates, Inc. Hillsdale.
38. INTROINI-COLLISON, I., D. SAGHAFI, G. NOVACK & J. L. McGAUGH. 1992. Brain Res. **572:** 81–86.
39. MATHIAS, C. J., N. CHRISTENSEN, J. CORBETT, H. FRANKEL & J. SPALDING. 1976. Circ. Res. **39:** 204–208.
40. KOLB, L. C., B. C. BURRIS & S. GRIFFITHS. 1984. *In* Post-traumatic Stress Disorder: Psychological and Biological Sequelae. B. A. Van der Kolk, Ed. American Psychiatric Press. Washington.
41. KOLB, L. C. 1987. Am. J. Psychiatry **144:** 989–995.

Stress-Activated Hormonal Systems and the Regulation of Memory Storage[a]

BENNO ROOZENDAAL,[b] GINA L. QUIRARTE,[b,d] AND
JAMES L. McGAUGH [b,c]

[b]Center for the Neurobiology of Learning and Memory, and

[c]Departments of Psychobiology and Pharmacology
University of California
Irvine, California 92697-3800

[d]Centro de Neurobiologia
Campus-UNAM-UAQ
Ap. Postal 1-1141
Juriquilla, Queretaro, Qro. Mexico

There is little doubt that all experiences are not equally well remembered. Most of our experiences are uneventful events that are generally quickly forgotten or, at best, poorly remembered. Extensive evidence indicates that experiences that are emotionally arousing tend to be well remembered. The strength of memories of events reflects the significance of the event. Although it might be argued that enhanced remembrance of emotionally arousing events results simply from increased attention to these situations or from subsequent thinking about or rehearsing the experiences, considerable evidence supports the hypothesis that emotional responses influence memory, at least in part, by modulating long-term memory storage.

Research in our laboratory has focused on the hormonal and brain systems that mediate the effects of emotional arousal on memory storage. This chapter reviews the findings of our experiments using laboratory animals to investigate the effects of stress-released hormones on memory storage. Our findings suggest that stress hormones influence memory storage by activating the amygdala, a brain system known to be involved in emotionally based memory (Davis, this volume; LeDoux, this volume). Furthermore, our findings suggest that the amygdala modulates memory storage in other brain regions. The findings have implications for understanding the role of emotional arousal, stress hormones, and brain systems in normal-human memory as well as pathological memory in patients with posttraumatic stress disorder (PTSD) (Cahill, this volume).[1]

MODULATION OF MEMORY STORAGE

It is well established that recently acquired information is susceptible to modulating influences for a period of time after learning. The hypothesis that memory traces

[a]This research was supported by an R. W. and L. Gerard Trust Fellowship (B.R.), a DGAPA-UNAM grant (G.L.Q.), and NIMH/NIDA research grant MH12526 (J.L.M.).

are initially fragile and subsequently become consolidated[2] is strongly supported by animal experimental as well as clinical findings, indicating that retention is impaired by conditions, such as brain trauma, electrical stimulation of the brain, or drugs, that interfere with normal brain functioning shortly after learning.[3] This evidence suggests that emotional arousal may enhance memory by activating systems involved in regulating the storage of newly acquired information. Thus, the susceptibility of memory storage processes to modulating influences occurring after learning provides the opportunity for emotional activation to regulate the strength of memory traces representing important experiences.[4]

HORMONAL SYSTEMS AND MEMORY STORAGE

During and immediately after emotionally arousing or stressful situations, several physiological systems are activated. Among them is the release of many hormones. Several of these substances, including adrenomedullary and adrenocortical hormones, adrenocorticotropin, prolactin, vasopressin, and opioid peptides are known to modulate memory storage.[5-7] This review focuses on two of the major hormonal systems: catecholamines and glucocorticoids. It is well established that in rats and mice, adrenal hormones are released during and immediately after stressful stimulation of the kind typically used in aversively motivated learning tasks.[8,9] Removal of adrenal hormones by adrenalectomy generally results in memory impairment.[10-13]

Catecholamines. Gold and van Buskirk[14] were the first to report that in adrenally intact rats trained in an inhibitory (passive) avoidance task, retention is enhanced by systemic posttraining injections of the adrenomedullary hormone epinephrine. The effects of epinephrine on retention were dose and time dependent: optimal enhancing effects on memory were seen at moderate doses, whereas higher or lower doses were less effective. Furthermore, the degree of enhancement was greatest when injections were administered shortly after training. Comparable effects were obtained in subsequent experiments using different types of training tasks, including inhibitory avoidance, active avoidance, discrimination learning, and appetitively motivated tasks.[15-18]

Glucocorticoids. Extensive evidence indicates that adrenocortical hormones, which are also released by stress, are involved in modulating memory storage as well. Like the catecholamines, glucocorticoids induce inverted-U shaped dose-response effects on memory storage. Large doses of glucocorticoids or chronic exposure to glucocorticoids generally results in memory impairment,[19,20] but single injections of moderate doses enhance memory storage.[21-23]

Interaction of Catecholamines and Glucocorticoids. Additional findings indicate that these two major hormonal stress systems, catecholamines and glucocorticoids, interact in influencing memory storage. Borrell and colleagues[10,11] showed that glucocorticoids can alter the sensitivity of epinephrine in influencing memory storage in adrenalectomized rats. To examine this issue further, we examined glucocorticoid-adrenergic interactions on memory storage in adrenally intact rats injected with metyrapone, an 11β-hydroxylase inhibitor,[24] a rate-limiting enzyme in the synthesis of corticosterone.[25] Although metyrapone treatment does not completely block the release of glucocorticoids, this drug greatly reduces the elevation of circulating corticosterone induced by emotionally arousing events.[26] In our experiment,[24] rats

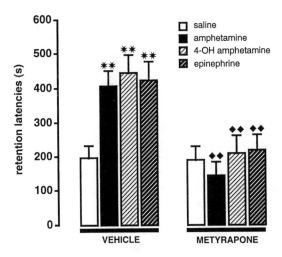

FIGURE 1. Step-through latencies (mean ± SEM) for a 48-hour inhibitory avoidance test. Effects of corticosteroid synthesis blockade with metyrapone (50 mg/kg) on the enhancement of memory produced by posttraining injections of amphetamine (1.0 mg/kg), 4-OH amphetamine (2.0 mg/kg), or epinephrine (0.1 mg/kg) in an inhibitory avoidance task.** $p < 0.01$ as compared with the corresponding saline group; ◆◆ $p < 0.01$ as compared with the corresponding vehicle pretreatment group. (Reprinted with permission from ref. 24.)

received systemic injections of metyrapone or a control solution 90 minutes before training in an inhibitory avoidance task, and epinephrine, amphetamine, or 4-OH amphetamine (a peripherally acting derivative of amphetamine) immediately after training. Retention was tested 48 hours later. Both amphetamine drugs are known to enhance memory, at least in part, by stimulating the release of epinephrine from the adrenal medulla.[27,28] As shown in FIGURE 1, all three adrenergic drugs enhanced retention of the training experience. Metyrapone administration alone did not affect memory, but completely blocked the memory-enhancing effects of the posttraining adrenergic drug treatments. These results indicate that stress-induced increases in plasma corticosterone are required to enable the memory-enhancing effects of epinephrine and amphetamine. Glucocorticoids are also known to influence the effects on memory storage of other neuromodulatory systems, including dopamine[29] and NMDA.[30]

INVOLVEMENT OF THE AMYGDALA

Emerging evidence indicates that epinephrine and glucocorticoid effects on memory are mediated by influences involving the amygdala. It is known that glucocorticoids readily enter the brain and bind directly to central adrenal steroid receptors.[31] However, catecholamines do not readily cross the blood-brain barrier, if at all; therefore, their influence on the amygdala *must* be mediated in an indirect way. Although these hormones differ in the way in which they influence the amygdala, a striking similarity exists in the neurobiological mechanism(s) involved. As discussed below, activation of the release of norepinephrine (NE) in the amygdala appears to be an essential step in mediating the memory-modulatory effects of both peripheral catecholamines and glucocorticoids on memory.

Catecholamines. The focus on the amygdala as a possible site of influence by epinephrine was guided by the evidence that posttraining stimulation of the amygdala can enhance as well as impair memory.[32,33] Furthermore, the amnestic effect typically produced by posttraining amygdala stimulation is not obtained in adrenal demedullated rats.[34] However, retrograde amnesia is produced if epinephrine is administered to adrenal demedullated rats shortly before brain stimulation.[35] Thus, influences induced by peripheral epinephrine appear to be essential for the memory-modulating effects of amygdala stimulation. Results from subsequent experiments indicate that epinephrine-induced enhancing effects on memory are blocked by lesions of the amygdala[36] or the stria terminalis, a major amygdala pathway.[37]

The finding that the memory-modulatory effects of epinephrine are blocked by the peripherally acting β-adrenergic antagonist sotalol[38] is consistent with evidence that the effects of epinephrine are initiated at peripheral sites. Several findings suggest that epinephrine activates β-adrenergic receptors located on vagal afferents[39] that project to the nucleus of the solitary tract (NTS) and that projections from the NTS release NE in the amygdala.[40] Consistent with this hypothesis, inactivation of the NTS with lidocaine blocks the effects of epinephrine on memory.[41] Furthermore, microinfusions of the β-adrenergic antagonist propranolol into the amygdala block the memory-modulatory effects of epinephrine.[42] These findings, considered together, strongly suggest that the effects of epinephrine on memory storage are mediated by the amygdala and that the effects involve activation of β-adrenergic mechanisms in the amygdala.

Thus, the release of NE in the amygdala appears to play a critical role in mediating the effects of epinephrine on memory. Several experiments provide evidence strongly supporting this implication. Posttraining intra-amygdala infusions of NE produce dose-dependent modulation of memory storage.[43,44] This hypothesis further implies that stimulation comparable to that used in inhibitory avoidance training should induce the release of NE in the amygdala. In experiments using *in vivo* microdialysis and high performance liquid chromatography (HPLC), we found that footshock stimulation of the kind typically used in inhibitory avoidance training induced NE release within the amygdala.[45] As shown in FIGURE 2, the release of NE in the amygdala after footshock stimulation depends on the level of stimulation: low-intensity footshock stimulation (0.30 mA for 3 s) induces a 41% increase in NE release, whereas a high-intensity footshock (1.20 mA for 3 s) induces a 96% increase in NE release.[46] NE release returns to baseline levels 30 minutes after footshock.

Glucocorticoids. Extensive evidence indicates that activation of adrenal steroid receptors in the hippocampus plays an important role in mediating the effects of glucocorticoids on memory storage.[5,31] Recent findings from our laboratory strongly indicate that glucocorticoids also affect memory storage through influences involving the amygdala. The findings of our studies on the effects of glucocorticoids on memory for inhibitory avoidance training are similar to those of our studies on the effects of epinephrine.[47] Lesions of the stria terminalis block the memory-enhancing effects of posttraining systemic injections of the synthetic glucocorticoid dexamethasone.[48]

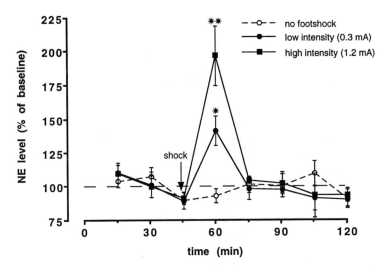

FIGURE 2. Effects of low- and high-intensity footshock on norepinephrine (NE) release in the amygdala assessed by *in vivo* microdialysis and HPLC. NE levels are represented as mean (± SEM) of basal levels prior to footshock.* $p < 0.05$; ** $p < 0.01$ as compared with the no footshock group. (Reprinted with permission from ref. 46.)

Furthermore, as shown in FIGURE 3A, lesions of the amygdala restricted selectively to the basolateral nucleus also block the memory-enhancing effects of posttraining systemic injections of dexamethasone.[22] As shown in FIGURE 3B, posttraining infusions of a specific glucocorticoid receptor (GR or type II) agonist (RU 28362) enhance retention in a dose-dependent fashion when administered into the basolateral nucleus, but are ineffective when administered into the central nucleus.[49] These findings indicate that (1) the basolateral and not the central nucleus is involved in modulating glucocorticoid effects on memory formation, and (2) the effects of glucocorticoids are mediated, at least in part, by direct binding to adrenal steroid receptors in the basolateral nucleus. Furthermore, as discussed below, the basolateral nucleus can also modulate or co-modulate the effects of activation of adrenal steroid receptors in the hippocampus.[50]

Recent findings also suggest that the memory-modulatory effects of glucocorticoids depend on the integrity of the amygdala β-adrenergic system. Microinfusions of the β-adrenergic antagonist propranolol administered into the basolateral nucleus block the memory-enhancing effects of posttraining systemic dexamethasone for inhibitory avoidance training.[51] In contrast, the finding that infusion of a noradrenergic blocker into the central nucleus does not block the memory-enhancing effect of dexamethasone provides additional evidence that the basolateral, and not the central nucleus, is involved in mediating glucocorticoid and possibly epinephrine effects on memory storage. Further evidence that activation of the noradrenergic system is required to obtain memory enhancement with glucocorticoids came from a study of the effects of infusion of a specific GR agonist (RU 28362) into the NTS. As discussed above, the NTS is a brainstem structure that provides noradrenergic input to the

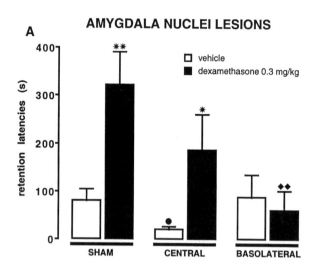

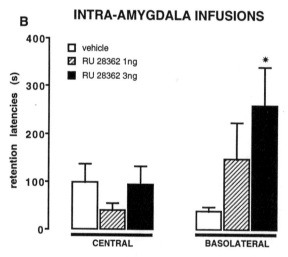

FIGURE 3. Step-through latencies (mean ± SEM) for a 48-hour inhibitory avoidance test. (A) Rats with sham, or lesions of either the central or basolateral nucleus of the amygdala had been treated with dexamethasone (0.3 mg/kg) or vehicle immediately after training. (B) Rats received posttraining microinfusions of the glucocorticoid receptor agonist RU 28362 (1.0 or 3.0 ng) in the central or basolateral nucleus. ✱ $p < 0.05$; ✱✱ $p < 0.01$ as compared with the corresponding vehicle group; ● $p < 0.05$ as compared with the corresponding sham lesion-vehicle group; ◆◆ $p < 0.01$ as compared with the corresponding sham lesion-dexamethasone group. (Reprinted with permission from refs. 22 and 49.)

amygdala.[40] The noradrenergic neurons of the NTS have high densities of GRs.[52] Posttraining administration of the GR agonist into the NTS dose-dependently enhanced memory for inhibitory avoidance training (Roozendaal, Williams & McGaugh, in preparation). Thus, the findings that both the catecholaminergic and glucocorticoid systems activate the noradrenergic system strongly support the hypothesis that the noradrenergic system is a locus of interaction of these systems in regulating long-term memory storage.

Interaction of the Noradrenergic System with Other Neuromodulatory Systems. The evidence just summarized suggests that epinephrine and glucocorticoid hormones modulate memory storage by influencing noradrenergic activity in the amygdala. Considerable evidence suggests that the effects on memory of other neuromodulatory systems, including opioid peptidergic and GABAergic systems, also involve activation of the noradrenergic system in the amygdala. It is known that posttraining systemic injections of opioid peptides and opiates generally impair memory and that opiate antagonists enhance memory.[53-55] Additionally, GABAergic antagonists and agonists enhance and impair retention, respectively.[56,57] Opioid peptidergic and GABAergic influences on memory storage are also blocked by lesions of the (basolateral) amygdala or stria terminalis.[58,59] Moreover, intra-amygdala infusions of opioid peptidergic and GABAergic drugs (including benzodiazepines) modulate retention of several tasks. When administered either systematically or intra-amygdally, opiate and GABAergic influences on memory are blocked by intra-amygdala injections of the β-adrenergic antagonist propranolol.[60,61] These interactions of neuromodulatory systems in modulating memory storage are summarized in FIGURE 4.

The foregoing evidence together with the finding that opioid peptides and opiates inhibit the release of NE in the cerebral cortex[62] suggest that opiate agonists and antagonists may influence memory storage by modulating the release of NE within the amygdala.[63] To examine this issue, we measured NE release in the amygdala in response to footshock stimulation followed by systemic injections of an opiate agonist (β-endorphin) or antagonist (naloxone). Post-footshock injections of β-endorphin reduced footshock induced release of NE in the amygdala, whereas naloxone potentiated NE release. Naloxone increased not only the magnitude, but also the duration of NE release. NE release following naloxone injections remained elevated 75 minutes postshock, whereas NE release in control-injected animals returned to baseline 30 minutes after footshock.[46]

ROLE OF THE AMYGDALA IN MEMORY STORAGE: INTERACTION WITH OTHER BRAIN SYSTEMS

Although the findings just summarized strongly suggest that the amygdala is a critical site for integrating the interactions of several neuromodulatory systems influencing memory storage, they do not identify the locus or loci of the influences. Evidence that long-term potentiation (LTP) can be induced in the amygdala,[64-66] as well as the findings that drugs that block LTP also attenuate fear based learning when administered into the amygdala prior to training suggest that neural changes mediating fear conditioning may be located within the amygdala.[67,68]

Findings from our laboratory, however, strongly suggest that the amygdala is not a site of memory storage. For example, lesions of the amygdala induced 1 week or

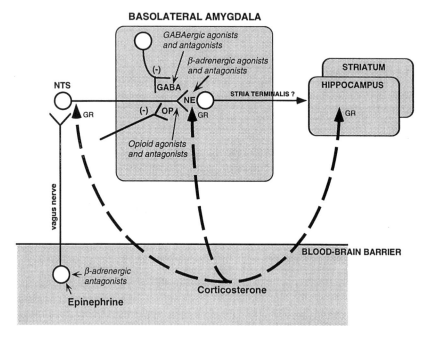

FIGURE 4. Schematic summarizing the interactions of neuromodulatory influences on memory storage as suggested by the findings of our experiments.

even 1 month after aversive training do not block retention.[69,70] Additionally, intra-amygdala infusions of the AMPA receptor antagonist CNQX before retention impair but do not block retrieval.[71]

In our view the role of the amygdala in memory storage involves activation of efferents mediated, at least in part, by the stria terminalis. The primary role of the amygdala in memory is to regulate memory storage in other brain structures. For example, recent findings indicate that the amygdala can modulate memory storage for either hippocampus-dependent or caudate nucleus-dependent learning tasks.[72] That study was based on evidence of a double dissociation between the hippocampus and caudate nucleus and two versions of a water-maze task.[73] Spatial learning in a water maze, in which rats have to learn to locate and swim to a submerged platform, is impaired following hippocampal lesions.[74-76] In contrast, although lesions of the caudate nucleus do not impair memory for this spatial task, memory for swimming to a visible platform (a cued task) is dramatically impaired after caudate nucleus lesions.[73] Furthermore, this cued version of the water-maze task is not affected by hippocampal lesions. In the Packard *et al.* study,[72] unilateral posttraining microinjections of amphetamine administered into the hippocampus immediately after a single training session enhanced memory storage for the spatial, but not the cued version of the water maze, whereas amphetamine injections into the caudate nucleus enhanced memory for the cued, but not the spatial version. However, and most importantly, amphetamine injected into the amygdala enhanced memory storage for both the spatial and the cued versions of the task. These findings clearly indicate that the amygdala can modulate memory storage processes for both hippocampus-dependent and caudate nucleus-dependent tasks. Other findings showing that an injection of *N*-methyl-D-aspartate (NMDA) into the amygdala induces expression of the proto-oncogene c-*fos* in the dentate gyrus of the dorsal hippocampus and the caudate nucleus suggest a functional connection between the amygdala and both brain structures.[40]

In another experiment we examined the interaction of the amygdala with the hippocampus in mediating glucocorticoid-induced memory effects. Intrahippocampal administration of the GR antagonist RU 38486 impaired retention performance for training based on spatial cues in the water maze, but this effect was completely blocked in animals with basolateral, but not central nuclei lesions.[50] These findings are consistent with recent evidence indicating that lesions of the basolateral nucleus attenuate the induction of LTP in the dentate gyrus *in vivo*.[77,78] Also consistent with our finding is evidence that lesions of the central nucleus did not affect hippocampal LTP.[77] These results indicate that an intact basolateral nucleus is required for neuroplasticity within the hippocampus, suggesting that the basolateral nucleus may provide the cofactor necessary for these processes. Moreover, high-frequency stimulation of the basolateral nucleus facilitates the induction of LTP in the dentate gyrus.[79] Thus, these findings support the idea that activation of the amygdala (by peripheral stress hormones) may strengthen memory storage in other brain structures.

POSSIBLE CONSEQUENCES FOR UNDERSTANDING POSTTRAUMATIC STRESS DISORDER

Our studies provide evidence that memory enhancement for emotionally arousing events involves activation of β-adrenergic mechanisms and the amygdala. In addition, the findings are consistent with evidence of involvement of β-adrenergic activation and the amygdala in emotionally enhanced memory in human subjects (Cahill, this volume). Our animal experiments suggest important new insights into the neurobiological mechanisms underlying the etiology of PTSD. As originally proposed by Pitman,[1] an extremely traumatic event may overstimulate the endogenous hormonal systems and neuromodulators, resulting in overconsolidation of the memory trace of that event. These deeply engraved traumatic memories may subsequently manifest themselves in intrusive recollections. Furthermore, during the recall of events, stress hormones are released, further enhancing the strength of the memory trace. This positive feedback loop may possibly explain the delayed onset in which subclinical PTSD ultimately becomes clinical. The fact that the noradrenergic system is overactivated in PTSD[80] supports this interpretation. Our findings from research using PET scanning, are also consistent with the evidence of high activity in the right amygdala of human patients with PTSD during thoughts about the traumatic events.[81] Generally, our findings provide insights into how significant events create lasting memories.

REFERENCES

1. PITMAN, R. K. 1989. Biol. Psychiatry **26:** 221-223.
2. MÜLLER, G. E. & A. PILZECKER. 1900. Z. Psychol. **1:** 1-288.

3. McGaugh, J. L. & M. J. Herz. 1972. Memory Consolidation. Albion Publishing Co. San Francisco, CA.
4. Gold, P. E. & J. L. McGaugh. 1975. *In* Short-Term memory. D. Deutsch & J. A. Deutsch, Eds.: 355-378, Academic Press. New York, NY.
5. Bohus, B. 1994. *In* The Memory System of the Brain. Advanced Series in Neuroscience. J. Delacour, Ed.: 337-364. World Scientific. New Jersey.
6. de Wied, D. 1991. *In* Peripheral Signaling of the Brain. Role in Neural-Immune Interactions, Learning and Memory. R. C. A. Frederickson, J. L. McGaugh & D. L. Felten, Eds.: 335-350. Hogrefe & Huber. Toronto.
7. Koob, G. F., C. Lebrun, R.-M. Bluthé, R. Dantzer, D. M. Dorsa & M. Le Moal. 1991. *In* Peripheral Signaling of the Brain: Role in Neural-Immune Interactions, Learning and Memory. R. C. A. Frederickson, J. L. McGaugh & D. L. Felten, Eds.: 351-363. Hogrefe & Huber. Toronto.
8. McCarty, R. & P. E. Gold. 1981. Horm. Behav. **15:** 168-182.
9. McGaugh, J. L. & P. E. Gold. 1989. *In* Psychoendocrinology. R. B. Brush & S. Levine, Eds.: 305-339. Academic Press. New York, NY.
10. Borrell, J., E. R. de Kloet, D. H. G. Versteeg & B. Bohus. 1983. Behav. Neural Biol. **39:** 241-258.
11. Borrell, J., E. R. de Kloet & B. Bohus. 1984. Life Sci. **34:** 99-107.
12. Oitzl, M. S. & E. R. de Kloet. 1992. Behav. Neurosci. **108:** 62-71.
13. Roozendaal, B., G. Portillo-Marquez & J. L. McGaugh. 1996. Behav. Neurosci. **110:** 1074-1083.
14. Gold, P. E. & R. van Buskirk. 1975. Behav. Biol. **13:** 247-260.
15. Liang, K. C., R. G. Juler, J. L. McGaugh. 1986. Brain Res. **368:** 125-133.
16. Sternberg, D. B., K. Isaacs, P. E. Gold & J. L. McGaugh. 1985. Behav. Neural Biol. **44:** 447-453.
17. Introini-Collison, I. B. & J. L. McGaugh. 1986. Behav. Neural Biol. **45:** 358-365.
18. Izquierdo, I. & R. D. Diaz. 1985. Psychoneuroendocrinology **10:** 165-172.
19. Luine, V., R. L. Spencer & B. S. McEwen. 1993. Brain Res. **616:** 65-70.
20. Newcomer, J. S., S. Craft, T. Hershey, K. Askins & M. E. Bardgett. 1994. J. Neurosci. **14:** 2047-2053.
21. Cottrell, G. A. & S. Nakajima. 1977. Pharmacol. Biochem. Behav. **7:** 277-280.
22. Roozendaal, B. & J. L. McGaugh. 1996. Neurobiol. Learning Memory **65:** 1-8.
23. Sandi, C. & S. P. R. Rose. 1994. Brain Res. **647:** 106-112.
24. Roozendaal, B., O. Carmi & J. L. McGaugh. 1996. Proc. Natl. Acad. Sci. USA **93:** 1429-1433.
25. Strashimirov, D. & B. Bohus. 1966. Steroids **7:** 171-180.
26. Roozendaal, B., B. Bohus & J. L. McGaugh. Psychoneuroendocrinology, in press.
27. Martinez, J. R., Jr., R. A. Jensen, R. B. Messing, B. J. Vasquez, B. Soumireu-Mourat, D. Geddes, K. C. Liang & J. L. McGaugh. 1980. Brain Res. **182:** 157-166.
28. Wiener, N. 1985. *In* The Pharmacological Basis of Therapeutics. A. G. Goodman, L. S. Goodman, T. W. Rall & F. Murad, Eds. Macmillian Publishing Co. New York, NY.
29. Cabib, S., C. Castellano, F. R. Patacchiolo, G. Cigliana, L. Angelucci & S. Puglisi-Allegra. 1996. Brain Res. **729:** 110-118.
30. Mondadori C. & L. Weiskrantz. 1993. Behav. Neural Biol. **60:** 205-210.
31. McEwen, B. S. & R. M. Sapolsky. 1995. Curr. Opin. Neurobiol. **5:** 205-216.
32. Kesner, R. P. & M. Wilburn 1974. Behav. Biol. **10:** 259-293.
33. McGaugh, J. L. & P. E. Gold. 1976. *In* Neural Mechanisms of Learning and Memory. M. R. Rosenzweig & E. L. Bennett, Eds.: 549-560. MIT Press. Cambridge, MA.
34. Bennett, C., K. C. Liang & J. L. McGaugh. 1985. Behav. Brain Res. **15:** 83-91.
35. Liang, K. C., C. Bennett & J. L. McGaugh. 1985. Behav. Brain Res. **15:** 93-100.
36. Cahill, L. & J. L. McGaugh. 1991. Psychobiology **19:** 206-210.
37. Liang, K. C. & J. L. McGaugh. 1983. Behav. Brain Res. **9:** 49-58.

38. INTROINI-COLLISON, I. B., D. SAGHAFI, G. NOVACK & J. L. MCGAUGH. 1992. Brain Res. **572:** 81-86.
39. SCHREURS, J., T. SEELING & H. SCHULMAN. 1986. J. Neurochem. **46:** 294-296.
40. PACKARD, M. G., C. L. WILLIAMS, L. CAHILL & J. L. MCGAUGH. 1995. *In* Neurobehavioral Plasticity: Learning, Development, and Response to Brain Insults. N. E. Spear, L. P. Spear & M. L. Woodruff, Eds.: 149-184. Lawrence Erlbaum. New Jersey.
41. WILLIAMS, C. L. & J. L. MCGAUGH. 1993. Behav. Neurosci. **107:** 1-8.
42. LIANG, K. C., R. G. JULER & J. L. MCGAUGH. 1986. Brain Res. **368:** 125-133.
43. LIANG, K. C., J. L. MCGAUGH & H.-Y. YAO. 1990. Brain Res. **508:** 225-233.
44. ROOZENDAAL, B., J. M. KOOLHAAS & B. BOHUS. 1993. Behav. Neurosci. **107:** 575-579.
45. GALVEZ, R., M. MESCHES & J. L. MCGAUGH. 1996. Neurobiol. Learning Memory **66:** 253-257.
46. GALVEZ, R., G. L. QUIRARTE & J. L. MCGAUGH. 1996. Soc. Neurosci. Abstr. **22:** 1869.
47. ROOZENDAAL, B., L. CAHILL & J. L. MCGAUGH. *In* Brain Processes and Memory. K. Ishikawa, J. L. McGaugh & H. Sakata, Eds.: 39-54. Elsevier. Amsterdam. In press.
48. ROOZENDAAL, B. & J. L. MCGAUGH. 1996. Brain Res. **709:** 243-250.
49. ROOZENDAAL, B. & J. L. MCGAUGH. 1997. Neurobiol. Learning Memory **67:** 176-179.
50. ROOZENDAAL, B. & J. L. MCGAUGH. 1997. Eur. J. Neurosci. **9:** 76-83.
51. QUIRARTE, G. L., B. ROOZENDAAL & J. L. MCGAUGH. 1996. Soc. Neurosci. Abstr. **22:** 1869.
52. HÄRFSTRAND, A., K. FUXE, A. CINTRA, L. F. AGNATI, I. ZINI, A. C. WIKSTRÖM, S. OKRET, Z. Y. YU, M. GOLDSTEIN, H. STEINBUSCH, A. VERHOFSTAD & J. Å. GUSTAFSSON. 1986. Proc. Natl. Acad. Sci. USA **83:** 9779-9783.
53. IZQUIERDO, I. & R. D. DIAZ. 1983. Psychoneuroendocrinology **8:** 81-87.
54. MCGAUGH, J. L. 1989. Ann. Rev. Neurosci. **12:** 255-287.
55. MCGAUGH, J. L., I. B. INTROINI-COLLISON & C. CASTELLANO. 1993. *In* Handbook of Experimental Pharmacology, Opioids. Part II. A. Herz, H. Akil & E. Simon. Eds.: 429-447. Springer-Verlag. Heidelberg.
56. BRIONI, J. D. & J. L. MCGAUGH. 1988. Psychopharmacology **96:** 505-510.
57. BRIONI, J. D., A. H. NAGAHARA & J. L. MCGAUGH. 1989. Brain Res. **487:** 105-112.
58. MCGAUGH, J. L., I. B. INTROINI-COLLISON, R. G. JULER & I. IZQUIERDO. 1986. Behav. Neurosci. **100:** 839-844.
59. AMMASSARI-TEULE, M., F. PAVONE, C. CASTELLANO & J. L. MCGAUGH. 1991. Brain Res. **551:** 104-109.
60. MCGAUGH, J. L., I. B. INTROINI-COLLISON & A. H. NAGAHARA. 1988. Brain Res. **446:** 37-49.
61. INTROINI-COLLISON, I. B., A. H. NAGAHARA & J. L. MCGAUGH. 1989. Brain Res. **476:** 94-101.
62. ARBILLA, S. & S. Z. LANGER. 1978. Nature **271:** 559-561.
63. MCGAUGH, J. L., I. B. INTROINI-COLLISON, L. CAHILL, M. KIM & K. C. LIANG. 1992. *In* The Amygdala: Neurobiological Aspects of Emotion, Memory, and Mental Dysfunction. J. P. Aggleton, Ed.: 431-451. Wiley-Liss. New York, NY.
64. CHAPMAN, P. F., E. W. KAIRISS, C. L. KEENAN & T. H. BROWN. 1990. Synapse **6:** 271-278.
65. CLUGNET, M. C. & J. E. LEDOUX. 1990. J. Neurosci. **10:** 1055-1061.
66. MAREN, S. & M. S. FANSELOW. 1995. J. Neurosci. **15:** 7548-7564.
67. FALLS, W. A., M. J. D. MISERENDINO & M. DAVIS. 1992. J. Neurosci. **12:** 854-863.
68. MISERENDINO, M. J. D., C. B. SANANES, K. R. MELIA & M. DAVIS. 1990. Nature **345:** 716-718.
69. PARENT, M. B., G. L. QUIRARTE & J. L. MCGAUGH. 1995. Behav. Neurosci. **109:** 803-807.
70. PARENT, M. B., M. WEST & J. L. MCGAUGH. 1994. Behav. Neurosci. **108:** 1080-1087.
71. MESCHES, M. H., M. BIANCHIN & J. L. MCGAUGH. 1996. Neurobiol. Learning Memory **66:** 324-340.
72. PACKARD, M. G., L. CAHILL & J. L. MCGAUGH. 1994. Proc. Natl. Acad. Sci. USA **91:** 8477-8481.
73. PACKARD, M. G. & J. L. MCGAUGH. 1992. Behav. Neurosci. **106:** 439-446.

74. MORRIS, R. G. M., P. GARRUD, J. N. P. RAWLINS & J. O'KEEFE. 1982. Nature **297:** 681-683.
75. MOSER, E., M.-B. MOSER & P. ANDERSEN. 1993. J. Neurosci. **13:** 3916-3925.
76. OLTON, D. S., J. T. BECKER & G. E. HANDELMANN. 1979. Behav. Brain Res. **2:** 313-365.
77. IKEGAYA, Y., H. SAITO & K. ABE. 1994. Brain Res. **656:** 157-174.
78. IKEGAYA, Y., H. SAITO & K. ABE. 1995. Brain Res. **671:** 351-354.
79. IKEGAYA, Y., H. SAITO & K. ABE. 1995. Neurosci. Res. **22:** 203-207.
80. SOUTHWICK, S. M., J. H. KRYSTAL, C. A. MORGAN, D. JOHNSON, L. M. NAGY, A. NICOLAOU, G. R. HENINGER & D. S. CHARNEY. 1993. Arch. Gen. Psychiatry **50:** 266-274.
81. RAUCH, S. L., B. A. VAN DER KOLK, R. E. FISLER, N. M. ALPERT, S. P. ORR, C. R. SAVAGE, A. J. FISCHMAN, M. A. JENIKE & R. K. PITMAN. 1996. Arch. Gen. Psychiatry. **53:** 380-387.

How the Brain Processes Emotional Information

JORGE L. ARMONY AND JOSEPH E. LeDOUX

Center for Neural Science
New York University
4 Washington Place
New York, New York 10003-6621

In recent years, much progress has been made in elucidating the neural system underlying classic fear conditioning, a well-defined behavioral model of emotional learning and memory processes. (For review, see refs. 1–5.) Although this body of work may not illuminate all aspects of all emotions, it is highly relevant to the emotion "fear" and its various manifestations, including psychopathological manifestations. In fact, the implications of work on fear conditioning have not escaped the attention of researchers who work on a variety of anxiety disorders including phobias, panic, and posttraumatic stress disorder (PTSD). (For reviews, see refs. 2 and 6.) We survey some of the major findings about the neural basis of fear conditioning and discuss some of the broader implications, including those for a neurobiological understanding of PTSD.

FEAR CONDITIONING

When a neutral stimulus co-occurs and becomes associated with a harmful event, it can itself acquire an aversive value. This phenomenon, originally studied by Pavlov,[7] is known as fear conditioning. It can be readily induced experimentally when the innocuous conditioned stimulus (CS), such as a light or a tone, is paired with the aversive unconditioned stimulus (US), usually a brief electric shock to the feet or air puff to the eye. As a result of the CS-US pairings, the CS will elicit innate reactions that are naturally elicited by threatening stimuli, such as the sight or sound of a predator. In rats, these responses usually include changes in the behavioral (e.g., immobility, or "freezing," and suppression of ongoing behavior), autonomic (e.g., heart rate and blood pressure), and hormonal systems as well as reduction in pain sensitivity (analgesia) and potentiation of reflexes (e.g., startle and eyeblink reflexes).[8–12] This form of Pavlovian conditioning is very robust; it can sometimes be induced with a single CS-US pairing and has been shown to operate in a wide variety of species, from flies to humans.[13]

NEURAL SYSTEM

Studies from several laboratories have helped elucidate in great detail the neural circuitry underlying fear conditioning. (For reviews, see refs. 1, 3, and 5.) Most of these studies involve experiments in which a rat is exposed to an auditory CS,

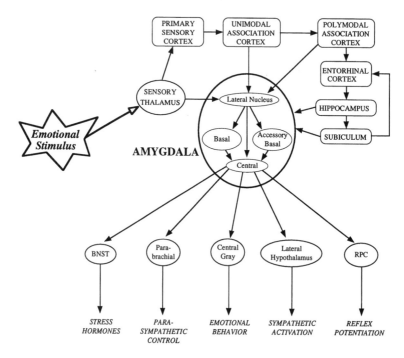

FIGURE 1. A hierarchical cascade of auditory information converges onto the lateral nucleus of the amygdala. After intraamygdala processing, information reaches the central nucleus, which controls effectors systems involved in the expression of the different emotional responses. Abbreviations: BNST = bed nucleus of the stria terminalis; RPC = nucleus reticularis pontis caudalis.

typically a single-frequency tone, paired with footshock. We will therefore focus on the networks in the rat brain involved in the processing of auditory conditioned stimuli. Nonetheless, several of these findings can be applied to other sensory modalities and species, including humans. A simplified diagram of the brain structures and pathways involved in fear conditioning is depicted in FIGURE 1.

It is now widely accepted that the amygdala is essential for the acquisition of conditioned fear as well as for the expression of innate and learned fear responses. Thus, it is believed that through the process of conditioning, the CS acquires the capacity to access and trigger the hard-wired fear response network in the amygdala, producing a cascade of innate defensive reactions. It becomes important then to understand how information about the CS is transmitted to and processed by the amygdala, and what cellular mechanisms are responsible for the changes in that processing as a consequence of conditioning.

Input Pathways

Processing an auditory CS involves transmission from the ear, through brainstem areas, to the auditory region of the thalamus, the medial geniculate body (MGB).[14]

From there, information is transmitted to the amygdala by way of two parallel pathways. A direct projection originates primarily in the medial division of the MGB (MGm) and the associated posterior intralaminar nucleus.[15] A second, indirect, pathway conveys information from all areas of the MGB to the auditory cortex, from where, and via several corticocortical links, it is transmitted to the amygdala.[16,17] Lesion studies have demonstrated that either pathway is sufficient for conditioning to a simple stimulus, such as a pure tone.[18] However, the different anatomical and physiological characteristics of these two pathways suggest that they may subserve different, and possibly complementary, functions, particularly when the conditioning involves more complex stimuli. The direct pathway transmits information to the amygdala through only one synapse and therefore it is fast, but physiological studies suggest that it may be limited in its capacity to represent complex auditory stimuli.[19] In contrast, the thalamo-cortico-amygdala pathway is longer and slower, but it has a much greater capacity to perform a detailed analysis and provide an accurate representation of the CS. In support of this view, lesion studies have shown that the auditory cortex may not be necessary for a simple frequency analysis of different tones,[20] but it becomes crucial for higher levels of stimulus processing such as pitch and temporal modulation.[21,22]

The subcortical and cortical pathways terminate in the lateral nucleus of the amygdala (LA),[15–17,23] often converging onto single neurons.[24] The thalamic and cortical afferent projections to the LA use the excitatory neurotransmitter glutamate. Whereas the cortical pathway acts only through fast AMPA receptors, the direct thalamic projections require the activation of both AMPA and NMDA receptors.[24,25] Interestingly, NMDA-mediated currents remain active for a longer time[26] and therefore could serve as a bridge for temporal integration of the information transmitted by the thalamic and cortical inputs. The existence of feedforward and feedback inhibitory circuits in LA provides another way in which the thalamic and cortical pathways may interact.[27]

Many cells in the LA respond to auditory stimuli, particularly high frequency signals, above 10 kHz.[28] A majority of these (about 90%) are also responsive to strong somatosensory stimulation.[29] Therefore, the lateral nucleus of the amygdala is a potential site for CS-US convergence at a single-cell level, along with the auditory thalamus.[28,30] (In the latter, however, the proportion of cells receiving convergent auditory-somatosensory input is less than 40%.) Such a neural intersection of pathways transmitting information about the CS and US has long been suspected to be a necessary mechanism for conditioning (e.g., see refs. 7, 31, and 32).

Information processed by the lateral nucleus is then transmitted, via intraamygdala connections,[33,34] to the basal and accessory basal nuclei and from there to the central nucleus. The central nucleus is the main output system of the amygdala; lesions of this structure abolish the expression of all conditioned responses.[1,4,5] Interestingly, the various modalities of conditioned responses are mediated by the central nucleus via separate output channels. It is possible to interfere with particular responses by lesioning areas to which the central nucleus projects. For example, lesions of the central gray disrupt conditioned motor activity, such as freezing;[35–37] lesions of the lateral hypothalamus interfere with conditioned sympathetic responses, such as blood pressure elevation,[35,38] and lesions of the bed nucleus of the stria terminalis abolish neuroendocrine responses.[39,40]

Contextual Conditioning

The particular environment in which the original fear conditioning takes place can play an important role in the responses to subsequent CS presentations. For example, fear responses are stronger when the CS is presented in the original conditioning context than when the presentation occurs in a different one.[41] Furthermore, the context in which conditioning takes place can, by itself, acquire aversive value.[42-44] Recent studies have determined that contextual conditioning, like conditioning to the CS, depends on the amygdala. However, unlike CS conditioning, contextual conditioning depends on the hippocampus.[41,45,46] Lesions of the hippocampus made prior to training selectively disrupt the contextual aspects of fear conditioning, without having any effect on conditioning to the CS.[41,44,46] In addition, lesions made after training impair the retention of contextual fear associations. This retrograde amnesia of contextual fear, however, is temporally graded; lesions made more than 2 weeks after training have no effect.[45] These findings are consistent with experimental studies[47] and computational models[48,49] that suggest that the hippocampus is essential for the formation and consolidation of declarative, or explicit memories, but not for their maintenance over long periods. The role of the hippocampus in the evaluation of contextual cues in fear conditioning is also consistent with theories of hippocampal spatial, configural, and/or relational processing proposed during the last two decades.[50-52] That is, the hippocampus would act as a high-level cognitive structure that supplies the fear system with a more complex stimulus representation than the sensory thalamus or cortices can provide. Although it is not clear yet how the hippocampus interacts with the fear network, anatomical evidence suggests a bidirectional flow of information between the hippocampal formation and the amygdala.[53-55] Moreover, recent studies have shown that connections between the hippocampus and the amygdala exhibit synaptic plasticity, suggesting a possible mode of interaction.[56]

Extinction of Conditioned Fear

If, after conditioning, the CS is repeatedly presented alone (in the absence of the US), reactions to the CS become weakened through a process known as extinction.[7] Extinction is not a passive forgetting of the original CS-US association, but an active process, possibly involving a new learning.[57] This is particularly apparent in situations when CS-elicited responses are spontaneously reinstated, particularly those after an unrelated traumatic experience.[7,58,59] For example, Pavlov's experimental dogs showed a reinstatement of their previously extinguished conditioned responses after they nearly drowned in the great flood of Petrograd in 1924. ("Any hypothesis of an irreparable destruction of the conditioned reflex [conditioned response] cannot possibly stand for a moment, since in every case of extinction the reflex invariably becomes spontaneously restored in a longer or shorter time.") Moreover, Bouton and colleagues[57,60] demonstrated that the extinction of conditioned responses to a CS is context dependent. In their experiments, rats that had showed extinction of their conditioned responses to the CS in a context different from the one in which they had received the CS-US pairings displayed a renewal of the conditioned reactions to the CS when placed back in the original conditioning chamber.

A growing body of evidence points towards the involvement of the prefrontal cortex in the extinction process. Lesions of the ventromedial prefrontal and/or medial orbitofrontal cortex in the rat, made before training, selectively retard the extinction of behavioral responses to the CS.[61,62] Lesions of sensory cortex also retard extinction.[63,64] In addition, neurons in the monkey orbitofrontal cortex can change their response properties to a stimulus whose reinforcement value is altered,[65–67] in contrast to amygdala cells, which tend to exhibit more persistent response patterns.[66,67] That is, cortical areas, particularly the prefrontal cortex, may be crucial in monitoring changes in the reinforcement value of external (and possibly internal as well) stimuli and inhibiting responses that are no longer appropriate. It is believed that the effect of the prefrontal cortex in extinction is mediated by its projections to the amygdala, as blockade of the NMDA receptors in the amygdala interferes with extinction of conditioned fear.[68] This finding further reinforces the view that extinction is an active form of learning, possibly through involvement of NMDA-dependent synaptic plasticity.

NEURAL PLASTICITY IN FEAR CONDITIONING

Neurons in several structures of the fear circuit develop changes in their response to the CS after conditioning. Specifically, cells in the MGm, auditory cortex, and amygdala show conditioning-induced plasticity. We focus on the changes observed in the amygdala, particularly its lateral nucleus, the sensory gateway to the amygdala, thus the site where amygdala plasticity would occur first.

As a result of the pairing of a tone with footshock, some cells in the lateral amygdala show an increase in response to the tone, which acquires aversive value as a predictor of the shock. The earliest changes in the response take place within 15 ms after the onset of the tone[69] (FIG. 2a). Based on the latency of response of the various structures in the circuit, it is possible to conclude that these changes reflect plasticity in the processing of information carried by the direct thalamo-amygdala pathway. In other words, the earliest plasticity observed in amygdala cells cannot be accounted for by projections from the cortex, as these signals take substantially longer to reach the amygdala (over 20 ms). It should be pointed out that although definitive evidence is still unavailable, previous studies seem to argue against amygdala plasticity as being just a reflection of active plastic changes occurring upstream in the circuit, that is, the auditory thalamus. Thalamic conditioned plasticity occurs later than that in the amygdala, typically around 20 ms following tone onset.[70–72] Plasticity in the lateral amygdala can, in turn, contribute to plasticity in other amygdala structures downstream, such as the basal and central nuclei, where conditioned increases in stimulus responses occur with latencies between 30 and 70 ms after CS onset.[73–75]

This conditioning-induced plasticity is frequency specific, as evidenced by shifts in the receptive fields of neurons in the lateral amygdala[76] towards the conditioned stimulus. This retuning of neural receptive fields results in an increase in the representation of the CS in the amygdala. Conditioned stimulus retuning was discovered and has been studied most thoroughly in the auditory thalamus and auditory cortex. (For a review, see ref. 77.) An example of an amygdala neuron's receptive-field retuning, after conditioning, is shown in FIGURE 2B.

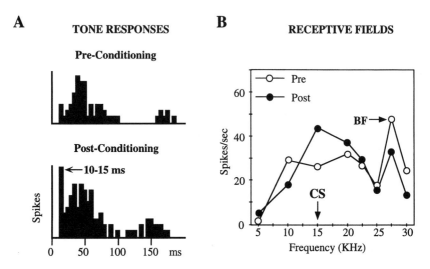

FIGURE 2. (**A**) Poststimulus time histogram showing the tone response of an amygdala neuron before and after conditioning. Note the increase in early responses (less than 15 ms) following CS-US pairings. Adapted from ref. 69. (**B**) Returning of auditory receptive field (RF) of an amygdala neuron. Prior to conditioning to an auditory CS, the neuron's receptive field (Pre) and best frequency (BF) were determined. Following conditioning, a shift in the RF resulted in the CS becoming the new best frequency. Adapted from ref. 20.

FEAR CONDITIONING IN HUMANS

Although most of the findings reported in previous sections were obtained from studies with experimental animals, particularly rats, some evidence is emerging suggesting that analogous brain regions and mechanisms are involved in human fear conditioning.

Patients with lesions that include the amygdala exhibited marked deficits on the acquisition of autonomic conditioned responses during a fear-conditioning paradigm[78,79] even though they were aware of the experimental reinforcement contingencies (that is, they realized that a particular stimulus, the CS, had been paired with the US). Interestingly, patients with an intact amygdala, but extensive hippocampal lesions, developed normal conditioned responses, but showed impairments in the declarative knowledge of the CS-US pairings: they were unable to determine which of the different stimuli presented had been paired with the aversive stimulus.[78] Furthermore, imaging studies revealed activation of the amygdala when subjects were presented with fearful stimuli.[80]

A COMPUTATIONAL MODEL OF THE FEAR NETWORK

To understand the neural mechanisms of fear processing it is important to have a comprehensive model that incorporates the experimental findings described so far.

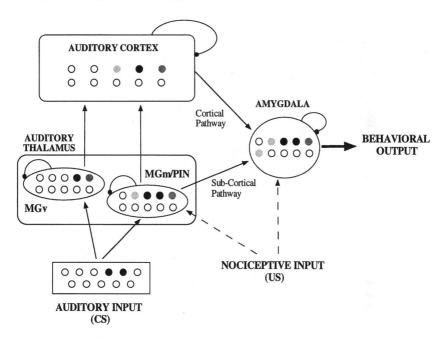

FIGURE 3. Diagram of the network used in the computer simulations of fear conditioning. Each module of self-inhibitory, nonlinear units represents a relevant structure in the fear-conditioning circuit. A typical pattern of activation is schematized by representing unit activity with *gray shadings* (*solid circles* = maximum activation; *open circles* = zero activation). Connections between modules are feedforward and excitatory and are a simplification of the corresponding pathways in the actual rat brain. The strengths of these connections are adjusted during learning through an extended Hebbian rule. *Dashed arrows* indicate excitatory, nonmodifiable connections. Adapted from ref. 20. Abbreviations: MGm = medial division of the medial geniculate body (MGB); MGv = ventral division of the MGB; PIN = posterior intralaminar nucleus.

Such a model could then be used to postulate hypotheses relating dysfunctions of specific elements in the circuit and various affective disorders observed in patients. Computational models are ideally suited for such a task, as they can be used to test the consistency of all the assumptions, explicit as well as implicit, that are present in the theory. Moreover, these models can be used to stimulate the effects of lesions of several brain regions in the processing of fear information. Some of the predictions made by the model can then be tested experimentally.

FIGURE 3 shows the schematic of a model of the fear circuit.[20,81] The network is constrained by some of the known anatomical connections of the fear-conditioning circuitry and captures several of the behavioral and physiological consequences of fear conditioning described in the previous sections. In particular, the model predicted that lesions of the auditory cortex would have no effect on the generalization of fear responses to frequencies other than the CS. This finding was later confirmed by performing the same study in experimental rats,[20] demonstrating that the direct tha-

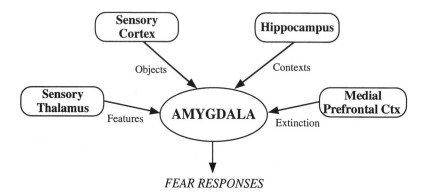

FEAR RESPONSES

FIGURE 4. The amygdala receives parallel inputs from a wide range of levels of sensory and cognitive processing. The thalamus conveys low-level stimulus features, whereas information about objects is provided by the cortex, especially the late stages of cortical processing. The hippocampus plays a crucial role in setting the emotional context. The medial prefrontal cortex has been implicated in the process of extinction of fear responses through its inputs to the amygdala. An imbalance between these input channels may lead to powerful, inappropriate fear responses, such as those seen in PTSD (see text for details).

lamo-amygdala pathway has greater stimulus-analysis capacity than previously thought.

INFORMATION PROCESSING IN THE FEAR NETWORK: A WORKING MODEL

The amygdala receives sensory information, as well as internally generated signals, through parallel and converging channels, each conveying a different aspect of the stimulus. For example, direct projections from the thalamus provide a fast, low-level representation of the external world. As just mentioned, these basic features can "prepare" the amygdala to process more highly processed information arriving from sensory cortices and the hippocampus. Unimodal association sensory cortices, in turn, may provide a conjunctive representation of a collection of features constituting an object. Furthermore, multimodal higher cortices and the hippocampus have the capacity to perform conjunctive encoding of complex stimuli and therefore could provide the amygdala with information about the context in which the stimulus is present.

FIGURE 4 provides a schematic of the different parallel channels converging onto the amygdala. The contribution of each of these inputs and their integration in the amygdala can be understood better with a simple example: a person is walking in the woods and sees a snake; the salient feature, a squiggly line, will be transmitted quickly to the amygdala by the direct thalamic pathway. Cells in the amygdala will be in an excited state, until further information arriving from the cortex confirms that it is indeed a snake, thus triggering the appropriate behavioral responses. If, however, a more detailed cortical analysis reveals that the stimulus is just a tree branch, further responses will be inhibited. If the same snake is now seen in the zoo, although both the thalamus and the cortex will signal information associated with danger, no fear responses will be elicited because the stimulus will be associated with a "safe" context, as determined by the hippocampal input to the amygdala.

It is important to note that even though the amygdala receives complex information from several structures, such as various neocortical areas and the hippocampus, this does not mean that the amygdala itself has to be capable of encoding and representing the information processed by those regions. For example, amygdala cells respond to faces.[66] Does this mean that the amygdala encodes and represents faces? No! Instead, the amygdala receives inputs from cortical areas that process faces. It "knows" the difference between inputs from the cortical area specialized for face processing and other specialized cortical areas. It also knows, on the basis of the inputs it receives, the differences between faces or different expressions on the same face. Thus, without encoding faces, the amygdala can still respond to faces and use the information about the difference between faces or different expressions on the same face. By pairing (associating) the cortical codes with aversive events (also encoded in this content-impoverished way), the amygdala can learn and participate in the storage of the emotional implications of complex environmental events. Although this hypothesis is at this point fairly speculative, it is consistent with a number of studies that address the processing of information by different structures in the circuit, using lesion or electrophysiological approaches, as described herein.

The present scheme suggests that if an imbalance occurs in the interaction between the different input channels to the amygdala, behaviors consistent with those observed in some anxiety disorders, such as simple phobias and PTSD, could result. For example, when a fear-conditioning experience takes place under severe stress, significant alterations may occur in various structures. First, since the hippocampus seems to shut down under severe stress,[82] it is conceivable that in some highly stressful situations, the context in which the conditioning takes place will not be fully encoded. This means that at later times, when the same conditioned stimulus is presented, it will elicit a fear response regardless of the current context. Second, high levels of the glucocorticoid corticosterone potentiate conditioned fear responses,[83] possibly through action on the CRF system in the central nucleus of the amygdala.[84] Third, the medial prefrontal cortex,[85] like the hippocampus,[86,87] is involved in negative feedback control of stress hormones. If the prefrontal cortex, like the hippocampus, proves to be susceptible to malfunction in traumatic situations, conditioning under stress could be equivalent to a functional disconnection of the prefrontal cortex from the amygdala, resulting in an increased resistance to extinction of the fear responses after the CS is no longer reinforced, as already described.

CONCLUSIONS

The neural system involved in the detection of dangerous stimuli has evolved very early in the phylogenetic scale and has remained essentially unchanged throughout evolution. The system involves transmission of information, through parallel and complementary channels, to the amygdala. The amygdala has the capacity to integrate this information (encoded in a content-impoverished manner) and, if appropriate, elicit a host of species-typical survival responses. However, this system can become maladaptive, such as when the balance between the components of the fear-conditioning system breaks down, leading to exaggerated fear responses.

One such case occurs when conditioning takes place under conditions of extreme stress. The combined effects of stress on the amygdala, hippocampus, and prefrontal cortex may result in context-independent, extinction-resistant, powerful fear responses to a CS. Furthermore, if the cortical input to the amygdala is disrupted, any stimulus that shares some feature with the CS will elicit a response through the thalamic pathway, resulting in a very strong stimulus overgeneralization of fear responses. Moreover, one need not be consciously aware of the processing of elementary features, and thus it may appear that one is having "spontaneous" (unprovoked) fear responses or fear responses to aspects of stimuli other than those one is attending to. Although some of these symptoms are reminiscent of those seen in emotional disorders, such as PTSD, much work remains to be done to elucidate the neural basis of these illnesses. Nevertheless, the extensive progress that has been made in characterizing the fear system and its learning and memory functions is an important step in this direction.

REFERENCES

1. LeDoux, J. E. 1995. Annu. Rev. Psychol. **46:** 209–235.
2. LeDoux, J. 1996. The Emotional Brain. Simon & Schuster. New York, NY.
3. Fanselow, M. S. 1994. Psychon. Bull. Rev. **1:** 429–438.
4. Davis, M. 1992. *In* The Amygdala: Neurobiological Aspects of Emotion, Memory, and Mental Dysfunction. J. P. Aggleton, Ed.: 255–306 Wiley-Liss. New York, NY.
5. Kapp, B. S., P. J. Whalen, W. F. Supple & J. P. Pascoe. 1992. *In* The Amygdala: Neurobiological Aspects of Emotion, Memory, and Mental Dysfunction. J. P. Aggleton, Ed.: Wiley-Liss. New York, NY.
6. Charney, D. S., A. Y. Deutch, S. M. Southwick & J. H. Krystal. 1995. *In* Neurobiological and Clinical Consequences of Stress: From Normal Adaptation to PTSD. M. J. Friedman, D. S. Charney & A. Y. Deutch, Eds.: 271–287. Lippincott-Raven Publishers. Philadelphia, PA.
7. Pavlov, I. P. 1927. Conditioned Reflexes. Dover. New York, NY.
8. Estes, W. K. & B. F. Skinner. 1941. J. Exp. Psychol. **29:** 390–400.
9. Blanchard, R. J. & D. C. Blanchard. 1969. J. Comp. Physiol. Psychol. **68:** 129–135.
10. McAllister, W. R. & D. E. McAllister. 1971. *In* Aversive Conditioning and Learning. F. R. Brush, Ed.: 105–179. Academic Press. New York, NY.
11. Schneiderman, N., J. Francis, L. D. Sampson & J. S. Schwaber. 1974. *In* Limbic and Autonomic Nervous System Research. L. V. DiCara, Eds.: 277–309. Plenum. New York, NY.
12. Bouton, M. E. & R. C. Bolles. 1980. Anim. Learn. Behav. **8:** 429–434.
13. LeDoux, J. E. 1994. Sci. Am. **270:** 32–39.
14. LeDoux, J. E., A. Sakaguchi & D. J. Reis. 1984. J. Neurosci. **4:** 683–698.
15. LeDoux, J. E., C. F. Farb & D. A. Ruggiero. 1990. J. Neurosci. **10:** 1043–1054.
16. Mascagni, F., A. J. McDonald & J. R. Coleman. 1993. Neuroscience **57:** 697–715.
17. Romanski, L. M. & J. E. LeDoux. 1993. Cereb. Cortex **3:** 515–532.
18. Romanski, L. M. & J. E. LeDoux. 1992. J. Neurosci. **12:** 4501–4509.
19. Bordi, F. & J. E. LeDoux. 1994. Exp. Brain Res. **98:** 261–274.
20. Armony, J. L., D. Servan-Schreiber, L. M. Romanski, J. D. Cohen & J. E. LeDoux. 1997. Cereb. Cortex **7:** 157–165.
21. Cranford, J. L. & M. Igarashi. 1977. Brain Res. **136:** 559–564.

22. WHITFIELD, I. C. 1980. J. Acoust. Soc. Am. **67:** 644-647.
23. TURNER, B. & M. HERKENHAM. 1991. J. Comp. Neurol. **313:** 295-325.
24. LI, X. F., G. E. STUTZMANN & J. E. LEDOUX. 1996. Learning & Memory **3:** 229-242.
25. LI, X., R. G. PHILLIPS & J. E. LEDOUX. 1995. Exp. Brain Res. **105:** 87-100.
26. HESTRIN, S., R. A. NICOLL, D. J. PERKEL & P. SAH. 1990. J. Physiol. **422:** 203-225.
27. LI, X. F., J. L. ARMONY & J. E. LEDOUX. 1996. Synapse **24:** 115-124.
28. BORDI, F. & J. LEDOUX. 1992. J. Neurosci. **12:** 2493-2503.
29. ROMANSKI, L. M., M. C. CLUGNET, F. BORDI & J. E. LEDOUX. 1993. Behav. Neurosci. **107:** 444-450.
30. CRUIKSHANK, S. J., J.-M. EDELINE & N. M. WEINBERGER. 1992. Behav. Neurosci. **106:** 471-483.
31. HEBB, D. O. 1949. The Organization of Behavior. John Wiley & Sons. New York, NY.
32. KONORSKI, J. 1967. *In* Integrative Activity of the Brain.: 490-505. University of Chicago Press, Chicago, IL.
33. PITKANEN, A., L. STEFANACCI, C. R. FARB, C.-G. GO, J. E. LEDOUX & D. G. AMARAL. 1995. J. Comp. Neurol. **356:** 288-310.
34. SAVANDER, V., C.-G. GO, J. E. LEDOUX & A. PITKANEN. 1995. J. Comp. Neurol. **361:** 345-368.
35. LEDOUX, J. E., J. IWATA, P. CICCHETTI & D. J. REIS. 1988. J. Neurosci. **8:** 2517-2529.
36. FANSELOW, M. S. 1991. *In* Fear, Avoidance, and Phobias: A Fundamental Analysis. M. R. Denny, Ed.: 61-86. Erlbaum. Hillsdale, NJ.
37. WILSON, A. & B. S. KAPP. 1994. Behav. Neural Biol. **62:** 73-76.
38. SMITH, O. A., C. A. ASTLEY, J. L. DEVITO, J. M. STEIN & R. E. WALSH. 1980. Fed. Proc. **39:** 2487-2494.
39. GRAY, T. S., M. E. CARNEY & D. J. MAGNUSON. 1989. Neuroendocrinology **50:** 433-446.
40. GRAY, T. S., R. A. PIECHOWSKI, J. M. YRACHETA, P. A. RITTENHOUSE, C. L. BETHA & L. D. VAN DER KAR. 1993. Neuroendocrinology **57:** 517-524.
41. SELDEN, N. R. W., B. J. EVERITT, L. E. JARRARD & T. W. ROBBINS. 1991. Neuroscience **42:** 335-350.
42. FANSELOW, M. S. & T. J. TIGHE. 1988. J. Exp. Psychol. Anim. Behav. Processes **14:** 187-199.
43. HELMSTETTER, F. 1992. Behav. Neurosci. **106:** 518-528.
44. PHILLIPS, R. G. & J. E. LEDOUX. 1994. Learn. Mem. **1:** 34-44.
45. KIM, J. J. & M. S. FANSELOW. 1992. Science **256:** 675-677.
46. PHILLIPS, R. G. & J. E. LEDOUX. 1992. Behav. Neurosci. **106:** 274-285.
47. SQUIRE, L. R., P. C. SLATER & P. M. CHACE. 1975. Science **187:** 77-79.
48. ALVAREZ, P. & L. R. SQUIRE. 1994. Proc. Natl. Acad. Sci. USA **91:** 7041-7045.
49. MCCLELLAND, J. L., B. L. MCNAUGHTON & R. C. O'REILLY. 1995. Psychol. Rev. **102:** 419-457.
50. COHEN, N. J. & H. EICHENBAUM. 1993. Memory, Amnesia, and the Hippocampal System. MIT Press. Cambridge, MA.
51. O'KEEFE, J. & L. NADEL. 1978. The Hippocampus as a Cognitive Map. Clarendon Press. Oxford, UK.
52. SUTHERLAND, R. J. & J. W. RUDY. 1989. Psychobiology **17:** 129-144.
53. AMARAL, D. G., J. L. PRICE, A. PITKANEN & S. T. CARMICHAEL. 1992. *In* The Amygdala: Neurobiological Aspects of Emotion, Memory, and Mental Dysfunction. J. P. Aggleton, Ed.: 1-66. Wiley-Liss. New York, NY.
54. CANTERAS, N. S., R. B. SIMERLY & L. W. SWANSON. 1992. J. Comp. Neurol. **324:** 143-179.
55. OTTERSEN, O. P. 1982. J. Comp. Neurol. **205:** 30-48.
56. MAREN, S. & M. S. FANSELOW. 1995. J. Neurosci. **15:** 7548-7564.
57. BOUTON, M. E. & D. SWARTZENTRUBER. 1991. Clin. Psychol. Rev. **11:** 123-140.
58. JACOBS, W. J. & L. NADEL. 1985. Psychol. Rev. **92:** 512-531.
59. RESCORLA, R. A. & C. D. HETH. 1975. J. Exp. Psychol. Anim. Behav. Processes **104:** 88-96.

60. BOUTON, M. E. 1994. J. Exp. Psychol. Anim. Behav. Processes **20:** 219-231.
61. MORGAN, M. A., L. M. ROMANSKI & J. E. LEDOUX. 1993. Neurosci. Lett. **163:** 109-113.
62. MORGAN, M. & J. E. LEDOUX. 1995. Behav. Neurosci. **109:** 681-688.
63. LEDOUX, J. E., L. M. ROMANSKI & A. E. XAGORARIS. 1989. J. Cognit. Neurosci. **1:** 238-243.
64. TEICH, A. H., P. M. McCABE, C. C. GENTILE, L. S. SCHNEIDERMAN, R. W. WINTERS, D.
     R. LISKOWSKY & N. SCHNEIDERMAN. 1989. Brain Res. **480:** 210-218.
65. THORPE, S. J., E. T. ROLLS & S. MADDISON, 1983. Exper. Brain Res. **49:** 93-115.
66. ROLLS, E. T. 1992. *In* The Amygdala: Neurobiological Aspects of Emotion, Memory,
     and Mental Dysfunction. J. P. Aggleton, Ed.: 143-165 Wiley-Liss. New York, NY.
67. ROLLS, E. T. 1995. *In* The Cognitive Neurosciences. M. S. Gazzaniga, Ed.: 1091-1106.
     The MIT Press. Cambridge, MA.
68. FALLS, W. A., M. J. D. MISERENDINO & M. DAVIS. 1992. J. Neurosci. **12:** 854-863.
69. QUIRK, G. J., J. C. REPA & J. E. LEDOUX. 1995. Neuron **15:** 1029-1039.
70. EDELINE, J.-M., N. NEUENSCHWANDER-EL MASSIOUI & G. DUTRIEUX. 1990. Behav. Brain
     Res.: 1076-1087.
71. OLDS, J., J. DISTERHOFT, M. SEGAL, C. KORNBLUTH & R. HIRSH. 1972. J. Neurophysiol.
     35: 202-219.
72. SUPPLE, W. F. & B. S. KAPP. 1989. Behav. Neurosci. **103:** 1276-1286.
73. MAREN, S., A. POREMBA & M. GABRIEL. 1991. Brain Res. **549:** 311-316.
74. MURAMOTO, K., T. ONO, H. NISHIJO & M. FUKUDA. 1993. Neuroscience **52:** 621-636.
75. PASCOE, J. P. & B. S. KAPP. 1985. Behav. Brain Res. **16:** 117-133.
76. BORDI, F., J. E. LEDOUX, M. C. CLUGNET & C. PAVLIDES. 1993. Behav. Neurosci. **107:**
     757-769.
77. WEINBERGER, N. M. 1995. *In* The Cognitive Neurosciences. M. S. Gazzaniga, Ed.: 1071-
     1090. The MIT Press. Cambridge, MA.
78. BECHARA, A., D. TRANEL, H. DAMASIO, R. ADOLPHS, C. ROCKLAND & A. R. DAMASIO.
     1995. Science **269:** 1115-1118.
79. LABAR, K. S., J. E. LEDOUX, D. D. SPENCER & E. A. PHELPS. 1995. J. Neurosci. **15:**
     6846-6855.
80. MORRIS, J. S., C. D. FRITH, D. I. PERRET, D. ROWLAND, A. W. YOUNG, A. J. CALDER &
     R. J. DOLAN. 1996. Nature **383:** 812-815.
81. ARMONY, J. L., D. SERVAN-SCHREIBER, J. D. COHEN & J. E. LEDOUX. 1995. Behav.
     Neurosci. **109:** 246-257.
82. STEIN-BEHRENS, B., M. P. MATTSON, I. CHANG, M. YEH & R. SAPOLSKY. 1994. J. Neurosci.
     14: 5373-5380.
83. CORODIMAS, K. P., J. E. LEDOUX, P. W. GOLD & J. SCHULKIN. 1994. N.Y. Acad. Sci.
     746: 392-393.
84. MAKINO, S., P. W. GOLD & J. SCHULKIN. 1994. Brain Res. **640:** 105-112.
85. DIORIO, D., V. VIAU & M. J. MEANEY. 1993. J. Neurosci. **13:** 3839-3847.
86. McEWEN, B. S. 1992. Biol. Psychiatry **31:** 177-199.
87. JACOBSON, L. & R. SAPOLSKY. 1991. Endocr. Rev. **12:** 118-134.

Stress Effects on Morphology and Function of the Hippocampus[a]

BRUCE S. McEWEN AND ANA MARIA MAGARINOS

Laboratory of Neuroendocrinology
Rockefeller University
New York, New York 10021

The hippocampal formation is an important brain structure in episodic and spatial learning as well as a component of the control of a variety of vegetative functions such as ACTH secretion.[1,2] It is also a plastic and vulnerable brain structure that is damaged by stroke and head trauma and susceptible to damage during aging and repeated stress.[3] In 1968, we showed that hippocampal neurons express receptors for circulating adrenal steroids,[4] and subsequent work in many laboratories has shown that the hippocampus has two types of adrenal steroid receptors which mediate a variety of effects on neuronal excitability, neurochemistry, and structural plasticity.[5]

Recent work in our laboratory indicates that adrenal steroids are involved in three types of plasticity in the hippocampal formation. First, they reversibly and biphasically modulate excitability of hippocampal neurons and influence the magnitude of long-term potentiation as well as producing long-term depression.[6-9] These effects may be involved in biphasic effects of adrenal secretion on excitability and cognitive function and memory during diurnal rhythm and after stress.[10-13] Second, adrenal steroids participate along with excitatory amino acids in regulating neurogenesis of dentate gyrus granule neurons, in which acute stressful experiences can suppress the ongoing neurogenesis.[14] We believe that these effects may be involved in fear-related learning and memory, because of the anatomical connections between the dentate gyrus and the amygdala, a brain area important in memory of aversive and fear-producing experiences.[15] Third, adrenal steroids participate along with excitatory amino acids in stress-induced atrophy of dendrites in the CA3 region of the hippocampus, a process that affects only the apical dendrites and results in cognitive impairment in the learning of spatial and short-term memory tasks.[16]

Because the atrophy does not affect the entire neuron and is reversible, we believe that it represents a physiological adaptive mechanism to severe and recurrent stress. However, it is unclear if atrophy is the first stage that leads to neuronal death or a mechanism that protects neurons at the expense of some cognitive function. Insofar as the atrophy seen in CA3 pyramidal neurons is the tip of the iceberg, so to speak, and represents atrophy occurring throughout the hippocampus, this model is relevant to atrophy of the human hippocampus that has been described in Cushing's syndrome, normal aging, dementia, recurrent depressive illness, schizophrenia, and posttraumatic

[a]This work was supported by grant MH41256, The Health Foundation (New York), and Servier (France).

TABLE 1. Atrophy of the Human Hippocampus

Condtion	References
Cushing's syndrome	65
Recurrent depressive illness	64
PTSD	66,67
Aging, preceding dementia	57,58
Dementia	68
Schizophrenia	69,70

stress disorder (PTSD) (TABLE 1). In these cases, the problem is to distinguish between reversible atrophy and permanent cell loss, because the former situation is potentially treatable at the time the atrophy is discovered, whereas the latter may be preventable with earlier intervention at the time the initial trauma is taking place. This chapter discusses the phenomenon of hippocampal atrophy and discusses possible mechanisms and therapeutic strategies.

RAPID PLASTICITY IN HIPPOCAMPAL PYRAMIDAL NEURONS

Hippocampal pyramidal neurons demonstrate considerable plasticity in the adult brain, including reversible synaptogenesis that is regulated by ovarian steroids and excitatory amino acids via NMDA receptors in female rats[17] and reversible atrophy of dendrites that is regulated by glucocorticoids and excitatory amino acids via NMDA receptors in males rats[16] and tree shrews.[18] Each type of plasticity is seen in different parts of the hippocampus; the ovarian cyclicity of synapses occurs mainly in the CA1 pyramidal neurons, whereas the dendritic atrophy takes place on the apical dendrites of CA3 pyramidal neurons that receive a powerful synaptic input from the dentate gyrus.

The CA1 synaptic plasticity is a rapid event, occurring during the female rats' 5-day estrus cycle, with the synapses taking several days to be induced under the influence of estrogens and endogenous glutamic acid and then disappearing within 12 hours under the influence of the proestrus surge of progesterone.[17] In contrast, the CA3 atrophy found in rats is a relatively slow process, taking normally at least 3 weeks to develop under daily stress and a week or so to disappear. However, a rapid example of dendritic atrophy in hibernating ground squirrels and hamsters also develops as fast as the hibernating state and can be reversed rapidly within several hours[19,20] (Magarinos, McEwen and Pevet, unpublished). Although anatomically similar to the stress-induced atrophy in rats and tree shrews, it is not yet clear if this process involves the same mechanisms; however, if this is the case, the question becomes what factors make the atrophy rapid in hibernation and slow in relation to repeated stress.

PHARMACOLOGICAL MANIPULATIONS OF DENDRITIC ATROPHY

In the hibernation and stress studies, dendritic length and branching are assessed by morphometry after silver staining neurons with the single section Golgi technique. More recently, electron microscopy has revealed that stress and glucocorticoids alter morphology of presynaptic mossy fiber terminals in the stratum lucidum region of CA3.[21] Initially, atrophy of apical dendrites of CA3 pyramidal neurons, and not dentate granule neurons or CA1 pyramidal neurons, was found after 21 days of daily corticosterone exposure and also after 21 days of 6 hours/day repeated restraint stress (reviewed in ref. 16). Psychosocial stress also cause apical dendrites of CA3 pyramidal neurons to atrophy in rats[22] and in an insectivore, the tree shrew.[18] Stress- and corticosterone-induced atrophy was prevented by the antiepileptic drug phenytoin (Dilantin), thus implicating the release and actions of excitatory amino acids, because phenytoin blocks glutamate release and antagonizes T-type calcium channels that are activated during glutamate-induced excitation. This result was consistent with evidence that stress induces release of glutamate in the hippocampus and other brain regions (see refs. 16 and 18). Recent work has shown that NMDA receptor blockade is also effective in preventing stress-induced dendritic atrophy (see ref. 16).

A model of the cellular and neurochemical interactions involved in dendritic atrophy is presented in FIGURE 1, and it emphasizes the interactions among neurons and neurotransmitters. The role of adrenal steroids will be discussed subsequently. Besides glutamate, other participating neurotransmitters include GABA and serotonin. Inhibitory interneurons have a significant role in controlling hippocampal neuronal excitability,[23] and involvement of the GABA-benzodiazepine receptor system is strongly suggested by the ability of a benzodiazepine, adinazolam, to block dendritic atrophy (Magarinos, unpublished). As for serotonin, repeated restraint stress in rats and psychosocial stress cause changes in hippocampal formation that include not only atrophy of dendrites of CA3c pyramidal neurons but also suppression of 5-HT1A receptor binding.[16,22]

Serotonin is released by stressors and tianeptine, an atypical tricyclic antidepressant that enhances serotonin reuptake and thus reduces extracellular 5HT levels, and prevented both stress- and corticosterone-induced dendritic atrophy of CA3c pyramidal neurons,[24] whereas several inhibitors of serotonin reuptake, fluoxetine and fluvoxamine, and desipramine, an inhibitor of noradrenaline uptake, failed to block atrophy (Magarinos, Watanabe, unpublished data). Thus, the effect of tianeptine on CA3 pyramidal neuron morphology is not due to its reported effects to reduce corticosterone secretion,[25] but may instead be related to its reported effects to enhance the reuptake of serotonin within the hippocampus.[26] Further evidence for serotonin involvement in dendritic atrophy comes from studies of psychosocial stress in rats, in that both dominant and subordinate rats show both dendritic atrophy as well as downregulation of 5HT transporter expression in the CA3 region, indicating either reduced density of serotonin terminals or reduced expression of the transporter (7186). However, dominant rats show a greater reduction in 5HT transporter sites than do subordinant ones, and dominant rats also show greater dendritic atrophy.[22]

Because both corticosterone- and stress-induced atrophy of CA3 pyramidal neurons are blocked by phenytoin as well as tianeptine (see ref. 16), serotonin released

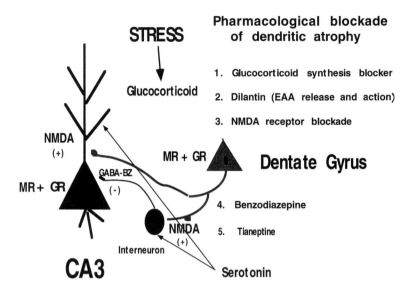

FIGURE 1. Schematic diagram showing relations and connections between major inputs to hippocampal CA3 pyramidal neurons that appear to be responsible for dendritic atrophy. Glucocorticoids interact with glucocorticoid (GR) and mineralocorticoid receptors (MR) expressed in pyramidal and granule cell neurons throughout the hippocampal formation. Mossy fiber input from granule neurons synapses on the base of apical dendrites of CA3 neurons and on inhibitory interneurons in the hilus of the dentate gyrus. Other excitatory input to the CA3 neurons converges on the dendritic tree. NMDA receptors are located in the apical dendritic tree and may also be present in the stratum lucidum where mossy fibers terminate, although at low concentrations. Serotonin fibers provide inputs to distal parts of the dendrites of CA3 neurons as well as to granule neurons of the dentate gyrus and interneurons of the dentate hilus. The final pathways of dendritic atrophy are the excitatory amino acids, which activate NMDA receptors and mobilize calcium. We believe that this increased calcium causes reversible depolymerization of the cytoskeleton through either second messenger systems or limited proteolysis. This conclusion is supported by the efficacy of both Dilantin and NMDA receptor blockade in preventing stress-induced dendritic atrophy. Empirical evidence summarized in the text also indicates that stress-induced dendritic atrophy is blocked by the following treatments given prior to daily stress: inhibiting glucocorticoid synthesis, enhancing serotonin uptake with tianeptine, and administering a benzodiazepine. A major question for studies of human hippocampal atrophy is whether such treatments are effective in either reversing the atrophy after it is established or preventing the development of the atrophy. Reversibility of hippocampal atrophy depends on whether it represents permanent cell loss or reversible atrophy of the dendrites of hippocampal neurons.

by stress or corticosterone may interact pre- or postsynaptically with glutamate released by stress or corticosterone, and the final common path may involve interactive effects between serotonin and glutamate receptors on the dendrites of CA3 neurons innervated by mossy fibers from the dentate gyrus. There is evidence for interactions between serotonin and NMDA receptors, indicating that serotonin potentiates NMDA receptor binding as well as the activity of NMDA receptors and may do so via 50-HT$_2$ receptors.[27,28]

The information on agents that block the stress-induced atrophy of dendrites in the hippocampus is summarized in FIGURE 1, showing also a schematic diagram of the principal inputs that are involved in modulating the atrophy of the apical dendrites of CA3 pyramidal neurons.

MECHANISM OF DENDRITIC ATROPHY AND THE ROLE OF ADRENAL STEROIDS

Glucocorticoid treatment causes dendritic atrophy, and stress-induced atrophy is blocked by treatment with an adrenal steroid synthesis blocker, cyanoketone.[16] What is the role of adrenal steroids in relation to the neurotransmitter involvement cited above? A primary site of action is the release of glutamate, because adrenalectomy markedly reduces the magnitude of the EAA release evoked by restraint stress.[29] In this connection, mossy fiber terminals from dentate granule neurons in the stratum lucidum of CA3 apical dendrites show morphological alterations as a result of chronic stress.[21] These changes involve reorganization of synaptic vesicles in the synaptic terminal, with a higher density occurring in regions adjacent to active synaptic zones.

The stratum lucidum zone of CA3 contains high levels of kainate receptors, as demonstrated by quantitative autoradiography, and, as noted above, these receptors are decreased in density by ADX and restored to normal by corticosterone replacement.[30] Because kainate receptors are feedforward autoreceptors for excitatory amino acids on presynaptic mossy fiber nerve endings (FIG. 1), the effects of adrenal steroids are consistent with the dependence of stress-induced glutamate release on the presence of the adrenal glands.[29]

Another possibility is that corticosterone or stress alters CA3 neuronal atrophy through regulation of GABAergic synaptic inhibition (FIG. 1). In support of this notion, low levels of corticosterone alter mRNA levels for specific subunits of GABAa receptors in CA3 and the dentate gyrus of adrenalectomized rats,[31] whereas stress levels of corticosterone have produced different effects on GABAa receptor subunit mRNA levels and receptor binding in hippocampal subregions including CA3 (Orchinik, Weiland, and McEwen, unublished data). Therefore, it appears that corticosterone may alter the excitability of hippocampal neurons through regulation of GABAa receptor expression, but it remains to be seen if the corticosteroid effects on neuronal morphology involve changes in the number or pharmacological properties of GABAa receptors.

Both stress and glucocorticoid treatment cause enhanced expression of NMDA receptors in the hippocampus,[32,33] and this is another potential mechanism by which adrenal steroids are involved in dendritic atrophy (FIG. 1). It is puzzling, however, that NMDA receptors are not expressed in very high concentrations in the stratum lucidum where mossy fibers terminate,[34] given the evidence cited herein for the importance of this innervation for dendritic atrophy. The presence of high levels of NMDA receptors on the more distal aspects of CA3 dendrites suggests that the mossy fiber activation of glutamate release triggers a much more widespread activity of excitatory amino acids affecting the entire dendritic tree of the CA3 pyramidal neurons.

Following upon the widespread activation of NMDA receptors, the increased levels of intracellular calcium may make the dendritic cytoskeleton become depolymerized or undergo proteolysis (see ref. 16 for discussion). Stress is also reported to alter the expression of the neurotrophins BDNF and NT-3 in the hippocampus.[35] Very little is known about the adrenal steroid receptor types involved in these effects or the localization of stress and adrenal steroid effects on neurotrophin expression within the hippocampus and their relation to the conditions of repeated stress that bring about morphological changes. However, conditions that cause dendritic atrophy, such as repeated restraint stress or psychosocial stress, do not appear to change neurotrophin expression in the hippocampus (Kuroda, unpublished data), indicating that neurotrophins are probably not directly involved in the mechanism of dendritic atrophy.

HIPPOCAMPAL NEURONAL DAMAGE RESULTING FROM CHRONIC STRESS AND AGING

Another important issue is the relation between the atrophy of CA3 neurons induced by repeated doses of corticosterone or by repeated restraint stress and the thinning and apparent loss of pyramidal neurons that have been reported after both 12 weeks of corticosterone treatment in rats and prolonged, severe psychosocial stress in vervet monkeys.[3] Indeed, we have seen that chronic psychosocial stress in tree shrews causes atrophy of CA3 pyramidal neurons, much as restraint stress does in rats.[18] However, the atrophy produced by stress in rats is reversible, within 7-14 days after the termination of stress (Magariños and McEwen, unpublished data). A possible link may be the fate of inhibitory interneurons that receive intense innervation from mossy fibers of dentate gyrus granule neurons and that are especially vulnerable to a variety of insults.[36] If some of these neurons were to die as a result of repeated restraint stress, then there might be a cumulative effect over time, in which repeated bouts of stress might progressively deplete the dentate gyrus of the buffering action that these inhibitory neurons appear to provide.

However, is a big gap in our understanding between neuronal atrophy and permanent cell loss of either interneurons or pyramidal neurons, and one of the most surprising and puzzling findings concerning glucocorticoids and neuronal damage in the hippocampus was the morphological changes resulting from prolonged exposure to stress or stress hormones that were interpreted as indicating neuronal damage and pyramidal cell loss. Aus der Muhlen and Ockenfels[37] reported that ACTH or cortisone administration in mature guinea pigs caused neurons in the hippocampus and other forebrain regions to stain darkly and appear necrotic, as if undergoing atrophy then perhaps also dying. Other investigators have described the appearance of ''darkly-stained'' CA3 pyramidal neurons following repeated cold swim stress in rats[38] and psychosocial stress in tree shrews.[39]

Whereas the interpretation of these findings may be questioned in light of the report that darkly-stained neurons can develop artifactually from physical trauma in fixing brains for histological analysis,[40] findings in the guinea pig were instrumental in stimulating the work of Landfield[41] and colleagues which showed that aging in the rat results in thinning of the pyramidal cell layer in the hippocampus and that this change was retarded by adrenalectomy in mid-life. Sapolsky[3] then demonstrated that 12 weeks of daily corticosterone injections into young adult rats mimicked the pyramidal neuron thinning seen in aging, and subsequent work on subordinate vervet monkeys revealed thinning and apparent necrosis of CA3 pyramidal neurons that implied some kind of stress-related hippocampal damage.

Dying cells, however, are rarely seen because they disappear rapidly, and evidence for neuronal loss depends on counting cells in histological material. This issue was raised recently,[42] using revised stereological procedures for estimated neuronal number, showing that aging rats that are cognitively impaired do not necessarily show reduced hippocampal neuron number. A similar conclusion was reached for cognitively impaired middle-aged rats without the use of elaborate neuronal counting methods,[43] and a recent study on rats with age-related spatial memory impairment revealed altered expression of markers of glial hypertrophy and oxidative stress that are interpreted as evidence for synaptic and dendritic pruning rather than neuronal loss.[44] However, none of these studies has directly looked for dendritic atrophy or synapse loss, and such studies are urgently needed. Moreover, current evidence is insufficient to exclude neuronal loss as a later stage of the aging process, and some evidence mentioned above can be interpreted either way.

Furthermore, the work of Sapolsky[3] just alluded to first showed thinning of pyramidal neuron number in both aging rats and rats treated for 12 weeks with daily corticosterone injections. Sapolsky then demonstrated that excitatory amino acids play an important role in cell loss by showing, first, that glucocorticoids exacerbate kainic acid-induced damage to the hippocampus as well as ischemic damage; and, second, that glucocorticoids potentiate excitatory amino acid-killing of hippocampal neurons in culture.[3] Recent work[45] has brought this issue full circle by demonstrating, using intracerebral microdialysis in the hippocampus, not only that restraint stress-induced glutamate release is exacerbated in aging rats, but also that it continues for some time after stress is terminated. Although this mechanism is consistent with enhanced dendritic atrophy and synapse loss in the aging hippocampus, it is also consistent with the possibility of enhanced rates of neuronal damage and loss by the same mechanisms that are implicated in ischemia- and trauma-induced hippocampal neuronal destruction.[3,46,47]

STRESS EFFECTS ON COGNITIVE PERFORMANCE IN RODENTS AND HUMANS

Stress and glucocorticoids are known to have specific effects on cognitive function in humans and animal models. Adrenal steroids and stressful experiences produce short-term and reversible deficits in episodic and spatial memory in animal models and in humans,[48] whereas repeated stress also impairs cognitive function in animal models and glucocorticoid elevation or treatment in humans is accompanied by cognitive dysfunction.[49] There are also declines in cognitive function in aging humans that are correlated with progressive elevations in HPA activity over 3–4 years.[50,51]

Acute effects of stress or glucocorticoid administration are evident within a time span of a few hours to a day and are generally reversible and selective to the task or particular situation.[48,52] Adrenal steroid effects are implicated in both selective attention as well as memory consolidation,[48] and such actions are consistent with the effects of adrenal steroids on the modulation of long-term potentiation and primed-burst potentiation (see above). However, some acute actions of stress may involve mechanisms other than glucocorticoids, including endogenous opioid neuropeptides in the case of painful stressors such as shock. (See ref. 16 for a summary.) With regard to nonpainful stressors, exposure of rats to a novel environment results in rapid and reversible impairment of plasticity *in vivo* in the CA1 region, and this effect may involve the actions of glucocorticoids.[13]

Longer-term stress that produces dendritic atrophy in the CA3 region of the hippocampus has also been shown to impair hippocampus-dependent learning. A recent study demonstrated impaired performance on an 8-arm radial maze in rats that received 21 days of restraint stress prior to maze training.[53] The stress effect is reversible, in that inhibition of the initial learning was evident when rats were trained and evaluated immediately after the end of stress but not 18 days after the termination of stress. This impairment was in the same direction, but not as great as, impairment found in aging rats; moreover, stress effects were prevented by prior treatment of rats with phenytoin or tianeptine under the same conditions in which phenytoin was able to prevent the stress-induced atrophy of CA3c pyramidal neurons.[24,53,54] A subsequent study showed that the same repeated restraint stress paradigm that causes dendritic atrophy impaired the short-term (4-hour) retention of a spatial recognition memory in a Y-maze, an action that was also prevented by tianeptine treatment during the stress regimen.[55]

Declines of hippocampally related cognitive functions, such as spatial and episodic memory, occur in human subjects and are correlated with increases in HPA activity over 3–4 years.[50,51] Recent evidence has revealed that the most severely impaired individuals have a significantly smaller hippocampal volume than that of the least impaired individuals.[56] This result is consistent with other findings of individual differences in cognitive function correlated with hippocampal volume reductions in elderly humans.[57,58]

LIFE-LONG IMPLICATIONS OF STRESSFUL EXPERIENCES

Long-term stress also accelerates many biological markers of aging in rats, including increasing the excitability of CA1 pyramidal neurons via a calcium-dependent mechanism and causing loss of hippocampal pyramidal neurons.[59] An important factor may be the enhancement by glucocorticoids of calcium currents in the hippocampus,[60] in view of the key role of calcium ions in destructive as well as plastic processes in hippocampal neurons (see above and chapter by Landfield). It is important to find out how learning processes may alter neural activity in such conditions as traumatic stress and recurrent depressive illness and how long-term changes in neural activity may alter structure and function of neurons, particularly in the hippocampus.

Another aspect of stressful experiences is the developmental influence of early stress and of neonatal handling on the life course of aging and age-related cognitive impairment. As discussed elsewhere,[61,62] such early experiences can either increase or decrease the rate of brain aging through a mechanism in which the activity of the HPA axis appears to be involved. Early experiences are believed to set the level of responsiveness of the HPA axis and autonomic nervous system in such a way that these systems either overreact in animals subject to early unpredictable stress or underreact in animals exposed to the neonatal handling procedure.

CONCLUSIONS

It has been known for some time that the human brain shows signs of atrophy as a result of elevated glucocorticoids and severe, traumatic stress (e.g., holocaust survivors[3]). Recent evidence indicates that the human hippocampus is particularly sensitive in this respect and tends to show greater changes than other brain areas, particularly in Cushing's syndrome, recurrent depressive illness, posttraumatic stress disorder, schizophrenia, and aging before overt dementia (TABLE 1). The diversity of conditions in which atrophy occurs raises the question of whether they all reflect a common mechanism and whether the atrophy is permanent or reversible.

Regarding mechanism, it is tempting to attribute the occurrence of hippocampal atrophy to glucocorticoids. However, glucocorticoids are elevated in Cushing's syndrome and may also be somewhat elevated in aging individuals, but this is probably not the case for any of the other disorders at the time they are studied, except as there are elevations in glucocorticoids associated with the diurnal rhythm and stressful experiences that take place on a daily basis. One example that is instructive in understanding how individual differences might play a role in brain changes is that some individuals who are exposed to repeated psychosocial stress (public speaking) fail to habituate their cortisol elevation; these individuals lack self-esteem and self-confidence.[63] It is therefore not difficult to imagine that individuals with a more reactive stress hormone profile will expose themselves to more cortisol and experience more stress-elevated neural activity than other persons who can more easily habituate to psychosocial challenges.

In disorders such as PTSD, we must learn more about stress responses and neurochemical changes accompanying the initial trauma, which usually take place months or years before, as well as the ongoing stress responsiveness and neurochemical activity (e.g., brain glucose metabolism) in traumatized individuals. For recurrent depressive illness, we are largely ignorant of the same type of history of the depressed individual as far as endocrine function and neurochemical activity as well as responses to stressful life experiences.

Regarding the role of adrenal steroids, we noted above, however, that glucocorticoids merely have to be present in moderate to stress levels for stress-induced atrophy of CA3 neurons to occur and that serotonin is involved along with excitatory amino acids acting via NMDA receptors as the final common path for such atrophy. Regarding reversibility, treatment with phenytoin or tianeptine, both of which block stress-induced atrophy, is a potential mean of both testing the mechanism and at the same time demonstrating the reversibility of human hippocampal atrophy. There is already some indication that hippocampal atrophy in Cushing's syndrome is reversible (Starkman, personal communication). If hippocampal atrophy in conditions such as recurrent depression and PTSD is reversible through the actions of agents such as tianeptine or phenytoin, then there must be sustained hyperactivity of the neurotransmitter systems involved or excessive activity of the HPA axis. On the other hand, there may be irreversible loss of hippocampal neurons, and some evidence in the MRI of recurrent depressive illness is consistent with this possibility.[64]

In conclusion, insofar as atrophy of the hippocampus and accompanying cognitive impairment are signs of reversible neuronal atrophy, they may be treatable with agents that block the actions of excitatory amino acids, serotonin, and adrenal steroids that are implicated in neuronal atrophy in animal models. Inasmuch as the decreased hippocampal volume is due to neuronal loss, treatment strategies should focus on the earlier traumatic or recurrent events, and it may be possible to devise strategies to reduce or prevent neuronal damage.

SUMMARY

The hippocampal formation, which contains high levels of adrenal steroid receptors, is vulnerable to insults such as stroke, seizures, and head trauma, and it is also sensitive and vulnerable to the effects of stress. We have discovered that the hippocampus of rodents and tree shrews shows atrophy of pyramidal neurons in the CA3 region. Psychosocial stress and restraint stress produce atrophy over approximately 3-4 weeks. Atrophy is blocked by inhibiting adrenal steroid formation and by blocking the actions of excitatory amino acids using Dilantin or NMDA receptor inhibitors. Glucocorticoid administration also blocks CA3 atrophy, but Dilantin administration blocks this as well, indicating that excitatory amino acid release mediates the atrophy, which likely involves disassembly of the dendritic cytoskeleton. Studies with *in vivo* microdialysis in several laboratories have shown that glutamate release in the hippocampus increases in stress and that stress-induced glutamate release is reduced by adrenalectomy. Recent electron microscopy of mossy fiber terminals on CA3 neurons has revealed a depletion of synaptic vesicles as a result of repeated stress. The mossy fiber terminals appear to be responsible for driving atrophy of CA3 neurons, which involves principally atrophy of the apical dendrites. These results are discussed in relation to data from MRI showing atrophy of the whole human hippocampus in Cushing's disease, recurrent depressive illness, PTSD, and normal aging as well as dementia.

REFERENCES

1. JACOBSON, L. & R. SAPOLSKY. 1991. The role of the hippocampus in feedback regulation of the hypothalamic-pituitary-adrenocortical axis. Endocr. Rev. **12:** 118-134.
2. EICHENBAUM, H. & T. OTTO. 1992. The hippocampus—what does it do? Behav. Neural. Biol. **57:** 2-36.
3. SAPOLSKY, R. 1992. Stress, the Aging Brain and the Mechanisms of Neuron Death.: 1-423. Cambridge MIT Press. Cambridge, MA.
4. McEWEN, B. S., J. WEISS & L. SCHWARTZ. 1968. Selective retention of corticosterone by limbic structures in rat brain. Nature **220:** 911-912.
5. DE KLOET, E. R., E. C. AZMITIA & P. W. LANDFIELD. 1996. Brain corticosteroid receptors: Studies on the mechanism, function, and neurotoxicity of corticosteroid action. Ann. N.Y. Acad. Sci., vol. 746.
6. PAVLIDES, C., A. KIMURA, A. M. MAGARINOS & B. S. McEWEN. 1994. Type I adrenal steroid receptors prolong hippocampal long-term potentiation. NeuroRep. **5:** 2673-2677.
7. PAVLIDES, C., A. KIMURA, A. M. MAGARINOS & B. S. McEWEN. 1995. Hippocampal homosynaptic long-term depression/depotentiation induced by adrenal steroids. Neuroscience **68:** 379-385.
8. PAVLIDES, C., Y. WATANABE, A. M. MAGARINOS & B. S. McEWEN. 1995. Opposing role of adrenal steroid Type I and Type II receptors in hippocampal long-term potentiation. Neuroscience **68:** 387-394.

9. PAVLIDES, C., S. OGAWA, A. KIMURA & B. S. McEWEN. 1996. Role of adrenal steroid mineralcorticoid and glucocorticoid receptors in long-term potentiation in the CA1 field of hippocampal slices. Brain Res. **738:** 229-235.

10. BARNES, C., B. McNAUGHTON, G. GODDARD, R. DOUGLAS & R. ADAMEC. 1977. Circadian rhythm of synaptic excitability in rat and monkey central nervous system. Science **197:** 91-92.

11. DANA, R. C. & J. L. MARTINEZ. 1984. Effect of adrenalectomy on the circadian rhythm of LTP. Brain Res. **308:** 392-395.

12. DIAMOND, D. M., M. C. BENNETT, M. FLESHNER & G. M. ROSE. 1992. Inverted-U relationship between the level of peripheral corticosterone and the magnitude of hippocampal primed burst potentiation. Hippocampus **2:** 421-430.

13. DIAMOND, D. M., M. FLESHNER & G. M. ROSE. 1996. Psychological stress impairs spatial working memory. Behav. Neurosci. **110:** 661-672.

14. CAMERON, H. A. & E. GOULD. 1996. The control of neuronal birth and survival. *In* Receptor Dynamics in Neural Development. C. A. Shaw, Ed.: 141-157. CRC Press. New York, NY.

15. LeDOUX, J. E. 1995. In search of an emotional system in the brain: Leaping from fear to emotion and consciousness. *In* The Cognitive Neurosciences. M. Gazzaniga, Ed.: 1049-1061. MIT Press. Cambridge.

16. McEWEN, B. S., D. ALBECK, H. CAMERON, H. M. CHAO, E. GOULD, N. HASTINGS, Y. KURODA, V. LUINE, A. M. MAGARINOS, C. R. McKITTRICK, M. ORCHINIK, C. PAVLIDES, P. VAHER, Y. WATANABE & N. WEILAND. 1995. Stress and the brain: A paradoxical role for adrenal steroids. *In* Vitamins and Hormones. G. D. Litwack, Ed.: 371-402. Academic Press, Inc. San Diego.

17. McEWEN, B. S., E. GOULD, M. ORCHINIK, N. G. WEILAND & C. S. WOOLLEY. 1995. Oestrogens and the structural and functional plasticity of neurons: Implications for memory, ageing and neurodegenerative processes. *In* Ciba Foundation Symposium #191. The Non-productive Actions of Sex Steroids. J. Goode, Ed.: 52-73. CIBA Foundation. London.

18. MAGARINOS, A. M., B. S. McEWEN, G. FLUGGE & E. FUCHS. 1996. Chronic psychosocial stress causes apical dendritic atrophy of hippocampal CA3 pyramidal neurons in subordinate tree shrews. J. Neurosci. **16:** 3534-3540.

19. POPOV, V. I. & L. S. BOCHAROVA. 1992. Hibernation-induced structural changes in synaptic contacts between mossy fibres and hippocampal pyramidal neurons. Neuroscience **48:** 53-62.

20. POPOV, V. I., & L. S. BOCHAROVA & A. G. BRAGIN. 1992. Repeated changes of dendritic morphology in the hippocampus of ground squirrels in the course of hibernation. Neuroscience **48:** 45-51.

21. MAGARINOS, A. M., J. M. VERDUGO GARCIA & B. S. McEWEN. 1996. Chronic restraint stress causes ultrastructural changes in rat mossy fiber terminals (Abstr.) Soc. Neurosci. **22:** 474.7, p 1196.

22. McKITTRICK, C. R., A. M. MAGARINOS, D. C. BLANCHARD, R. J. BLANCHARD & B. S. McEWEN. 1996. Chronic social stress decreases binding to 5HT transporter sites and reduces dendritic arbors in CA3 of hippocampus (Abstr.) Soc. Neurosci. **22:** 809.18, p 2060.

23. FREUND, T. F. & G. BUZASKI. 1996. Interneurons of the hippocampus. Hippocampus **6:** 345-470.

24. WATANABE, Y., E. GOULD, H. CAMERON, D. DANIELS & B. S. McEWEN. 1992. Stress and antidepressant effects on hippocampus. Eur. J. Pharmacol. **222:** 157-162.

25. DELBENDE, C., V. CONTESSE, E. MOCAER, A. KAMOUN & H. VAUDRY. 1991. The novel antidepressant, tianeptine, reduces stress-evoked stimulation of the hypothalamo-pituitary-adrenal axis. Eur. J. Pharmacol. **202:** 391-396.

26. WHITTON, P., G. SARNA, M. O'CONNELL & G. CURZON. 1991. The effect of the novel antidepressant tianeptine on the concentration of 5-hydroxytryptamine in rat hippocampal dialysates in vivo. Psychopharmacology **104:** 81-85.

27. MENNINI, T. & A. MIARI. 1991. Modulation of 3H glutamate binding by serotonin in rat hippocampus: An autoradiographic study. Life Sci. **49:** 283-292.

28. RAHMANN, S. & R. S. NEUMANN. 1993. Activation of 5-HT2 receptors facilitates depolarization of neocortical neurons by N-methyl-D-aspartate. Eur. J. Pharmacol. **231:** 347-354.

29. LOWY, M. T., L. GAULT & B. K. YAMAMOTO. 1993. Adrenalectomy attenuates stress-induced elevations in extracellular glutamate concentrations in the hippocampus. J. Neurochem. **61:** 1957-1960.

30. WATANABE, Y., N. G. WEILAND & B. S. MCEWEN. 1995. Effects of adrenal steroid manipulations and repeated restraint stress on dynorphin mRNA levels and excitatory amino acid receptor binding in hippocampus. Brain Res. **680:** 217-225.

31. ORCHINIK, M., N. G. WEILAND & B. S. MCEWEN. 1994. Adrenalectomy selectively regulates GABAa receptor subunit expression in the hippocampus. Molec. Cell. Neurosci. **5:** 451-458.

32. BARTANUSZ, V., J. M. AUBRY, S. PAGLIUSI, D. JEZOVA, J. BAFFI & J. Z. KISS. 1995. Stress-induced changes in messenger RNA levels of N-methyl-D-aspartate and ampa receptor subunits in selected regions of the rat hippocampus and hypothalamus. Neuroscience **66:** 247-252.

33. WEILAND, N. G., M. ORCHINIK & B. S. MCEWEN. 1995. Corticosterone regulates mRNA levels of specific subunits of the NMDA receptor in the hippocampus but not in cortex of rats (Abstr.) Soc. Neurosci. **21:** 502.

34. MONAGHAN, D. T., V. R. HOLETS, D. W. TOY & C. W. COTMAN. 1983. Anatomical distributions of four pharmacologically distinct 3H-L-glutamate binding sites. Nature **306:** 176-179.

35. SMITH, M. A., S. MAKINO, R. KVETNANSKY & R. M. POST. 1995. Stress and glucocorticoids affect the expression of brain-derived neurotrophic factor and neurotrophin-3 mRNAs in the hippocampus. J. Neurosci. **15:** 1768-1777.

36. HSU, M. & G. BUZSAKI. 1993. Vulnerability of mossy fiber targets in the rat hippocampus to forebrain ischemia. J. Neurosci. **13:** 3964-3979.

37. AUS DER MUHLEN, K. & H. OCKENFELS. 1969. Morphologische Veranderungen im Diencephalon und Telencephalon: Storungen des Regelkreises adenohypophysenebennierenrinde. Z. Zellforsch. Mikrosck. Anat. **93:** 126-141.

38. MIZOGUCHI, K., T. KUNISHITA, D. H. CHUI & T. TABIRA. 1992. Stress induces neuronal death in the hippocampus of castrated rats. Neurosci. Letts. **138:** 157-160.

39. FUCHS, E., H. UNO & G. FLUGGE. 1995. Chronic psychosocial stress induces morphological alterations in hippocampal pyramidal neurons of the tree shrew. Brain Res. **673:** 275-282.

40. CAMMERMEYER, J. 1978. Is the solitary dark neuron a manifestation of postmortem trauma to the brain inadequately fixed by perfusion? Histochemistry **56:** 97-115.

41. LANDFIELD, P. 1987. Modulation of brain aging correlates by long-term alterations of adrenal steroids and neurally-active peptides. Prog. Brain Res. **72:** 279-300.

42. RASMUSSEN, T., T. SCHLIEMANN, J. C. SORENSEN, J. ZIMMER & M. J. WEST. 1996. Memory impaired aged rats: No loss of principal hippocampal and subicular neurons. Neurobiol. Aging **14:** 143-147.

43. ISSA, A., W. ROWE, S. GAUTHIER & M. MEANEY. 1990. Hypothalamic-pituitary-adrenal activity in aged, cognitively impaired and cognitively unimpaired rats. J. Neurosci. **10:** 3247-3254.

44. SUGAYA, K., M. CHOUINARD, R. GREENE, M. ROBBINS, D. PERSONETT, C. KENT, M. GALLAGHER & M. MCKINNEY. 1996. Molecular indices of neuronal and glial plasticity in the hippocampal formation in a rodent model of age-induced spatial learning impairment. J. Neurosci. **16:** 3427-3443.

45. LOWY, M. T., L. WITTENBERG & B. K. YAMAMOTO. 1995. Effect of acute stress on hippocampal glutamate levels and spectrin proteolysis in young and aged rats. J. Neurochem. **65:** 268–274.

46. CHOI, D. 1988. Calcium-mediated neurotoxicity: Relationship to specific channel types and role in ischemic damage. TINS **11:** 465–469.

47. SIESJO, B. & F. BENGTSSON. 1989. Calcium fluxes, calcium antagonists and calcium-related pathology in brain ischemia, hypoglycemia and spreading depression: A unifying hypothesis. J. Cereb. Blood Flow Metab. **9:** 127–140.

48. LUPIEN, S. J. & B. S. MCEWEN. 1996. The acute effects of corticosteroids on cognition: Integration of animal and human model studies. Brain Res. Rev., in press.

49. MCEWEN, B. S. & R. M. SAPOLSKY. 1995. Stress and cognitive function. Curr. Opin. Neurobiol. **5:** 205–216.

50. LUPIEN, S., A. R. LECOURS, I. LUSSIER, G. SCHWARTZ, N. P. V. NAIR & M. J. MEANEY. 1994. Basal cortisol levels and cognitive deficits in human aging. J. Neurosci. **14:** 2893–2903.

51. SEEMAN, T. E., B. S. MCEWEN, B. H. SINGER, M. S. ALBERT & J. W. ROWE. 1996. Increase in urinary cortisol excretion and memory declines: MacArthur studies of successful aging. J. Clin. Exp. Endocrinol. in press.

52. KIRSCHBAUM, C., O. T. WOLF, M. MAY, W. WIPPICH & D. H. HELLHAMMER. 1996. Stress- and treatment-induced elevations of cortisol levels associated with impaired verbal and spatial declarative memory in healthy adults. Life Sci. **588:** 1475–1483.

53. LUINE, V., M. VILLEGAS, C. MARTINEZ & B. S. MCEWEN. 1994. Repeated stress causes reversible impairments of spatial memory performance. Brain Res. **639:** 167–170.

54. WATANABE, Y., E. GOULD, H. A. CAMERON, D. C. DANIELS & B. S. MCEWEN. 1992. Phenytoin prevents stress- and corticosterone-induced atrophy of CA3 pyramidal neurons. Hippocampus **2:** 431–436.

55. CONRAD, C. D., L. A. M. GALEA, Y. KURODA & B. S. MCEWEN. 1996. Chronic stress impairs rat spatial memory on the Y-maze and this effect is blocked by tianeptine pretreatment. Behav. Neurosci. **110:** 1321–1334.

56. LUPIEN, S., M. DELEON, S. DESANTI, A. CONVIT, B. M. TANNENBAUM, N. P. V. NAIR, B. S. MCEWEN, R. L. HAUGER & M. J. MEANEY. 1996. Longitudinal increase in cortisol during human aging predicts hippocampal atrophy and memory deficits (Abstr.) Soc. Neurosci. In press.

57. GOLOMB, J., A. KLUGER, M. J. DE LEON, S. H. FERRIS, A. CONVIT, M. S. MITTELMAN, J. COHEN, H. RUSINEK, S. DE SANTI & A. E. GEORGE. 1994. Hippocampal formation size in normal human aging: A correlate of delayed secondary memory performance. Neurobiol. Learn. Mem. **1:** 45–54.

58. CONVIT, A., M. J. DE LEON, C. TARSHISH, S. DE SANTI, A. KLUGER, H. RUSINEK & A. J. GEORGE. 1995. Hippocampal volume losses in minimally impaired elderly. The Lancet **345:** 266.

59. KERR, S., L. CAMPBELL, M. APPLEGATE, A. BRODISH & P. LANDFIELD. 1991. Chronic stress-induced acceleration of electrophysiologic and morphometric biomarkers of hippocampal aging. J. Neurosci. **1:** 1316–1324.

60. KERR, D. S., L. W. CAMPBELL, O. THIBAULT & P. W. LANDFIELD. 1992. Hippocampal glucocorticoid receptor activation enhances voltage-dependent Ca2+ conductances: Relevance to brain aging. Proc. Natl. Acad. Science USA **89:** 8527–8531.

61. MEANEY, M., D. AITKEN, H. BERKEL, S. BHATNAGER & R. SAPOLSKY. 1988. Effect of neonatal handling of age-related impairments associated with the hippocampus. Science **239:** 766–768.

62. MEANEY, M. J., B. TANNENBAUM, D. FRANCIS, S. BHATNAGAR, N. SHANKS, V. VIAU, D. O'DONNELL & P. M. PLOTSKY. 1994. Early environmental programming hypothalamic-pituitary-adrenal responses to stress. Semin. Neurosci. **6:** 247–259.

63. KIRSCHBAUM, C., J. C. PRUSSNER, A. A. STONE, I. FEDERENKO, J. GAAB, D. LINTZ, N. SCHOMMER & D. H. HELLHAMMER. 1995. Persistent high cortisol responses to

repeated psychological stress in a subpopulation of healthy men. Psychosom. Med. **57:** 468-474.

64. SHELINE, Y. I., P. W. WANG, M. H. GADO, J. C. CSERNANSKY & M. W. VANNIER. 1996. Hippocampal atrophy in recurrent major depression. Proc. Natl. Acad. Sci. USA **93:** 3908-3913.

65. STARKMAN, M., S. GEBARSKI, S. BERENT & D. SCHTEINGART. 1992. Hippocampal formation volume, memory dysfunction, and cortisol levels in patients with Cushing's syndrome. Biol. Psychiatry **32:** 756-765.

66. BREMNER, D. J., P. RANDALL, T. M. SCOTT, R. A. BRONEN, J. P. SEIBYL, S. M. SOUTHWICK, R. C. DELANEY, G. MCCARTHY, D. S. CHARNEY & R. B. INNIS. 1995. MRI-Based measurement of hippocampal volume in patients with combat-related posttraumatic stress disorder. Am. J. Psychiatry **152:** 973-981.

67. GURVITS, T. V., M. E. SHENTON, H. HOKAMA, H. OHTA, N. B. LASKO, S. P. ORR, R. KIKINIS, F. A. JOLESZ, R. W. MCCARLEY & R. K. PITMAN. 1996. Reduced hippocampal volume on magnetic resonance imaging in chronic post-traumatic stress disorder. Biol. Psychiatry **40:** 1091-1099.

68. DE LEON, M. J., J. GOLOMB, A. E. GEORGE, A. CONVIT, C. Y. TARSHISH, T. MCRAE, S. DE SANTI, G. SMITH, S. H. FERRIS, M. NOZ & H. RUSINEK. 1993. The radiologic prediction of Alzheimer disease: The atrophic hippocampal formation. Am. J. Neuroradiol. **14:** 897-906.

69. BOGERTS, B., J. A. LIEBERMAN, M. ASHTAIR, R. M. BILDER, G. DE GREEF, G. LERNER, C. JOHNS & S. MASIAR. 1993. Hippocampus-amygdala volumes and psychopathology in chronic schizophrenia. Biol. Psychiatry **33:** 236-246.

70. FUKUZAKO, H., T. FUKUZAKO, T. HASHIGUCHI, Y. HOKAZONO, K. TAKEUCHI, K. HIRAKAWA, K. UEYAMA, M. TAKIGAWA, Y. KAJIYA, M. NAKAJO & T. FUJIMOTO. 1996. Reduction in hippocampal formation volume is caused mainly by its shortening in chronic schizophrenia: Assessment by MRI. Biol. Psychiatry **39:** 938-945.

Kindling versus Quenching

Implications for the Evolution and Treatment of Posttraumatic Stress Disorder[a]

ROBERT M. POST,[b] SUSAN R. B. WEISS,
MARK SMITH, HE LI, AND UNA McCANN

Biological Psychiatry Branch
National Institute of Mental Health
National Institute of Health
Bethesda, Maryland 20892-1272

Two animal paradigms, behavioral sensitization and kindling, help to illustrate two different models of memory, wherein behavioral output increases, rather than decreases, with repetition of the inducing event.[1] As in these models, although posttraumatic stress disorder (PTSD) may be induced by a single intense stimulus, recurrent or repeated severe stressors appear to be associated with more pernicious forms of the illness.[2,3] Yehuda and Antelman[4] have further discussed the homologies between single stress sensitization (time-dependent sensitization) and stress-induced PTSD symptoms.

In the repeated or multiple stress sensitization paradigms, there appears to be a progressive evolution in the biochemical and neuroanatomical substrates crucially involved. For example, different neurotransmitter systems mediate the development versus the expression of stimulant sensitization,[5-7] and lesions of the amygdala, which are sufficient to block conditioned sensitization in a single exposure paradigm, become ineffective following multiple exposures.[8] Taken together, these data suggest that different neuroanatomical and neurotransmitter systems may be successively introduced in the early and late phases of stress sensitization and that these may provide differential targets for intervention, concepts that are spelled out in more detail elsewhere.[8]

In this article we focus on the neurobiology of the kindling paradigm not only because of its easily measurable endpoints, but also because of the opportunity to attempt to alter the development and persistence of these memory-like traces with quenching procedures. In our discussions of the caveats of the sensitization and kindling models as applied to neuropsychiatric disorders,[9] we stressed that although the neuroanatomy, biochemistry, and pharmacology of kindling to a seizure endpoint were likely different from those of PTSD (and other illnesses in which seizures are

[a]We would like to thank the Stanley Foundation for its generous supplemental support of this work of the National Institute of Mental Health.

[b]Address for correspondence: Robert M. Post, M.D., Biological Psychiatry Branch, NIMH, Bldg. 10, Room 3N212, 10 Center Drive MSC 1272, Bethesda, MD 20892-1272.

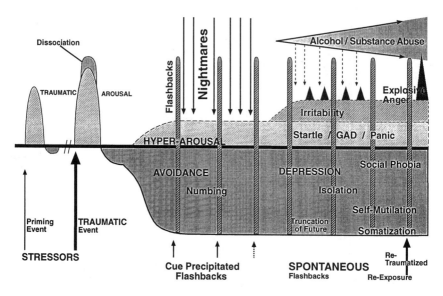

FIGURE 1A. Schematic illustration of emerging symptoms of posttraumatic stress disorder (PTSD). GAD = generalized anxiety disorder.

not involved), the kindling model may nevertheless have heuristic value. The evolution of full-blown seizure episodes in response to repeated subthreshold stimulation, and their eventual spontaneous emergence in the absence of obvious electrophysiological stimulation, bear at least some temporal similarity to the ability of the memory-like PTSD episodes to replay and eventually emerge in initially triggered and then spontaneous flashbacks. In this way, it might be conceptualized that kindling represents the evolution of a motor memory (increasingly consolidated on a pathological basis), whereas PTSD, in a parallel fashion, may be the quintessential expression of emotional memory utilizing partially overlapping but also different circuits.

Some of the key symptomatic elements of PTSD are schematized in FIGURE 1A. This schema focuses first on triggered primary symptoms and flashbacks and then on the eventual autonomous occurrence of flashbacks and psychopathology.

NEUROBIOLOGY OF KINDLING: PATHOLOGICAL VS ADAPTIVE CHANGES IN GENE EXPRESSION

Elsewhere we outlined some of the neurobiological events that could underlie the unfolding of amygdala-kindled seizures and their progression to spontaneity.[8,10–12] We postulated that amygdala kindling evolution involves a complex spatiotemporal cascade of neurobiological events involving changes in gene expression. We further hypothesized that changes in a gene transcription program involve a series of neurobiological events that could be roughly conceptualized into two groups. The first group relates to the primary pathological process of the kindled seizures or their accumulated memory trace, whereas the second group represents secondary, compensatory, potentially adaptive changes that may dampen or "quench" the kindled hyperexcitability.[13]

This potential separation into primary and secondary adaptations is based on the empirical observations that kindled seizures themselves leave behind not only a memory trace progressing towards increased severity and spontaneity, but also, at the same time, a more transient set of compensatory adaptations. These secondary adaptations are revealed by the observation that drugs such as carbamazepine and diazepam are more effective if a seizure has recently occurred than after 4 or 10 seizure-free days, respectively.[13,14] Moreover, the same time-course is associated with a decrease in the amygdala-kindled seizure threshold, further indicating that endogenous adaptations have been programmed following seizures and that these decay after several days.[14] Thus, it is evident that these putative endogenous anticonvulsant mechanisms are relatively short lasting, whereas the kindled memory trace appears relatively permanent.

Recent evidence suggests that not only are a host of transcriptional regulators induced with kindled seizures, but also neurotrophic factors,[15,16] neuropeptides,[17,18] and genes involved in preprogrammed cell death (apoptosis),[19] suggesting that the microstructure of the brain and potentially the survival, sprouting, or death of neural elements could be reprogrammed as part of the kindled memory trace.[20,21]

In this regard it is of considerable interest that we observed that the transcription factor *c-fos* initially and then bilaterally was induced ipsilaterally in the amygdala and piriform cortex during kindling evolution;[22] however, following a spontaneous seizure *c-fos* was induced on the side contralateral to the electrode placement (Clark *et al.*, unpublished observations). These observations suggest that the spontaneous seizure could be generated by a secondary or mirror focus, a well-recognized phenomenon in epileptogenesis.[23] To the extent that these observations prove replicable and are pertinent to the evolution of triggered and then spontaneous flashbacks, they suggest that the spontaneous variety could involve triggering from a different brain region or hemisphere than the flashbacks provoked by specific stimuli. This postulate could be directly tested using positron emission tomography (PET) or functional magnetic resonance imaging (fMRI) in patients with PTSD.

POTENTIAL RELEVANCE OF KINDLING PRINCIPLES TO PTSD: A SCHEMA FOR EVOLVING NEUROBIOLOGY

If this preliminary schema proves useful for uncovering some of the neurobiological principles involved in the evolution of emotional memory traces and their replay in PTSD, it behooves us to develop a parallel schema for mapping the evolution of PTSD symptoms over time. Such a preliminary attempt, as illustrated in FIGURE 1A, can be modified according to the frequency, magnitude, and interval between inducing traumatic stimuli and their ultimate relation to PTSD symptoms. Events above the time line are representative of arousal states of a chronic nature (hyperstartle and insomnia) or a paroxysmal nature (flashbacks, dissociative events, and nightmares); below the time line are the withdrawal and numbing events and their associated proclivity to depression, irritability, anger attacks, and substance abuse.

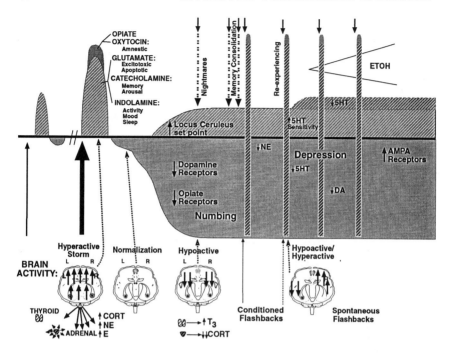

FIGURE 1B. Hypothetical neurobiological correlates of PTSD symptom evolution.

In FIGURE 1B, we present an even more speculative set of potential neurobiological correlates of some of these processes. We do this on the basis of both the minimal clinical empirical data involved to date[24,25] and the postulated involvement of some of these neurotransmitter and peptide systems from animal models. For example, hyperstartle can be induced with partial amygdala kindling[26] or expressed in the transgenic mouse model of deficient glucocorticoid receptors.[27] Therefore, the highly provisional nature of FIGURE 1B deserves reemphasis and is presented only to begin the dialogue towards a more accurate and detailed portrayal of potential correlates of this type of symptomatology. This exercise is therefore only an effort to suggest the importance of completing the major elements of this puzzle at this level of analysis.

FIGURE 1B also supports the view, as in kindling, that the complexity and spatio-temporal evolution of these changes are likely to occur at multiple levels of neurobiological events, potentially involving hundred of millions,[28] if not billions, of the cellular elements of the brain. How these postulated events at a molecular level become coordinated and evocative of the emergent properties of emotional memory, its replay, and the behavioral manifestations of PTSD, most likely awaits the next generation of molecular and cognitive neuroscience exploration.

Nonetheless, such a schema is presented here to raise the possibility that inherent in some of these postulated neurobiological changes are potential targets for therapeutics. As suggested elsewhere,[13] one would postulate not only the utility of inhibiting some changes that convey the hyperexcitability or memory trace of the pathological state (PTSD), but also of enhancing some of the secondary or compensatory adaptations as targets for therapeutic intervention.

TARGETS FOR THERAPEUTICS

Thyrotropin-releasing hormone (TRH), for example, is transiently induced after amygdala-kindled seizures,[18] and in light of its anticonvulsant properties in a variety of animal models we postulated that it is a putative endogenous anticonvulsant adaptation.[13,14] In a parallel fashion, TRH appears hypersecreted in depression based on evidence of its elevation in the cerebrospinal fluid (CSF) of patients in some studies,[29,30] the concomitant approximately 30% blunting of the thyrotropin-stimulating hormone (TSH) response to TRH in severe depression,[31] and evidence of relatively higher thyroid function during depression and subsequent lowering of peripheral thyroid indices with recovery from depression.[32–34] As both parenteral[35,36] and intrathecal[37] TRH have been shown to induce transient antidepressant and antianxiety effects in depressed patients, TRH now also represents a putative endogenous antidepressant candidate. Recent evidence implicates TRH in amygdala kindling and in startle,[38] therefore, we would postulate that enhancement of TRH could be a potential therapeutic maneuver in PTSD as well, and such clinical trials are in progress (McCann *et al.*, 1996, unpublished data).

The postulated spatiotemporal unfolding of neurobiological changes also highlights the idea that interfering with neurobiological events before or immediately after the kindled process may involve one set of neurotransmitter systems initially, but later, a very different set of neurochemical events. This idea is reflected by the findings that the induction of both long-term potentiation (LTP) and kindling (two prominently used neurobiological models of memory) involves NMDA receptors, whereas expression of LTP or completed kindled seizures does not.[39] In contrast, AMPA receptors may be involved in the expression of LTP.[40] Therefore, for later interventions in an already "evolved" PTSD process, very different pharmacological interventions from those that are effective early on may be required.

The potential separation of therapeutic targets into those that should be enhanced versus those that should be suppressed, and the likely possibility that these same targets will change as a function of time, is the basis for presenting the preliminary schema in FIGURE 1B, so that these principles and their predictive validity can be tested.

In other areas of medicine, therapeutics are targeted at eliminating or minimizing the long-term consequences of an acute pathological event. For example, massive doses of steroids are used in spinal cord injury, and thrombolytic substances followed by longer-term repair processes such as angioplasty or bypass surgery are administered after myocardial infarction and stroke. The window of opportunity for these interventions has been relatively well delineated. Treatments at this time are very different from the later, often more protracted and recalcitrant remedial interventions required, once the consequences of a full-blown myocardial infarction, stroke, or spinal cord injury have unfolded.

In a parallel fashion, we suggest the utility of conceptualizing acute emergency interventions to limit traumatic impact and develop a preventive view towards PTSD evolution. This possibility is supported by the literature involving stroke, wherein interventions immediately after the trauma can make a substantial difference including, for example, the preservation of hippocampal CA1 neurons and the prevention of associated memory loss, even if substances are applied several hours after a stroke induced experimentally by a ligated artery.[41] What the optimal therapeutic interventions would be in an immediate acute posttraumatic phase are currently speculative; however, substances that interfere with the development of long-term memory traces, such as high-potency benzodiazepines, are obvious candidates, although they are of dubious value in the late, fully developed phases of the syndrome. Another possibility was proposed by Adamec[42] who demonstrated that the CCK_B antagonists PD 135158 and LY 288 313 can be administered to rats 30 minutes after exposure to a cat to prevent the delayed increase in anxiety behaviors typically produced by this experience. This beta-blocker propranolol may also be useful, because Cahill et al.[43] have demonstrated its ability to disrupt memory when given to people following exposure to an emotionally charged story.

THE POSSIBILITY OF QUENCHING

Similar processes may also be achievable by nonpharmacological means. Weiss and associates[44] discovered that if the daily high-frequency 1-second stimulation, which normally results in the development of fully kindled seizures after several weeks, is followed by 15 minutes of low-frequency "quenching" stimulation (1 Hz appears optimal), animals never develop kindled seizures. Moreover, if animals are fully kindled and having seizures consistently following each stimulation, a series of seven once-daily 15-minute quenching sessions (again with 1 Hz stimulation) markedly and long-lastingly raises the amygdala afterdischarge and seizure thresholds. These animals no longer experience seizures when the initial kindling stimulation is resumed. This effect persists for weeks to months following a single 1-week administration of quenching stimulation. Thus, quenching appears capable of blocking both the development and the expression of kindled seizures through increases in the seizure or afterdischarge threshold.[44,45]

These data raise the possibility that quenching-like stimulation, applied immediately after a trauma or even in the fully developed PTSD syndrome, could inhibit PTSD evolution or suppress its manifestations by raising the threshold for PTSD flashbacks, nightmares, and paroxysmal components of the syndrome. Obviously, some of the first questions to be asked are: What are the critical areas of brain to be quenched in the PTSD syndrome, and can quenching be achieved without the use of a depth electrode as in the amygdala-kindled seizure paradigm? These questions become even more important in relation to the availability of extracranial modes of brain stimulation, such as repeated transcranial magnetic stimulation (rTMS), which allows noninvasive, relatively localized stimulation of the brain.[46–48] For example, rTMS over the left frontal cortex has been shown to be antidepressant in a series of clinical trials,[46,49] whereas stimulation over the motor cortex evokes movement, and over the occipital cortex, visual images or phosphenes.

Given the recent demonstration of the ability to image PTSD experiences as evoked by scripts of the original trauma while utilizing PET methodology,[25] it may be possible to ascertain what areas of brain are hyper- and hypofunctional during different phases of the PTSD syndrome and change their threshold for activation with rTMS accordingly. Such a study is ongoing at the National Institute of Mental Health (McCann *et al.*, unpublished data, 1997). Nonrepetitive transcranial magnetic stimulation has also been reported by Belmaker *et al.* (personal communication, June 1996) to have transient positive effects in patients with PTSD.

On the assumption that quenching would be most effective when applied to the anatomical sites most directly involved (such as the amygdala in amygdala kindling), one could speculate whether a combination of modalities might not be most effective in attempting to prevent, inhibit, or partially erase the traumatic memory trace in PTSD. For example, in psychotherapy, prolonged, intensive consoling, support, and holding after an assault trauma appear to resemble some of the optimal parametrics of quenching. As reported by Foa and Riggs,[50] when a rape victim is acutely assaulted verbally, psychically, and physically, the therapist and a friend or spouse can engage in soothing reassurance and physical holding and stroking in an attempt to counter the acute characteristics of the traumatic event with more chronic, low-level stimulation, and minimize the potential for the longer-term evolution of the PTSD syndrome. Perhaps such processes combined with appropriately timed and targeted pharmacotherapies can ultimately reduce the incidence of posttraumatic syndromes in many emergency room situations.

If the temporal characteristics of the intervention proved critical, perhaps some type of emergency management could be provided, and such measures be made available either in the emergency room itself or in a specialized trauma treatment facility to which the patient could also be briefly admitted. In patients with already fully evolved PTSD syndromes, it is possible that other psychotherapeutic, electrophysiological, and pharmacological quenching techniques could be more systematically applied (like the quenching of fully developed kindled seizures) to attempt to change the threshold for these experiences.

Although it currently may be premature to conceptualize such treatment efforts in the relative absence of a strong empirical database, it would nonetheless appear useful in beginning to bring together all of the information and conceptual frameworks for such a potential integrative therapy. These might involve PET (as in the epilepsies to localize a seizure focus) to localize and assess the degree of regional hypo- or hyperfunction during a PTSD event and then have the appropriate rTMS parameters (in terms of frequency, duration, and location of stimulation) designed accordingly on an individual basis. Similarly, as some of the molecular neurobiological substrates of quenching become available, it may be possible to target some of the alterations directly with appropriate pharmacological, neurotransmitter, or peptide therapies as well. Finally, there would appear to be a crucial role for the therapeutic interaction and evocation of the traumatic memories, as the appropriate bringing ''on line'' of the traumatic events may facilitate their ultimate quenching.[45] That is, activity-dependent mechanisms of synaptic plasticity may be required to optimally affect activity-dependent engrams.

CONCLUSION

That the quenching process, through the same amygdala electrode used for kindling, can suppress the development and manifestation of kindling to a seizure endpoint suggests the potential that the appropriate pharmacotherapeutic and psychotherapeutic maneuvers might, in a parallel fashion, be capable of providing equally dramatic impacts on PTSD symptoms in its different phases of evolution. A key issue in psychotherapy has been how to evoke aspects of the PTSD experience without retraumatizing or rekindling the individual. The quenching paradigm may thus indirectly facilitate the exploration and development of more specific psychotherapeutic techniques that enable the patient and therapist to remain under threshold for activation of the traumatic experiences based on the characteristics necessary for quenching, that is, low frequency and more sustained interaction.

The reciprocal potentiation and inhibition of synaptic excitability with LTP and LTD and of behavioral and convulsive syndromes with kindling and quenching certainly raise the possibility of more successful and targeted interventions for even fully developed PTSD syndromes based on some of the principles uncovered in these models of long-term memory. As alluded to here in a most preliminary fashion, this whole area of therapeutic endeavor appears to be ideal for exploration and integration of clinical trials experimentation, as they might interact with appropriate preclinical laboratory investigation. In this manner, there may be an ideal marriage of the molecular genetics of learning, memory, and experience with the long-term consequences and treatment of PTSD syndromes.

REFERENCES

1. Post, R. M. 1992. Transduction of psychosocial stress into the neurobiology of recurrent affective disorder. Am. J. Psychiatry **149:** 999–1010.
2. Bremner, J. D., S. M. Southwick, D. R. Johnson, R. Yehuda & D. S. Charney. 1993. Childhood physical abuse and combat-related posttraumatic stress disorder in Vietnam veterans. Am. J. Psychiatry **150:** 235–239.
3. Yehuda, R., B. Kahana, J. Schmeidler, S. M. Southwick, S. Wilson & E. L. Giller. 1995. The impact of cumulative lifetime trauma and recent stress on current posttraumatic stress disorder symptoms in Holocaust survivors. Am. J. Psychiatry **152:** 1815–1818.
4. Yehuda, R. & S. M. Antelman. 1993. Criteria for rationally evaluating animal models of posttraumatic stress disorder. Biol. Psychiatry **33:** 479–486.
5. Weiss, S. R. B., R. M. Post, A. Pert, R. Woodward & D. Murman. 1989. Context-dependent cocaine sensitization: Differential effect of haloperidol on development versus expression. Pharmacol. Biochem. Behav. **34:** 655–661.
6. Post, R. M., S. R. B. Weiss, D. Fontana & A. Pert. 1992. Conditioned sensitization to the psychomotor stimulant cocaine. Ann. N.Y. Acad. Sci. **654:** 386–399.
7. Pert, A., R. M. Post & S. R. B. Weiss. 1990. Conditioning as a critical determinant of sensitization induced by psychomotor stimulants. *In* Neurobiology of Drug Abuse: Learning and Memory, NIDA Research Monograph 97. L. Erinoff, Ed.: 208–241. U.S. Government Printing Office. Washington, DC.
8. Post, R. M., S. R. B. Weiss & M. Smith. 1995. Sensitization and kindling: Implications for the evolving neural substrate of PTSD. *In* Neurobiology and Clinical Consequences of Stress: From Normal Adaptation to PTSD. M. J. Friedman, D. S. Charney & A. Y. Deutch, Eds. Chap. **12:** 203–224. Lippincott-Raven. Philadelphia, PA.

9. WEISS, S. R. B. & R. M. POST. 1995. Caveats in the use of the kindling model of affective disorders. J. Toxicol. Indust. Health **10:** 421-447.

10. POST, R. M., S. R. B. WEISS & G. S. LEVERICH. 1994. Recurrent affective disorder: Roots in developmental neurobiology and illness progression based on changes in gene expression. *In* Development and Psychopathology. D. Cicchetti & D. Tucker, Eds. Vol. **6:** 781-813. Cambridge University Press. New York, NY.

11. POST, R. M., S. R. B. WEISS, G. S. LEVERICH, M. S. GEORGE, M. FRYE & T. A. KETTER. 1996. Developmental psychobiology of cyclic affective illness: Implications for early therapeutic intervention. *In* Development and Psychopathology. D. Cicchetti & D. Tucker, Eds. Vol. **8:** 273-305. Cambridge University Press. New York, NY.

12. POST, R. M. & S. R. B. WEISS. 1996. A speculative model of affective illness cyclicity based on patterns of drug tolerance observed in amygdala-kindled seizures. Mol. Neurobiol. **12:** 39-66.

13. POST, R. M. & S. R. B. WEISS. 1992. Endogenous biochemical abnormalities in affective illness: Therapeutic vs. pathogenic. Biol. Psychiatry **32:** 469-484.

14. WEISS, S. R. B., M. CLARK, J. B. ROSEN, M. A. SMITH & R. M. POST. 1995. Contingent tolerance to the anticonvulsant effects of carbamazepine: Relationship to loss of endogenous adaptive mechanisms. Brain Res. Rev. **20:** 305-325.

15. SMITH, M. A., S. MAKINO, R. KVETNANSKY & R. M. POST. 1995. Stress and glucocorticoids affect the expression of brain-derived neurotropic factor and neurotrophin-3 mRNAs in the hippocampus. J. Neurosci. **15:** 1768-1777.

16. SMITH, M. A. 1996. Hippocampal vulnerability to stress and aging: Possible role of neurotrophic factors. Behav. Brain Res. **78:** 25-36.

17. SMITH, M., S. R. B. WEISS, T. ABEDIN, R. M. POST & P. GOLD. 1991. Effects of amygdala-kindling and electroconvulsive seizures on the expression of corticotropin releasing hormone (CRH) mRNA in the rat brain. Mol. Cell. Neurosci. **2:** 103-116.

18. ROSEN, J. B., C. J. CAIN, S. R. B. WEISS & R. M. POST. 1992. Alterations in mRNA of enkephalin, dynorphin and thyrotropin releasing hormone during amygdala kindling: An in situ hybridization study. Brain Res. Mol. Brain Res. **15:** 247-255.

19. ZHANG, L. X., L. ZHANG, M. A. SMITH, J. C. REED, M. CLARK, A. N. FELDMAN, D. R. RUBINOW & R. M. POST. 1995. Ratio of BCL-2 and bax during development and apoptosis of neurons in the CNS (abstr). Abstr. Soc. Neurosci. Mtng. **21** (part 1): 559.

20. CAVAZOS, J. E. & T. P. SUTULA. 1990. Progressive neuronal loss induced by kindling: A possible mechanism for mossy fiber synaptic reorganization and hippocampal sclerosis. Brain Res. **527:** 1-6.

21. SUTULA, T. P. 1991. Reactive changes in epilepsy: Cell death and axon sprouting induced by kindling. Epilepsy Res. **10:** 62-70.

22. CLARK, M., R. M. POST, S. R. B. WEISS & T. NAKAJIMA. 1992. Expression of c-fos mRNA in acute and kindled cocaine seizures in rats. Brain Res. **592:** 101-106.

23. MORRELL, F. 1985. Secondary epileptogenesis in man. Arch. Neurol. **42:** 318-335.

24. CHARNEY, D. S., A. Y. DEUTCH, J. H. KRYSTAL, S. M. SOUTHWICK & M. DAVIS. 1993. Psychobiologic mechanisms of posttraumatic stress disorder. Arch. Gen. Psychiatry **50:** 294-305.

25. VAN DER KOLK, B. A., J. A. BURBRIDGE & J. SUZUKI. 1995. Current status of the psychobiology of posttraumatic stress disorder. Acta Neuropsychiatrica 7(Suppl. 3): S34-S37.

26. ROSEN, J. B., E. HAMERMAN, M. SITCOSKE, J. R. GLOWA & J. SCHULKIN. 1996. Hyperexcitability: Exaggerated fear-potentiated startle produced by partial amygdala kindling. Behav. Neurosci. **110:** 43-50.

27. BEAULIEU, S., I. ROUSSE, A. GRATTON, N. BARDEN & J. ROCHFORD. 1994. Behavioral and endocrine impact of impaired type II glucocorticoid receptor function in a transgenic mouse model. Brain corticosteroid receptors: Studies on the mechanism, function and neurotoxicity of corticosteroid action. Ann. N.Y. Acad. Sci. **748:** 388-391.

28. JOHN, E. R., Y. TANG, A. B. BRILL, R. YOUNG & K. ONO. 1986. Double-labeled metabolic maps of memory. Science **233:** 1167-1175.

29. KIRKEGAARD, C., J. FABER, L. HUMMER & P. ROGOWSKI. 1979. Increased levels of TRH in cerebrospinal fluid from patients with endogenous depression. Psychoneuroendocrinology **4:** 227-235.

30. BANKI, C. M., G. BISSETTE, M. ARATO & C. B. NEMEROFF. 1988. Elevation of immunoreactive CSF TRH in depressed patients. Am. J. Psychiatry **145:** 1526-1531.

31. LOOSEN, P. T. 1985. The TRH-induced TSH response in psychiatric patients: A possible neuroendocrine marker. Psychoneuroendocrinology **10:** 237-260.

32. WINOKUR, A. 1993. The thyroid axis and depressive disorders. *In* The Biology of Depressive Disorders. J. J. Mann & D. J. Kupfer, Eds.: 155-170. Plenum Press. New York, NY.

33. JOFFE, R. T. & T. H. SOKOLOV. 1994. Thyroid hormones, the brain, and affective disorders. Crit. Rev. Neurobiol. **8:** 45-63.

34. BAUER, M. S. & P. C. WHYBROW. 1991. Rapid cycling bipolar disorder. Clinical features, treatment, and etiology. *In* Advances in Neuropsychiatry and Psychopharmacology, Vol. **2:** Refractory Depression. J. D. Amsterdam, Ed.: 191-208. Raven Press. New York, NY.

35. PRANGE, A. J., JR., P. P. LARA, I. C. WILSON, L. B. ALLTOP & G. R. BREESE. 1972. Effects of thyrotropin-releasing hormone in depression. Lancet **2:** 999-1002.

36. CALLAHAN, A. M., M. A. FRYE, L. B. MARANGELL, M. S. GEORGE, T. A. KETTER, T. L'HERROU & R. M. POST. 1996. Comparative antidepressant effects of intravenous and intrathecal thyrotropin-releasing hormone: Confounding effects of tolerance and implications for therapeutics. Biol. Psychiatry **41:** 264-272.

37. MARANGELL, L. B., M. S. GEORGE, A. M. CALLAHAN, T. A. KETTER, P. J. PAZZAGLIA, T. A. L'HERROU & R.M. POST. 1996. Effects of protirelin (thyrotropin-releasing hormone) in refractory depressed patients. Arch. Gen. Psychiatry **54:** 212-214.

38. SMURTHWAITE, S., J. B. ROSEN, S. R. B. WEISS & R. M. POST. 1995. An assessment of the behavioral effects of thyrotropin-releasing hormone (abstract). Abstr. Soc. Neurosci. Mtng. **21**(part 1): 757.

39. CAIN, D. P., F. BOON & E. L. HARGREAVES. 1992. Evidence for different neurochemical contributions to long-term potentiation and to kindling and kindling-induced potentiation: Role of NMDA and urethane-sensitive mechanisms. Exp. Neurol. **116:** 330-338.

40. COSTA, E., J. AUTA, J. M. THOMPSON & A. GUIDOTTI. 1996. Positive allosteric modulation of AMPA or GABA, receptors antagonize alprazolam induced learning impairment in monkeys (abstr.). J. Eur. Coll. Neuropsychopharmacol. **6:** 152.

41. YASUI, M. & K. KAWASAKI. 1995. CCKB receptor activation protects CA1 neurons from ischemia-induced dysfunction in stroke-prone spontaneously hypertensive rats hippocampal slices. Neurosci. Lett. **191:** 99-102.

42. ADAMEC, R. 1995. Mechanisms of initiation and maintenance of increased generalized anxiety following traumatic stress. Presented at the Society for Neuroscience Meeting, 1995.

43. CAHILL, L., B. PRINS & J. L. MCGAUGH. 1994. Beta-adrenergic activation and memory for emotional events. Nature **371:** 702-704.

44. WEISS, S. R. B., X. L. LI, J. B. ROSEN, H. LI, T. HEYNEN & R. M. POST. 1995. Quenching: Inhibition of development and expression of amygdala kindled seizures with low frequency stimulation. NeuroReport **6:** 2171-2176.

45. WEISS, S. R. B., X.-L. LI, E. C. NOGUERA, T. HEYNEN, H. LI, J. B. ROSEN & R. M. POST. 1997. Quenching: Persistent alterations in seizure and afterdischarge threshold following low-frequency stimulation. *In* Kindling. V. M. Corcoran & S. Moshe, Eds. Plenum. New York, NY. In press.

46. GEORGE, M. S., E. M. WASSERMANN, W. A. WILLIAMS, A. CALLAHAN, T. A. KETTER, P. BASSER, M. HALLETT & R. M. POST. 1995. Daily repetitive transcranial magnetic stimulation (rTMS) improves mood in depression. NeuroReport **6:** 1853-1856.

47. PASCUAL-LEONE, A., J. GRAFMAN, L. G. COHEN, B. J. ROTH & M. HALLETT. 1997. Transcranial magnetic stimulation: A new tool for the study of higher cognitive functions

in man. *In* Handbook of Neuropsychology. J. Grafman & E. Boller, Eds. Vol. 10. Elsevier. Amsterdam. In press.

48. HALLETT, M. 1996. Transcranial magnetic stimulation: A useful tool for clinical neurophysiology. Unpublished manuscript.

49. PASCUAL-LEONE, A., B. RUBIO, F. PALLARDO & M. D. CATALA. 1996. Rapid-rate transcranial magnetic stimulation of left dorsolateral prefrontal cortex in drug-resistant depression. Lancet **348:** 233–237.

50. FOA, E. B. & D. S. RIGGS. 1993. Posttraumatic stress disorder and rape. *In* American Psychiatric Press Review of Psychiatry. J. M. Oldham, M. B. Riba & A. Tasman, Eds. Vol. **12:** 273–303. American Psychiatric Press. Washington, D.C.

Stressor-Induced Oscillation

A Possible Model of the Bidirectional Symptoms in PTSD[a]

SEYMOUR M. ANTELMAN,[b,f]
ANTHONY R. CAGGIULA,[c,e] SAMUEL GERSHON,[b]
DAVID J. EDWARDS,[d] MARK C. AUSTIN,[b]
SUSAN KISS,[b] AND DONNA KOCAN [b]

[b]Department of Psychiatry
Western Psychiatric Institute and Clinic
University of Pittsburgh School of Medicine

[c]Department of Psychology
University of Pittsburgh

[d]Department of Pharmacology
University of Pittsburgh School of Pharmacy and

[e]University of Pittsburgh Cancer Institute
Pittsburgh, Pennsylvania 15213

The central feature of PTSD is that the survivor reexperiences elements of the trauma.... Alternately, the victim feels numb ... The reexperiencing of the trauma and the emotional constrictedness are assumed to coexist in the same individual and may occur in cycles, although one phase may predominate in a given individual or time period.

> Green et al., Trauma and its Wake, 1985[1]

... after reexperiencing begins (hours, months or years later), avoidance alternates with reexperiencing, apparently with a frequency and to a degree which allows the reexperiencing to be tolerated.

> Arnold, The Trauma of War, 1985[2]

Although it is not thought of as such, posttraumatic stress disorder (PTSD) may, to some extent, be an example of a cycling illness. It is characterized by the bidirectional symptom clusters of intrusive, involuntary reexperiencing of an initiating trauma through nightmares, flashbacks, and unwanted memories, on one hand, and avoidance/ numbing, on the other.[3] Reexperiencing may alternate with avoidance symptoms[2] or coexist with them. These observations suggest that any attempt to construct a

[a]This work was supported by grant DA09163 from the National Institute on Drug Abuse at the National Institutes of Health.

[f]Address for correspondence: S. M. Antelman, Ph.D., Western Psychiatric Institute and Clinic, University of Pittsburgh School of Medicine, 3811 O'Hara St., Pittsburgh, PA 15213 (tel: (412) 624-4523; fax: (412) 624-1772).

296

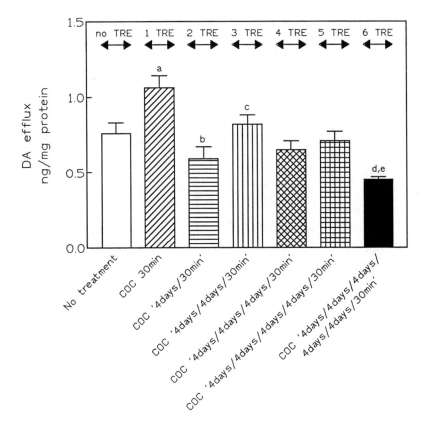

FIGURE 1. Dopamine efflux from rat brain striatal slices evoked by 10 μM amphetamine following ip administration of 15 mg/kg cocaine (COC) 30 minutes/20 days before sacrifice. Overall ANOVA $F_{(6,53)} = 8.47$, $p < 0.0001$; [a]$p < 0.005$ vs No Treatment (amphetamine alone); [b]$p < 0.001$ vs COC at 30 minutes; [c]$p < 0.02$ vs COC '4 days/30 min'; [d]$p < 0.006$ vs COC '4 days/4 days/4 days/4 days/30 min'; [e]$p < 0.003$ vs No Treatment. TRE = number of COC pretreatments; $n = 7$-9.

comprehensive model of PTSD must account for the alternation or cycling between bidirectional symptoms.[4] Unidirectional models of a bidirectional disorder such as PTSD must, at best, be considered incomplete.

Recent findings from our laboratory have shown that repeated, intermittent exposure to either pharmacological or nondrug stressors can induce both a neurochemical and a behavioral oscillation or cycling, that is, an alternating pattern of decreases and increases in the response to each subsequent treatment.[5-7] Oscillation appears to occur when a highly sensitized neurochemical, physiological, or endocrine system reaches or approaches its physiological boundaries or limits. In other words, oscillation follows sensitization and may represent an attempt by individual or multiple systems to prevent "overload" and reestablish a form of dynamic homeostasis.[8] Similarly,

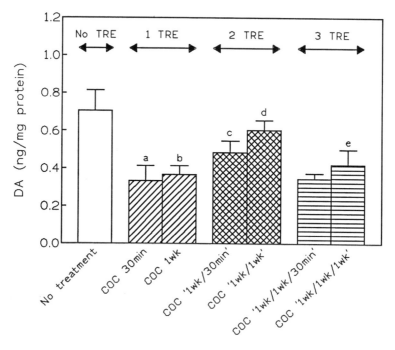

FIGURE 2. Dopamine efflux from rat brain striatal slices evoked by 10 μM amphetamine following repeated ip administration of 15 mg/kg cocaine (COC) with the last injection given 30 minutes or 1 week before sacrifice. Overall ANOVA $F_{(6,53)} = 3.784$, $p = 0.003$. [a]$p < 0.001$ vs No Treatment (amphetamine alone); [b]$p = 0.01$ vs No Treatment; [c]$p = 0.023$ vs COC at 30 minutes; [d]$p = 0.028$ vs COC at 1 week; [e]$p = 0.046$ vs COC '1 wk/1 wk'. TRE = number of COC pretreatments; $n = 8$–9.

the switch to avoidance symptoms in PTSD is thought to signify a coping attempt by the organism, allowing it to better tolerate intrusive reexperiencing.[2] Stressor-induced oscillation is a ubiquitous phenomenon, having been demonstrated with treatments such as cocaine, ethanol, amphetamine, morphine, nicotine, and psychological stress and immobilization and for endpoints as diverse as efflux of striatal and nucleus accumbens dopamine, hippocampal serotonin, frontal cortical aspartate, hypothalamic CRF, pituitary ACTH, heart norepinephrine and acetylcholine, plasma levels of corticosterone and glucose, and a behavioral measure, stressor-induced hypoalgesia (refs. 5-7 and unpublished observations). Such diversity suggests that the oscillation phenomenon described is likely to represent a general principle of biological functioning. That is to say, further attempts to drive an already highly sensitized neurochemical or physiological system will result in oscillation or cycling of that system. Because the biological findings of PTSD are consistent with those of a sensitization disorder,[4,8–12] and given the extreme nature of the traumas that precipitate this disorder, it is not unlikely that some biological systems would be sensitized near the limits of their functioning and thus susceptible to making the transition to an oscillatory pattern of responding.

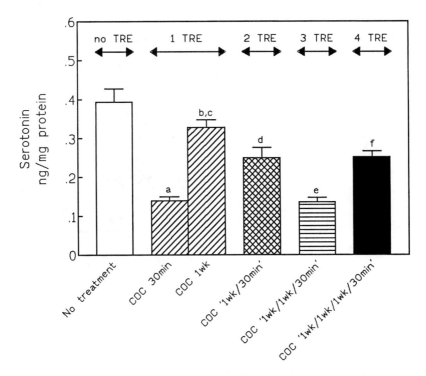

FIGURE 3. Serotonin efflux from hippocampal slices of female rats evoked by 10 μM amphetamine following 1-4 cocaine (COC; 15 mg/kg) treatments at weekly intervals with the last treatment 30 minutes before sacrifice. Overall ANOVA $F(5,46) = 22.387$, $p < 0.0001$. [a]p <0.001 vs No Treatment (amphetamine alone); [b]$p = 0.032$ vs No Treatment; [c]$p <0.001$ vs COC at 30 minutes; [d]$p = 0.015$ vs COC at 1 week; [e]$p = 0.001$ vs COC '1 wk/30 min'; [f]$p <0.001$ vs COC '1 wk/1 wk/30 min'. TRE = number of COC pretreatments; $n = 8-9$.

The oscillation phenomenon is illustrated in FIGURE 1. In this experiment, separate groups of 7-9 rats received from 1-6 cocaine pretreatments, with 4-day intervals between treatments. Following sacrifice, dopamine efflux from striatal slices evoked by 10 μM amphetamine was measured using the method of Snyder *et al.*[13] Saline, the vehicle for cocaine, could not legitimately be used as a "control" in these experiments, because we have shown repeatedly in our sensitization work that drug vehicles are stressors,[8,14] and inasmuch as oscillation appears to be a stress-induced phenomenon,[5,7] vehicle would not be a "control" but rather another experimental condition. More directly relevant, we have shown that saline can sometimes substitute for cocaine in inducing oscillation.[5] Interestingly, the same point has also been raised by others studying sensitization.[15,16] Although saline may not always elicit all of the neurochemical and behavioral consequences associated with drug-induced sensitization or oscillation, the differences may be more the result of its being a relatively low-intensity stressor rather than a functionally discrete stimulus.

A single intraperitoneal injection of 15 mg/kg cocaine 30 minutes before sacrifice significantly increased *in vitro* measurement of amphetamine-induced dopamine ef-

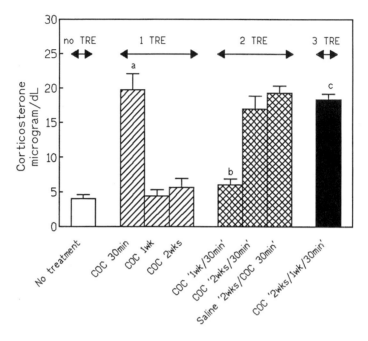

FIGURE 4. Plasma corticosterone following ip administration of 15 mg/kg cocaine (COC) 30 minutes/2 weeks before sacrifice. Overall ANOVA $F(7,65) = 30.34$, $p < 0.001$; [a]$p < 0.001$ vs No Treatment (No TRE = basal levels of corticosterone); [b]$p < 0.001$ vs COC at 30 minutes; [c]$p < 0.001$ vs COC '1 wk/30 min'. TRE = number of COC pretreatments; $n = 9$-10. From Antelman *et al.*,[5] with permission.

flux from striatal slices when compared to non-cocaine-treated controls (FIG. 1). The increase was significantly reversed in animals that had received two cocaine treatments at 4 days and 30 minutes before sacrifice (cocaine "4 days/30 min"). This oscillatory pattern continued through six cocaine treatments and was statistically significant for four of the six comparisons. Most importantly, the direction of cocaine's effect was completely reversed over the course of the six treatments. Whereas cocaine significantly increased dopamine efflux by 39% when given only once, dopamine efflux was significantly decreased by 41% in animals receiving six cocaine treatments. This cannot be explained as simply due to tolerance, because six injections produced an effect significantly below control levels, whereas tolerance, by definition, can only bring the organism back to control levels. Depletion of dopamine is also an unlikely explanation of these results, because they were not seen with five injections, and a period of 4 days between treatments is more than adequate time for a depleted system to have repleted itself.

Oscillation following sequential cocaine is not an isolated phenomenon, limited to a particular neurotransmitter, site, or a constrained set of experimental circumstances. Thus, FIGURE 2 illustrates oscillation of striatal dopamine in response to cocaine in animals sacrificed either 30 minutes or 1 week following the last injection.

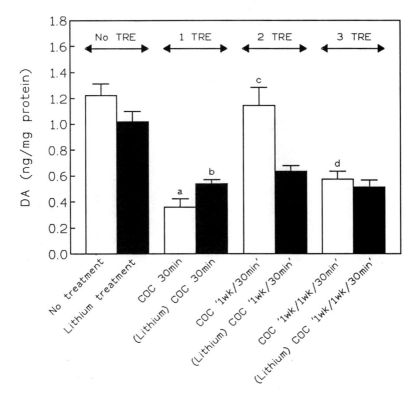

FIGURE 5. Dopamine efflux from nucleus accumbens slices evoked by 10 μM amphetamine following 1–3 cocaine (COC; 15 mg/kg) treatments at weekly intervals with the last treatment 30 minutes before sacrifice. Dark bars = rats receiving lithium chloride 15 mEq/L in their drinking water 1 week before the beginning of the experiment and continuing until sacrifice. [a]p <0.001 vs No Treatment (amphetamine alone); [b]p <0.001 vs lithium treatment; [c]p <0.001 vs COC at 30 minutes; [d]p <0.001 vs COC '1 wk/30 min'. TRE = number of COC pretreatments; $n = 10$.

This finding also suggests that it is a long-lasting phenomenon. As noted in the introduction, oscillation has been observed in many neurotransmitter systems. FIGURE 3 illustrates it for cocaine-induced serotonin efflux from hippocampal slices of female rats. (FIGURES 1 and 2 were from males.) Moreover, in addition to being obtained using evoked efflux, oscillation is also observed in hormonal systems, such as corticosterone measured in plasma (FIG. 4), an index requiring neither an evocative agent such as amphetamine nor the use of an isolated, *in vitro* tissue preparation.

To the extent that the oscillation phenomenon described may serve as a model of one or more cyclic neuropsychiatric disorders, we should expect it to respond to the same pharmacological "treatments" as do those syndromes. Because lithium has long been the treatment of choice in one such illness, bipolar affective disorder (i.e., manic-depressive disorder), and has also been effective in controlling feelings

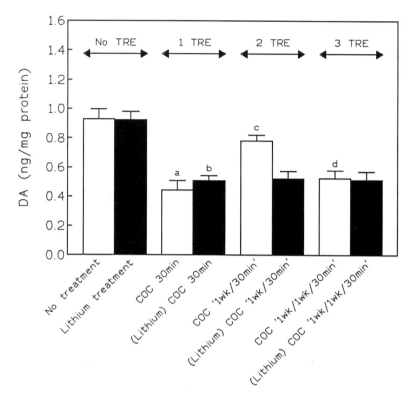

FIGURE 6. Dopamine efflux from striatal slices evoked by 10 μM amphetamine following 1–3 cocaine (COC; 15 mg/kg) treatments at weekly intervals with the last treatment 30 minutes before sacrifice. Dark bars = rats receiving lithium chloride 15 mEq/L in their drinking water 1 week before the beginning of the experiment and continuing until sacrifice. [a] $p < 0.001$ vs No Treatment (amphetamine alone); [b] $p < 0.001$ vs lithium treatment; [c] $p < 0.001$ vs COC at 30 minutes; [d] $p = 0.001$ vs COC '1 wk/30 min'. TRE = number of COC pretreatments; $n = 10$.

of explosive anger and irritibility in otherwise treatment-resistant veterans with PTSD,[17–19] we tested it against our oscillation model.

As indicated in FIGURES 5 and 6, prophylactic lithium chloride (15 mEq/L), added to the drinking water of rats starting 5 days before the administration of sequential injections of cocaine (15 mg/kg, ip) at 1-week intervals, completely prevented oscillation of amphetamine-evoked dopamine efflux from both nucleus accumbens and striatal slices. This represents a complete replication of the same experiment performed earlier (Antelman *et al.,* submitted for publication).

Although (as already noted) the data on PTSD are consistent with those of a sensitization disorder, sensitization as presently understood is a unidirectional process. Alone, it cannot account for the bidirectional symptoms that constitute the diagnostic hallmark of this illness. However, when it is understood that all biological systems have their limits or "boundaries" and therefore cannot sensitize indefinitely but, instead, at a certain point begin to oscillate, then we move closer to answering some of the questions that this disease raises. For instance, we can see how symptoms might alternate between predominantly intrusive and avoidance/numbing. Moreover, because neurochemical and physiological systems appear to manifest a hierarchy in terms of their susceptibility to making the transition from sensitization to an oscillatory mode of responding to stressors, one relevant system could still be in the sensitization mode, whereas another is already oscillating. Thus, a sensitization-oscillation model even permits us to understand how these symptoms can coexist concurrently. Finally, oscillation in response to sequential stressors would have predicted (Fig. 4) the otherwise odd finding by Yehuda *et al.*[20] that women who have been raped twice have half the cortisol levels of those raped once. It may also explain the hypocortisolemia in PTSD.[21]

REFERENCES

1. GREEN, B. L., J. P. WILSON & J. D. LINDY. 1985. Conceptualizing post-traumatic stress disorder: A psychosocial framework. *In* Trauma and Its Wake: The Study and Treatment of Post-Traumatic Stress Disorder. C. R. Figley, Ed.: 55. Brunner/Mazel. New York, NY.

2. ARNOLD, A. L. 1985. Diagnosis of post-traumatic stress disorder in Viet Nam veterans. *In* The Trauma of War: Stress and Recovery in Viet Nam Veterans. S. M. Sonnenberg, A. S. Blank, Jr. & J. A. Talbott, Eds.: 99-123. American Psychiatric Press, Inc. Washington, DC.

3. AMERICAN PSYCHIATRIC ASSOCIATION. 1994. Diagnostic and Statistical Manual of Mental Disorders, 4th Ed. Washington, DC.

4. YEHUDA, R. & S. M. ANTELMAN. 1993. Criteria for rationally evaluating animal models of posttraumatic stress disorder. Biol. Psychiatry **33**: 479-486.

5. ANTELMAN, S. M., A. R. CAGGIULA, S. KISS, D. J. EDWARDS, D. KOCAN & R. STILLER. 1995. Neurochemical and physiological effects of cocaine oscillate with sequential drug treatment: Possibly a major factor in drug variability. Neuropsychopharmacology **12**: 297-306.

6. CAGGIULA, A. R., S. M. ANTELMAN, A. M. PALMER, S. KISS, D. J. EDWARDS & D. KOCAN. 1996. The effects of ethanol on striatal dopamine and frontal cortical D-[³H]aspartate efflux oscillate with repeated treatment: Relevance to individual differences in drug responsiveness. Neuropsychopharmacology **15**: 125-132.

7. ANTELMAN, S. M. & A. R. CAGGIULA. 1996. Oscillation follows drug sensitization: Implications. Crit. Rev. Neurobiol. **10**: 101-117.

8. ANTELMAN, S. M. 1988. Time-dependent sensitization as the cornerstone for a new approach to pharmacotherapy: Drugs as foreign/stressful stimuli. Drug Dev. Res. **14**: 1-30.

9. POST, R. M. & S. R. B. WEISS. 1988. Sensitization and kindling: Implications for the evolution of psychiatric symptomatology. *In* Sensitization in the Nervous System. P. W. Kalivas & C. D. Barnes, Eds.: 257-291. The Telford Press. Caldwell, NJ.

10. CHARNEY, D. S., A. DEUTCH, J. KRYSTAL, S. M. SOUTHWICK & L. NAGY. 1993. Psychobiological mechanisms of post-traumatic stress disorder. Arch. Gen. Psychiatry **50**: 294-305.

11. ANTELMAN, S. M. & R. YEHUDA. 1994. Time-dependent change following acute stress: Relevance to the chronic and delayed aspects of PTSD. *In* Catecholamine Function in Posttraumatic Stress Disorder: Emerging Concepts. M. M. Murburg, Ed.: 87-98. American Psychiatric Press. Washington, DC.

12. YEHUDA, R. & A. C. MCFARLANE. 1995. Conflict between current knowledge about posttraumatic stress disorder and its original conceptual basis. Am. J. Psychiatry **152**: 1705-1713.

13. SNYDER, G. L., R. W. KELLER, JR. & M. J. ZIGMOND. 1990. Dopamine efflux from striatal slices after intracerebral 6-hydroxydopamine: Evidence for compensatory hyperactivity of residual terminals. J. Pharmacol. Exp. Ther. **253:** 867-876.

14. ANTELMAN, S. M., A. R. CAGGIULA, S. KNOPF, D. J. KOCAN & D. J. EDWARDS. 1992. Amphetamine or haloperidol 2 weeks earlier antagonized the plasma corticosterone response to amphetamine; evidence for the stressful/foreign nature of drugs. Psychopharmacology **107:** 331-336.

15. ROBINSON, T. E., J. B. BECKER, E. A. YOUNG, H. AKIL & E. CASTANEDA. 1987. The effects of footshock stress on regional brain dopamine metabolism and pituitary beta-endorphin release in rats previously sensitized to amphetamine. Neuropharmacology **26:** 679-691.

16. ZAHNISER, N. R. & J. PERIS. 1992. Neurochemical mechanisms of cocaine-induced sensitization. *In* Cocaine: Pharmacology, Physiology, and Clinical Strategies. J. M. Lakoski, M. P. Galloway & F. J. White, Eds.: 229-260. CRC Press. Boca Raton, FL.

17. VAN DER KOLK, B. A. 1983. Psychopharmacological issues in posttraumatic stress disorder. Hosp. Community Psychiatry **34:** 683-684, 691.

18. KITCHNER, I. & R. GREENSTEIN. 1985. Low dose lithium carbonate in the treatment of post traumatic stress disorder: Brief communication. Mil. Med. **150:** 378-381.

19. FORSTER, P. L., F. B. SCHOENFELD, C. R. MARMAR & A. JANNA LANG. Lithium for irritability in post-traumatic stress disorder. J. Traumatic Stress **8:** 143-149.

20. YEHUDA, R., H. RESNICK, B. KAHANA & E. L. GILLER. 1993. Long-lasting hormonal alterations to extreme stress in humans: Normative or maladaptive? Psychosom. Med. **55:** 287-297.

21. YEHUDA, R., S. M. SOUTHWICK, J. H. KRYSTAL, D. BREMNER, D. S. CHARNEY & J. W. MASON. 1993. Enhanced suppression of cortisol following dexamethasone administration in posttraumatic stress disorder. Am. J. Psychiatry **150:** 83-86.

Roles of the Amygdala and Bed Nucleus of the Stria Terminalis in Fear and Anxiety Measured with the Acoustic Startle Reflex

Possible Relevance to PTSD[a]

MICHAEL DAVIS,[b] DAVID L. WALKER, AND
YOUNGLIM LEE

Ribicoff Research Facilities of the Connecticut Mental
Health Center
Department of Psychiatry
Yale University School of Medicine
34 Park Street
New Haven, Connecticut 06508

Over the last several years, our laboratory has been studying how a simple reflex, the acoustic startle reflex, can be modified by prior emotional learning. Thus far, most of our work has concentrated on an experimental paradigm called the *fear-potentiated startle effect,* in which the amplitude of the startle reflex can be modified by a state of fear. More recently, however, we are trying to develop experimental methods to measure both fear and anxiety using changes in the acoustic startle reflex. Fear is a natural, adaptive change in an organism elicited by a potentially threatening stimulus which prepares the organism to cope with the provocation. Fear generally is elicited by a clearly identifiable stimulus and subsides shortly after its offset. Anxiety also is a change in the state of an organism which has many of the same signs and symptoms of fear. However, it may not be clearly associated with a single eliciting stimulus, may last a long time once activated, and may lack clear adaptive significance.

[a] Research reported in this chapter was supported by National Institute of Mental Health grants MH-25642, MH-47840, Research Scientist Development Award MH-00004, a grant from the Air Force Office of Scientific Research, and the State of Connecticut. This same chapter will be published as "Amygdala and bed nucleus of the stria terminalis: Differential roles in fear and anxiety measured with the acoustic startle reflex. *In* Biological and Psychological Perspectives on Memory and Memory Disorders, L. Squire & D. Schacter, Eds. American Psychiatric Association Press. Washington, DC. In press.

[b] Tel: (203)789-7450; fax: (203)562-7079.

FEAR-POTENTIATED STARTLE AS A MEASURE OF EXPLICIT CUE CONDITIONING

The Fear-Potentiated Startle Test

Although fear is a complex emotion, it can be objectively measured in the laboratory using classic conditioning procedures in which a neutral stimulus, such as a light (conditioned stimulus, CS), is consistently paired with an aversive stimulus, such as a shock (unconditioned stimulus, US). Following a small number of pairings, the light now comes to elicit a constellation of behaviors that are typically used to define a state of fear in animals. These may include a change in heart rate, an increase in blood pressure, pupil dilation, labored respiration, vocalization, cessation of ongoing behavior, and hyperresponsivity to sensory stimuli.

Our laboratory measures conditioned fear in rats using changes in the amplitude of the acoustic startle response, a short-latency reflex that can be elicited in all mammals.[1,2] In our typical paradigm, rats are placed into a chamber specially designed to elicit and measure the amplitude of the acoustic startle reflex and are presented with a small number of startle-eliciting stimuli. The average startle amplitude across the last several stimuli (once habituation has occurred so that startle has reached a relatively stable level) is used as a measure of the basal startle amplitude (baseline startle). The next day, the rats are returned to the same chamber and presented with light-shock pairings. No startle stimuli are given on this training day. At later times (1–30 days) the rats are returned to the test chamber and presented with acoustic startle stimuli alone as well as in the presence of the light previously paired with shock. Under these conditions, startle amplitude is significantly increased when elicited by the same auditory stimulus in the presence of the light.[3,4] The difference in startle amplitude elicited in the presence versus the absence of the light or versus the original baseline level of startle is used to define the magnitude of conditioned fear (fear-potentiated startle). When startle is elicited at various times during testing, it increases almost immediately after light onset and returns to its baseline level shortly after the light goes off.[5] Hence, fear-potentiated startle is highly time-locked to the presence of the emotionally significant stimulus, making it an example of explicit cue conditioning. Drugs that reduce or increase fear in humans selectively reduce or increase fear-potentiated startle in rats.[6]

Role of the Amygdala in Fear-Potentiated Startle

A great deal of data now indicate that the amygdala is critically involved in explicit cue conditioning.[7-15] The natural pattern of behaviors produced by conditioned fear can be blocked by lesions of the amygdala and produced by electrical stimulation of the amygdala. Anatomical data indicate that the central nucleus of the amygdala projects directly to hypothalamic and brainstem target areas critically involved in specific signs and symptoms of fear. Lesions of the amygdala completely block fear-potentiated startle,[16,17] and low-level electrical stimulation of the amygdala increases startle.[18] Both conditioned fear and electrical stimulation of the amygdala appear to increase startle amplitude by ultimately altering transmission at a particular point along the acoustic startle pathway called the nucleus reticularis pontis caudalis, which receives a direct monosynaptic connection from the central nucleus of the amygdala.[19] Finally, local infusion of NMDA antagonists into the amygdala blocks the acquisition but not the expression of conditioned fear,[20,21] whereas pretest infusion of non-NMDA receptor antagonists blocks the expression of fear-potentiated startle.[22]

FEAR VERSUS ANXIETY

Although a good deal is known about the neural circuitry involved in explicit cue conditioning, much less is known about the closely related, but somewhat different emotion of anxiety. For example, in explicit cue conditioning, a state of fear is clearly elicited by a very specific stimulus that has previously been associated with an aversive event. In fact, much progress has been made in precisely tracing out the exact pathways to the amygdala that allow an auditory stimulus previously paired with a footshock to produce a state of fear using either freezing[23] or potentiated startle[24,25] as a measure of conditioned fear. With anxiety, however, it is often difficult to specify the actual sensory event that triggers anxiety or to predict exactly when this change in emotion will subside. Moreover, certain animal tests purported to measure anxiety because of their sensitivity to drugs that reduce anxiety clinically are not always affected by lesions of the amygdala. For example, benzodiazepines have consistently been shown to have anxiolytic effects in the elevated plus maze, yet lesions of the amygdala fail to have an anxiolytic effect in this test.[26] We believe that observations such as these are extremely important because they suggest that different areas of the brain may be involved in different types of aversive emotional states, which ultimately may lead to a distinction between brain areas involved in fear versus anxiety. Because anxiety rather than stimulus-specific fear is a major problem in many types of psychiatric disorders, identifying separate neural substrates for fear versus anxiety could ultimately lead to more effective anxiety treatments. Because the acoustic startle reflex offers several advantages as a marker for aversive emotional states,[6] we are trying to develop procedures that use the acoustic startle response to assess anxiety and brain areas involved in anxiety.

LIGHT-ENHANCED STARTLE

The Light-Enhanced Startle Effect

Although fear-potentiated startle offers several advantages as an animal model of fear and anxiety, one disadvantage, common to all procedures that rely on conditioning, is that treatment effects cannot unambiguously be attributed to effects on fear versus memory. It is difficult to say, for example, whether a given drug that reduces fear-potentiated startle does so because the drug is anxiolytic or, alternatively, because the drug has a more general effect on memory retrieval. Consequently, it would be valuable to develop a procedure that preserves the benefits of fear-potentiated startle, but that relies on unconditioned stimuli to elicit anxiety.

Previous reports suggest that bright light may be an anxiety-provoking stimulus for rats and mice. For example, open field activity is decreased by high illumination,[27–33] and this effect has been attributed by some to an activity-suppressing influence of fear.[28] An anxiogenic influence of light is also suggested by work from File and Hyde[34] who have shown that social interactions among rat pairs are significantly reduced in high- versus low-illumination environments, particularly if the environment is an unfamiliar one. This group has also reported that plasma corticosterone concentrations of rats placed for 20 minutes in a brightly lit and unfamiliar environment are almost twice those of rats placed in a dimly lit unfamiliar environment[35] and that both the behavioral and physiological effects are blocked by chlordiazepoxide.[34,35] The tendency of rodents to spend more time in the darkened side of a two-chambered dark-light box also suggests that light is aversive,[36,37] and consistent with this view, anxiolytic compounds such as diazepam, chlordiazepoxide, and buspirone decrease this preference and other indices of anxiety (i.e., suppression of activity, transitions between the two compartments) in this paradigm.[37–39]

If, as would seem to be the case, high illumination levels are indeed anxiogenic, then illumination might also elevate the amplitude of acoustic startle. In fact, previous reports suggest that the unconditioned effects of light on startle are biphasic, with inhibition being reported at very short light-onset to startle-elicitation intervals, as short as 40 ms[40] and facilitation occurring at somewhat longer intervals, 400 ms[40] to at least as long as 52 seconds.[5] Flashing lights also have been reported to "sensitize" startle responding[41–43] and to do so for as long as the visual stimuli are presented, up to 30 minutes.[43]

Recently, we tested the effects of sustained illumination on the startle reflex and the possible role of the amygdala versus the bed nucleus of the stria terminalis on the facilitatory effects of light on the startle reflex.[44] Twenty-four rats were randomly divided into three groups of eight rats each. In each group, the effect on startle of either an 8, 70, or 700 footlambert light source was evaluated. Each animal was tested on two separate days. On one day, startle was measured in the dark during Phase I and in the light during Phase II. On a second day, the light remained off during both phases. These two session types were counterbalanced such that half of the rats in each illumination group began the experiment with a dark→light session type and half the rats began the experiment with a dark→dark session type. For both session types, a difference score (startle amplitude during Phase II minus startle amplitude during Phase I) was obtained.

FIGURE 1 shows the mean startle amplitude over successive blocks of three stimuli during Phase I, combined across all groups, and during Phase II, shown separately for the different groups that were tested in Phase II in the dark or with 8, 70, or 700 footlamberts of light. In both phases, startle responses habituated over the course of testing. Superimposed on this habituation was a general increase of startle amplitude which was directly related to light intensity and which remained relatively stable for the duration of the 20-minute test. FIGURE 2 shows these same data in terms of difference scores, indicating that light-enhanced startle was directly related to the intensity of the light in Phase II with significant increases occurring at the 700- and 70-footlambert intensities but not with the 8-footlambert light intensity.

These results indicate that high levels of sustained illumination produce an increase in the amplitude of the acoustic startle response which persists for at least 20 minutes after placement into the illuminated test chamber. It is possible, however, that the elevation in startle was produced simply by the change in illumination (e.g., dishabitua-

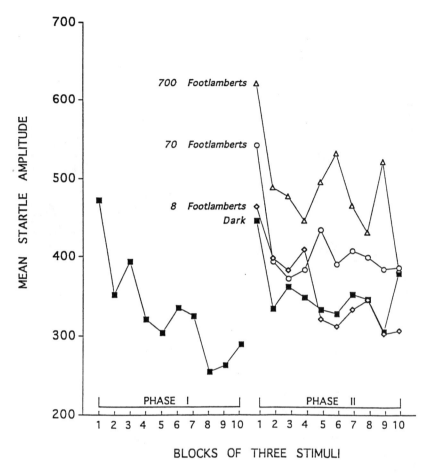

FIGURE 1. Mean startle amplitude over successive blocks of three stimuli during Phase I, combined across all groups, and during Phase II shown separately for the different groups that were tested in Phase II in the dark or with 8, 70, or 700 footlamberts of light in Phase II.

tion) rather than the continued presence of the very bright light. If so, then decreasing the level of illumination should also increase startle amplitude. To evaluate this possibility the same animals were retested using the procedure just described with the exception that rats were tested initially in the presence of the light (Phase I) and subsequently in the absence of the light (Phase II). The results showed that when illumination levels were decreased from Phase I to Phase II, the mean amplitude of acoustic startle also decreased. These results could not be accounted for by dishabituation and confirm that the amplitude of acoustic startle is greater when elicited in an illuminated as opposed to a darkened environment.

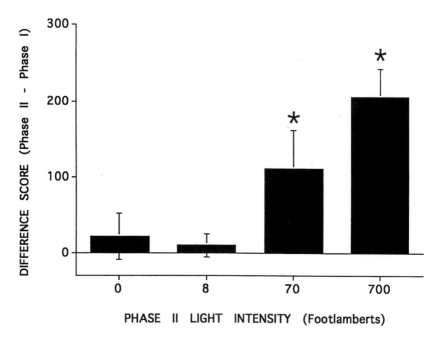

FIGURE 2. Mean change in startle amplitude from Phase I to Phase II as a function of the light intensity in Phase II. *Significantly different from dark-dark.

Effects of Buspirone on Light-Enhanced Startle

Treatments that increase the amplitude of acoustic startle are often associated with aversive or anxiogenic properties. For example, cues previously paired with footshock increase the amplitude of acoustic startle,[3] as does footshock itself,[45] and drugs that produce anxiety in humans increase the amplitude of acoustic startle in rats.[46,47] Perhaps, then, the effects of light shown here reflect an unconditioned anxiogenic effect of high illumination levels. As an initial test of this hypothesis, we assessed the susceptibility of the unconditioned light effect to the compound buspirone, a clinically used anxiolytic that also blocks fear-potentiated startle in rats.[48–50] Sixteen rats were tested under each of four conditions (dark→light saline, dark→light buspirone, dark→dark saline, and dark→dark buspirone). The ordering of session type and treatment was counterbalanced across animals. During each phase, startle responses were elicited by 30 noise bursts, 10 at each of three intensities (90, 95, and 105 dB). Light intensity was set at 700 footlamberts. Immediately prior to Phase I, buspirone (5 mg/kg) or saline solution (1 ml/kg) was injected subcutaneously in the neck.

FIGURE 3 shows that the effect of light was blocked by buspirone. However, consistent with previous results,[49,51] buspirone itself increased the amplitude of baseline startle. Although this effect appears to be independent of buspirone's anxiolytic effects on fear-potentiated startle because buspirone can still block fear-potentiated startle under conditions in which it has no effect on baseline startle,[49] the unusually

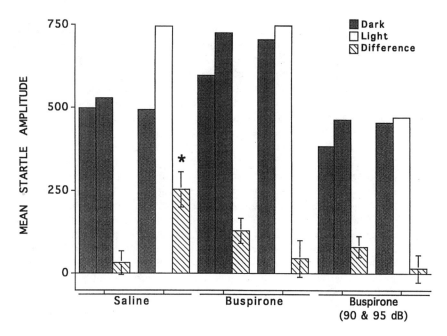

FIGURE 3. *Left* and *middle panels* show mean startle amplitude in dark-dark or dark-light conditions following injection of saline solution or buspirone. *Hatched bars* represent the difference between Phase I and Phase II in either the dark-dark or dark-light conditions. *Right panel* shows the same data only at the 90- and 95-dB test stimuli following injection of buspirone. *Significantly different from dark-dark.

large effect on baseline startle seen in the present experiment may have prevented measurement of any further increases of startle amplitude by light because of a ceiling effect. To address this possibility, the buspirone data were reanalyzed using only those startle responses elicited by the lower intensity noise bursts (i.e., 90 and 95 dB). When these data were compared with the data from saline-treated animals (i.e., 90-, 95-, and 105-dB noise bursts), this time across comparable baselines, similar results were obtained (FIG. 3).

These data show that the elevation of startle amplitude by light is blocked by buspirone. Response amplitude in the dark was not decreased, but instead showed a moderate increase. As such, the effect of buspirone cannot be attributed to a general suppression of startle amplitude but reflects instead a specific blockade of the light-induced increase. As previously indicated, buspirone is clinically used in the treatment of anxiety and has also been shown to block the effects of conditioned fear on startle.[48-50] Thus, these results are consistent with the view that the effects of light reflect anxiogenic properties of high illumination levels.

Recently, we found that humans show a significant increase of startle amplitude (i.e., the eyeblink response) in the dark.[52] The opposite effects of illumination in rats versus humans may be attributable to the fact that rats are nocturnal whereas humans are diurnal. Interestingly, Grillon *et al.*[52] also reported that dark-enhanced startle only occurred in those subjects who rated the experiment as more unpleasant in the dark than in the light and was correlated with the subjects' self-ratings of how fearful they were of the dark when they were young. Again, these results are consistent with the view that the effects of light on startle are related to fear or anxiety.

Overall, we believe that there are sufficient grounds for attributing the effects of light on startle to increased anxiety and that this paradigm may be a useful model for the study of anxiety in animals. In general, animal models not involving conditioning may afford significant benefits,[53] and, indeed, several such models have been proposed.[54–57] When evaluating the effects of various treatments on conditioned fear, for example, it is difficult to distinguish drug effects on anxiety from drug effects on memory. Because light-enhanced startle does not involve conditioning, treatment effects may be more confidently attributed to the former. Also, because tests of conditioned behavior generally lead to either an increase or a decrease of response strength (depending on whether the conditioned stimulus or response is or is not reinforced during testing), separate groups of animals are usually required when evaluating multiple treatments in order to avoid the potential contamination of baseline responding by previous tests and treatments. Because light-enhanced startle is not reinforced and does not markedly habituate across sessions (Walker and Davis, unpublished observations), this paradigm may be particularly suitable for studies in which repeated testing is desirable.

Effects of Glutamate Antagonists Infused into the Bed Nucleus of the Stria Terminalis versus the Amygdala on Light-Enhanced Startle

Because local infusion of glutamate antagonists into the central nucleus of the amygdala completely blocks the expression of fear-potentiated startle,[22] we wondered whether this treatment would also block light-enhanced startle. As a control, we measured the effects of local infusion of glutamate antagonists into the bed nucleus of the stria terminalis. The bed nucleus of the stria terminalis is considered to be part of the so-called extended amygdala, because it is highly similar to the central nucleus of the amygdala in terms of its transmitter content, cell morphology, and efferent connections.[58] However, lesions of the bed nucleus of the stria terminalis fail to block either fear-potentiated startle[59] or conditioned freezing using an explicit cue,[60] suggesting that it may not be involved in explicit cue conditioning. On the other hand, several ongoing studies in our laboratory suggest that the bed nucleus of the stria terminalis might be involved in elevations of startle that were more long-lasting than explicit cue conditioning. For example, lesions of the bed nucleus of the stria terminalis blocked long-term sensitization of the startle reflex[61] or conditioned freezing using the experimental context as the conditioned stimulus rather than an explicit cue.[62] It also blocked the excitatory effect of the peptide corticotropin releasing hormone on startle[63] (see below).

To evaluate the role of the bed nucleus of the stria terminalis versus the amygdala in light-enhanced startle, animals were implanted with bilateral cannulas in either the bed nucleus of the stria terminalis, the basolateral complex of the amygdala (i.e., lateral and basolateral nuclei), or the central nucleus of the amygdala. One week later animals were tested for light-enhanced startle using the procedures just described.

During Phase I, animals were placed into the darkened chamber and presented with startle stimuli over a 20-minute period. They were then removed from the chamber, handled, and placed back into the brightly illuminated chamber and startled for another 20 minutes. Before being placed into the chamber during Phase II, half of the animals were infused with the AMPA/kainate antagonist 6-nitro-7-sulfamoylben-zo(f)quinoxaline-2-3-dione (NBQX–3 μg/side) and the other half with its vehicle, phosphate-buffered saline solution (PBS). Two days later these procedures were repeated except that animals previously infused with NBQX were now infused with PBS and vice-versa.

FIGURE 4 shows the results. Consistent with previous results in noninfused rats, light increased the amplitude of the startle reflex when animals were shifted from the darkened chamber in Phase I to the brightly illuminated chamber in Phase II after infusion of PBS into each of the three brain structures. Infusion of the glutamate antagonist NBQX into the central nucleus of the amygdala had no effect on light-enhanced startle. On the other hand, infusion of NBQX into either the lateral/basolateral amygdala complex or the bed nucleus of the stria terminalis significantly decreased light-enhanced startle.

These data indicate an important role for both the lateral/basolateral amygdala complex and the bed nucleus of the stria terminalis in light-enhanced startle. It is possible, however, that infusion of NBQX into the bed nucleus of the stria terminalis or the basolateral amygdala caused a depressant effect on startle that simply subtracted from the expected excitatory effect of testing in the brightly illuminated chamber. Previous studies in our laboratory had shown that local infusion of NBQX into the basolateral amygdala did not depress startle (Walker and Davis, unpublished observations), so that this explanation could not account for the basolateral amygdala results. To address this issue with regard to the bed nucleus of the stria terminalis, other animals were implanted with cannulas into the bed nucleus of the stria terminalis and then tested for startle in the darkened chamber at the same time after infusion of NBQX that occurred during Phase II in the light-enhanced experiment just described. NBQX had no depressant effect on startle when testing took place in the darkened chamber at the same time after infusion when it decreased light-enhanced startle (data not shown). These data strengthen the conclusion that the bed nucleus of the stria terminalis and the basolateral amygdala, which receives visual input and projects to the bed nucleus of the stria terminalis, are critically involved in light-enhanced startle, whereas the central nucleus of the amygdala is not.

It is possible however that the cannulas in the central nucleus of the amygdala were misplaced and that this accounted for the lack of an effect of inactivation of the central nucleus on light-enhanced startle. As mentioned earlier, previous studies have shown that local infusion into the central nucleus of the amygdala blocks the expression of fear-potentiated startle.[22] If the central nucleus implants in the present study were located properly, then infusion of NBQX into these animals should also block fear-potentiated startle. To evaluate this, rats used in the light-enhanced startle experiment were trained and tested for fear-potentiated startle after infusion of NBQX into either the amygdala or bed nucleus of the stria terminalis. During training, animals were placed into a darkened chamber and 5 minutes later were presented with the first of 10 light shock pairings using a 3.7-second light which coterminated with an 0.5-second, 0.6-mA footshock. Light shock pairings were presented at an

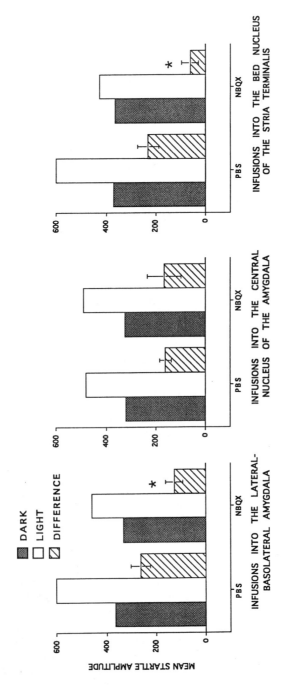

FIGURE 4. Mean amplitude startle in the dark (Phase I)-light (Phase II) conditions after local infusion of either phosphate-buffered saline solution (PBS) or the glutamate antagonist NBQX into either the basolateral amygdala (*left panel*), the central nucleus of the amygdala (*middle panel*), or the bed nucleus of the stria terminalis (*right panel*). The difference between the two phases defines the amount of light-enhanced startle. *Significantly different from PBS.

average intertrial interval of 4 minutes (range 3-5 minutes). These same procedures were repeated 24 hours later, creating a total of 20 light shock pairings. Two days later the animals were placed back into a darkened startle chamber and 5 minutes later were presented with a total of 60 startle stimuli, half of which occurred 3.2 seconds after the onset of the light and half of which occurred in darkness. Three different noise burst intensities were used (90, 95, or 105 dB), creating a total of 10 occurrences of each of six test trial types.

FIGURE 5 shows the mean startle amplitude, collapsed over the three test-intensities, when startle was elicited in darkness (Noise-Alone trials: black bars) or 3.2 seconds after the onset of light (Light-Noise trials: white bars). Consistent with previous results, infusion of the glutamate antagonist into the central nucleus of the amygdala completely blocked the expression of fear-potentiated startle. This was also true after an infusion of NBQX into the basolateral nucleus of the amygdala. In contrast, infusion of NBQX into the bed nucleus of the stria terminalis had no effect on fear-potentiated startle. These data indicate, therefore, that the location of the cannulas into the central nucleus of the amygdala was adequate to allow infusion of NBQX to totally block fear-potentiated startle. Hence, the ineffectiveness of NBQX infused into the central nucleus of the amygdala to block light-enhanced startle cannot be attributed to misplaced cannulas. Moreover, these data show a double dissociation between inactivation of glutamate receptors in the central nucleus of the amygdala versus the bed nucleus of the stria terminalis in relation to fear-potentiated versus light-enhanced startle.

CORTICOTROPIN RELEASING HORMONE-ENHANCED STARTLE AS A MEASURE OF ANXIETY

In addition to evaluating the role of the amygdala versus the bed nucleus of the stria terminalis in fear-potentiated startle and light-enhanced startle, we are testing how these same brain areas might be involved in the excitatory effect of the peptide corticotropin releasing hormone (CRH) on the startle reflex. Intraventricular administration of CRH produces a variety of behavioral and neuroendocrine effects similar to those seen during fear and anxiety, whereas intraventricular administration of the CRH antagonist alpha-helical CRH_{9-41} blocks the behavioral and neuroendocrine effects of natural stressors or conditioned fear.[64] Swerdlow *et al.*[65] reported that intraventricular administration of CRH increased the acoustic startle reflex and that this effect could be blocked by the benzodiazepine chlordiazepoxide, suggesting that the excitatory effect of CRH on startle reflected an anxiogenic effect of the hormone. We have confirmed and extended this work showing that intraventricular infusion of CRH (0.1-1.0 µg) produced a pronounced, dose-dependent enhancement of the acoustic startle reflex in rats.[66]

Recently, we attempted to determine the primary receptor site upon which CRH acts after intraventricular administration to increase startle amplitude. Three criteria were used to evaluate whether a given structure represented a primary receptor site for CRH-enhanced startle. First, lesions of the structure should block the excitatory effects of CRH on startle. Second, local infusion of CRH into the structure should elevate startle at doses considerably smaller than those required to increase startle

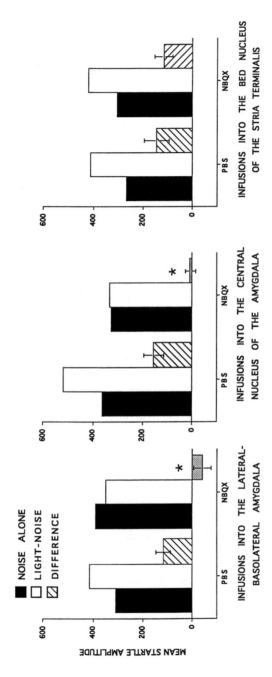

FIGURE 5. Mean amplitude startle on the Noise-Alone and Light-Noise Trials after local infusion of either phosphate-buffered saline solution (PBS) or the glutamate antagonist NBQX into either the basolateral amygdala (*left panel*), the central nucleus of the amygdala (*middle panel*), or the bed nucleus of the stria terminalis (*right panel*). The difference between the two trial types defines the amount of fear-potentiated startle.

after intraventricular infusion. Third, local infusion of a CRH antagonist directly into the structure should block the excitatory effects of CRH given intraventricularly.

Effects of Lesions of the Septal Area on CRH-Enhanced Startle

The first brain area examined was the septal nucleus. The lateral septal nucleus contains a high density of CRH receptors and is adjacent to the lateral ventricle. Lesions of the lateral septal nucleus are known to increase startle amplitude,[67] and this effect can be prevented by concomitant lesions of the amygdala,[68] suggesting that septal lesions increase startle via disinhibition of the amygdala. Perhaps intraventricular CRH might functionally inhibit the lateral septum and thereby increase startle via disinhibition of the amygdala. This hypothesis seemed plausible, because previous data had shown that large electrolytic lesions of the amygdala attenuated CRH-enhanced startle even though local infusion of CRH into the amygdala did not significantly elevate startle.[69] Thus, the amygdala seemed to be part of the neural circuitry required for CRH to elevate startle, but it did not appear to be the primary receptor area where CRH acts.

To test the role of the septal area in CRH-enhanced startle, animals were implanted with intraventricular cannulas and at the same time given electrolytic lesions of either the medial septum, lateral septum, medial and lateral septum together, or sham lesions. Two weeks later, when the excitatory effects of septal lesions on startle had dissipated,[70] all animals were placed into a startle test chamber and given a pretest consisting of presentation of 60 startle stimuli at a 30-second interstimulus interval. The animals were then removed from the chambers and infused intraventricularly with either CRH or its vehicle, artificial cerebrospinal fluid. Immediately thereafter they were presented with the first of 240 startle stimuli at a 30-second interstimulus interval, creating a 2-hour postinfusion test session. Two days later these same procedures were repeated except that animals previously infused with CRH were now infused with artificial cerebrospinal fluid and vice versa.

FIGURE 6 shows the results. Consistent with previous reports, intraventricular infusion of CRH caused a marked elevation of startle that began approximately 20 minutes after infusion and reached a stable plateau from 60-120 minutes thereafter in the sham-lesioned animals. Electrolytic lesions of either the medial septum or whole septum completely blocked CRH-enhanced startle. On the other hand, counter to expectation, electrolytic lesions of the lateral septum did not block CRH-enhanced startle.

These data suggested an important role for fibers or cell bodies in the medial septum in CRH-enhanced startle. To evaluate the role of cell bodies versus fibers of passage, other animals were given either chemical lesions of the medial septum or sham lesions and then tested for CRH-enhanced startle as described earlier. FIGURE 7 shows that chemical lesions of the medial septum failed to block CRH-enhanced startle in contrast to the total ablation of CRH-enhanced startle following electrolytic lesions of the same structure. These data indicate that fibers passing through the medial septum most likely are involved in CRH-enhanced startle, whereas cell bodies within the medial nucleus themselves appear not be involved. Further studies showed that local infusion of CRH into the medial septum also failed to increase startle (data

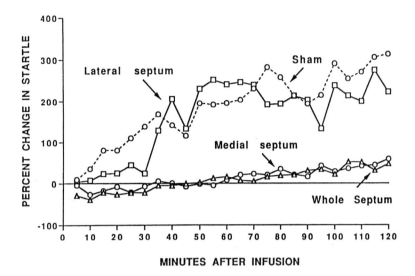

FIGURE 6. Mean percent change in startle amplitude, relative to the preinfusion baseline, after intraventricular infusion of corticotropin releasing hormone in animals previously given either sham lesions, electrolytic lesions of the lateral septum, electrolytic lesions of the medial septum, or electrolytic lesions of the whole septum.

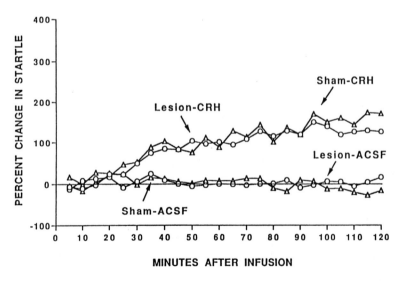

FIGURE 7. Mean percent change in startle amplitude, relative to the preinfusion baseline, after intraventricular infusion of corticotropin releasing hormone (CRH) or artificial CSF (ACSF) in animals previously given either sham lesions of the medial septum or chemical lesions of the medial septum.

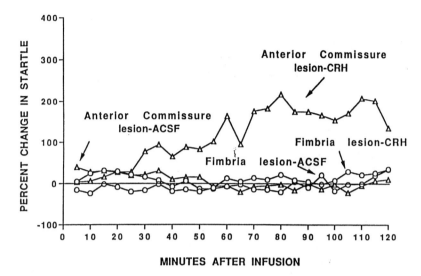

FIGURE 8. Mean percent change in startle amplitude, relative to the preinfusion baseline, after intraventricular infusion of either corticotropin releasing hormone (CRH) or artificial CSF (ACSF) in animals previously given either electrolytic lesions of the anterior commissure or transections of the fimbria.

not shown), indicating once again that receptors within the medial septal area do not seem to be involved in CRH-enhanced startle.

Effects of Transection of the Fimbria on CRH-Enhanced Startle

The most prominent fiber tract traversing the medial septum is the fornix which connects the hippocampus to the bed nucleus of the stria terminalis as well as carrying fibers from the medial septum to the hippocampus itself.[71] Hence, we hypothesized that blockade of CRH-enhanced startle produced by electrolytic lesions of the medial septum resulted from destruction of the fornix. To test this, other animals were given transections of the fimbria, the fiber bundle outside of the medial septum that forms the fornix, so as to evaluate the role of the fornix without concomitant damage to cell bodies in the medial septum. As a control, other animals sustained lesions of another major fiber bundle, the anterior commissure. FIGURE 8 shows that transections of the fimbria completely blocked CRH-enhanced startle, whereas electrolytic lesions of the anterior commissure had no significant effect. Taken together with the electrolytic lesion data of the medial septum these results strongly implicate the fornix as being critical for the expression of CRH-enhanced startle.

Effects of Lesions of the Amygdala, Hippocampus, or Bed Nucleus of the Stria Terminalis on CRH-Enhanced Startle

At the present time the exact role of the fornix in CRH-enhanced startle is not clear. FIGURE 9 shows a schematic diagram indicating possible connections between

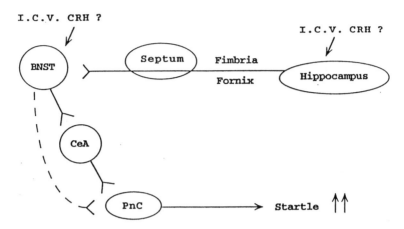

FIGURE 9. Schematic diagram showing the connections between the hippocampus and the bed nucleus of the stria terminalis via the fimbria fornix, which passes through the septum. Outputs of the bed nucleus of the stria terminalis project to the nucleus reticularis pontis caudalis in the brainstem, critical for startle, either directly or indirectly via the central nucleus of the amygdala.

limbic structures that may be involved in CRH-enhanced startle. The fornix is known to connect the hippocampus to the bed nucleus of the stria terminalis,[71-73] which in turn projects either directly to the startle pathway (Lee, Shi, and Davis, unpublished observations) or indirectly via the central nucleus of the amygdala.[74] Hence, the first question was whether chemical lesions of the hippocampus, bed nucleus of the stria terminalis, or amygdala would block the excitatory effect of CRH on startle after intraventricular administration. FIGURE 10 shows that NMDA-induced lesions of the ventral hippocampus or bed nucleus of the stria terminalis completely blocked CRH-enhanced startle. In contrast, chemical lesions of either the central nucleus of the amygdala or the basolateral/lateral amygdala nuclei had no significant effect on CRH-enhanced startle. However, the lack of an effect of chemical lesions of the amygdala to block CRH-enhanced startle might have resulted from inaccurate or incomplete lesions of these structures. To evaluate this, the same animals were trained for the fear-potentiated startle effect as described previously and then tested 1 week later.

FIGURE 11 shows that chemical lesions of either the central or basolateral amygdala nuclei completely blocked fear-potentiated startle, consistent with prior results.[25,75] In contrast, chemical lesions of the bed nucleus of the stria terminalis, which completely blocked CRH-enhanced startle, failed to block fear-potentiated startle. Like the difference between light-enhanced startle and fear-potentiated startle, chemical lesions of the bed nucleus of the stria terminalis and amygdala also resulted in a double dissociation in relation to CRH-enhanced startle.

These data strongly implicate the hippocampus and bed nucleus of the stria terminalis, but not the amygdala, in CRH-enhanced startle. The prior findings that large electrolytic lesions of the central nucleus of the amygdala blocked CRH-enhanced startle is still not resolved by these data. However, our suspicion is that

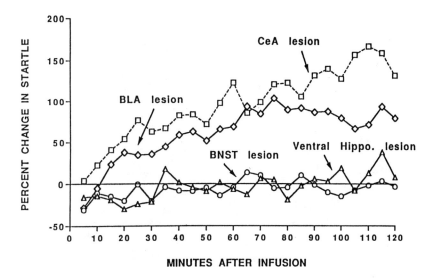

FIGURE 10. Mean percent change in startle amplitude, relative to the preinfusion baseline, after intraventricular infusion of corticotropin releasing hormone in animals previously given chemical lesions of either the central nucleus of the amygdala (CeA), the basolateral nucleus of the amygdala (BLA), the bed nucleus of the stria terminalis (BNST), or the ventral hippocampus (Ventral Hippo.).

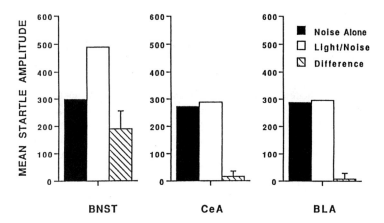

FIGURE 11. Mean startle amplitude on the Noise Alone and Light/Noise trials and the difference between these two trial types in animals previously given NMDA lesions of either the bed nucleus of the stria terminalis (BNST), the central nucleus of the amygdala (CeA), or the basolateral nucleus of the amygdala (BLA).

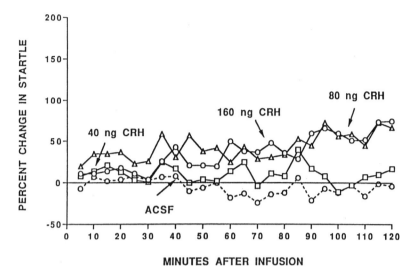

FIGURE 12. Percent change in startle amplitude, relative to the preinfusion baseline, after local infusion into the bed nucleus of the stria terminals of various doses of corticotropin releasing hormone (CRH) or artificial CSF (ACSF).

the electrolytic lesions destroyed fibers projecting from the bed nucleus of the stria terminalis to the startle pathway. Further studies using electrolytic lesions in combination with retrograde or anterograde tracing techniques will be required to address this issue.

Effects of Local Infusion of CRH into the Hippocampus or the Bed Nucleus of the Stria Terminalis on Startle

To further evaluate the role of the hippocampus and the bed nucleus of the stria terminalis in CRH-enhanced startle, other groups of animals were implanted with bilateral cannulas in either the ventral hippocampus or the lateral division of the bed nucleus of the stria terminalis. One week later they were infused with various doses (40, 80, or 160 ng) of CRH or artificial cerebrospinal fluid and tested for startle in the usual way. Local infusion of CRH into the hippocampus failed to increase startle at any of the test doses (data not shown). On the other, local infusion of CRH into the bed nucleus of the stria terminalis caused a dose-dependent elevation in startle that mimicked to some extent the excitatory effect of CRH given intraventricularly (Fig. 12). However, the excitatory effect of CRH given locally into the bed nucleus of the stria terminalis was never as large as that seen after intraventricular administration. Nonetheless, these data suggest that the bed nucleus of the stria terminalis may be at least one of the primary receptor areas critical for CRH-enhanced startle.

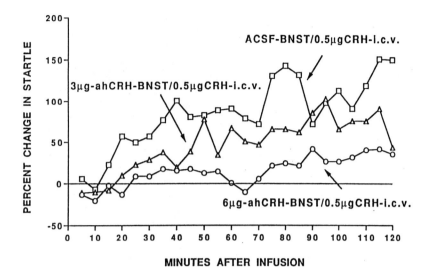

FIGURE 13. Mean percent change in startle amplitude, relative to the preinfusion baseline, after intraventricular infusion of corticotropin releasing hormone (CRH) 5 minutes after local infusion into the bed nucleus of the stria terminalis of either artificial CSF (ACSF), 3 μg of the CRH antagonist α-helical CRH, or 6 μg of α-helical CRH.

Effects of Local Infusion of the CRH Antagonist Alpha-Helical CRH$_{9-41}$ into the Bed Nucleus of the Stria Terminalis on CRH-Enhanced Startle

To evaluate the role of the bed nucleus of the stria terminalis more fully, other animals were implanted with bilateral cannulas into the bed nucleus of the stria terminalis along with a single cannula into the fourth ventricle. Previous data had shown that both the time course and the magnitude of CRH-enhanced startle were similar when infusions were made in the lateral or fourth ventricle.[66] This arrangement allowed us to test whether local infusion of a CRH antagonist into the bed nucleus of the stria terminalis could block the ability CRH given intraventricularly to elevate startle. Placement of the intraventricular cannula into the fourth ventricle, rather than the lateral ventricle, was necessary because there was not enough space to allow implantation of both an intraventricular cannula and bilateral cannulas into the bed nucleus of the stria terminalis. One week after surgery, animals were infused with 0.5 μg of CRH intraventricularly 5 minutes after local infusion into the bed nucleus of the stria terminalis of 1.5 or 3 μg/side of the CRH antagonist alpha-helical CRH$_{9-41}$. FIGURE 13 shows that intraventricular infusion of CRH using the fourth ventricle produced the usual excitatory effect on startle after infusion of artificial CSF into the bed nucleus of the stria terminalis. However, infusion the CRF antagonist alpha-helical CRH$_{9-41}$ into the bed nucleus of the stria terminalis caused a dose-dependent attenuation of CRH-enhanced startle. These data strongly suggest that CRH receptors in the bed nucleus of the stria terminalis are importantly involved in CRH-enhanced startle. Further studies indicated that the ability of 6 μg of alpha-

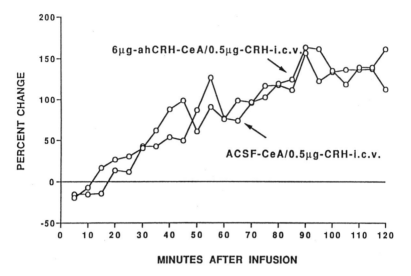

FIGURE 14. Mean percent change in startle amplitude, relative to the preinfusion baseline, after intraventricular infusion of corticotropin releasing hormone (CRH) 5 minutes after local infusion into the central nucleus of the amygdala of either artificial CSF (ACSF) or 6 μg of the CRH antagonist α-helical CRH.

helical CRH_{9-41} infused locally into the bed nucleus of the stria terminalis to block CRH-enhanced startle could not be attributed to leakage into the ventricular space, because the same dose of alpha-helical CRH_{9-41} given directly intraventricularly had no effect on CRH-enhanced startle. Furthermore, the effect was anatomically specific, because of 6 μg of alpha-helical CRH_{9-41} infused directly into the central nucleus of the amygdala failed to block CRH-enhanced startle (FIG. 14).

In summary, these data suggest that the bed nucleus of the stria terminalis may well be a primary receptor site involved in CRH-enhanced startle. Chemical lesions of the bed nucleus of the stria terminalis blocked CRH-enhanced startle. Microinfusion of CRH into the bed nucleus of the stria terminalis mimicked, at least partially, the excitatory effects of CRH on startle given intraventricularly. Finally, local infusion of a CRH antagonist directly into the bed nucleus of the stria terminalis blocked CRH-enhanced startle. In contrast, the amygdala does not seem to be involved in CRH-enhanced startle because (1) chemical lesions of the amygdala fail to block CRH-enhanced startle; (2) local infusion of CRH into the amygdala does not mimic CRH-enhanced startle; and (3) local infusion into the amygdala of a CRH antagonist does not block CRH-enhanced startle.

DIFFERENTIAL ROLES OF THE AMYGDALA VERSUS THE BED NUCLEUS OF THE STRIA TERMINALIS IN FEAR VERSUS ANXIETY

The series of experiments just outlined shows a clear distinction between the central nucleus of the amygdala and the bed nucleus of the stria terminalis in relation to fear-potentiated startle versus CRH-enhanced and light-enhanced startle. Lesions or chemical inactivation of the central nucleus of the amygdala completely block the expression of fear-potentiated startle but have no effect whatsoever on either light-enhanced startle or CRH-enhanced startle. Conversely, lesions or chemical inactivation of the bed nucleus of the stria terminalis significantly attenuated either light-enhanced startle or CRH-enhanced startle without having any effect whatsoever on fear-potentiated startle. It is currently still unclear why these two structures separate so completely in relation to fear-potentiated startle versus light-enhanced and CRH-enhanced startle. It is especially interesting, for example, that the basolateral amygdala appears to be involved in light-enhanced startle as well as fear-potentiated startle, but not in CRH-enhanced startle. Visual information is known to reach the bed nucleus of the stria terminalis via projections from the perirhinal cortex to the basolateral nucleus. Because light-enhanced startle eventually must depend on visual information getting to the bed nucleus of the stria terminalis, the ability of chemical inactivation of the basolateral nucleus of the amygdala to block light-enhanced startle may reflect interruption of visual information passing through the basolateral nucleus of the amygdala to the bed nucleus of the stria terminalis. On the other hand, chemical lesions of the basolateral nucleus of the amygdala did not block CRH-enhanced startle. This may make sense, because CRH-enhanced startle would not require visual input to the bed nucleus of the stria terminalis, and hence interruption of the visual pathway to the bed nucleus of the stria terminalis would not be expected to block CRH-enhanced startle. It should be emphasized that the very same light is used in both fear-potentiated test and the light-enhanced startle test. The only difference is that in fear-potentiated startle the light is previously paired with a shock and is presented for a brief time, whereas in light-enhanced startle the light is not paired with a shock and is presented for a relatively long time. The necessity of the central nucleus of the amygdala in fear-potentiated startle is likely dependent on prior classical fear conditioning because a great deal of data show that the amygdala is critically involved in both the acquisition and the expression of stimulus associations. This does not seem to be the case for the bed nucleus of the stria terminalis because lesions of this structure fail to block changes in behavior produced by prior aversive conditioning. It is considerably less clear, however, why sustained activation of the central nucleus of the amygdala via a very bright light source does not seem to be involved in light-enhanced startle. Similarly, the prolonged increase of startle produced by intraventricular administration of CRH also seemed not to involve the amygdala but instead involve the bed nucleus of the stria terminalis. It is possible, therefore, that in addition to differences between the two structures as they relate to prior classical conditioning, differences in the ability of neural networks in the two areas to respond in a sustained way to sensory activation could also explain the differences between these two areas in fear-potentiated startle versus light-enhanced startle. For example, perhaps the amygdala is especially able to respond to the onset of an aversive stimulus but then rapidly adapts to such activation so as to be prepared for subsequent presentation of another aversive stimulus. On the other hand, the bed nucleus of the stria terminalis may be arranged in such a way that networks within this nucleus can respond in a much more sustained way to aversive stimulation, leading to long-lasting changes in various behavioral responses via projections from the bed nucleus of the stria terminalis to different target areas in the hypothalamus

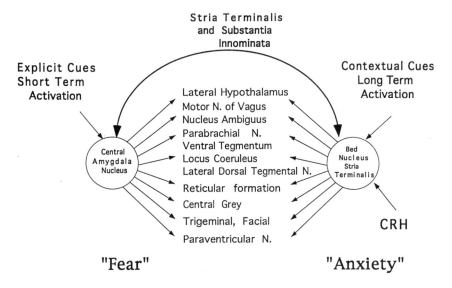

"Fear"   "Anxiety"

FIGURE 15. Hypothetical schematic suggesting that the central nucleus of the amygdala and the bed nucleus of the stria terminalis may be differentially involved in fear versus anxiety, respectively. Both brain areas have highly similar hypothalamic and brainstem targets known to be involved in specific signs and symptoms of fear and anxiety. However, the stress peptide corticotropin releasing hormone (CRH) appears to act on receptors in the bed nucleus of the stria terminalis rather than the amygdala, at least in terms of an increase in the startle reflex. Furthermore, the bed nucleus of the stria terminalis seems to be involved in the anxiogenic effects of a very bright light presented for a long time but not when that very same light was previously paired with a shock. Just the opposite is the case for the central nucleus of the amygdala, which is critical for fear conditioning using explicit cues such as a light or tone paired with aversive stimulation (i.e., conditioned fear).

and brain stem. This could also explain why the bed nucleus is more prominently involved in the excitatory effects of CRH on startle compared to the central nucleus of the amygdala. That is, the long-lasting behavioral effects of CRH given intraventricularly would require activation of a structure that could respond in a continuous fashion to receptor occupation by CRH compared to a structure that only could respond in a phasic way. In fact, it might make sense to have separate brain areas respond phasically and tonically to aversive stimulation so as to register both the immediate onset of an aversive experience as well as its prolonged presence, while maintaining a system such as the amygdala to allow responding in a phasic way to another aversive stimulus. Otherwise, if the "fear system" were completely saturated, then subsequent presentation of a threatening stimulus might not be fully processed, severely comprising survival of the organism.

We suggest, therefore, that the bed nucleus of the stria terminalis may be a system that responds to signals more akin to anxiety than to fear, whereas the amygdala is clearly involved in fear and perhaps not as much in anxiety (FIG. 15). Both these structures have very similar efferent connections to various hypothalamic and brainstem target areas known to be involved in specific signs and symptoms of fear and anxiety cf.[76] Both receive highly processed sensory information from the basolateral nucleus of the amygdala and hence are in a position to respond to emotionally significant stimuli. CRH is known to be released during stress or anxiety, some of which may come from CRH-containing neurons in the amygdala which project to the bed nucleus of the stria terminalis and act on CRH receptors there. Thus, phasic activation of the amygdala by certain stressors could lead to long-term activation of the bed nucleus of the stria terminalis via CRH. If so, then compounds that specifically block CRH receptors in the bed nucleus of the stria terminalis might be especially effective in the treatment of anxiety while leaving the fear response largely intact. Indeed, as our colleague George Heninger once remarked, "One would like to develop drugs to reduce anxiety but not prevent you from jumping out of the way of the on coming car." CRH antagonists designed to specifically bind to receptors in the bed nucleus of the stria terminalis might be especially effective in this regard.

REFERENCES

1. DAVIS, M. 1984. The mammalian startle response. *In* Neural Mechanisms of Startle Behavior. R. C. Eaton, Ed.: 287-351. Plenum Publishing Corp. New York.
2. LANDIS, C. & W. HUNT. 1939. The Startle Paradigm. Farrar & Rinehart. New York.
3. BROWN, J. S., H. I. KALISH & I. E. FARBER. 1951. Conditional fear as revealed by magnitude of startle response to an auditory stimulus. J. Exp. Psychol. **41:** 317-328.
4. DAVIS, M. & D. I. ASTRACHAN. 1978. Conditioned fear and startle magnitude: Effects of different footshock or backshock intensities used in training. J. Exp. Psychol. Anim. Behav. Processes **4:** 95-103.
5. DAVIS, M., L. S. SCHLESINGER & C. A. SORENSON. 1989. Temporal specificity of fear-conditioning: Effects of different conditioned stimulus-unconditioned stimulus intervals on the fear-potentiated startle effect. J. Exp. Psychol. Anim. Behav. Processes **15:** 295-310.
6. DAVIS, M. 1986. Pharmacological and anatomical analysis of fear conditioning using the fear-potentiated startle paradigm. Behav. Neurosci. **100:** 814-824.
7. DAVIS, M. 1992. The role of the amygdala in fear and anxiety. Ann. Rev. Neurosci. **15:** 353-375.
8. ELLIS, M. E. & R. P. KESNER. 1983. The noradrenergic system of the amygdala and aversive information processing. Behav. Neurosci. **97:** 399-415.
9. GLOOR, P., A. OLIVIER & L. F. QUESNEY. 1981. The role of the amygdala in the expression of psychic phenomena in temporal lobe seizures. *In* The Amygdaloid Complex. Y. Ben-Ari, Ed.: 489-507. Elsevier/North Holland. New York.
10. HENKE, P. G. 1980. The centromedial amygdala and gastric pathology in rats. Physiol. Behav. **25:** 107-112.
11. KAPP, B. S., J. P. PASCOE & M. A. BIXLER. 1984. The amygdala: A neuroanatomical systems approach to its contribution to aversive conditioning. *In* The Neuropsychology of Memory. N. Butters & L. S. Squire, Ed.: 473-488. The Guilford Press. New York.
12. LEDOUX, J. E. 1987. Emotion. *In* Handbook of Physiology, Sec. 1, Neurophysiology: Vol. 5. Higher Functions of the Brain. F. Plum, Ed.: 416-459. American Psychological Society. Bethesda, MD.
13. LIANG, K. C., R. G. JULER & J. L. MCGAUGH. 1986. Modulating effects of post-training epinephrine on memory: Involvement of the amygdala noradrenergic systems. Brain Res. **368:** 125-133.
14. MISHKIN, M. & J. AGGLETON. 1981. Multiple function contributions of the amygdala in the monkey. *In* The Amygdaloid Complex. Y. Ben-Ari, Ed.: 409-420. Elsevier/North Holland. New York.

15. SARTER, M. & H. J. MARKOWITSCH. 1985. Involvement of the amygdala in learning and memory: A critical review, with emphasis on anatomical relations. Behav. Neurosci. **99:** 342–380.

16. HITCHCOCK, J. M. & M. DAVIS. 1986. Lesions of the amygdala, but not of the cerebellum or red nucleus, block conditioned fear as measured with the potentiated startle paradigm. Behav. Neurosci. **100:** 11–22.

17. KIM, M. & M. DAVIS. 1993. Lack of a temporal gradient of retrograde amnesia in rats with amygdala lesions assessed with the fear-potentiated startle paradigm. Behav. Neurosci. **107:** 1088–1092.

18. ROSEN, J. B. & M. DAVIS. 1988. Enhancement of acoustic startle by electrical stimulation of the amygdala. Behav. Neurosci. **102:** 195–202.

19. ROSEN, J. B., J. M. HITCHCOCK, C. B. SANANES, M. J. D. MISERENDINO & M. DAVIS. 1991. A direct projection from the central nucleus of the amygdala to the acoustic startle pathway: Anterograde and retrograde tracing studies. Behav. Neurosci. **105:** 817–825.

20. CAMPEAU, S., M. J. D. MISERENDINO & M. DAVIS. 1992. Intra-amygdala infusion of the N-methyl-D-aspartate receptor antagonist AP5 blocks acquisition but not expression of fear-potentiated startle to an auditory conditioned stimulus. Behav. Neurosci. **106:** 569–574.

21. MISERENDINO, M. J. D., SANANES, C. B., MELIA, K. R. & DAVIS, M. 1990. Blocking of acquisition but not expression of conditioned fear-potentiated startle by NMDA antagonists in the amygdala. Nature **345:** 716–718.

22. KIM, M., S. CAMPEAU, W. A. FALLS & M. DAVIS. 1993. Infusion of the non-NMDA receptor antagonist CNQX into the amygdala blocks the expression of fear-potentiated startle. Behav. Neural Biol. **59:** 5–8.

23. LEDOUX, J. E. 1992. Emotion and the amygdala. In The Amygdala: Neurobiological Aspects of Emotion, Memory, and Mental Dysfunction. J. P. Aggleton, Ed.: 339–352. Wiley-Liss. New York.

24. CAMPEAU, S. & M. DAVIS. 1995. Involvement of subcortical and cortical afferents to the lateral nucleus of the amygdala in fear conditioning measured with fear-potentiated startle in rats trained concurrently with auditory and visual conditioned stimuli. J. Neurosci. **15:** 2312–2327.

25. CAMPEAU, S. & M. DAVIS. 1995. Involvement of the central nucleus and basolateral complex of the amygdala in fear conditioning measured with fear-potentiated startle in rats trained concurrently with auditory and visual conditioned stimuli. J. Neurosci. **15:** 2301–2311.

26. TREIT, D., C. PESOLD & S. ROTZINGER. 1993. Dissociating the anti-fear effects of septal and amygdaloid lesions using two pharmacologically validated models of rat anxiety. Behav. Neurosci. **107:** 770–785.

27. CANDLAND, D. K. & Z. M. NAGY. 1969. The open-field: Some comparative data. Ann N.Y. Acad. Sci. **159:** 831–851.

28. DEFRIES, J. C., J. P. HEGMANN & M. W. WEIR. 1966. Open-field behavior in mice: Evidence for a major gene effect mediated by the visual system. Science **154:** 1577.

29. LIVESEY, P. J. & G. J. EGGER. 1970. Age as a factor in open-field responsiveness in the white rat. J. Comp. Physiol. Psychol. **73:** 93–99.

30. MCLEARN, G. E. 1960. Strain differences in activity in mice: Influence of illumination. J. Comp. Physiol. Psychol. **53:** 142–143.

31. NAGGY, Z. & D. N. GLASER. 1970. Open-field behavior of C57BL/6J mice: Effect of illumination, age, and number of test day. Psychon. Sci. **19:** 143–145.

32. VALLE, F. P. 1970. Effects of strain, sex, and illumination on open-field behavior of rats. Am. J. Psychol. **83:** 103–111.

33. WALSH, R. N. & R. A. CUMMINS. 1976. The open-field test: A critical review. Psychol. Bull. **83:** 482–504.

34. FILE, S. E. & J. R. G. HYDE. 1978. Can social interaction be used to measure anxiety. Br. J. Pharmacol. **62:** 19-24.
35. FILE, S. E. & L. A. PEET. 1980. The sensitivity of the rat corticosterone response to environmental manipulations and to chronic chlordiazepozide treatment. Physiol. Behav. **25:** 753-758.
36. CRAWLEY, J. & F. K. GOODWIN. 1980. Preliminary report of a simple animal behavior model for the anxiolytic effects of benzodiazipines. Pharmacol. Biochem. Behav. **13:** 167.
37. CRAWLEY, J. N. 1981. Neuropharmacologic specificity of a simple animal model for the behavioral actions of benzodiazepines. Pharmacol. Biochem. Behav. **15:** 695-699.
38. COSTALL, B., B. J. JONES, M. E. KELLY, R. J. NAYLOR & D. M. TOMKINS. 1989. Exploration of mice in a black and white test box: Validation as a model of anxiety. Pharmacol. Biochem. Behav. **32:** 777-785.
39. ONAIVI, E. S. & B. R. MARTIN. 1989. Neuropharmacological and physiological validation of a computer-controlled two-compartment black and white box for the assessment of anxiety. Prog. Neuro-Psychopharmacol. Biol. Psychiatry **13:** 963-976.
40. ISON, J. R. & G. HAMMOND. 1971. Modification of the startle reflex in the rat by changes in the auditory and visual environment. J. Comp. Physiol. Psychol. **75:** 435-452.
41. GROVES, P. M. & R. F. THOMPSON. 1970. Habituation: A dual process theory. Psychol. Rev. **77:** 419-450.
42. RUSSO, J. M. & J. R. ISON. 1979. Sensitization of the rat's acoustic startle response by repetition of a photic stimulus. Physiol. Psychol. **7:** 102-106.
43. WEDEKING, P. & P. L. CARLTON. 1979. Habituation and sensitization in the modulation of reflex amplitude. Physiol. Behav. **22:** 57-62.
44. WALKER, D. & M. DAVIS. 1996. Inactivation of the bed nucleus of the stria terminalis (BNST), but not the central nucleus of the amygdala (CNA) disrupts light-enhanced startle: A novel paradigm for the assessment of anxiety in rats (Abstr.). Soc. Neurosci. **22:** 1117.
45. DAVIS, M. 1989. Sensitization of the acoustic startle reflex by footshock. Behav. Neurosci. **103:** 495-503.
46. DAVIS, M. 1980. Neurochemical modulation of sensory-motor reactivity: Acoustic and tactile startle reflexes. Neurosci. Biobehav. Rev. **4:** 241-263.
47. DAVIS, M. 1990. Animal models of anxiety based on classical conditioning: The conditioned emotional response (CER) and the fear-potentiated startle effect. Pharmacol. & Ther. **47:** 147-165.
48. DAVIS, M., J. V. CASSELLA & J. H. KEHNE. 1988. Serotonin does not mediate anxiolytic effects of buspirone in the fear-potentiated startle paradigm: Comparison with 8-OH-DPAT and ipsapirone. Psychopharmacology **94:** 14-20.
49. KEHNE, J. H., J. V. CASSELLA & M. DAVIS. 1988. Anxiolytic effects of buspirone and gepirone in the fear-potentiated startle paradigm. Psychopharmacology **94:** 8-13.
50. MANSBACH, R. S. & M. A. GEYER. 1988. Blockade of potentiated startle responding in rats by 5-hydroxytryptamine 1A receptor ligands. Eur. J. Pharmacol. **156:** 375-383.
51. EISON, A. S., M. S. EISON, M. STANLEY & L. A. RIBLET. 1986. Serotonergic mechanisms in the behavioral effects of buspirone and gepirone. Pharmacol. Biochem. Behav. **24:** 701-707.
52. GRILLON, C., M. PELLOWSKI, K. R. MERIKANGAS & M. DAVIS. 1997. Darkness facilitates the acoustic startle reflex in humans. Am. J. Psychiatry. In press.
53. LISTER, R. G. 1990. Ethologically-based animal models of anxiety disorders. Pharmacol. Ther. **46:** 321-340.
54. GARDNER, C. R. 1985. Distress vocalization in rat pups. A simple screening method for anxiolytic drugs. J. Pharmacol. Methods **14:** 181-187.
55. HOGG, S. & S. E. FILE. 1994. Responders and nonresponders to cat odor do not differ in other tests of anxiety. Pharmacol. Biochem. Behav. **49:** 219-222.

56. PELLOW, S., P. CHOPIN, S. E. FILE & M. BRILEY. 1985. Validation of open > closed arm entries in an elevated plus-maze as a measure of anxiety in the rat. J. Neurosci. Methods **14:** 149-167.
57. TREIT, D. & M. FUNDYTUS. 1989. Thigmotaxis as a test for anxiolytic activity in rats. Pharmacol. Biochem. Behav. **31:** 959-962.
58. ALHEID, G., J. S. DEOLMOS & C. A. BELTRAMINO. 1995. Amygdala and extended amygdala. *In* The Rat Nervous System. G. Paxinos, Ed.: 495-578. New York.
59. HITCHCOCK, J. M. & M. DAVIS. 1991. The efferent pathway of the amygdala involved in conditioned fear as measured with the fear-potentiated startle paradigm. Behav. Neurosci. **105:** 826-842.
60. LEDOUX, J. E., J. IWATA, P. CICCHETTI & D. J. REIS. 1988. Different projections of the central amygdaloid nucleus mediate autonomic and behavioral correlates of conditioned fear. J. Neurosci. **8:** 2517-2529.
61. DAVIS, M., K., MCNISH, J. GEWIRTZ & M. KIM. 1995. The roles of the amygdala and bed nucleus of the stria terminalis (BNST) in the acquisition of fear-potentiated startle using both explicit and contextual cues (Abstr.). Soc. Neurosci. **21:** 1224.
62. MCNISH, K., J. C. GEWIRTZ & M. DAVIS. 1996. Lesions of the dorsal hippocampus or bed nucleus of the stria terminalis (BNST) block freezing not enhancement of the startle reflex in a context previously paired with shock (Abstr.). Soc. Neurosci. **22:** 1381.
63. LEE, Y. & M. DAVIS. 1995. The role of the ventral hippocampus and the bed nucleus of the stria terminalis in the excitatory effect of corticotropin releasing hormone on the acoustic startle reflex (Abstr.). Soc. Neurosci. **21:** 1697.
64. DUNN, A. J. & C. W. BERRIDGE. 1990. Physiological and behavioral responses to corticotropin-releasing factor administration: Is CRF a mediator of anxiety or stress responses. Brain Res. Rev. **15:** 71-100.
65. SWERDLOW, N. R., M. A. GEYER, W. W. VALE & G. F. KOOB. 1986. Corticotropin-releasing factor potentiates acoustic startle in rats: Blockade by chlordiazepoxide. Psychopharmacology **88:** 147-152.
66. LIANG, K. C., K. R. MELIA, M. J. D. MISERENDINO, W. A. FALLS, S. CAMPEAU & M. DAVIS. 1992. Corticotropin-releasing factor: Long-lasting facilitation of the acoustic startle reflex. J. Neurosci. **12:** 2303-2312.
67. LEE, E. H. Y., Y. P. LIN, & T. H. YIN. 1988. Effects of lateral and medial septal lesions on various activity and reactivity measures in the rat. Physiol. Behav. **42:** 97-102.
68. MELIA, K. R., C. B. SANANES & M. DAVIS. 1992. Lesions of the central nucleus of the amygdala block the excitatory effects of septal ablation on the acoustic startle reflex. Physiol. Behav. **151:** 175-180.
69. LIANG, K. C., K. R. MELIA, S. CAMPEAU, W. A. FALLS, M. J. D. MISERENDINO & M. DAVIS. 1992. Lesions of the central nucleus of the amygdala, but not of the paraventricular nucleus of the hypothalamus, block the excitatory effects of corticotropin releasing factor on the acoustic startle reflex. J. Neurosci. **12:** 2313-2320.
70. MELIA, K. R. & M. DAVIS. 1991. Effects of septal lesions on fear-potentiated startle, and on the anxiolytic effects of buspirone and diazepam. Physiol. Behav. **49:** 603-611.
71. AMARAL, D. G. & M. P. WITTER. 1995. Hippocampal formation. *In* The Rat Nervous System. G. Paxinos, Ed.: 443-494. Academic Press. New York.
72. CANTERAS, N. & L. SWANSON. 1992. Projections of the ventral subiculum to the amygdala, septum, and hypothalamus: A PHAL anterograde tract-tracing study in the rat. J. Comp. Neurol. **324:** 180-194.
73. CULLINAN, W. E., J. P. HERMAN & S. J. WATSON. 1993. Ventral subicular interaction with the hypothalamic paraventricular nucleus: Evidence for a relay in the bed nucleus of the stria terminalis. J. Comp. Neurol. **332:** 1-20.
74. DEOLMOS, J., G. F. ALHEID & C. A. BELTRAMINO. 1985. Amygdala. *In* The Rat Nervous System. G. Paxinos, Ed.: 223-334. Academic Press. Orlando.

75. SANANES, C. B. & M. DAVIS. 1992. *N*-Methyl-D-aspartate lesions of the lateral and basolateral nuclei of the amygdala block fear-potentiated startle and shock sensitization of startle. Behav. Neurosci. **106:** 72-80.

76. DAVIS, M. 1992. The role of the amygdala in conditioned fear. *In* The Amygdala: Neurobiological Aspects of Emotion, Memory and Mental Dysfunction. J. Aggleton, Ed.: 255-305. John Wiley & Sons, Inc. New York.

Animal Models of Relevance to PTSD

ANN M. RASMUSSON [a] AND DENNIS S. CHARNEY

Psychiatry Service
Connecticut VA Healthcare System
950 Campbell Ave.
West Haven, Connecticut 06516

Posttraumatic stress disorder or PTSD[1] is a psychiatric disorder of considerable prevalence and morbidity and can affect persons of any age and ethnic or socioeconomic background.[2–10] It is, unfortunately, a far too common outcome of participation in war, affecting 15.2% of Vietnam theater veterans 20 years after the war.[11] Its prevalence may be even higher in inner city communities exposed to compound community trauma. In one small northeastern city, it was found to affect 67% of adolescents frequenting a community medical clinic for routine preventive health care.[12]

Reducing exposure to trauma would obviously be the most effective and immediate means of controlling the induction of PTSD and should be given the highest social priority. Beyond such efforts, understanding the means by which the extreme stress of trauma is neurobiologically transduced to produce PTSD may help in its prevention and treatment. Clinical studies have yielded, thus far, important empiric findings on ways in which the neurobiology of persons with PTSD differs from that of normal controls and from that of individuals with other psychiatric disorders. The most robust findings include apparent increased baseline activation of the noradrenergic system[13] and exaggerated noradrenergic responses to pharmacologic perturbation of that system,[14] decreased 24-hour urine cortisol levels,[15–19] opiate antagonist-sensitive increases in stress-induced analgesia,[20] apparent enhanced negative feedback in the hypothalamic-pituitary-adrenal axis system,[21] increased circulating thyroid hormone levels,[22] increased cerebrospinal fluid corticotropin-releasing factor,[23] and diminished hippocampal volume as measured by magnetic resonance imaging.[24–26]

These findings are invaluable in guiding further scientific studies. For example, it would be useful to know if these neurobiologic characteristics are sequelae of threshold trauma in all individuals or only in those individuals predisposed in some way to the development of PTSD. It would also be useful to know if any of these characteristics could be premorbid and thereby predispose to PTSD symptom formation on exposure to trauma. It is also not clear whether or how these findings relate to specific symptoms of PTSD. Also, are they early manifestations of PTSD or do they develop over time? Indeed, if these neurobiological stigmata of PTSD can be

[a] Address for correspondence: Ann M. Rasmusson, M.D., Psychiatry Service/116A, Connecticut VA Healthcare System, West Haven Campus, 950 Campbell Avenue, West Haven, CT 06516 (tel: (203)932-5711, ext. 2483; fax: (203)937-3886; page: (203)867-3132).

altered, will the manifestation of symptoms and the course of the disorder be altered? These questions can and should be answered in carefully designed clinical studies.

However, it is important to appreciate that the delineation of specific neurobiologic changes associated with PTSD in humans has been limited by the means available for probing human neurobiologic processes. For instance, numerous animal studies suggest that function of the dopaminergic, serotonergic, and excitatory amino acid systems is altered in particular parts of the brain during stress or from previous exposure to stress. However, alterations in these systems are generally more challenging to detect in humans.[27] Clinical inquiries are also limited by logistical difficulties in organizing human studies of the scale and prospective design needed to answer many of the important scientific questions just outlined. Thus, animal studies have been and remain important in guiding inquiries into the nature of the interactions between stress and potential neurobiologic systems involved in the induction and symptomatic manifestations of PTSD.

Therefore, this chapter sets forth a broad range of animal models that have potential for studying neurobiologic processes of apparent relevance to PTSD. Some of these models have already generated hypotheses of demonstrated clinical relevance to PTSD and other neuropsychiatric disorders. We then suggest a means of integrating these apparently disparate models to more effectively study neurobiologic endpoints of postulated significance to PTSD. We take into account several clinically observed phenomena that appear to influence the development of PTSD as well as consider previous recommendations regarding important characteristics to be possessed by valid animal models of PTSD.[28-31] Conversely, because progress in understanding and treating human disease largely depends on an iterative interplay between knowledge gained on the basic and clinical research fronts, we make recommendations regarding future directions for clinical inquiries based on data from the animal models discussed.

STRESS AND HIPPOCAMPAL NEURODEGENERATION IN ANIMALS AS A MODEL OF HIPPOCAMPAL PATHOLOGY IN PTSD

Potential Role of Glucocorticoids

Findings of hippocampal pathology in PTSD can be credited to one of the most fruitful, converging epistemologic exchanges yet between basic researchers investigating the effects of stress on the neural substrate and clinical researchers investigating the neurobiology of PTSD. First, multiple lines of evidence from primate and human research had indicated the importance of the intact hippocampus to memory function.[32-35] It had also long been observed that trauma victims frequently have fragmented memory for the details of traumatic events or even complete amnesia.[36,37] Then in the mid-1980s, researchers demonstrated the toxic effects of glucocorticoids to hippocampal neurons of rats and primates and postulated that stress may be deleterious to the structure and function of the hippocampus.[38-40] Subsequent animal studies indeed confirmed that chronic physical stress, such as restraint, or psychosocial stress, such as daily exposure to the aggression of a dominant conspecific, causes hippocampal damage. More recently, persons with PTSD were found to have deficits in hippocampus-dependent tests of immediate recall.[41] Finally, as noted in the introduction, magnetic resonance imaging was used to demonstrate decreases in the volume of the hippocampus of subjects with PTSD secondary to combat and civilian trauma.[24–26]

However, there is work yet to be done. The material substance of the hippocampal volume deficits in PTSD is not yet clear; human postmortem studies will be necessary for specification. Also, the precise etiology of the neuroanatomic and cognitive changes in PTSD has not yet been confirmed. It is possible that hippocampal pathology precedes and predisposes to the development of PTSD and associated cognitive deficits. Prospective, longitudinal clinical studies will be necessary to explore this possibility. Also, although extensive animal research suggests that stress-induced increases in circulating corticosteroids, relative glucoprivation or hypoxia in the presence of increased metabolic demand, and changes in hippocampal excitatory amino acids, cytosolic calcium, and serotonin may all contribute to hippocampal degeneration,[38–40,42–46] the results of clinical research raise questions about the relevance of these findings to PTSD.

In the animal models typically used to study the effects of stress on hippocampal morphology, significant hippocampal cell death resulted only from exposure to *chronic* restraint, *chronic* psychosocial stress, or *chronic, high* levels of corticosterone. Clinical observation, on the other hand, indicates that PTSD may result from exposure to even a single, brief, traumatic event.[31] However, this discrepancy may not be important because chronic stress appears to occur in individuals with PTSD due to physiologic, psychologic, and behavioral reexperiencing of the initial stress state when exposed to trauma reminders.[20,47–50] Indeed, animal studies of aversive conditioning suggest that such reexperiencing may include a recapitulation of the central neurochemical and peripheral neuroendocrine responses previously stimulated by the unconditioned stressor.[51]

A potential second discrepancy involves the role of high glucocorticoids in the mediation of hippocampal damage in PTSD. Several clinical studies, although not all, have found 24-hour urine free cortisol levels to be *low* in PTSD, rather than high.[15–19] However, hippocampal damage in animals has been shown to result from an adrenalectomy-induced low glucocorticoid state as well as from high glucocorticoid states.[52] The relevance of this finding to PTSD may be questionable because the hippocampal neuron drop-out due to adrenalectomy could be prevented by minimal corticosterone replacement. However, animals receiving corticosterone in these experiments were not subjected to stress; it is possible that the neuroprotective capacity of minimal glucocorticoid replacement would have been overcome under conditions of stress.

It is also important to note, however, that glucocorticoid levels measured during exposure to unconditioned trauma such as combat have been high.[53] It is therefore possible that significant hippocampal damage results from the neurobiologic responses to index traumatic events. Studies of the hippocampal volume of individuals with and without PTSD immediately after trauma exposure would address this possibility. However, if animal studies to date are relevant, they suggest that *repeated* exposure to unconditioned stress, as may occur in warfare, chronic domestic abuse, or cities plagued by community violence, would be necessary to engender measurable hippocampal volume deficits. Thus, it might be expected that hippocampal volume deficits would not be seen immediately after a single trauma exposure, even if acute symptoms of PTSD were present.

To further improve the fidelity of the match between animal models of stress-induced hippocampal damage and the clinical syndrome of PTSD, the neuroendocrine status of persons with PTSD needs to be further clarified. We do not yet know, for instance, if the low glucocorticoid output observed in individuals with PTSD is a static or a phasic phenomenon. If phasic, it would be important to know if this state relates to the presence of particular symptoms or to general periods of increased or decreased symptoms.[54] It would also be important to know if low cortisol output and the apparent increase in negative feedback in the HPA axis system appear early or late in the course of PTSD.

A Potential Role for Neuronal Growth Factors?

Of possible relevance to the hippocampal volume deficits seen in PTSD and other stress-related disorders are recent findings that brain-derived neurotrophic factor (BDNF) mRNA decreases in the hippocampus of rats exposed to acute restraint stress or chronic exogenous corticosterone.[55,56] BDNF is one of a family of central nervous system growth factors found at high levels in the hippocampus. It is essential to long-term potentiation (LTP),[57,58] a cellular process that underlies learning and memory,[59] and that thereby contributes to the maintenance of neuron viability via "activity-dependent neuronal competition."[60] In genetically altered mice with half the normal complement of BDNF ("heterozygous BDNF knock-outs"), LTP is impaired; when BDNF levels are restored to normal, LTP processes normalize.[61]

BDNF mRNA in the hippocampus of rats also decreases significantly in response to relatively moderate levels of footshock; in addition, it decreases when animals are *reexposed* to stimuli previously paired with footshock (A. Rasmusson and R. Duman, unpublished observations). Thus, decreases in BDNF levels in response to unconditioned and conditioned stress may underly the memory disturbances that immediately follow trauma as well as contribute to the long-term deficits in memory and hippocampal morphology observed in PTSD. If so, this may have treatment implications. The chronic administration of several antidepressants, including fluoxetine, which has clinical efficacy in the treatment of civilian but not combat trauma-related PTSD,[62] blocks the restraint stress-induced downregulation of hippocampal BDNF mRNA.[56] This suggests that it may be beneficial to prescribe antidepressants prior to trauma exposure (e.g., combat) to prevent neuropathologic changes in the hippocampus or other brain areas. It might also prove to be useful to treat patients with PTSD with antidepressants before exposure therapies in order to enhance cognitive processing and the therapeutic response. Or, as we come to better understand the molecular genetic regulation of potentially relevant neural substrates such as BDNF, it may be possible to develop new pharmacologic or molecular biologic strategies for preventing the neurodegenerative effects of stress.

Of course, at this point, it is not clear to what extent, if any, stress-induced decreases in BDNF in the hippocampus are deleterious. As suggested by Magarinos *et al.,*[46] apparently deleterious acute reactions to stress may ultimately prove to be neuroprotective; for instance, they may reduce metabolic demand. At another level of scrutiny, decrements in memory formation due to decreases in BDNF during trauma may advantageously "protect" an individual from remembering overwhelming traumatic material. On the other hand, fragmented and indistinct traumatic memories can be the source of severe psychic and physiologic dysequilibrium when triggered by conditioned stimuli or when they spontaneously intrude upon consciousness. Indeed, organization of such fragments under controlled treatment conditions is believed to be the therapeutic action of some PTSD exposure therapies.[63]

Further study of the behavioral, memory, and anatomic effects of stress-induced changes in hippocampal BDNF and other growth factors using animal models of controllable and uncontrollable stress or animal models of fear conditioning and extinction may help to clarify the contribution of these phenomena to stress-related psychopathology and to the neurodegenerative changes associated with PTSD. It would also be helpful to be able to measure BDNF levels in humans. It would be of interest to know whether CSF levels of BDNF are low in subjects with PTSD and/or whether CSF BDNF rises in parallel with symptom relief in response to antidepressants.

SENSITIZATION MODELS AND PTSD

PTSD has been characterized as a disorder resulting from sensitization,[64,65] a phenomenon whereby the response to a stressor becomes stronger on exposure to subsequent stressors of the same or lesser intensity. Up to this point, animal models used to study sensitization have largely focused on the capacity of psychostimulants to "cross-sensitize" with unconditioned stressors such as footshock or restraint stress to activate central monoamine systems and enhance behaviors such as locomotion or grooming. These studies of cross-sensitization between psychostimulants and nonpharmacologic stressors raise an interesting question regarding whether exposure to psychostimulants such as cocaine or amphetamine could facilitate the development of PTSD. Although this has not been demonstrated, the high prevalence of substance abuse and PTSD among combat participants in the Vietnam war suggests that the relationship between drug use and the development of PTSD bears closer investigation.

Other studies of sensitization have focused on the effects of nonpharmacologic stressors on behavioral or neurochemical responses to subsequent milder or simply different nonpharmacologic stressors. For example, Finlay et al.[66] showed a decrease in baseline noradrenergic system activation and an increase in shock-induced noradrenergic system activation in rats initially exposed to chronic cold stress. Kalivas and Duffy[67] showed sensitization of prefrontal cortical dopamine responses to repeated footshock. Pynoos et al.[68] repeatedly reexposed animals to a context near which they previously received footshock, while preventing the animals from directly encountering the chamber where footshock occurred. These animals developed an increased acoustic startle reflex as well as increased aggressivity, compared to animals that were shocked, but not reexposed to the shock context. This is the only demonstration of apparent sensitization of a behavioral response similar to a symptom of PTSD.

Investigators have generally demonstrated psychostimulant or nonpharmacologic stressor-induced sensitization of neurotransmitter release. This has been demonstrated in the dopaminergic[66,67,69–72] and noradrenergic[66,73–76] systems innervating several brain regions, including the prefrontal cortex, nucleus accumbens, hippocampus, and hypothalamus. Repeated stress has also been shown to increase the behavioral responses to a serotonin agonist[77] and to increase 5-HT$_2$ binding sites in the frontal cortex.[78]

The neurobiological mechanisms underlying sensitization have only partially been delineated. For instance, sensitization of the dopamine system appears to depend on activation of D$_1$, dopamine receptors in the ventral tegmental area, the site of the dopaminergic neuronal cell bodies that project to the nucleus accumbens and the medial prefrontal cortex. It has also been established that initiation of sensitization is critically dependent on normal fluctuating levels of cortisol as well as on increases in corticosterone associated with administration of psychostimulant drugs or other nonpharmacological stressors.[65] However, it is not yet clear how fluctuations in corticosterone contribute to sensitization and whether other neural factors may contribute.

It is also important to note that sensitization, strictly defined, has not been clearly demonstrated in clinical studies of PTSD, although it appears *en face* to account for the intensity of affect and physiological responses noted in patients with PTSD. Indeed, it may be difficult to ascertain whether a given stress reaction represents a stronger response to a previous stressor or simply the expression of a conditioned response to what was formerly a neutral and therefore apparently milder stimulus. Clarification of such issues will be helpful in ascertaining the relevance of the growing animal literature on sensitization to PTSD.

FEAR CONDITIONING AS A MEANS OF EXPLORING PROCESSES RELEVANT TO REEXPERIENCING, AVOIDANCE, AND HYPERAROUSAL SYMPTOMS IN PTSD

Results of research using animal models of aversive conditioning have led previous authors to suggest that the neural processes underlying fear conditioning and failure of extinction are important to the production of reexperiencing symptoms in PTSD.[79] Work by LeDoux *et al.*[80,81] and others[51,82] suggests that sensory cues associated with an unconditioned physical stressor become indelibly linked to that stressor via synaptic connections in the amygdala; such previously neutral stimuli then become capable of independently stimulating defensive responses formerly triggered by the unconditioned stressor. Normally, repeated reexposure to conditioned stressors in the absence of the unconditioned stressor reduces and eventually "extinguishes" the expression of defensive responses. This is thought to be due to the formation of new, more complex associations that compete with or actively inhibit expression of the original response-producing association.[79,83] Conversely, once a conditioned defense reaction is extinguished, it can be "reinstated" by even a single reexposure to the initial unconditioned stimulus.[84] In addition, extinction has been shown to be context specific, in that reexposure of an animal to the conditioned stressor in a context other than that in which extinction previously occurred results in reactivation of the conditioned stress response.[85,86]

It is important to note, however, that animal research has delineated the neural events underlying fear conditioning and extinction in presumably normal laboratory animals. Such work suggests that a resurgence of traumatic memories of the deaths of fellow soldiers is to be expected in combat veterans faced with the death of family members 20 years later. Similarly, a resurgence of distrust of authority figures may be expected to occur with job changes, if a perceived betrayal by an authority figure was "indelibly" linked to an earlier trauma. How then can the reexperiencing symptoms of PTSD be considered pathologic?

Foa et al.[30] suggest that in PTSD, stress responses to conditioned stimuli become overgeneralized; indeed, in more extreme cases of PTSD, reexperiencing appears to occur persistently without regard to the presence of definable conditioned triggers. Others have suggested that failures of extinction and/or of conditioned inhibition account for the persistence of reexperiencing symptoms in PTSD (M. Davis, this volume). We additionally suggest that the amplitude of autonomic, behavioral, neuroendocrine, and central neurochemical responses linked to conditioned stimuli is exaggerated in PTSD so that these responses interfere to a greater degree with daily function. We also suggest that the exaggerated amplitude of these responses may not necessarily depend on sensitization, but relate instead to the amplitude of the initial trauma reaction.

Increases in prefrontal cortical dopamine, serotonin, and norepinephrine release[51,87-89] as well as increases in serum corticosterone, hypervigilance and freezing[51,80,89,90] have consistently been observed during conditioning using inescapable footshock. When animals are subsequently reexposed to the tone and/or context previously associated with footshock, increases in freezing, ultrasonic vocalization, serum corticosterone, and prefrontal cortical norepinephrine, serotonin, and dopamine utilization are duplicated.[51,88,89,91,92] Of note, preconditioning amygdalectomy blocks unconditioned stress-induced defense responses,[51,80,93] while postconditioning amygdalectomy blocks conditioned stress-induced responses, including activation of the mesoprefrontal cortical monoamine systems.[51]

It has also been observed that freezing and prefrontal cortical dopamine utilization increase with increasing footshock levels during conditioning and tend to correlate with each other during both conditioning and reexposure of animals to stimuli previously paired with footshock. In addition, within individual animals, a strong correlation exists between the amount of time spent freezing during conditioning and during subsequent reexposure to conditioned stimuli (Rasmusson et al., unpublished observations). This is consistent with the finding that the medial prefrontal cortical dopamine response is regulated in parallel with the freezing response by the amygdala[51] and/or suggests that the mesoprefrontal cortical dopamine response directly influences the expression of defensive behaviors such as freezing; indeed previous studies have demonstrated that local application of a dopamine antagonist to the prefrontal cortex increases locomotion.[94] These findings also indicate that unconditioned and conditioned stress-induced central neurochemical and behavioral responses relate not only to the intensity of the index trauma, but also to the innate stress reactivity of individual animals.

These findings may relate to purported extinction deficits in PTSD. A large body of animal data now suggests that deficits as well as increases in prefrontal cortical dopamine and norepinephrine are detrimental to prefrontal cortical functioning.[95-99] Medial prefrontal cortical lesions, in turn, increase stress reactivity and novelty avoidance[100-102] as well as decrease the rate of extinction of conditioned behavioral defense responses.[103] Also, of particular relevance to the findings of increased noradrenergic system activation in PTSD,[13,14] transient inactivation of frontal cortex causes an increase in the firing of locus coeruleus neurons, consistent with a strong frontal cortical inhibitory influence on the tonic activity of these neurons.[104]

The capacity for attention and "working memory" provided by the prefrontal cortex allows the assimilation of relevant cues from the immediate external environment and from memory,[105,106] which may then be brought to bear on subcortically coordinated defense responses via direct neuronal projections from the medial prefrontal cortex to the amygdala[107,108] as well as from the medial prefrontal cortex to more distal neuronal centers involved in the execution of specific aspects of the conditioned stress response.[109–114] Morgan *et al.,*[103] reflecting on their finding that medial prefrontal cortical lesions decrease the rate of extinction of freezing in an aversive conditioning model, suggest that the medial prefrontal cortex promotes extinction by inhibiting amygdala-mediated conditioned stress responses during nonreinforcement. Clinical studies of prefrontal cortical function at baseline and in response to psychological or physical stress or to pharmcological perturbation will be important in empirically ascertaining the applicability of such frontal cortical deficit models to the behavioral and cognitive deficits in PTSD.

FEAR-POTENTIATED STARTLE AS A MODEL OF AROUSAL SYMPTOMS IN PTSD

Exaggerated startle is one of several symptoms of hyperarousal characteristic of PTSD.[1] However, clinical studies of startle in PTSD have yielded variable results. Although some clinical studies have reported exaggerated *baseline* startle in PTSD,[115] others have not.[116,117] Fear-potentiated startle, on the other hand, appears to be more unequivocally increased in this population.[118] Work based on animal fear-potentiated startle paradigms[82] has since led to a more careful look at the means by which increases in fear might contribute to variable findings in baseline startle studies. For instance, Grillon *et al.*[119] recently ascertained that subjects with PTSD may be more susceptible to the effects of contextual fear than are normal controls. Thus, to the extent that previous study populations were unfamiliar with the testing environment and thereby anticipated danger, "baseline" startle may have been inadvertently potentiated. This work further suggests that dysfunction of the bed nucleus of the stria terminalis or hippocampus may be involved in the pathology of PTSD based on animal studies of contextually conditioned fear.[120,121] Thus, further weight is added to other clinical studies implicating hippocampal dysfunction in this disorder.[24–26,41]

LEARNED HELPLESSNESS AS A MODEL OF ATTENTION AND CONCENTRATION DEFICITS IN PTSD

In "learned helplessness" models, rats are initially exposed to inescapable stress, usually consisting of repeated tailshock or footshock. In later sessions, animals are reexposed to footshock in a shuttlebox which allows the animal to escape by crossing over either once or twice to the other side. After exposure to the initial inescapable stress session, animals tend to separate into two groups, one that subsequently learns and one that fails to learn to escape footshock in a shuttlebox when the complexity of the task is increased so that two crossings are necessary to inactivate the shock (i.e., developed ''learned helplessness''). Of interest, membership in these two groups remains stable when animals are retested several weeks later.[122] In addition, central neurochemical correlates of membership in the ''fail to learn'' group include depletion of norepinephrine measured after testing,[123] increased hippocampal norepinephrine release when the animals are reexposed to mild restress,[76] and decreased prefrontal cortical intracellular serotonin stores after shuttlebox testing.[124]

We suggest that findings obtained with learned helplessness models may be more informative and useful in understanding PTSD if interpreted within an aversive conditioning framework. First, both models use inescapable footshock, although the level and duration of footshock used in the aversive conditioning studies discussed are substantially less than that typically used in learned helplessness models. This suggests that learned helplessness may not be a passive state, but rather result from the production of a competing, active freezing response. In addition, a state of learned helplessness is likely associated with marked increases in prefrontal cortical monoamine release, which may account for the previously noted finding of Petty *et al.*[124] on the depletion of prefrontal serotonin stores in animals that previously exhibited learned helplessness.

Of note, Foa *et al.*[30] previously suggested that the escape deficit seen in learned helplessness models may be attributable to ''increased fear and anxiety produced by unpredictable-uncontrollable shock [which] may compete for *limited attentional resources* and, thereby, reduce the processing capacity for [complex] task performance.'' We alternatively suggest that central neurochemical correlates of fear and anxiety (i.e., marked increases in prefrontal cortical monoamine release) produced by unpredictable-uncontrollable shock may actively limit attentional resources by compromising prefrontal cortical function and thereby reduce the processing capacity for [complex] tasks such as extinction in aversive conditioning models *and* shuttlebox escape in learned helplessness models.

IS THERE AN ANIMAL MODEL FOR PERITRAUMATIC DISSOCIATION?

Several clinical studies now suggest that peritraumatic dissociation is associated with an increase in the subsequent development of PTSD[125-128] and that peritraumatic dissociation in predicted, to some extent, by the magnitude of the index trauma.[125,129,130] In Vietnam veterans, for instance, peritraumatic dissociation predicts the development of PTSD better than does combat exposure, total time in Vietnam, and substance abuse while in Vietnam.[125] Subsequent dissociative symptoms and flashbacks in response to stressful events were also more frequent in those subjects who dissociated during the index traumatic event.[128] An understanding of the neural state underlying dissociation may thus provide clues as to what factors facilitate the development of PTSD. Unfortunately, few neurobiologic studies of dissociation have been done besides that of Demitrick *et al.*[131] who demonstrated a correlation between degree of dissociation and CSF levels of homovanillic acid, the major metabolite of dopamine, as well as 5-hydroxyindole-acetic acid, the major metabolite of serotonin. Given the anxiety typically observed in subjects having spinal taps, these findings may reflect stress-induced increases in central nervous system monoamine release. Indeed, research in nonhuman primates suggests that CSF homovanillic acid levels may largely reflect cortical dopaminergic activity.[132] Thus, a parallel with the stress state characterized in animals using aversive conditioning models is suggested.

EARLY DEVELOPMENTAL EXPERIENCE VERSUS GENETIC ENDOWMENT AS DETERMINANTS OF STRESS SENSITIVITY

That there may be a relatively stable variance among rats of the same outbred species in the magnitude of unconditioned and conditioned stress-induced behavioral and central neurochemical responses is consistent with a large body of human developmental data supporting the idea that individuals, even infants, differ in their response to anxiety-provoking situations and that these differences are relatively stable.[133,134] These data have led some investigators to invoke the concept of emotional intelligence as a stable individual trait that influences emotional receptivity as well as expressivity.[135] One might concretize these concepts to suggest that relatively stable biologic factors regulate the central neurochemical stress responses that underly emotional reactivity and related information-processing capacities. It is possible that such factors are genetic; for instance, it has been observed that parents with anxiety disorders are more likely to have children with early behavioral inhibition when confronted with the unfamiliar, a trait that in turn is associated with the later development of anxiety disorders.[134]

Over the last several years, however, an impressive body of animal data has emerged illustrating the tremendous influence of early developmental experience on later behavioral manifestations of emotional reactivity as well as on central neurochemical and neuroendocrine responses to stress. In one case, macaque monkey mothers were subjected to variable, unpredictable foraging conditions when their infants were between the ages of 3 and 6 months. These infants grew into adults that were markedly more timid, less social, and more subordinate than control monkeys whose mothers were subjected to low, constant foraging conditions.[136] The affected monkeys also exhibited emotional reactions to yohimbine[137] that qualitatively compared with the responses of inhibited children who withdraw when faced with the unfamiliar, exhibit excessive autonomic arousal in response to a challenge or novelty, and show a predisposition to the later development of anxiety disorders.[134,138–140] Of note, the period of variable foraging was imposed during the neurodevelopmental period when infant monkeys first exhibit a capacity for prefrontal cortex-dependent working memory tasks, wherein internal and external stimuli can be held together "in mind" and used to direct action. This neurodevelopmental epoch in monkeys also happens to correspond to the age of 9–10 months in human infants, when object permanence begins to evidence itself.

Interestingly, monkeys raised by mothers subjected to variable foraging also had increased cerebrospinal fluid corticotropin-releasing factor levels as adults.[141] Studies in rats have also demonstrated differences in hypothalamic-pituitary-adrenal axis functioning associated with differences in early experience. For instance, rats handled in the postnatal period so that increased maternal attention is elicited, show attenuated neuroendocrine, anatomical, and cognitive impairments usually related to the aged hippocampus[142]; this appears to result from the development of enhanced negative feedback control over hypothalamic-pituitary-adrenal axis function due to increased glucocorticoid receptor density in the hippocampus.[143] Compared to rats that were handled as infants, adult rats subjected to prolonged maternal separation or early nonhandling showed increased corticosterone release during restraint stress. Hypothalamic corticotropin-releasing factor messenger RNA was also highest in rats subjected to maternal separation, next highest in the nonhandled rats, and lowest in the handled rats.[144] In another study,[145] adult rats previously isolated from their mothers had increases in median eminence and parabrachial nucleus CRF, findings that parallel increased CSF CRF levels in PTSD subjects.[23] The rats with a history of maternal separation also had increases in basal and stress-induced ACTH concentrations.

These studies in animals suggest that early childhood experiences, such as neglect, may induce individual stress reaction profiles that contribute to the later development of PTSD in response to trauma. This has also been suggested by clinical studies. For instance, Bremner et al.[146] report a relatively high frequency of childhood physical abuse in a cohort of subjects with combat-related PTSD. The incidence of childhood neglect in this sample was not explored. Lipschitz et al.[147,148] found that of 70 consecutive adolescents admitted to an inner city inpatient psychiatric unit, 50% had a diagnosis of PTSD. Eighty percent of the group with PTSD had a history of sexual abuse. Of all patients who had a history of sexual abuse, including some without PTSD, 50% reported emotional neglect, whereas 61% reported physical neglect. It would therefore be interesting and important to investigate in this sample to what extent neglect may have been associated with the development of PTSD among those who had been traumatized, whether sexually or otherwise.

CONSTRUCTION OF AN "IDEAL" ANIMAL MODEL OF PTSD?

Previous authors have addressed several issues regarding essential characteristics of a valid animal model of PTSD. Earlier discussions focused on characteristics of the stressor that influence manifestations of PTSD symptom-like sequelae in animals.[28-30] In an incisive review and reanalysis of a complex body of earlier animal research literature, Foa et al.[30] note that animals exposed to uncontrollable and/or unpredictable stressors are much more likely to develop behavioral and biochemical manifestations similar to core PTSD symptoms.[1] Animals so treated developed more pronounced (a) contextual fear (related to symptoms of "increased arousal"); (b) fear to explicitly conditioned aversive stimuli (related to symptoms of "reexperiencing"); (c) opioid-mediated stress-induced analgesia (related to symptoms of "numbing"); (d) impairments in active avoidance—influenced by the complexity of cognition required, dependent on limited-capacity attentional resources, mediated in part by the opioid system, and mitigated by antianxiety drugs (related to "difficulties with attention and concentration"); and (e) enhanced passive avoidance, mitigated by antianxiety drugs (related to "avoidance of stimuli previously associated with trauma").

Yehuda and Antelman[31] subsequently proposed five criteria to be met by models meant to address the induction rather than the symptom manifestations of PTSD: (1) even very brief stressors should be capable of inducing biological and behavioral sequelae of PTSD; (2) the stressor should be capable of producing PTSD sequelae in a dose-dependent manner; (3) the stressor should produce biological alterations that persist over time or become more pronounced with time; (4) the stressor should induce biobehavioral alterations that have the potential for bidirectional expression; and (5) interindividual variability in response to a stressor should be present as a function of either experience (e.g., stress history and poststressor adaptations) or genetics, or an interaction of the two. These authors diminished the potential utility of such models as "inescapable shock" or "learned helplessness," stating that they make use of relatively prolonged exposures to stress (violating their first criterion). They also argued that the behavioral deficits induced by these models had not been demonstrated to be dependent on the intensity of the initial stressor. These authors, in turn, proposed that "time-dependent sensitization" meets the criteria for a model that addresses processes critical to the induction of PTSD. In time-dependent sensitization, "one exposure to a stressor (e.g., injection of a pharmacologic agent or immobilization stress) is associated with an extremely long-lasting alteration in the subsequent responsiveness of the organism to pharmacological or nonpharmacological stressors."

We, in turn, suggest that a melding of these two points of view would be most beneficial in developing an understanding of the neurobiologic events necessary to induce or promulgate the core symptoms of PTSD. First, biobehavioral responses selected for measurement in any animal model of PTSD should have arguable relevance to the clinical manifestations of the disorder. For instance, measurement of activation of the central and peripheral noradrenergic systems would be logical, because aberrations in this system have already been noted in clinical studies. Measurement of the stress-induced activation of the prefrontal cortical dopamine system is of plausible relevance because prefrontal cortical dopamine levels have been shown to influence attention and concentration, processes that are impaired in PTSD. In contrast, it would be difficult to argue that measurement of cocaine-induced increases in striatal or accumbens dopamine, although subject to time-dependent sensitization, is of interest, unless it can be shown that monoamine reuptake blockers predispose to the development of PTSD. Secondly, investigations should focus on whether biobehavioral responses selected for measurement are governed by phenomena that appear to influence the development of PTSD; namely, the duration, intensity, controllability, and predictability of the unconditioned stressor. In addition, the expression of these responses should be subject to the opposing processes of extinction and sensitization.[28,30,31,65,79]

Thus, we propose that no single animal model will address the myriad facets of PTSD or the myriad factors that may conspire to produce a PTSD-like syndrome. Any experimental approach to modeling PTSD should therefore involve an exploration of the impact of a range of experimental manuevers on animal behavior or biochemical endpoints with plausible or proven face validity. To take, as an example, the question of whether hippocampal BDNF might play a role in the development of hippocampal volume deficits in PTSD, one might ask if the degree or duration of the stress-induced decrease in hippocampal BDNF is subject to the duration or intensity of the unconditioned stressor, whether controllability and predictability of the stressor influence this response, and whether this response can be conditioned to contextual or explicit cues previously paired with the unconditioned stressor. One might also investigate whether the conditioned stress-induced decrease in hippocampal BDNF can be extinguished, whether its extinction can be interfered with, and whether it can be sensitized. For example, the animal model of sensitization developed by Pynoos *et al.*[68] may be reasonable in which to test whether decreases in hippocampal BDNF sensitize in parallel with the behavioral responses measured. One would also want to explore whether interindividual differences in this response occur, either using genetically disparate strains of animals with measureably different behavioral stress responses or looking for individual differences within single strains. The variations in the BDNF response should then predict the induction of PTSD-compatible behavioral or anatomic sequelae.

In summary, we do not believe that there is a single ideal animal model of PTSD for the purposes of scientific inquiry. Control of the experimental procedures used to induce stress of varying kinds, patterns, and intensity and measurement of the number of endpoint variables likely to be relevant to the induction and subsequent manifestations of a range of PTSD-like sequelae require that many different and complementary approaches be pursued. Based on the discussion in this chapter, we also suggest that any number of vulnerabilities may predispose to the development of PTSD; however, a predisposition towards enhanced reactivity of the mesocortico-limbic monoamine systems, by whatever mechanism(s), may be of central significance.

REFERENCES

1. AMERICAN PSYCHIATRIC ASSOCIATION. 1994. Diagnostic and Statistical Manual of Mental Disorders, Fourth Edition. Washington, DC. American Psychiatric Association.
2. TERR, L. 1985. Psychic trauma in children and adolescents. Psychiatr. Clin. North Am. **8:** 815-835.
3. HELZER, J., L. ROBINS & L. MCEVOY. 1987. Post-traumatic stress disorder in the general population. Findings of the epidemiologic catchment area survey. N. Engl. J. Med. **317:** 1630-1634.
4. PYNOOS, R., C. FREDERICK, K. NADER, W. ARROYO, A. STEINBERG, S. ETH, F. NUNEZ & L. FAIRBANKS. 1987. Life threat and posttraumatic stress in school-age children. Arch. Gen. Psychiatry **44:** 1057-1063.
5. COONS, P., E. BOWMAN, T. PELLOW & P. SCHNEIDER. 1988. Post-traumatic aspects of the treatment of victims of sexual abuse and incest. Psychiatr. Clin. North Am. **11:** 581-590.
6. SONNENBERG, S. 1988. Victims of violence and post-traumatic stress disorder. Psychiatr. Clin. North Am. **11:** 581-590.
7. BRESLAU, N., G. C. DAVIS & P. ANDRESKI. 1991. Traumatic events and post traumatic stress disorder in an urban population of young adults. Arch. Gen. Psychiatry **48:** 216-222.
8. DAVIDSON, J., D. HUGHES, D. BLAZER & L. GEORGE. 1991. Posttraumatic stress disorder in the community: An epidemiological study. Psychol. Med. **21:** 713-721.
9. NADER, K. & R. PYNOOS. 1993. A preliminary study of PTSD and grief among the children of Kuwait following the Gulf crisis. Br. J. Clin. Psychol. **32:** 407-413.
10. GOENJIAN, A. 1993. A mental health relief programme in Armenia after the 1988 earthquake. Br. J. Psychiatry **163:** 230-239.
11. KULKA, R., W. SCHLENGER, J. FAIRBANK, R. HOUGH, B. JORDAN, C. MARMOR & WEISS. 1990. Trauma and the Vietnam War Generation. Brunner/Mazel. New York.
12. HOROWITZ, K., S. WEINE & J. JEKEL. 1995. PTSD symptoms in urban adolescent girls: Compounded community trauma. J. Am. Acad. Child Adolesc. Psychiatry **34:** 1353-1361.
13. KOSTEN, T., J. MASON, E. GILLER, R. OSTROFF & L. HARKNESS. 1987. Sustained urinary norepinephrine and epinephrine elevation in post-traumatic stress disorder. Psychoneuroendocrinology. **12:** 13-20.

14. SOUTHWICK, S., J. KRYSTAL, C. MORGAN, D. JOHNSON, L. NAGY, A. NICOLAOU, G. HENINGER & D. CHARNEY. 1993. Abnormal noradrenergic function in posttraumatic stress disorder. Arch. Gen. Psychiatry **50:** 266-274.

15. MASON, J. W., E. L. GILLER, T. R. KOSTEN, R. B. OSTROFF & L. RODD. 1986. Urinary-free cortisol levels in post-traumatic stress disorder patients. J. Nerv. Ment. Dis. **174:** 145-159.

16. PITTMAN, R. & S. ORR. 1990. Twenty-four hour urinary cortisol and catecholamine excretion in combat-related posttraumatic stress disorder. Biol. Psychiatry **27:** 245-247.

17. YEHUDA, R., S. M. SOUTHWICK, G. NUSSBAUM, V. WAHBY, E. L. GILLER & J. W. MASON. 1990. Low urinary cortisol excretion in patients with posttraumatic stress disorder. J. Nerv. Ment. Dis. **178:** 366-369.

18. YEHUDA, R., D. BOISONEAU, J. W. MASON & E. L. GILLER. 1993. Relationship between lymphocyte glucocorticoid receptor number and urinary-free cortisol excretion in mood, anxiety, and psychotic disorder. Biol. Psychiatry **34:** 18-25.

19. YEHUDA, R., B. KAHANA, K. BINDER-BRYNES, S. SOUTHWICK, S. ZEMELMAN, J. MASON & W. GILLER. 1995. Low urinary cortisol excretion in Holocaust survivors with posttraumatic stress disorder. Am. J. Psychiatry **152:** 982-986.

20. PITTMAN, R., B. VAN DER KOLK, S. ORR & M. GREENBERG. 1990. Naloxone-reversible analgesic response to combat-related stimuli in posttraumatic stress disorder. Arch. Gen. Psychiatry **47:** 541-544.

21. YEHUDA, R., E. GILLER, R. LEVENGOOD, S. SOUTHWICK & L. SIEVER. 1995. Hypothalamic-pituitary-adrenal functioning in posttraumatic stress disorder. *In* Neurobiological and Clinical Consequences of Stress: From Normal Adaptation to PTSD. M. J. Friedman, D. S. Charney & A. Y. Deutch, Eds. Lippincott-Raven, Philadelphia, pp. 351-365.

22. MASON, J., S. SOUTHWICK, R. YEHUDA, S. WANG, S. RINEY, D. BREMNER, D. JOHNSON, H. LIBIN, D. BLAKE, G. ZHOU, F. GUSMAN & D. CHARNEY. 1995. Elevation of serum free T3, total T3, TBG, and total T4 levels in combat-related posttraumatic stress disorder. Arch. Gen. Psychiatry **51:** 629-641.

23. BREMNER, J., J. LICINIO, A. DARNELL, J. KRYSTAL, M. OWENS, S. SOUTHWICK, C. NEMEROFF & D. CHARNEY. 1997. Elevated CSF corticotropin-releasing factor concentrations in posttraumatic stress disorder. Am. J. Psychiatry, in press.

24. BREMNER, J., P. RANDALL, T. SCOTT, R. BRONEN, J. SEIBYE, S. SOUTHWICK, R. DELANEY, G. MCCARTHY, D. CHARNEY & R. INNIS. 1995. MRI-based measurement of hippocampal volume in combat-related posttraumatic stress disorder. Am. J. Psychiatry **152:** 973-981.

25. STEIN, M., C. HANNAH, C. KOVEROLA & B. MCCLARTY. 1995. Neuroanatomic and cognitive correlates of early abuse. Am. Psychiatric Assoc. Syllabus Proc. Summary **148:** 113.

26. GURVITS, T., M. SHENTON, H. HOKAMA, H. OHTA, N. LASKO, M. GILBERTSON, S. ORR, R. KIKINIS, F. JOLESZ, R. MCCARLEY & R. PITMAN. 1996. Magnetic resonance imaging study of hippocampal volume in chronic, combat-related posttraumatic stress disorder. Biol. Psychiatry **40:** 1091-1099.

27. RASMUSSON, A. M., M. A. RIDDLE, J. F. LECKMAN, G. M. ANDERSON & D. J. COHEN. 1990. Neurotransmitter assessment in neuropsychiatric disorders of childhood. *In* Application of Basic Neuroscience to Child Psychiatry. S. I. Deutsch, A. Weizman & R. Weizman, Eds. pp. 41-47. Plenum Publishers. New York.

28. VAN DER KOLK, B., M. GREENBERG, H. BOYD & J. H. KRYSTAL. 1985. Inescapable shock, neurotransmitters, and addiction to trauma: Toward a psychobiology of post traumatic stress. Biol. Psychiatry **20:** 314-325.

29. KRYSTAL, J. H. 1990. Animal models for posttraumatic stress disorder. *In* Biological Assessment and Treatment of Posttraumatic Stress Disorder, Progress in Psychiatry. Giller, E. L. Ed. American Psychiatric Press, Inc. Washington, DC. pp. 1-26.

30. FOA, E., R. ZINBARG & B. ROTHBAUM. 1992. Uncontrollability and unpredictability in post-traumatic stress disorder: An animal model. Psychol. Bull. **112:** 218-238.

31. YEHUDA, R. & S. ANTELMAN. 1993. Criteria for rationally evaluating animal models of posttraumatic stress disorder. Biol. Psychiatry **33:** 479-486.

32. SCOVILLE, W. & B. MILNER. 1957. Loss of recent memory after bilateral hippocampal lesions. J. Neurol. Psychiatry **20:** 11-21.

33. DELANEY, R., A. ROSEN, R. MATTSON & R. NOVELLY. 1980. Memory function in focal epilepsy: A comparison of non-surgical, unilateral temporal lobe and frontal lobe samples. Cortex **16:** 103-117.

34. ZOLA-MORGAN, S. & L. SQUIRE. 1990. The primate hippocampal formation: Evidence for a time-limited role in memory storage. Science **250:** 288-290.

35. SQUIRE, L. & S. ZOLA-MORGAN. 1991. The medial temporal lobe memory system. Science **253:** 1380-1386.

36. GRINKER, R. & J. SPIEGEL. 1943. War Neuroses in North Africa. Josiah Macy Jr. Foundation. New York.

37. HENDERSON, J. & M. MOOR. 1944. The psychoneurosis of war. N. Engl. J. Med. **230:** 274-278.

38. SAPOLSKY, R. 1985. A mechanism for glucocorticoid toxicity in the hippocampus: Increased neuronal vulnerability to metabolic insults. J. Neurosci. **5:** 1228-1232.

39. MCEWEN, B., E. DE KLOET & W. ROSTENE. 1986. Adrenal steroid receptors and actions in the nervous system. Phys. Rev. **66:** 1121-1189.

40. SAPOLSKY, R. 1986. Glucocorticoid toxicity in the hippocampus: Synergy with an excitotoxin. Neuroendocrinology **43:** 440-446.

41. BREMNER, J., T. SCOTT, R. DELANEY, S. SOUTHWICK, J. MASON, D. JOHNSON, R. INNIS, G. MCCARTHY & D. CHARNEY. 1993. Deficits in short-term memory in post-traumatic stress disorder. Am. J. Psychiatry **150:** 1015-1019.

42. MOGHADDAM, B., M. BOLINAO, B. STEIN-BEHRENS & R. SAPOLSKY. 1994. Glucocorticoids mediate the stress-induced extracellular accumulation of glutamate. Brain Res. **655:** 251-254.

43. SAPOLSKY, R., S. BROOKE & B. STEIN-BEHRENS. 1995. Methodologic issues in studying glucocorticoid-induced damage to neurons. J. Neurosci. Methods **58:** 1-15.

44. DASH, R., M. LAWRENCE, D. HO & R. SAPOLSKY. 1996. A herpes simplex virus vector overexpressing the glucose transporter gene protects the rat dentate gyrus from an antimetabolite toxin. Exp. Neurol. **137:** 43-48.

45. SAPOLSKY, R. 1996. Why stress is bad for your brain. Science **273:** 749-750.

46. MAGARINOS, A., B. MCEWEN, G. FLUGGE & E. GUCHS. 1996. Chronic psychosocial stress causes apical dendritic atrophy of hippocampal CA3 pyramidal neurons in subordinate tree shrews. J. Neurosci. **16:** 3534-3540.

47. MALLOY, P., J. FAIRBANK & T. KEANE. 1983. Validation of a multimethod assessment of posttraumatic stress disorders in Vietnam veterans. J. Consult. Clin. Psychol. **51:** 488-494.

48. BLANCHARD, E., L. KOLB, R, GERARDI, P. RYAN & T. PALLMEYER. 1986. Cardiac response to relevant stimuli as an adjunctive tool for diagnosing post-traumatic stress disorder in Vietnam veterans. Behav. Ther. **17:** 592-606.

49. SOLOMON, Z., R. GARB, A. BLEICH & D. GRUPPER. 1987. Reactivation of combat-related posttraumatic stress disorder. Am. J. Psychiatry. **144:** 51-55.

50. PITTMAN, R., S. ORR, D. FORGUE, J. DE JONG & J. CLAIBORN. 1987. Psychophysiologic assessment of post-traumatic stress disorder imager in Vietnam combat veterans. Arch. Gen. Psychiatry **44:** 970-975.

51. GOLDSTEIN, L., A. RASMUSSON, B. BUNNEY & R. ROTH. 1996. Role of the amygdala in the coordination of behavioral, neuroendocrine, and prefrontal cortical monoamine responses to psychological stress in the rat. J. Neurosci. **16:** 4787-4798.

52. SAPOLSKY, R., B. BEHRENS & M. ARMANINI. 1991. Long-term adrenalectomy causes loss of dentate gyrus and pyramidal neurons in the adult hippocampus. Exp. Neurobiol. 114: 246-249.

53. HOWARD, J., J. OLNEY, J. FRAWLEY, R. PETERSON, L. SMITH, J. DAVIS, S. GUERRA & W. DIBRELL. 1955. Studies of adrenal function in combat and wounded soldiers. Ann. Surg. 141: 314-320.

54. WANG, S., J. WILSON & J. MASON. 1996. Stages of decompenmsation in combat-related posttraumatic stress disorder: A new conceptual model. Integr. Physiol. Behav. Sci. 31: 237-253.

55. SMITH, M., S. MAKINO, R. KVETNANSKY & R. POST. 1995. Stress alters the expression of brain-derived neurotrophic factor and neurotrophin-3 mRNAs in the hippocampus. J. Neurosci. 15: 1768-1777.

56. NIBUYA, M., S. MORINOBU & R. DUMAN. 1995. Regulation of BDNF and trkB mRNA in rat brain by chronic electroconvulsive seizure and antidepressant drug treatments. J. Neurosci. 15: 7539-7547.

57. KANG, H., E. SCHUMAN. 1995. Long-lasting neurotrophin-induced enhancement of synaptic transmission in the adult hippocampus. Science 267: 1658-1662.

58. FIGUROV, A., L. POZZO-MILLER, P. OLAFSSON, T. WANG & B. LU. 1996. Regulation of synaptic responses to high-frequency stimulation and LTP by neurotrophins in the hippocampus. Nature 381: 706-709.

59. BLISS, T. & G. COLLINGRIDGE. 1993. A synaptic model of memory: Long-term potentiation in the hippocampus. Nature 361: 31-39.

60. SHATZ, C. 1990. Competitive interactions between retinal ganglion cells during prenatal development. J. Neurobiol. 21: 197-211.

61. PATTERSON, S., T. ABEL, T. DEUEL, K. MARTIN, J. ROSE & E. KANDEL. 1996. Recombinant BDNF rescues deficits in basal synaptic transmission and hippocampal LTP in BDNF knockout mice. Neuron 16: 1137-1145.

62. VAN DER KOLK, B., D. DREYFUSS, M. MICHAELS, D. SHERA, R. BERKOWITZ, R. FISLER & G. SAXE. 1994. Fluoxetine in posttraumatic stress disorder. J. Clin. Psychiatry 55: 517-522.

63. SHAPIRO, F. 1995. Eye Movement Desensitization and Reprocessing: Basic Principles, Protocols, and Procedures. Guilford Press. New York.

64. ANTELMAN, S. 1988. Stressor-induced sensitization to subsequent stress: implications for the development and treatment of clinical disorders. In Sensitization in the Central Nervous System. P. W. Kalivas & C. D. Barnes, Eds.: 227-259. Academic Press. New York.

65. SORG, B. & P. KALIVAS. 1995. Stress and neuronal sensitization. In Neurobiological and Clinical Consequences of Stress: From Normal Adaptation to PTSD. M. Friedman, D. Charney & A. Deutch, Eds.: 83-102. Lippincott-Raven Publishers. Philadelphia.

66. FINLEY, J., M. ZIGMOND & E. ABERCROMBIE. 1995. Increased dopamine and norepinephrine release in medial prefrontal cortex induced by acute and chronic stress: effects of diazepam. Neuroscience 64: 619-628.

67. KALIVAS, P. & P. DUFFY. 1989. Similar effect of daily cocaine and stress on mesocorticolimbic dopamine neurotransmission in the rat. Biol. Psychiatry 25: 913-928.

68. PYNOOS, R., R. RITZMANN, A. STEINBERG, A. GOENJIAN & I. PRISECARU. 1996. A behavioral animal model of posttraumatic stress disorder featuring repeated exposure to situational reminders. Biol. Psychiatry 39: 129-134.

69. BLANC, G., D. HERVE, H. SIMON, A. LISOPRAWSKI, J. GLOWINSKI & J.-P. TASSIN. 1980. Response to stress of mesocortical-frontal dopaminergic neurons after long-term isolation. Nature 284: 265-276.

70. CAGGIULA, A., S. ANTELMAN, E. AUL, S. KNOPF & D. EDWARDS. 1989. Prior stress attenuates the analgesic response but sensitizes the corticosterone and cortical dopamine responses to stress 10 days later. Psychopharmacology 99: 233-237.

71. SORG, B. & P. KALIVAS. 1991. Effects of cocaine and footshock stress on extracellular dopamine levels in the ventral striatum. Brain Res. **559:** 29-36.

72. GRESCH, P., A. AVED, M. ZIGMOND & J. FINLAY. 1994. Stress-induced sensitization of dopamine and norepinephrine efflux in medial prefrontal cortex of the rat. J. Neurochem. **63:** 575-583.

73. KVETNANSKY, R., M. PALKOVITS, A. MITRO, T. TORDA & L. MIKULAJ. 1977. Catecholamines in individual hypothhalamic nuclei of acutely and repeatedly stressed rats. Neuroendocrinology **23:** 257-267.

74. ADELL, A., C. GARCIA-MARQUEZ, A. ARMARIO & E. GELPI. 1988. Chronic stress increases serotonin and noradrenaline in rat brain and sensitizes their responses to a further acute stress. J. Neurochem. **50:** 1678-1681.

75. NISENBAUM, L., M. SIGMOND, A. SVED & E. ABERCROMBIE. 1991. Prior exposure to chronic stress results in enhanced synthesis and release of hippocampal norepinephrine in response to a novel stressor. J. Neurosci. **11:** 1478-1484.

76. PETTY, F., Y.-L. CHAE, G. KRAMER, S. JORDAN & L. WILSON. 1994. Learned helplessness sensitizes hippocampal norepinephrine to mild restress. Biol. Psychiatry **35:** 903-908.

77. OHI, K., M. MIKUNI & K. TAKAHASHI. 1989. Stress adaptation and hypersensitivity in 5-HT neuronal systems after repeated foot shock. Pharmacol. Biochem. Behav. **34:** 603-608.

78. TORDA, T., J. CULAMAN, E. CECHOVA & K. MURGAS. 1988. 3H-ketanserin (serotonin type 2) binding in rat frontal cortex: effect of immobilization stress. Endocrinol. Exp. **22:** 99-105.

79. CHARNEY, D., A. DEUTCH, J. KRYSTAL, S. SOUTHWICK & M. DAVIS. 1993. Psychobiologic mechanisms of posttraumatic stress disorder. Arch. Gen. Psychiatry **50:** 294-305.

80. LEDOUX, J., L. ROMANSKI & A. XAGORARIS. 1989. Indelibility of subcortical emotional memories. J. Cognit. Neurosci. **1:** 238-243.

81. LEDOUX, J., P. CICCHETTI, A. XAGORARIS & L. ROMANSKI. 1990. The lateral amygdaloid nucleus: sensory interface of the amygdala in fear conditioning. J. Neurosci. **10:** 1062-1069.

82. DAVIS, M. 1986. Pharmacological and anatomical analysis of fear conditioning using the fear-potentiated startle paradigm. Behav. Neurosci. **100:** 814-824.

83. KONORSKI, J. 1948. Conditioned Reflexes and Neuronal Organization. Cambridge University Press. London, England.

84. MCALLISTER, W. & D. MCALLISTER. 1988. Reconditioning of extinguished fear after a one-year delay. Bull. Psychonomic Soc. **26:** 463-466.

85. BOUTON, M. & R. BULLES. 1985. Contexts, event memories, and extinction. *In* Context & Learning. P. Balsam & K. Tomic, Eds.: 133-166. Lawrence Erlbaum Associates. Hillsdale, NJ.

86. BOUTON, M. & D. KING. 1986. Effect of context with mixed histories of reinforcement and nonreinforcement. J. Exp. Psychol. Anim. Behav. **12:** 4-15.

87. ABERCROMBIE, E., K. KEEFE, F. DIFRISCHIA & M. ZIGMOND. 1989. Differential effects of stress on *in vivo* dopamine release in striatum, nucleus accumbens, and medial prefrontal cortex, J. Neurochem. **52:** 1655-1658.

88. INOUE, T., T. KOYAMA & I. YAMASHITA. 1993. Effect of conditioned fear stress on serotonin metabolism in the rat brain. Pharmacol. Biochem. Behav. **44:** 371-374.

89. GOLDSTEIN, L., A. RASMUSSON, B. BUNNEY & R. ROTH. 1994. The NMDA glycine site antagonist (+)-HA-966 selectively regulates conditioned stress-induced metabolic activation of the mesoprefrontal cortical dopamine but not serotonin systems: A behavioral, neuroendocrine, and neurochemical study in the rat. J. Neurosci. **14:** 4937-4950.

90. FANSELOW, M. 1980. Conditional and unconditional components of post-shock freezing. J. Biol. Sci. **15:** 177-182.

91. HERMAN, J. P., D. GUILLONNEAU, R. DANTZER, B. SCATTON, L. SEMERDJIAN-ROUGUIER & M. LEMOAL. 1982. Differential effects of inescapable footshocks and of stimuli

previously paired with inescapable footshocks on dopamine turnover in cortical and limbic areas of the rat. Life Sci. **30:** 2207-2214.

92. DEUTCH, A. Y., S.-Y. TAM & R. H. ROTH. 1985. Footshock and conditioned stress increase in 3,4-dihyroxyphenylacetic acid (DOPAC) in the ventral tegmental area but not substantia nigra. Brain Res. **333:** 143-146.

93. DAVIS, M., J. M. HITCHCOCK, M. B. BOWERS, C. W. BERRIDGE, K. R. MELIA & R. H. ROTH. 1994. Stress-induced activation of prefrontal cortex dopamine turnover: blockade by lesions of the amygdala. Brain Res. **664:** 207-210.

94. MORENCY, M., R. STEWART & R. BENINGER. 1985. Effects of unilateral microinjections of sulpiride into the medial prefrontal cortex on circling behavior of rats. Prog. Neuro-Psychopharmacol. Biol. Psychiatry **9:** 735-738.

95. ARNSTEN, A., J. CAI & P. GOLDMAN-RAKIC. 1988. The alpha-2 adrenergic agonist guanfacine improves memory in aged monkeys without sedative or hypotensive side effects: evidence for alpha-2 receptor subtypes. J. Neurosci. **8:** 4287-4298.

96. WILLIAMS, G. & P. GOLDMAN-RAKIC. 1995. Modulation of memory fields by dopamine D1 receptors in prefrontal cortex. Nature **376:** 572-575.

97. VERMA, A. & B. MOGHADDAM. 1996. NMDA receptor antagonists impair prefrontal cortex function as assessed via spatial delated alternation performance in rats: Modulation by dopamine. J. Neurosci. **16:** 373-379.

98. MURPHY, B., A. ARNSTEN, J. JENTSCH & R. ROTH. 1996. Dopamine and spatial working memory in rats and monkeys: Pharmacological reversal of stress-induced impairment. J. Neurosci. **16:** 7768-7775.

99. MURPHY, B., A. ARNSTEN, P. GOLDMAN-RAKIC & R. ROTH. 1996. Increased dopamine turnover in the prefrontal cortex impairs spatial working memory performance in rats and monkeys. Proc. Natl. Acad. Sci. USA **93:** 1325-1329.

100. DIVAC, I., J. MOGENSON, R. BLANCHARD & D. BLANCHARD. 1984. Mesial cortical lesions and fear behavior in the wild rat. Physiol. Psychol. **12:** 271-274.

101. HOLSON, R. 1986. Mesial prefrontal cortical lesions and timidity in rats. I. Reactivity to aversive stimuli. Physiol. Behav. **37:** 221-230.

102. HOLSON, R. 1986. Mesial prefrontal cortical lesions and timidity in rats. III. Behavior in a semi-natural environment. Physiol. Behav. **37:** 239-247.

103. MORGAN, M. A., L. M. ROMANSKI & J. E. LEDOUX. 1993. Extinction of emotional learning: Contribution of medial prefrontal cortex. Neurosci. Lett. **163:** 109-113.

104. SARA, S. & A. HERVE-MINVIELLE. 1995. Inhibitory influence of frontal cortex on locus coeruleus neurons. Proc. Natl. Acad. Sci. USA **92:** 6032-6036.

105. GOLDMAN-RAKIC, P. 1987. Circuitry of the primate prefrontal cortex and regulation of behavior by representational memory. *In* Handbook of Physiological Soc., The Nervous System: Higher Functions of the Brain. Vol. 5, sec. 1. F. Plum & V. Mountcastle, Eds. American Physiological Society. Bethesda, MD.

106. GOLDMAN-RAKIC, P. 1991. Prefrontal cortical dysfunction in schizophrenia: The relevance of working memory. *In* Psychopathology and the Brain. B. J. Carroll & J. E. Barrett, Eds.: 1-23. Raven Press. New York.

107. CASSELL, M. & D. WRIGHT. 1986. Topography of projections from the medial prefrontal cortex to the amygdala in the rat. Brain Res. Bull. **17:** 321-333.

108. SESACK, S. R., A. Y. DEUTCH, R. H. ROTH & B. S. BUNNEY. 1989. Topographical organization of the efferent projections of the medial prefrontal cortex in the rat: An anterograde tract-tracing study with *Phaseolus vulgaris* leukoagglutinin. J. Comp. Neurol. **290:** 213-242.

109. TERREBERRY, R. & E. NEAFSEY. 1987. The rat medial frontal cortex projects directly to autonomic regions of the brainstem. Brain Res. Bull. **19:** 639-649.

110. TERREBERRY, R. & E. NEAFSEY. 1983. Rat medial frontal cortex: a visceral motor region with a direct projection to the solitary nucleus. Brain Res. **278:** 245-249.

111. VAN DER KOOY, D., L. KODA, J. McGINTY, C. GERFEN & F. BLOOM. 1984. The organization of projections from the cortex, amygdala, and hypothalamus to the nucleus of the solitary tract in rat. J. Comp. Neurol. **224:** 1–24.

112. CHRISTIE, M., S. BRIDGE, L. JAMES & P. BEART. 1985. Excitotoxin lesions suggest an aspartatergic projection from rat medial prefrontal cortex to ventral tegmental area. Brain Res. **333:** 169–172.

113. HURLEY, K., H. HERBERT, M. MOGA & C. SAPER. Efferent projections of the infralimbic cortex of the rat. J. Comp. Neurol. **308:** 249–276.

114. BERENDSE, H. Y. GALIS-DE GRAFF & H. GROENEWEGEN. 1992. Topographical organization and relationship with ventral striatal compartments of prefrontal corticostriatal projections in the rat. J. Comp. Neurol. **316:** 314–347.

115. BUTLER, R., D. BRAFF, J. RAUSCH, M. JENKINS, J. SPROCK & M. GEYER. 1990. Physiological evidence of exaggerated startle response in a subgroup of Vietnam Veterans with combat-related PTSD. Am. J. Psychiatry **147:** 1308–1312.

116. ORNITZ, E. & R. PYNOOS. 1989. Startle modulation in children with posttraumatic stress disorder. Am. J. Psychiatry **146:** 866–870.

117. GRILLON, C., C. MORGAN, S. SOUTHWICK, M. DAVIS & D. CHARNEY. 1996. Baseline startle amplitude and prepulse inhibition in Vietnam veterans with PTSD. Psychiatry Res. **64:** 169–178.

118. MORGAN, C., C. GRILLON, S. SOUTHWICK, M. DAVIS & D. CHARNEY. 1995. Fear-potentiated startle in posttraumatic stress disorder. Biol. Psychiatry **38:** 378–385.

119. GRILLON, C., C. MORGAN, M. DAVIS & S. SOUTHWICK. 1996. Preliminary report presented at the Annual Meeting of the Society for Biological Psychiatry. May 1996. New York, NY.

120. DAVIS, M., J. GEWIRTZ, K. McNISH & M. KIM. 1995. The roles of the amygdala and bed nucleus of the stria terminalis (BNST) in the acquisition of fear potentiated startle using both explicit and contextual cues. Soc. Neurosci. **21:** 1224.

121. PHILLIPS, R. & J. LEDOUX. 1992. Different contribution of amygdala and hippocampus to cued and contextual fear conditioning. Behav. Neurosci. **106:** 274–285.

122. DRUGAN, R., P. SKOLNICK, S. PAUL & J. CRAWLEY. 1989. A pretest procedure reliably predicts performance in two animal models of inescapable stress. Pharmacol. Biochem. Behav. **33:** 649–654.

123. WEISS, J., P. GOODMAN, B. LOSITO, S. CORRIGAN, J. CHARRY & W. BAILEY. 1981. Behavioral depression produced by an uncontrollable stressor: relationship to norepinephrine, dopamine, serotonin levels in various regions of rat brain. Brain Res. Rev. **3:** 167–205.

124. PETTY, F., G. KRAMER & L. WILSON. 1992. Prevention of learned helplessness: *in vivo* correlation with cortical serotonin. Pharmacol. Biochem. Behav. **43:** 361–367.

125. BREMNER, J., S. SOUTHWICK, E. BRETT, A. FONTANA, R. ROSENHECK & D. CHARNEY. 1992. Dissociation and posttraumatic stress disorder in Vietnam combat veterans. Am. J. Psychiatry **149:** 328–333.

126. KOOPMAN, C., C. CLASSEN & D. SPIEGEL. 1994. Predictors of posttraumatic stress symptoms among survivors of the Oakland/Berkeley, Calif., firestorm. Am. J. Psychiatry **151:** 888–894.

127. MARMAR, C., D. WEISS, D. SCHLENGER, J. FAIRBANK, B. JORDAN, R. KULKA & R. HOUGH. 1994. Peritraumatic dissociation and posttraumatic stress in male Vietnam theater veterans. Am. J. Psychiatry **151:** 902–907.

128. BREMNER, J. & E. BRETT. 1997. Trauma-related dissociative states and long-term psychopathology in posttraumatic stress disorder. J. Traumatic Stress **10:** 37–49.

129. CHU, J. & D. DILL. 1990. Dissociative symptoms in relation to childhood physical and sexual abuse. Am. J. Psychiatry **147:** 887–892.

130. KIRBY, J., J. CHU & D. DILL. 1992. Correlates of dissociative symptomatology in patients with physical and sexual abuse histories. Comp. Psychiatry **34:** 258–263.

131. DEMITRACK, A., F. PUTNAM, D. RUBINOW, T. PIGOTT, M. ALTEMIUS, D. KRHAN & P. GOLD. 1993. Relation of dissociative phenomena to levels of cerebral spinal fluid monoamine metabolites and Bendorphin in patients with eating disorders: A pilot study. Psychiatry Res. **49:** 1-10.

132. ELLSWORTH, J., D. LEAHY, R. ROTH *et al.* 1987. Homovanillic acid concentrations in brain, CSF and plasma as indicators of central dopamine function in primates. J. Neural Trans. **68:** 51-62.

133. IZARD, C., D. LIBERO, P. PUTNAM & O. HAYNES. 1993. Stability of emotion experiences and their relations to traits of personality. J. Pers. Soc. Psychol. **64:** 847-860.

134. BIEDERMAN, J., J. ROSENBAUM, E. BOLDUC-MURPHY, S. FARAONE, J. CHALOFF, D. HIRSHFELD & J. KAGAN. 1993. A 3-year follow-up of children with and without behavioral inhibition. J. Am Acad. Child Adolesc. Psychiatry **32:** 814-821.

135. MAYER, J., M. DIPAOLO & P. SALOVEY. 1990. Perceiving affective content in ambiguous visual stimuli: a component of emotional intelligence. J. Pers. Assess. **54:** 772-781.

136. ANDREWS, M. & L. ROSENBLUM. 1991. Dominance and social competence in differentially reared bonnet macaques. *In* Primatology Today. A. Ehara, T. Kimura, O. Takenako & M. Iwqamoto. Eds.: 347-50. Elsevier. Amsterdam.

137. ROSENBLUM, L., J. COPLAN, S. FRIEDMAN, T. BASSOFF, J. GORMAN & M. ANDREWS. 1994. Adverse early experiences affect noradrenergic and serotonergic functioning in adult primates. Biol. Psychiatry **35:** 221-227.

138. KAGAN, J., J. S. REZNICK & N. SNIDMAN. 1988. Biological bases of childhood shyness. Science **240:** 167-171.

139. KAGAN, J., J. S. REZNICK, N. SNIDMAN & M. JOHNSON. 1988. Childhood derivatives of inhibition and lack of inhibition to the unfamiliar. Child Dev. **59:** 1580-1589.

140. ROSENBERG, A. & J. KAGAN. 1989. Physical and physiological correlates of behavioral inhibition. Dev. Psychobiol. **22:** 753-770.

141. COPLAN, J., M. ANDREWS, L. ROSENBLUM, M. OWENS, S. FRIEDMAN, J. GORMAN & C. NEMEROFF. 1996. Persistent elevations of cerebrospinal fluid concentrations of corticotropin releasing factor in adult nonhuman primates exposed to early-life stressors: Implications for the pathophysiology of mood and anxiety disorders. Proc. Natl. Acad. Sci. USA **93:** 1619-1623.

142. MEANEY, M., D. AITKEN, S. BHATNAGAR, C. VAN BERKEL & P. SAPOLSKY. 1988. Postnatal handling attenuates neuroendocrine, anatomical, and cognitive impairments related to the aged hippocampus. Science **238:** 766-768.

143. VIAU, V., S. SHARMA, P. PLOTSKY & M. MEANY. 1993. Increased plasma ACTH responses to stress in nonhandled compared with handled rats require basal levels of corticosterone and are associated with increased levels of ACTH secretagoges in the median eminence. J. Neurosci. **13:** 1097-1105.

144. PLOTSKY, P. & M. MEANEY. 1993. Early, postnatal experience alters hypothalamic corticotropin-releasing factor (CRF) mRNA, median eminence CRF content and stress-induced release in adult rats. Mol. Brain. Res. **18:** 195-200.

145. LADD, C, M. OWENS & C. NEMEROFF. 1996. Persistent changes in corticotropin-releasing factor neuronal systems induced by maternal deprivation. Endocrinology **137:** 1212-1218.

146. BREMNER, J., S. SOUTHWICK, D. JOHNSON, R. YEHUDA & D. CHARNEY. 1993. Childhood physical abuse in combat-related posttraumatic stress disorder. Am. J. Psychiatry **150:** 235-239.

147. LIPSCHITZ, D., S. SOUTHWICK, A. NICOLAU, R. WINEGAR & E. HARTNICK. 1996. Abuse and neglect as risk factors for suicide in adolescents. Abstract presented at the 149th annual meeting of the American Psychiatric Association. New York, May 1996.

148. LIPSCHITZ, D., R. WINEGAR, E. HARTNICK & S. SOUTHWICK. 1996. Comorbidity and correlates of post traumatic stress disorder in hospitalized adolescents. Poster presented at the 43rd Annual Meeting of the American Academy of Child & Adolescent Psychiatry. Philadelphia, October, 1996.

The Psychobiology of Posttraumatic Stress Disorder: An Overview

M. MICHELE MURBURG

University of Washington
Seattle, Washington
and
Department of Veterans Affairs
Puget Sound Health Care System
American Lake Division
Mail Stop 116
Tacoma, Washington 98493

Not long ago, when inquiries into the biology of posttraumatic stress disorder (PTSD) were first being made, many rejected the notion that a disorder for which the etiology was thought to be mainly experiential could possibly involve any significant neurobiological alterations. Yet, those who chose to study the psychobiology of PTSD reasoned that because stress exposure in animals is associated with profound alterations in multiple neurobiological systems,[1–3] exposure to traumatic stressors might cause similar (or perhaps different) changes in humans.

Today the number of studies investigating biological alterations in PTSD is large, and together with data derived from basic scientific inquiries into the effects of stress in animals, the findings from those studies are beginning to help us to construct a useful, if still incomplete, picture of what happens to persons exposed to extreme stress. Among the important lessons that we have learned so far are several concepts that are expanded upon by many of the contributors to this book, but I would like to highlight them here.

First, it is now quite clear that *stress* and probably nearly any experience of significance to which an organism is exposed *alters neurobiological systems.* Stress-induced alterations may range from molecular changes that have an impact on learning and memory to disruption of complex functions such as sleep, information processing, and emotions. Second, *prior stress exposure,* acting via neurobiological changes, *alters a variety of behavioral and physiological responses to subsequent experiences.* These altered responses are not necessarily pathological, and some in fact may be adaptive. Thus, "stress-induced alterations" are not necessarily identical to the biological processes that underlie the pathophysiology of PTSD, although the two sets of phenomena may be related and in part overlap. Third, on the other hand, *neurobiological responses that allow short-term survival of acute stress situations may have detrimental effects.* Fourth, to come full circle, *if traumatic experiences can induce neurobiological changes* that produce pathology, it is not incomprehensible that *other experiences may result in neurobiological changes that may mitigate or compensate for those induced by stress.* Exploring what these mitigating experiences might be could create new and effective methods for treating PTSD.

STRESS ALTERS NEUROBIOLOGICAL SYSTEMS

Post and colleagues, as well as others,[4-10] have shown that even minor stressors can alter neuronal biology at the genomic level, initially inducing immediate early genes, such as c-fos. The activation of c-fos and other transcription factors may be the first step in a series of biological events, leading to the induction or suppression of other genes whose products allow for changes in neurobiological systems.[11] It has been noted that the relative proportions of various oncogenes change over time in response to prior experiences, altering the "oncogene milieu," interacting in complex ways with other experientially altered systems and thereby providing for differential cellular responses to subsequent stimuli.[11] (See ref. 11 for a review.)

At the neuroendocrine level, stress-induced alterations are found in many systems, some of which have now been studied quite extensively in PTSD. The HPA axis alterations in PTSD are well described by Dr. Yehuda (this volume) and will not be discussed here. Central and peripheral catecholaminergic systems appear to have undergone complex modifications in PTSD, as described by Dr. Southwick (this volume). Taken as a whole, the literature suggests that relative basal quiescence of these systems with enhanced responsivity to stimulation may provide for enhancement of "signal to noise ratios" in neuronal and other systems. Such enhancement may facilitate selective attention and selective responding to the most strongly determined inputs (as has been described in animal species),[12] potentially contributing to symptoms including hypervigilance, insomnia, flashbacks, intrusive memories, panic, physiologic hyperreactivity, and startle.

Catecholaminergic and other systems involved in cardiovascular regulation appear to be strongly influenced by stress-induced "learning" or conditioning, undoubtedly mediated by as yet incompletely elucidated neurobiological processes in patients with significant PTSD. As shown by the work of Dr. Orr and colleagues (Orr, this volume), physiologic hyperreactivity is not seen in all patients with PTSD and may be seen in patients who no longer meet criteria for PTSD, but patients with more severe PTSD nearly always show this hyperreactivity. The work of McGaugh and colleagues[13] prompts the question of whether this physiological hyperreactivity, which may also involve the release of peripheral epinephrine,[14] may actually contribute to the further consolidation of traumatic memories and to the progressive worsening of PTSD symptoms.

At the functional anatomic level, it is fascinating that the act of visualizing traumatic events is associated with increased blood flow in the right amygdala and anterior cingulate cortex in PTSD patients and decreased blood flow in the left inferior frontal cortex (Rauch and Shin, this volume). As it has been shown that exposure to stimuli that are reminiscent of the original trauma can prompt the release of peripheral epinephrine[14] and because peripheral epinephrine is thought to participate in the consolidation of memory via activation of amygdalar structures,[13] it is possible that this blood flow change is indirectly influenced by peripheral epinephrine release. The blood flow changes furthermore likely reflect the anatomy of the PTSD patient's memory activation per se and possibly also the patient's selective attention, under the circumstances of the study, to the most meaningful current neural input (in this case a strong emotional memory arising from the amygdala in comparison with which the mere cognitions supplied by left cerebral inputs have little attentional valence).

At the organismic level, traumatic stress disrupts important functions ranging from sleep to the ability to process information. As Dr. Mellman points out (Mellman, this volume), PTSD patients tend to have interrupted sleep, particularly disrupted REM sleep, and may experience an increased "pressure" for REM. Moreover, because REM may be involved in the processing of stressful events and in the consolidation of learning, the continued sleep disturbance may contribute to perpetuation of the disorder by interfering with the occurrence of compensatory processes.

PRIOR STRESS EXPOSURE ALTERS RESPONSES TO SUBSEQUENT EXPERIENCES

Stress exposure in the generic sense, then, can be viewed broadly as causing a series of cellular changes that modify neuronal and other cellular biology,[11] ultimately contributing to altered systemic and organismic responses to subsequent stimuli. Antelman et al.[15–19] have shown that a single exposure to a stressor, whether physiological or psychological in nature, can cause enduring alterations in physiological and behavioral responses to subsequent stimuli. Moreover, the neurochemical and behavioral changes caused by stress may intensify over time[15,19–21] and may be bidirectional (Antelman et al., this volume). Thus, the neurobiological responses to subsequent stressors may be expected to be quite different from the neurobiological response to the initial stressor. Moreover, as Post[11] has pointed out, the experience of responding to a stressor, including an episode of psychiatric illness (such as an affective disorder or perhaps an exacerbation of PTSD), may itself leave behind molecular "memory traces" that so alter involved neural pathways as to predispose them to be more readily activated in the future. Such mechanisms may be involved in the genesis and perpetuation of the physiological hyperreactivity seen in PTSD (Orr, this volume) and perhaps other PTSD symptoms as well.

Not all exposure to stressors, however, results in sensitization of all neurobiological responses to further stress. For example, repeatedly immobilized animals release smaller amounts of catecholamines into plasma than do acutely stressed rats in response to single short intervals of immobilization, suggesting adaptation of the stress response under these circumstances (for review, see Stone and McCarty.[21]) The cortisol response to repeated exposure to the same stressor decreases in a number of experimental paradigms (see Yehuda et al.[22] for a review). Early postnatal handling of rats results in the development of a more efficient HPA response to stress[23] paralleled by enduring increases in glucocorticoid binding in the hippocampus and frontal cortex.[24]

In human studies, Resnick et al.[25] showed that women previously sexually assaulted had lower plasma cortisol levels shortly following an index episode of sexual assault than did women not previously assaulted. As the work of Yehuda has established, patients with PTSD show increased numbers of glucocorticoid receptors on circulating lymphocytes, with increased cortisol suppression in response to low doses of dexamethasone. A parallel increase in hippocampal and/or hypothalamic glucocorticoid receptor number strongly suggested by the finding of enhanced cortisol suppression in response to low doses of exogenous glucocorticoids in PTSD, may help to explain the lower levels of cortisol seen at many times during the circadian cycle and a higher circadian HPA axis "signal to noise" ratio in PTSD patients.[26,27] (See also Yehuda *et al.*, this volume.) This altered state of HPA axis functioning may also help to explain the lower cortisol response of previously assaulted women to subsequent rape.[25]

NEUROBIOLOGICAL RESPONSES THAT ALLOW SHORT-TERM SURVIVAL OF ACUTE STRESS SITUATIONS MAY ULTIMATELY BE DETRIMENTAL

In an acutely stressful situation, the CNS release of norepinephrine allows for the direction of attention to relevant stimuli and participates in the activation of pathways for sympathoadrenal responses. Sympathoadrenal activation releases peripheral norepinephrine and epinephrine which alter heart rate and blood pressure and mobilize energy substrates also made more available by cortisol. The body is thus prepared for "fight or flight" in response to a stressor. But, as seen in animal studies, high rates of central norepinephrine release may lead to at least a transient depletion of central norepinephrine levels, associated with behavioral depression.[28] In humans, high circulating catecholamine levels may be associated with cardiac stress and hypertension. Chronic elevations in glucocorticoids may be associated with osteoporosis,[29] muscle wasting,[30] and reproductive dysfunction.[31] Even transient elevations in plasma cortisol have been found to damage the hippocampus in nonhuman species, resulting in loss of neurons.[32,33] Therefore, it is not surprising that recent studies such as that of Stein *et al.* (this volume) have reported smaller hippocampal volumes in traumatized patients. Although PTSD may not be associated with elevated circulating cortisol levels, initial exposures to traumatic stress are almost certainly accompanied by plasma cortisol elevation, which may translate into hippocampal damage.

It is fortunate that PTSD patients do not typically suffer from the extensive deleterious physiological changes associated with chronic stress in many animal studies. As demonstrated by Dr. Yehuda (this volume), the increased glucocorticoid responsivity seen in PTSD appears to dampen ultradian plasma cortisol excursions and stress-induced increases in circulating cortisol. Thus, the patient with PTSD theoretically has some protection from the potential neurotoxicity associated with further stress-induced elevations in circulating glucocorticoid levels. Similarly, as shown by our group,[34] basal sympathetic nervous system activity, including the basal rate of norepinephrine release into plasma, is not increased, but rather may be suppressed, in PTSD,[34] thus affording PTSD patients with at least some protection from the potential detrimental sequelae of chronically increased sympathetic nervous system activity which has been reported in some animal studies.

IF TRAUMATIC EXPERIENCES CAN INDUCE PATHOGENIC NEUROBIOLOGICAL CHANGES, OTHER EXPERIENCES MAY CAUSE COMPENSATORY NEUROBIOLOGICAL CHANGES

The study of the psychobiology of PTSD has, in a sense, brought about a revolution in our thinking about the brain and experience. We can no longer think of some types of experiences, or some types of psychological states, including psychiatric illnesses, as being "biological," while others are somehow independent of the brain. All human perceptions, thoughts, emotions, and actions are mediated by the brain and, in turn, impact on the brain. It stands to reason, then, that at least some types of experiences have salutary, and perhaps even compensatory, effects on the "traumatized" nervous system. Mellman (this volume) suggests, for example, that consolidated sleep may help to protect traumatized persons from developing PTSD. Other types of potentially helpful experiences, including carefully defined and selected types of psychotherapy, should continue to be investigated for potential roles in preventing and treating PTSD.

Clearly it is not possible to "undo" a traumatic experience, and it is likely that some neurobiological alterations seen in PTSD, such as hippocampal damage, will not be modifiable via a "corrective experience." However, although it may not be possible to reverse cellular loss, it may be possible to compensate for it. Other stress-induced changes may be more easily counterbalanced. Furthermore, it is likely that some of the biological changes induced in PTSD, such as the upregulation of glucocorticoid receptors or the enhancement of central and peripheral catecholamine responsivity, have adaptive functions. The adaptive aspects of stress-induced changes, including some that are associated with PTSD and others that may not be, need to be better understood.

In this volume the findings of many clinical investigations into the psychobiology and treatment of PTSD have been summarized as have basic studies of numerous relevant phenomena ranging from the biology of neuronal sensitization to the anatomy of memory and startle. Many findings in the field have contradicted our initial hypotheses, with some even having the nerve to be downright counterintuitive, and yet highly replicable, forcing us to relinquish long-cherished ideas about stress, adaptation, pathology, and PTSD. Clearly the psychobiology of PTSD is not identical to the neurobiology of stress, and the more PTSD is investigated, the more we learn to appreciate in new ways the profound and multiple effects of experience on neural systems and human beings.

REFERENCES

1. STRATAKIS, C. A. & G. P. CHROUSOS. 1995. Neuroendocrinology and pathophysiology of the stress system. *In* Stress: Basic Mechanisms and Clinical Implications. Chrousos, R. McCarty, K. Pacák, G. Ciźza, E. Sternberg, P. W. Gold & R. Kvetňanský. G. P., Eds. Ann. N.Y. Acad. Sci. **771:** 1-18.
2. KOPIN, I. J. 1995. Definitions of stress and sympathetic neuronal Responses. *In* Stress: Mechanisms and Clinical Implications. Chrousos, G. P. *et al.,* Eds. Ann. N.Y. Acad. Sci. **771:** 19-30.
3. MURBURG, M. M., M. E. MCFALL & R. C. VEITH. 1990. Catecholamines, stress, and post-traumatic stress disorder. *In* Biological Assessment and Treatment of Posttraumatic Stress Disorder. Giller, E. L., Ed.: 27-64. American Psychiatric Press, Inc. Washington, DC.
4. NAKAJIMA, T., J. L. DAVAL, C. H. GLEITER, J. DECKAERT, R. M. POST & P. J. MARANGOS. 1989. c-Fos mRNA expression following electrical-induced seizure and acute nociceptive stress in mouse brain. Epilepsy Res. **4:** 156-159.

5. NAKAJIMA, T., R. M. POST, S. R. B. WEISS, A. PERT & T. A. KETTER. 1989. Perspectives on the mechanism of action of electroconvulsive therapy: Anticonvulsant, dopaminergic, and c-fos oncogene effects. Convulsive Ther. **5:** 274-295.

6. DAVAL, J. L., T. NAKAJIMA, C. H. GLEITER, R. M. POST & P. J. MARANGOS. 1989. Mouse brain c-fos mRNA distribution following a single electroconvulsive shock. J. Neurochem. **52:** 1954-1957.

7. DRAISCI, G. & M. J. IADAROLA. 1989. Temporal analysis of increases in c-fos, preprodynorphin and preproenkephalin mRNAs in rat spinal cord. Brain Res. Mol. Brain Res. **6:** 31-37.

8. CECCATELLI, S., M. J. VILLAR, M. GOLDSTEIN & T. HOKFELT. 1989. Expression of c-fos immunoreactivity in transmitter-characterized neurons after stress. Proc. Natl. Acad. Sci. USA **86:** 9569-9573.

9. BULLITT, E. 1989. Induction of c-fos-like protein within the lumbar spinal cord and thalamus of the rat following peripheral stimulation. Brain Res. **493:** 391-397.

10. SMITH, M., S. R. B. WEISS, T. ABEDIN, R. M. POST & P. GOLD. 1991. Effects of amygdala-kindling and electroconvulsive seizures on the expression of corticotrophin releasing hormone (CRH) mRNA in the rat brain. Mol Cell Neurosci. **2:** 103-116.

11. POST, R. M. 1992. Transduction of psychosocial stress into the neurobiology of recurrent affective disorder. Am. J. Psychiatry **149:** 999-1010.

12. ASTON-JONES, G., R. J. VALENTINO, E. J. VAN BOCKSTAELE & A. T. MEYERSON. 1994. Locus coeruleus, stress, and PTSD: Neurobiological and clinical parallels. *In* Catecholamine Function in PTSD: Emerging Concepts. Murburg, M. M., Ed.: 17-62. American Psychiatric Press. Washington, DC.

13. MCGAUGH, J. L. 1997. Emotional activation, neuromodulatory systems and memory. *In* Memory Distortion. D. Schachter, Ed. Harvard University Press. Boston. In press.

14. MCFALL, M. E., M. M. MURBURG, G. N. KO & R. C. VEITH. 1990. Autonomic responses to stress in Vietnam combat veterans with posttraumatic stress disorder. Biol. Psychiatry **27:** 1165-1175.

15. ANTELMAN, S. M., D. KOCAN, D. J. EDWARDS *et al.* 1986. Behavioral effects of a single neuropeptide treatment grow with the passage of time. Brain Res. **385:** 58-67.

16. ANTELMAN, S. M., D. KOCAN, D. J. EDWARDS *et al.* 1987. A single injection of diazepam induces long-lasting sensitization. Psychopharmacol. Bull. **23:** 430-434.

17. ANTELMAN, S. M. 1988. Time-dependent sensitization as the cornerstone for a new approach to pharmacotherapy: Drugs as foreign/stressful stimuli. Drug Dev. Res. **14:** 1-30.

18. ANTELMAN, S. M., L. A. DEGIOVANNI & D. KOCAN. 1989. A single exposure to cocaine or immobilization stress provides extremely longlasting selective protection against sudden cardiac death from tetracaine. Life Sci. **44:** 201-207.

19. ANTELMAN, S. M., S. KNOPF, D. KOCAN *et al.* 1988. One stressful event blocks multiple actions of diazepam for up to at least a month. Brain Res. **445:** 380-385.

20. ANTELMAN, S. M., D. KOCAN, D. J. EDWARDS *et al.* 1989. Anticonvulsants and other effects of diazepam grow with the time after single treatment: Pharmacol. Biochem. Behav. **33:** 31-39.

21. STONE, E. A. & MCCARTY R. 1983. Adaptation to stress: Tyrosine hydroxylase activity and catecholamine release. Neurosci. Biobehav. Rev. **7:** 29-34.

22. YEHUDA, R., E. L. GILLER, S. M. SOUTHWICK, M. T. LOWY & J. W. MASON. 1991. Hypothalamic-pituitary-adrenal dysfunction in posttraumatic stress disorder. Biol. Psychiatry **30:** 1031-1048.

23. ADER, R. 1970. The effect of early experience on the adrenocortical response to different magnitudes of stimulation. Physiol. Behav. **5:** 837-840.

24. MEANEY, M. J., D. H. AITKEN, S. R. BODNOFF, L. J. INY, J. E. TATAREWICZ & R. M. SAPOLSKY. 1985. Early postnatal handling alters glucocorticoid receptor concentrations in selected brain regions. Behav. Neurosci. **99:** 765-770.

25. RESNICK, H. S., R. YEHUDA, R. K. PITMAN & D. W. FOY. 1995. Effect of previous trauma on acute plasma cortisol level following rape. Am. J. Psychiatry **152:** 1675-1677.

26. YEHUDA, R., M. T. LOWY, S. M. SOUTHWICK, D. SHAFFER & E. L. GILLER. 1991. Lymphocyte glucocorticoid receptor number in posttraumatic stress disorder. Am. J. Psychiatry **148:** 499-503.

27. YEHUDA, R., D. BOISONEAU, M. T. LOWY & E. L. GILLER. 1995. Dose-response changes in plasma cortisol and lymphocyte glucocorticoid receptors following dexamethasone administration in combat veterans with and without posttraumatic stress disorder. Arch. Gen. Psychiatry **52:** 583-593.

28. MAIER, S. F. 1983. Learned helplessness, depression, analgesia, and endogenous opiates. Psychopharmacol. Bull. **19:** 531-536.

29. REID, I. 1989. Pathogenesis and treatment of steroid osteoporosis. Clin. Endocrinol. **30:** 83.

30. KAPLAN, S. & C. NATAREDA SHIMIZI. 1963. Effects of cortisol on amino acids in skeletal muscle and plasma. Endocrinology **72:** 267.

31. SLUTER, D. & N. SCHWARTZ. 1985. Effects of glucocorticoids on secretion of luteinizing hormone and follicle-stimulating hormone by female rat pituitary cells in vitro. Endocrinology **117:** 849.

32. CHAN, R. S., E. D. HUEY, H. L. MAECKER, K. M. CORTOPASSI, S. A. HOWARD, A. M. IYER, L. J. McINTOSH, O. A. AJILORE, S. M. BROOKE & R. M. SAPOLSKY. 1996. Endocrine modulators of necrotic neuron death. Brain Pathol. **6:** 481-491.

33. SAPOLSKY, R. M. 1996. Why stress is bad for your brain. Science **273** (5276): 749-750.

34. MURBURG, M. M., M. E. McFALL & R. C. VEITH. 1995. Plasma norepinephrine kinetics in patients with post-traumatic stress disorder. Biol. Psychiatry **38:** 819-825.

Drug Treatment for PTSD

Answers and Questions

MATTHEW J. FRIEDMAN

National Center for PTSD
White River Junction, Vermont 05009
and
Departments of Psychiatry and Pharmacology
Dartmouth Medical School
Hanover, New Hampshire 03755

The first randomized clinical trial of a drug treatment for posttraumatic stress disorder (PTSD) was published in 1988 (ref. 1, later expanded to ref. 2). It was a promising beginning. Good results were obtained with both a monoamine oxidase inhibitor (MAOI) and a tricyclic antidepressant (TCA) in Vietnam veterans with PTSD. Since that time, however, only eight additional clinical trials have been published and only two drugs have been tested more than once. This paucity of drug studies contrasts unfavorably with the proliferation of studies on the neurobiology and psychophysiology of PTSD.

During this same period, a number of neurobiological abnormalities have been detected among PTSD patients, and it appears that we may have only scratched the surface in appreciating the complex pathophysiology of this disorder. Furthermore, unlike the situation with most psychiatric disorders, a number of promising animal models for PTSD provide an opportunity to conduct extensive laboratory testing on potentially useful pharmacological agents before initiating clinical trials.[3]

Although recent findings with fluoxetine[4] have revived hopeful interest in pharmacotherapy for PTSD, we must ask ourselves why progress has been so slow and why success has been so elusive in drug treatment for PTSD. There are a number of related questions: (1) Have we been testing drugs on the wrong clinical populations? (2) Have we optimized our clinical trials with respect to design and instrumentation? (3) Have we been testing the wrong drugs? (4) Are there different subtypes or stages of PTSD that may require different treatments at different times? (5) Is there a magic bullet for PTSD? Before considering these questions, we need to review the current literature on pharmacotherapy for PTSD.

LITERATURE REVIEW

Overview

TABLE 1 presents information from the nine published randomized clinical trials on drug treatment for PTSD. It shows that most studies have tested antidepressants (TCAs, MAOIs, and selective serotonin reuptake inhibitors [SSRIs]), most investigations have been conducted on military veterans, and most outcomes have been assessed with the Impact of Events Scale (IES). Results have been mixed. If you accept the

TABLE 1. Randomized Clinical Trials of PTSD: Drug vs Placebo Treatment[a]

Drug Class	Study[b]	n	Subjects	Length (wk)	Outcome	Drugs	Effect Size
TCA	8	46	Military	8	IES Total	Amitriptyline	.38
TCA	20	18	Military	4	IES Avoidance	Desipramine	.04
TCA	20	18	Military	4	IES Intrusion	Desipramine	.16
TCA	2	60	Military	8	IES Total	Imipramine	.39
MAOI	2	60	Military	8	IES Total	Phenelzine	.70
MAOI	5[c]	13	Mil./Civ.	4	IES Total	Phenelzine	-.41
MAOI/SSRI	6	113	Mil./Civ.	10	CAPS Total	Brofaromine	.13
MAOI/SSRI	7	45	Mil./Civ.	14	CAPS Total	Brofaromine	.71
SSRI	4	24	Military	5	PTSD Interview	Fluoxetine	.38
SSRI	4	23	Adult CSA	5	PTSD Interview	Fluoxetine	1.12
BZD	23	10	Mil./Civ.	5	IES Total	Alprazolam	.42
2nd Mess.	28[c]	13	Mil./Civ.	4	IES Total	Inositol	.28

ABBREVIATIONS: TCA = tricyclic antidepressant; MAOI = monoamine oxidase inhibitor; SSRI = selective serotonin reuptake inhibitor; BZD = benzodiazepine; 2nd Mess = second messenger; IES = Impact of Events Scale; CAPS = Clinician Administered PTSD Scale; Mil./Civ. = military and civilian; CSA = childhood sexual abuse.

[a] Augmented and modified from Friedman and Schnurr (1995): Unpublished VA Cooperative Study Research Proposal.

[b] See references.

[c] Cross-over design.

proposition that the minimum effect size necessary for a clinically noticeable difference between an active treatment and a placebo is .5 standard deviations, most drug trials do not exceed this threshold (TABLE 1). This is in marked contrast to randomized clinical psychotherapy trials which have tested exposure therapy or cognitive-behavioral treatments for PTSD in which effect sizes for most studies range between .68 and 1.29 standard deviations (Friedman and Schnurr, 1995, unpublished VA Cooperative Study research proposal).

The three studies with clinically meaningful effect sizes involve an MAOI, phenelzine, an SSRI, fluoxetine, and the novel SSRI/reversible MAO-A inhibitor brofaromine. Even here, however, results are far from unambiguous. Whereas phenelzine had an effect size of .70 in one study,[2] it was less efficacious than placebo (effect size −.41) in another investigation.[5] Whereas fluoxetine had an effect size of 1.12 in adult (mostly female) PTSD patients who had been exposed to childhood sexual abuse, its effect size was only .38 when administered by the same investigators in the same study[4] to adult male Vietnam veterans with war-related PTSD. Finally, whereas brofaromine had an effect size of .71, in one study the effect size was only .13 in a larger multicenter study in which the same protocol was followed.[6,7]

Furthermore, clinical trials with imipramine[2] and amitriptyline[8] demonstrated statistically significant results that may not be clinically meaningful because the effect sizes were only .39 and .38, respectively.

In summary, dramatic responses to medication have been the exception rather than the rule. MAOIs alone or in combination with SSRIs appear more efficacious than other drugs, but serious questions remain about the best way to interpret these positive results.

Selective Serotonin Reuptake Inhibition

SSRIs have revolutionized pharmacotherapy and have replaced TCAs and MAOIs as first line drugs in the treatment of depression, panic disorder, and obsessive compulsive disorder. They also are beginning to emerge as the first choice of clinicians treating PTSD patients despite the few published open trials and only one published randomized clinical trial with an SSRI. In addition, some pharmaceutical companies have begun to show an interest in PTSD treatment as indicated by a large multicenter randomized trial of sertraline currently in progress in both civilian patients and military veterans with PTSD.

In the previously mentioned randomized clinical trial of fluoxetine, van der Kolk and associates[4] observed a marked reduction in overall PTSD symptoms, especially with respect to numbing and arousal symptoms. These results could not be attributed to fluoxetine's antidepressant actions. A particularly important finding (shown in TABLE 1) was the large effect size on adult (mostly female) survivors of childhood sexual abuse (1.12) as compared to a much smaller effect size on military veterans with PTSD (.38). I will return to this point subsequently.

In addition, open trials and case reports on fluoxetine, sertraline, and fluvoxamine have appeared (see ref. 9 for references). Investigators have generally been impressed by the capacity of SSRIs to reduce the numbing symptoms of PTSD, because other drugs tested thus far do not have this property.

A second unique property of SSRIs may make them an attractive choice for PTSD patients, given the high comorbidity rates between PTSD and alcohol abuse/dependence among treatment-seeking patients.[10] Because SSRI treatment has produced significant reductions in alcohol consumption among heavy drinkers and alcohol-dependent subjects.[11] Brady and associates[12] conducted an open trial of sertraline with nine subjects who were comorbid for PTSD and alcohol dependence. They observed significant reductions in both PTSD symptoms and alcohol consumption. This is clearly an important finding that requires more extensive and systematic investigation.

Finally, SSRIs may be clinically useful because a number of symptoms associated with PTSD may be mediated by serotonergic mechanisms. These include rage, impulsivity, suicidal intent, depressed mood, panic symptoms, obsessional thinking, and behaviors associated with alcohol or drug abuse/dependency.[13]

Monoamine Oxidase Inhibitors

Phenelzine produced excellent reduction of PTSD symptoms (effect size .70) during an 8-week randomized clinical trial,[2] but it was less effective than placebo (effect size −.41) in a 4-week cross-over study.[5] The negative findings in the latter study may be explained by differences in study design, differences in duration of treatment, or the unusually high response to placebo[5] which may partially be due to the cross-over design of this study. In addition to these two randomized clinical trials are two successful open trials of phenelzine[14,15] and many positive case reports on MAOI treatment for PTSD (see ref. 16 for references). With one exception, all published results concern phenelzine administration to American or Israeli military veterans with PTSD. The exception is an interesting case report on successful MAOI treatment of five Indochinese refugees with tranylcypromine or isocarboxazid in which remission of PTSD symptoms was invariably associated with amelioration of depressive symptoms.[16]

Southwick et al.[17] reviewed all published findings (randomized trials, open trials, and case reports) on MAOI (phenelzine) treatment for PTSD. They found that MAOIs produced moderate to good global improvement in 82% of all patients, primarily because of a reduction in reexperiencing symptoms such as intrusive recollections, traumatic nightmares, and PTSD flashbacks. Insomnia also improved. No improvement was found, however, in PTSD avoidant/numbing, PTSD hyperarousal, depressive, or anxiety/panic symptoms.

In summary, with the exception of Shestatzky et al.'s[5] findings in a study that may have been methodologically flawed (see below), MAOIs have effectively reduced PTSD symptoms. Legitimate concerns about the risk of administrating these drugs to patients who may ingest alcohol or certain illicit drugs or who may not adhere to necessary dietary restrictions may be allayed in the future by the use of reversible inhibitors of MAO-A such as moclobemide. The oxidizing action of these drugs is restricted to norepinephrine and serotonin; they are free of hepatotoxicity, and they have a low risk of producing hypertension when combined with tyramine-containing foods.[18]

Brofaromine

Given the favorable results with fluoxetine and phenelzine, a medication that contains the properties of both drugs might be expected to prove effective in PTSD treatment. Brofaromine is such a drug. It is an investigational drug that is both an SSRI and a reversible MAO-A inhibitor. Two multicenter trials have been conducted with brofaromine in which a total of 158 patients were randomized to active drug or placebo groups and in which treatment was continued for 10-14 weeks. Collectively, this is the largest number of patients to have ever received any specific drug and the longest duration of treatment in any randomized clinical trial with PTSD patients. Unfortunately, results with brofaromine have been disappointing. In one study,[6] (n = 113), there were essentially no differences between drug and placebo groups after 10 weeks of treatment (effect size was only .13). A better outcome was found in the second study[7] (n = 45) in which the effect size was .71 but findings fell short of statistical significance for the overall sample (p ≤ 0.08). (Results were significant, however [p ≤ 0.05], when analysis was restricted to patients who had had PTSD for 1 year or more.) Katz and associates[7] argued that their findings should be considered clinically, if not statistically significant, because 55% of patients receiving brofaromine, in contrast to only 26% of those receiving a placebo, no longer met full diagnostic criteria for PTSD following 14 weeks of treatment. They also point out that brofaromine's efficacy was obscured because approximately 30% of placebo patients in both studies exhibited improvement. This contrasts markedly with the low placebo response rates generally observed during randomized clinical trials with PTSD; usually only 5-17% of patients show improvement following placebo treatment.

Tricyclic Antidepressants

There have been three randomized clinical trials with tricyclic antidepressants involving 124 patients as well as numerous case reports and open trials (see ref. 19 for references). As shown in TABLE 1, results have been mixed. Imipramine produced statistically significant global improvement and reductions in reexperiencing symptoms following an 8-week trial, but the effect size was only .39.[2] Amitryptyline significantly reduced avoidant/numbing but not reexperiencing or arousal symptoms after 8 weeks of treatment, but the effect size was only .38.[8] Finally, desipramine was no better than placebo following a 4-week trial.[20] In their analysis of 15 randomized trials, open trials, and case reports involving TCA treatment for PTSD, Southwick and associates[17] found that 45% of patients showed moderate to good global improvement following treatment, whereas MAOIs produced global improvement in 82% of patients who received them. As with MAOIs, most improvement was due to reductions in reexperiencing rather than avoidant/numbing or arousal symptoms. It also appeared that a minimum of 8 weeks of treatment with either TCAs or MAOIs was necessary to achieve positive clinical results. Of interest is a single report on an open trial of clomipramine, a TCA that acts like an SSRI, in which reduction of PTSD reexperiencing symptoms was accompanied by a marked decrease in obsessional symptoms.

To summarize, TCAs appear to reduce PTSD reexperiencing symptoms but have not demonstrated the efficacy of SSRIs or MAOIs.

Benzodiazepines

Although there are theoretical reasons why benzodiazepines might be effective in PTSD[21] and clinical reports that they have been prescribed widely for PTSD patients in some clinical settings,[22] there are only three publications on benzodiazepine treatment for PTSD. In a randomized clinical trial, Braun *et al.*[23] found that alprazolam was no better than placebo in reducing core PTSD symptoms (effect size .42); however, modest reductions in generalized anxiety were observed.

An open trial with alprazolam produced similar results in which PTSD patients reported reduced insomnia, anxiety, and irritability.[24] Finally, Lowenstein,[25] observed that clonazepam successfully reduced insomnia, nightmares, and panic attacks in PTSD patients who also had Dissociative Identity Disorder, but it did not produce improvement in avoidance or dissociative symptoms. In summary, there is little reason to select a benzodiazepine before other treatment alternatives. I have suggested elsewhere[9] three possible clinical indications for clonazepam: (1) acute stress reactions; (2) episodically in chronic PTSD when extreme anxiety interferes with the patient's participation in treatment; and (3) in carefully selected patients with comorbid alcohol or substance abuse (see also ref. 21).

Inositol

Inositol is a second messenger precursor that has been used successfully to treat both depression[26] and panic disorder[27] in randomized clinical trials. For those reasons, Kaplan and coworkers[28] conducted a randomized double-blind 4-week crossover study of inositol in 13 Israelis with PTSD related to military and civilian exposure to trauma. No difference was found between inositol and placebo (effect size .28), but some patients exhibited a reduction in depressive symptoms.

Antiadrenergic Agents: Propranolol and Clonidine

It is well established that adrenergic dysregulation is associated with chronic PTSD (see refs. 3 and 29 for details and references). Therefore, it is surprising that so few reports on PTSD treatment with clonidine or propranolol have been published despite the fact that positive findings with both drugs were reported as early as 1984.[30] Indeed, although there are no randomized clinical trials with either drug, there is one report[31] in which the beta-adrenergic blocking agent propranolol was administered to 11 physically and/or sexually abused children with PTSD in an A-B-A design (6 weeks off-6 weeks on-6 weeks off medication). Significant reductions in reexperiencing and arousal symptoms were observed during drug treatment, but symptoms relapsed to pretreatment severity following discontinuation of medication. In addition to Kolb *et al.*'s[30] open trial in which propranolol successfully reduced reexperiencing and arousal symptoms in Vietnam veterans, the only other relevant report is an unsuccessful open trial of propranolol in Cambodian refugees with PTSD.[32]

Three open trials have shown that the alpha$_2$-adrenergic agonist clonidine has produced successful outcomes in PTSD patients by reducing traumatic nightmares, intrusive recollections, hypervigilance, insomnia, startle reactions, and angry outbursts, and by improving mood and concentration. It is noteworthy that each of these trials involved three different clinical populations with PTSD: Vietnam veterans,[30] abused children,[33] and Cambodian refugees.[34] In the latter study, a clonidine/imipramine combination was more effective than either drug alone.

Anticonvulsants

It has been proposed that following exposure to traumatic events, limbic nuclei become kindled or sensitized so that, henceforth, they exhibit excessive responsivity to less intense trauma-related stimuli. Post and associates[35] have written the most comprehensive and elegant review of this model. Arguing from this theoretical perspective, Lipper and associates[36] conducted an open trial of the anticonvulsant/ antikindling agent carbamazepine with Vietnam veterans and observed significant reductions in traumatic nightmares, flashbacks, intrusive recollections, and insomnia. Since that time, positive results have been obtained in many open trials with anticonvulsant/antikindling drugs in PTSD patients. In five studies, carbamazepine produced reductions in reexperiencing and arousal symptoms, whereas in three studies, valproate produced reductions in avoidant/numbing and arousal (but not reexperiencing) symptoms (see ref. 21 for references).

An interesting recent clinical report described the effectiveness of a different anticonvulsant which was prescribed for a different theoretical reason. Vigabatrin, a specific gamma aminobutyric acid (GABA) transaminase inhibitor, is an effective anticonvulsant[37] that has been used to treat startle disease (hyperekplexia) of neonates.[38] Since fear-potentiated startle has been proposed as a psychobiologic mechanism for PTSD,[39] MacLeod[40] prescribed vigabatrin to five PTSD patients whose persistent startle and hypervigilance had not responded to other medications. In all cases, vigabatrin produced marked relief of these distressing symptoms.

It is always exciting when hypothesis-driven experiments yield successful results. It will be even more exciting if these open trials and case reports with anticonvulsants pass the test of randomized clinical trials.

Other Drugs

A number of other drugs have been the focus of one or two reports. Almost every kind of psychoactive drug has been represented and, as is usually the case with uncontrolled trials that get published, results have generally been positive. For the sake of completeness, I will mention each drug briefly. (The reader is referred to refs. 9 and 21 for further details and literature citations.)

Buspirone, an anxiolytic that is a 5-HT1A partial agonist, reduced reexperiencing and arousal symptoms in three patients. Cyproheptidine, a 5-HT antagonist, selectively suppressed traumatic nightmares without improving other PTSD symptoms. Lithium appeared to reduce hyperarousal symptoms in two open trials, with no therapeutic effect on reexperiencing or avoidant/numbing symptoms. One case report on phenothiazine treatment has appeared in which thioridazine reduced reexperiencing and arousal symptoms in one patient. Finally, the narcotic antagonist nalmefene markedly reduced numbing symptoms in some patients but worsened anxiety and panic symptoms in others, whereas the narcotic antagonist naltrexone suppressed PTSD flashbacks in one patient.

These are interesting findings in view of current hypotheses about the pathophysiology of PTSD, but these drugs must be tested more rigorously before they can command our attention.

ANSWERS AND QUESTIONS

As stated at the outset, the answers provided by randomized clinical trials raise some important questions that must be addressed in subsequent research.

Have we been testing drugs on the wrong clinical populations? We have argued elsewhere (ref. 21, page 475) that:

> American Vietnam veterans who have served as subjects in most published randomized clinical trials may be the most severely impaired, chronic, and treatment-refractory patient cohorts. The reason why they remain the most available patients for drug trials is because they are still enrolled in VA treatment programs. . . [and] constitute a self-selected cohort of chronic patients with multiple levels of impairment who may be most refractory to drug (or any other) treatment.

TABLE 1 supports this conclusion. Considering an effect size of .5 standard deviations as the minimum effect size necessary for a clinically meaningful difference, every study that failed to exceed that threshold was conducted on military veterans. Comparing the civilian and veteran cohorts in the fluoxetine trial conducted by van der Kolk and coworkers,[4] the effect size for civilian (mostly female adult survivors of childhood sexual abuse) subjects was 1.12, whereas it was only .38 for military veterans who participated in the same protocol. The two brofaromine studies in which the same protocol was followed suggest the same conclusion. In the American trial[6] in which there was no difference between groups (effect size was only .13), 60% of the subjects were military veterans. In the mostly European trial,[7] considerably fewer (9% brofaromine and 26% placebo) subjects were military veterans;[7] results were nearly significant ($p \leq 0.08$) and the effect size was .71. In fact, the only study with military veterans that was both significant and clinically meaningful (effect size .70) was the trial of phenelzine conducted by Kosten and associates.[2] As the investigators in that study excluded all veterans with major depression, they may have inadvertently screened out the most treatment-refractory patients as well.

It is important to emphasize that I am not suggesting that there is anything about military trauma or male gender that is inherently refractory to pharmacotherapy. I am stating, however, that it would be premature to write off any drug as a potential treatment for PTSD until it has been tested on an appropriate clinical sample. Therefore, future studies should be conducted on a variety of patient cohorts to insure that lack of clinical success of a specific drug is genuinely due to lack of pharmacological efficacy rather than to the testing of a particularly refractory group of patients.

Have we optimized our clinical trials with respect to design and instrumentation? Kudler and associates[41] were the first to suggest that methodological factors such as differences in experimental design, duration of treatment, and instrumentation might account for differences in results from one clinical trial to the next. They emphasized that the most successful trials (with MAOIs and TCAs) tended to last at least 8 weeks. This is generally true of the data shown in TABLE 1 with the notable exception of the 5-week fluoxetine trial on nonveteran subjects.[4]

Kudler et al.[41] also questioned the use of the Impact of Events Scale (IES) as the best instrument for assessing PTSD. The IES has served honorably in PTSD research, but it is a self-rating scale that neglects a whole category of PTSD symptoms (hyperarousal symptoms). There are many newer and more comprehensive self-report and observer rating scales that may be more sensitive for assessing weekly changes during a drug trial which are being used in the most current drug trials.[42] In fact, the IES itself was recently revised to correct some of its deficiencies.[43]

Research designs should also include adequate controls for psychiatric disorders frequently comorbid with PTSD, such as alcohol abuse/dependence, depression, and other anxiety disorders.[41] In this regard, the study by Brady et al.[12] is particularly noteworthy because it was designed to investige the efficacy of sertraline on patients comorbid for both PTSD and alcohol dependence.

Finally, all clinical trials have focused on reduction of PTSD symptoms as the major outcome measure. Although it is obviously important to monitor symptoms, other clinical domains such as social/vocational function or clinical utilization may be important outcomes, especially in patients with severe and chronic PTSD. It is conceivable that successful treatment with some cohorts might be indicated by improved marital, family, social, or vocational function or by lower inpatient or outpatient clinical service utilization, rather than by a reduction in PTSD symptoms.

Have we been testing the wrong drugs? Almost every drug tested in PTSD was developed as an antidepressant and has shown efficacy against panic and other anxiety disorders. Given high comorbidity rates between PTSD and such disorders and given the symptomatic overlap between PTSD, major depression, panic disorder, and generalized anxiety disorder,[44] it seems reasonable to test such drugs in PTSD. On the other hand, PTSD appears to be distinctive in a number of ways. First, it seems to be more complex than affective or other anxiety disorders; abnormalities have already been detected in at least seven unique neurobiological systems.[3] Second, its underlying pathophysiology appears to be different. For example, abnormalities in the hypothalamic-pituitary-adrenocortical (HPA) system, as shown by Yehuda and associates,[45] are markedly different from those present in major depressive disorder despite similarities in clinical phenomenology. In short, the time has come to develop and test drugs that have been developed specifically for PTSD rather than to recycle pharmacological agents that have been developed to treat affective or other anxiety disorders.

We have stated elsewhere that PTSD is the neurobiological and clinical consequence of failure of humans to cope with catastrophic stressors. During such exposure persons attempt to use the same neurobiological mechanisms that are activated by any stressful event. In contrast to a successful coping response which is followed by restoration of normal homeostatic balance, however, the unsuccessful coping that precipitates PTSD results in a steady state that deviates significantly from normal homeostasis. We have invoked McEwen's[46] concept of "allostasis" to describe this abnormal neurobiological steady state which we hypothesize to be present in PTSD patients.[47]

From this perspective, the best way to understand the pathophysiology of PTSD is by investigating the human stress response. Such an approach would focus attention on neuropeptides rather than biogenic amines. Because corticotropin-releasing factor (CRF) appears to play such a central role in the stress response,[48] it seems that drugs that block or modify the actions of CRF might prove efficacious in treating PTSD patients. This might include CRF antagonists such as alpha-helical CRF. Another approach is to enhance the actions of neuropeptide Y, a peptide that may act as an endogenous anxiolytic and that may diminish the actions of CRF.[48] Once we shift our focus from traditional antidepressants and anxiolytics to the complex human stress response, many other targets can be considered for potential anti-PTSD drugs. Hopefully, such a shift in focus will occur in the near future.

Are there different subtypes or stages of PTSD that may require different treatments at different times? Some evidence indicates that there may be different neurobiological subtypes of PTSD. For example, Southwick *et al.*[49] have shown that yohimbine may precipitate panic and flashbacks in some PTSD patients, whereas others are more likely to respond to *m*-chloro-phenyl-piperazine. This suggests that adrenergic dysregulation may be more prominent in some PTSD patients, whereas serotonergic sensitization is more prominent in others. This has obvious implications for pharmacotherapy.

Diagnostically we know that some traumatized patients develop borderline personality disorder or dissociative identity disorder or what Herman[50] has named, "complex PTSD," with or without PTSD itself. In the future we must determine if these also represent different subtypes of PTSD with a somewhat different pattern of neurobiological abnormalities that may require different pharmacotherapeutic strategies.

Finally, we must consider whether PTSD is a dynamic rather than a static disorder that evolves over time. Post and associates[35] presented such a model of PTSD which is based on mechanisms underlying sensitization and kindling. Sensitization and kindling evolve neurobiologically over time, and pharmacological responsivity to a drug (such as carbamezepine) may vary at different stages of evolution. Therefore, it would be essential to identify these different stages accurately in order to know when to prescribe a neuroleptic, an anticonvulsant, or some other drug. Extrapolating from this model, Post and associates[35] suggest that PTSD may also progress through different stages and that it may be necessary to identify these stages to know when to prescribe the most effective drug. One clinical vignette that is consistent with this theoretical approach was the finding by Katz *et al.*[7] that brofaromine was more effective in patients who had had PTSD for at least 12 months than in those who had developed PTSD within the last year.

Is there a magic bullet for PTSD? We concluded elsewhere[21] that no magic bullet for PTSD is in sight. Instead, we previously suggested that a combination of drugs, each targeting a specific cluster of symptoms, might provide the best approach at this time. For example, we recommended that MAOIs or TCAs might be best for reexperiencing, SSRIs for avoidant/numbing, and antiadrenergic agents (such as clonidine and propranolol) for hyperarousal symptoms.

Although that approach may be a reasonable for the time being, it is clear that we have just begun to conduct a systematic evaluation of drugs for PTSD. It is still an open question whether there is a specific drug or class of drugs that might provide effective treatment for all three clusters of PTSD symptoms. The few randomized clinical trials that have been published have generated more questions than answers. We may not have tested drugs on the right clinical cohorts. We may not have used the best experimental protocols or assessment instruments. We may not have tested the most effective drugs. And we may not have understood how different subtypes or states of PTSD might affect the efficacy of different medications at different times.

In short, rather than feeling discouraged we should intensify our search for a magic bullet, fortified by recent gains in our emerging understanding of the pathophysiology of PTSD.

REFERENCES

1. FRANK, J. B. *et al.* 1988. A randomized clinical trial of phenelzine and imipramine for post-traumatic stress disorder. Am. J. Psychiatry **145:** 1289-1291.
2. KOSTEN, T. R. *et al.* 1991. Pharmacotherapy for post-traumatic stress disorder using phenelzine or imipramine. J. Nerv. Ment. Dis. **179:** 366-370.
3. FRIEDMAN, M. J. *et al.* 1995. Neurobiological and Clinical Consequences of Stress: From Normal Adaptation to PTSD. Lippincott-Raven Press. Philadelphia, PA.
4. VAN DER KOLK, B. A. *et al.* 1994. Fluoxetine in post-traumatic stress disorder. J. Clin. Psychiatry **55:** 517-522.
5. SHESTATZKY, M. *et al.* 1988. A controlled trial of phenelzine in post-traumatic stress disorder. Psychiatry Res. **24:** 149-155.
6. BAKER, D. G. *et al.* 1995. A double-blind, randomized, placebo-controlled, multicenter study of brofaromine in the treatment of post-traumatic stress disorder. Psychopharmacology **122:** 386-389.
7. KATZ, R. J. *et al.* 1994/1995. Pharmacotherapy of post-traumatic stress disorder with a novel psychotropic. Anxiety **1:** 169-174.
8. DAVIDSON, J. *et al.* 1990. Treatment of post-traumatic stress disorder with amitriptyline and placebo. Arch. Gen. Psychiatry **47:** 259-266.
9. FRIEDMAN, M. J. 1996. Biological alterations in PTSD: Implications for pharmacotherapy. *In* Baillière's Clinical Psychiatry: International Practice and Research: Post-Traumatic Stress Disorder, Vol. 2(2). E. Giller & L. Weisaeth, Eds.: 245-262. Baillière Tindall. London.
10. KOFOED, L. *et al.* 1993. Alcoholism and drug abuse in patients with PTSD. Psychiatr. Q. **64:** 151-169.
11. NARANJO, C. A. & E. M. SELLARS. 1989. Serotonin uptake inhibitors attenuate ethanol intake in problem drinkers. Recent Dev. Alcohol **7:** 255-266.
12. BRADY, K. T. *et al.* 1995. Sertraline treatment of comorbid posttraumatic stress disorder and alcohol dependence. J. Clin. Psychiatry **56:** 502-505.
13. FRIEDMAN, M. J. 1990. Interrelationships between biological mechanisms and pharmacotherapy of post-traumatic stress disorder. *In* Post-Traumatic Stress Disorder: Etiology, Phenomenology, and Treatment. M. E. Wolfe & A. D. Mosnaim, Eds.: 204-225. American Psychiatric Press. Washington, DC.
14. DAVIDSON, J. *et al.* 1987. A pilot study of phenelzine in posttraumatic stress disorder. Br. J. Psychiatry **150:** 252-255.
15. LERER, B. *et al.* 1987. Posttraumatic stress disorder in Israeli combat veterans. Arch. Gen. Psychiatry **44:** 976-981.
16. DEMARTINO, R. *et al.* 1995. Monoamine oxidase inhibitors in posttraumatic stress disorder. J. Nerv. Ment. Dis. **183:** 510-515.
17. SOUTHWICK, S. M. *et al.* 1994. Use of tricyclics and monoamine oxidase inhibitors in the treatment of PTSD: A quantitative review. *In* Catecholamine Function in Post-Traumatic

Stress Disorder: Emerging Concepts. M. M. Murburg, Ed.: 293-305. American Psychiatry Press. Washington, DC.

18. DaPRADA, M. *et al.* 1990. Some basic aspects of reversible inhibitors of monoamine oxidase-A. Acta Psychiatr. Scand. Suppl. **360:** 7-12.

19. VER ELLEN, P. & D. P. VAN KAMMEN. 1990. The biological findings in post-traumatic stress disorder: A review. J. Appl. Soc. Psychol. **20**(21,pt1):1789-1821.

20. REIST, C. *et al.* 1989. A controlled trial of desipramine in 18 men with post-traumatic stress disorder. Am. J. Psychiatry **146:** 513-516.

21. FRIEDMAN, M. J. & S. M. SOUTHWICK. 1995. Towards pharmacotherapy for PTSD. *In* Neurobiological and Clinical Consequences of Stress: From Normal Adaptation to PTSD. M. J. Friedman *et al.,* Eds.: 465-481. Lippincott-Raven Press. Philadelphia, PA.

22. CICCONE, P. E. *et al.* 1988. [Letter]. Am. J. Psychiatry **145:** 1484-1485.

23. BRAUN, P. *et al.* 1990. Core symptoms of posttraumatic stress disorder unimproved by alprazolam treatment. J. Clin. Psychiatry **51:** 236-238.

24. FELDMAN, T. B. 1987. Alprazolam in the treatment of post-traumatic stress disorder [letter]. J. Clin. Psychiatry **48:** 216-217.

25. LOWENSTEIN, R. J. 1991. Rational psychopharmacology in the treatment of multiple personality disorder. Psychiatr. Clin. N. Am. **14:** 721-740.

26. LEVINE, J. *et al.* 1995. A double-blind controlled trial of inositol treatment of depression. Am. J. Psychiatry **152:** 792-794.

27. BENJAMIN, J. *et al.* 1995. Inositol treatment for panic disorder. Am. J. Psychiatry **152:** 1084-1086.

28. KAPLAN, Z. *et al.* 1996. Inositol treatment of PTSD. Anxiety **2:** 51-52.

29. MURBURG, M. M., Ed. 1994. Catecholamine Function in Post-Traumatic Stress Disorder: Emerging Concepts. American Psychiatric Press. Washington, DC.

30. KOLB, L. C. *et al.* 1984. Propranolol and clonidine in the treatment of the chronic post-traumatic stress disorders of war. *In* Post-Traumatic Stress Disorder: Psychological and Biological Sequelae. B. A. van der Kolk, Ed.: 97-107. American Psychiatric Press. Washington, DC.

31. FAMULARO, R. *et al.* 1988. Propranolol treatment for childhood post-traumatic stress disorder, acute type: A pilot study. Am. J. Dis. Child. **142:** 1244-1247.

32. KINZIE, J. D. 1989. Therapeutic approaches to traumatized Cambodian refugees. J. Trauma Stress **2:** 207-228.

33. PERRY, B. D. 1994. Neurobiological sequelae of childhood trauma: PTSD in children. *In* Catecholamine Function in Post-Traumatic Stress Disorder: Emerging Concepts. M. M. Murburg, Ed.: 233-255. American Psychiatric Press. Washington, DC.

34. KINZIE, J. D. & F. LEUNG. 1989. Clonidine in Cambodian patients with post-traumatic stress disorder. J. Nerv. Ment. Dis. **177:** 546-550.

35. POST, R. M. *et al.* 1995. Sensitization and kindling: Implications for the evolving neural substrate of PTSD. *In* Neurobiological and Clinical Consequences of Stress: From Normal Adaptation to PTSD. M. J. Friedman *et al.,* Eds.: 203-224. Lippincott-Raven Press. Philadelphia, PA.

36. LIPPER, S. *et al.* 1986. Preliminary study of carbamazepine in post-traumatic stress disorder. Psychosomatics **27:** 849-854.

37. KURLAND, A. H. & T. R. BROWNE 1994. Review: Vigabatrin (Sabril). Clin. Neuropharmacol. **17:** 560-568.

38. STEPHENSON, J. B. P. 1992. Vigabatrin for startle disease with altered cerebrospinal fluid free gamma-aminobutyric acid. Lancet **340:** 430-431.

39. CHARNEY, D. S. *et al.* 1993. Psychobiologic mechanisms of post-traumatic stress disorder. Arch. Gen. Psychiatry **50:** 294-305.

40. MacLEOD, A. D. 1996. Letter: Vigabatrin and posttraumatic stress disorder. J. Clin. Psychopharmacol. **16:** 190-191.

41. KUDLER, H. *et al.* 1987. The DST and post-traumatic stress disorder. Am. J. Psychiatry **144:** 1068-1071.

42. WILSON, J. & T. M. KEANE, Eds. 1997. Assessing Psychological Trauma and PTSD. Guilford. New York.

43. WEISS, D. 1997. Psychometric review of the Impact of Events Scale—Revised. *In* Measurement of Stress, Trauma and Adaptation. B. H. Stamm, Ed. Sidran Press. Lutherville, MD. In press.

44. FRIEDMAN, M. J. & R. YEHUDA. 1995. PTSD and co-morbidity: Psychobiological approaches to differential diagnosis. *In* Neurobiological and Clinical Consequences of Stress: From Normal Adaptation to PTSD. M. J. Friedman *et al.*, Eds.: 429-446. Lippincott-Raven Press. Philadelphia, PA.

45. YEHUDA, R. *et al.* 1993. Enhanced suppression of cortisol following dexamethasone administration in posttraumatic stress disorder. Am. J. Psychiatry **150:** 83-86.

46. McEWEN, B. S. 1995. Adrenal steroid actions on brain: Dissecting the fine line between protection and damage. *In* Neurobiological and Clinical Consequences of Stress: From Normal Adaptation to PTSD. M. J. Friedman *et al.*, Eds.: 135-147. Lippincott-Raven Press. Philadelphia, PA.

47. FRIEDMAN, M. J. *et al.* 1995. Preface. *In* Neurobiological and Clinical Consequences of Stress: From Normal Adaptation to PTSD. M. J. Friedman *et al.*, Eds.: xix-xx. Lippincott-Raven Press. Philadelphia, PA.

48. STOUT, S. C. *et al.* 1995. Neuropeptides and stress: Preclinical findings and implications for pathophysiology. *In* Neurobiological and Clinical Consequences of Stress: From Normal Adaptation to PTSD. M. J. Friedman *et al.*, Eds.: 103-123. Lippincott-Raven Press. Philadelphia, PA.

49. SOUTHWICK, S. M. *et al.* 1995. Clinical studies of neurotransmitter alterations in posttraumatic stress disorder. *In* Neurobiological and Clinical Consequences of Stress: From Normal Adaptation to PTSD. M. J. Friedman *et al.*, Eds.: 335-350. Lippincott-Raven Press. Philadelphia, PA.

50. HERMAN, J. L. 1992. Trauma and Recovery. Basic Books. New York.

Treatment Failure in Acute PTSD

Lessons Learned about the Complexity of the Disorder[a]

ARIEH Y. SHALEV

Department of Psychiatry
Hadassah University Hospital
P.O. Box 12000
Jerusalem, 91120, Israel

The treatment of chronic posttraumatic stress disorder (PTSD) often fails to achieve the desired results, and the treatment of acute PTSD does not fare much better. Possibly, we simply do not know how to treat the disorder, and better treatment methods are the proper response to the current shortcoming. Yet this may not be the entire story. Other reasons include (1) difficulties in properly identifying survivors at risk; (2) the finding that many factors that lead to PTSD precede trauma and are not affected by treatment; (3) lack of the proper definition of a "critical period" during which the neurobiological processes that lead to PTSD can be reversed; and (4) treatment methods that target the overt expression of the disorder rather than its pathogenesis. This chapter reviews the treatment of PTSD, and addresses the foregoing propositions, reporting data from prospective studies of trauma survivors conducted in the author's laboratory in Jerusalem.

COURSE AND TREATMENT OF PTSD

PTSD is a pervasive anxiety disorder that follows exposure to extreme stress. Symptoms resembling those of PTSD are expressed by most trauma survivors during the days that follow the trauma.[1] In most trauma survivors, however, the intensity of these symptoms declines with time. Yet, a few others continue to have chronic PTSD, often for the rest of their lives. Spontaneous recovery from chronic PTSD is the exception and may not occur at all after 6 years of illness.[2] Moreover, the results of treatment intervention in chronic PTSD are limited.[3,4] Neither recovery nor sustained remission have been reported in controlled studies[5–20] (TABLES 1 and 2).

The limited effect of treatment in chronic PTSD may simply reflect the duration of the disorder. Prolonged arousal produces significant alteration in neuronal functioning, which treatment interventions may fail to redress. Treatment resistance in chronic PTSD may also result from the presence of comorbid disorders (identified in up to 88% of males and 79% of females with PTSD[2]). Finally, the population identified by current diagnostic criteria for PTSD may still be heterogeneous, as suggested by

[a]This work was supported by a research grant from the Ministry of Labor, Israel, and by US Public Health Service research grant MH-50379.

TABLE 1. Controlled Studies of Pharmacological Treatment in PTSD

Authors and Year	Drug and Dose (mg/day)	Population and Number	Results and Conclusions
Shestazki et al.,[5] 1987	Phenelzine (45–75) vs placebo	Miscellaneous trauma, 13	Decrease in PTSD and anxiety symptoms. No difference between active drug and placebo
Frank et al.,[b] 1988	Phenelzine (71) Imipramine (240) Placebo	Veterans, 34	Phenelzine and imipramine superior to placebo. Improved intrusion but not avoidance
Reist et al.,[7] 1989	Desipramine (200)	Veterans, 18	Improvement in depression, no change in anxiety and PTSD symptoms
Braun et al.,[8] 1990	Alprazolam vs placebo (2.5–6)	Miscellaneous PTSD, 10	Improvement in anxiety, no effect on PTSD symptoms
Davidson et al.,[9] 1990	Amitriptyline (50–300) vs placebo	Miscellaneous PTSD, 40	Reduction in depression on week 4. Additional effect on PTSD symptoms on week 8
Kosten et al.,[10] 1991	Phenelzine (60–79) Imipramine (50–300) Placebo	Veterans, 60	44% improvement w/phenelzine & 25% with imipramine. Avoidance symptoms not improved
Davidson et al.,[11] 1993	Amitriptyline (160)	War veterans, 55	Significant effect on depression. Trend towards improvement in PTSD symptoms
Van der Kolk et al.,[12] 1994	Fluoxetine (20) vs placebo	War veterans and civilian PTSD, 24	Reduction in arousal, numbing, and depression. Not in intrusion dissociation and hostility. Better effect on recent PTSD

TABLE 2. Controlled Studies of Psychological Treatment of PTSD

Authors and Year	Treatment	Population and Number	Results and Conclusions
Peniston,[13] 1986	Desensitization & biofeedback vs no treatment	War veterans, 16	Reduction in nightmares, flashbacks, muscle tension, and re-admissions rate in active treatment group
Resick et al.,[14] 1988	Stress-inoculation, assertion-training; supportive psychotherapy	Rape victims, 37	Improvement across measures; no difference between treatment protocols at 3- and 6-month follow-up
Brom et al.,[15] 1989	Desensitization, hypnotherapy, psychodynamic therapy, and waiting list	Miscellaneous trauma, 112	60% improvement in active treatment vs 26% in controls; no difference between treatment modalities
Keane et al.,[16] 1989	Flodding vs waiting list	War veterans, 24	Improved reexperiencing, anxiety, and depression, no effect on numbing and avoidance
Boudewyns et al.,[17] 1990	Direct exposure (DTE) vs counseling	War veterans, 58	DTE superior to counseling
Foa et al.,[18] 1991	Stress-inoculation (SIT); prolonged exposure (PE); supportive counseling (SC); and wait-list (WL)	Rape victims, 45	All active conditions produced improvement. SIT> SC & WL immediately after treatment. PE> all others on 3.5-month follow-up
Resick & Schnicke,[19] 1992	Cognitive processing vs waiting list	Sexual assault, 19	Improved PTSD and depression in active treatment group maintained for 6 months
Richards et al., 1994	Imaginal vs live exposure	Miscellaneous trauma, 14	Improvement in measures of PTSD and depression in both protocols; more improvement of avoidance in live exposure

a recent report of selective responsiveness to either norepinephrine or serotonin activation in subgroups of PTSD patients.[21]

Hence, treatment failure in chronic PTSD can hardly lead to specific neurobiological hypotheses. A closer look at the results of early treatment may therefore be more informative. Indeed, it had been hoped that early treatment would effectively prevent PTSD. The following vignettes, however, illustrate that such is often not the case.

CLINICAL VIGNETTES[b]

Case I. The patient (D.), a 32-year-old male storekeeper from Jerusalem, was in his shop when he heard terrorist shooting. He immediately pushed the customers who were close to the door into the safety of the shop, then peered out to see what was going on. Seconds later he was lying on the sidewalk, injured by a gunshot to his leg. He would later say that he had seen two young individuals with red ribbons on their foreheads, one of them pointing a semiautomatic gun to his chest. Before yielding to the pain, he managed to run a few steps which, he thought, had saved his life.

While in the hospital, he had intrusive memories of the event, yet still complimented himself for having reacted to the incident in a "reasonable and respectable" way. He would repeatedly imagine what could have happened if the bullet had hit him in the head. Intrusive images of the young terrorist aiming his rifle would assail his sleep. Media coverage of the survivors left him with penetrating fear that the attackers or their "associates" could identify and follow him. Recently married, he tried to protect his younger wife from knowing "too much," dismissing her questions in a brief "never mind." His agitation growing, he was recognized as having acute stress disorder, was promptly educated about the nature of his condition, and was partially relieved by the support and the clarification. Upon his release from the hospital he returned to his work.

In the following days, however, he could not concentrate. He avoided the sidewalk where he had been wounded. When one of his clients got into an argument with him, he was suddenly overwhelmed by fear and promptly left the shop. He started to believe that he could not "hold the whole thing together" and that others were observing him, witnessing his fear. In business meetings, he would experience panic and fail to defend his own interests, often leaving the place humiliated and ashamed. Coming home he would scan the staircase for armed assailants, double lock the door, draw the curtains, and spend more and more time alone, protected from noise and people.

Six weeks after the incident he was referred to a trauma clinic, where he started a treatment program in which the generalization of his fears, his obsessive expectation of another terrorist act, his sense of helplessness, and his avoidance were systematically addressed. Nevertheless, his irritability, sleep problems, and anger continued to grow. He was, therefore, put on long-acting benzodiazepines. Later, his depressed

---

[b] Subjects whose cases are presented here have agreed to have them published, with some modification in details concerning their personal identification.

mood was treated with specific serotonine reuptake inhibitors (SSRIs), and when this treatment failed, a reversible MAO inhibitor was prescribed with the idea that his symptoms resembled social phobia.

He strictly complied with medication, steadily attended the treatment sessions, and did not abuse alcohol. His wife was seen in supportive treatment and educated about PTSD. Self-referral to an eye movement desensitization and reprocessing program has temporarily reactivated the trauma. Consultations with a spiritual leader of his community increased his ability to accept his condition but did not affect it. In the long run it was clear that treatment had failed, leaving D with chronic and disabling PTSD, self-depreciation, isolation, and fearful avoidance.

Case II. The patient (Mrs. S.) a 54-year-old woman who had recently immigrated to Israel from Russia, witnessed a terrorist shooting in a bus in which she was traveling to work. Two passengers were killed and several others wounded. Mrs. S. was evacuated to a general hospital in a state of panic, yet without physical injury. She has been seen by a Russian-speaking psychiatric registrar, who replied to her panic by reassuring her and helped her to regain some level of self-control. Upon release from the emergency room she was given a contact telephone number in case she needed more help. She did call after 2 days, during which she could not sleep and was literally dysfunctional. She was seen by the same physician in a state of extreme agitation. Clonazepam (4 mg per day) was prescribed and supportive psychotherapy started. Mrs S. slept better, but remained agitated, experiencing intrusive images of the trauma and pervasive insecurity.

Mrs. S.'s past history was one of deprived social background, painful separation from friends and relatives in Russia, and immigration to Israel. Throughout her life she had been working in unskilled jobs, and right before the trauma she was holding two jobs, being the main income provider for her family. Despite 2 years of treatment, however, Mrs. S never returned to work again. One month after her trauma, Mrs. S. met DSM III-R PTSD criteria, which she still meets 3 years later.

Case III. The patient (Mr. D.), a 55-year-old construction supervisor, was buried under a landslide in which another worker died. He was referred to a trauma unit 8 weeks later, with insomnia and intrusive images of the dying worker's face. This dedicated worker, who had been involved in major construction projects in Jerusalem, was again seen regularly since his trauma in interpersonal therapy, family therapy, and pharmacotherapy (clonazepam, lithium, and paroxetine) with the only gain being successful withdrawal from opiate analgesics and a level of tolerance to suffering, now, from previously unknown outbursts of anger, hypervigilence, memory and concentration problems, and a pervasive sense of guilt. Brain imaging and neuropsychological workup did not reveal any structural or functional brain dysfunction.

These vignettes illustrate what has become a frequent observation in our trauma center, the trauma survivor, seen very shortly after the event, who develops PTSD despite intensive treatment. Although these observations may reflect the shortcomings of a treatment strategy, the current literature suggests that the problem is more general.

PREVENTION OF PTSD IN RECENT TRAUMA SURVIVORS

Prospective treatment studies are difficult to carry out; hence most studies of early treatment are retrospective. Front-line treatment of combat stress reactions has been systematically conducted by the Israel Defense Force during the 1982 Lebanon War. The effect of such treatment was measured retrospectively by Solomon et al.[22] In that study, combat stress reaction casualties 1 year after the war rated the degree to which their frontline therapist had adhered to principles of frontline treatment (i.e., proximity to the site of combat, immediacy of the response, and explicit expectations of recovery). The results have shown that adherence to these principles correlated with lower levels of PTSD symptoms and a lower incidence of PTSD. This work is often cited to support the beneficial effects of early treatment. However, Solomon et al.'s larger follow-up study, from which the foregoing subsample was taken, offers a very different perspective:[23] An astonishing 59% of 382 combat stress reaction casualties who had been evacuated from their units to *specialized treatment facilities of the Israel Defense Force* (an inclusion criterion for the study) had PTSD 1 year after the war and 42% had PTSD 3 years later.

In a similar vein, a study of postcombat debriefing in the British Armed Forces during Operation Desert Shield[24] failed to show a significant effect of postcombat debriefing on the incidence and severity of PTSD. Deahl et al.[25] studied 62 British soldiers whose duties included the handling and identification of dead bodies during the Gulf War and found that psychological debriefing upon completion of their mission did not appear to make any difference in subsequent psychiatric morbidity. Yet, the largest psychological manipulation, designed to reduce psychological traumatization during war, namely, the systematic implementation of a 1-year tour of duty in the Vietnam War and strict adherence to a frontline treatment routine,[26] were associated with 30% lifetime and 15.2% chronic PTSD 20 years later.[27]

Several studies evaluated the effect of early treatment on survivors of civilian trauma. Brom et al.[28] studied the effects of early counseling for motor traffic accidents victims and found that that although counseling was appreciated by victims, it could not be proven to be effective in preventing PTSD 6 months later. Kenardy et al.[29] studied the effects of stress debriefing on the rate of recovery of 195 helpers following an earthquake in Newcastle, Australia. They found no evidence of an improved rate of recovery among 62 helpers who had been debriefed. Finally, Gelpin et al.[30] compared 13 civilians who received high-potency benzodiazepines within 2-18 days of trauma with 13 survivors matched for age, gender, and symptom severity. They found no difference in the course of PTSD symptoms between the groups and a higher incidence of PTSD in the treated group. Their data were interpreted in reference to Hebert et al.'s study[31] in which diazepam, administered to male hamsters following a defeat by an aggressive male, increased subsequent fearfulness and avoidance.

As a whole, these data point to major weaknesses in preventing PTSD by early treatment interventions. Such problems may reflect poor treatment strategies, and reports of individual treatment programs are often more positive. Yet, the consistency of the findings across populations and traumatic events suggests that improving the quality of early treatment may not be the only key for preventing PTSD. Indeed, Kessler et al.[2] compared individuals who had received treatment within 6 years of trauma with those who had not and found no difference in the prevalence of PTSD between the groups.[2] Alternative explanations include: (1) problems identifying subjects at risk for developing PTSD; (2) the amount of variance in the total causation of PTSD left for early interventions; and (3) missing the ''critical period'' during which treatment can reverse the neurobiological processes that lead to PTSD. Prospective studies at the Center for Traumatic Stress at Hadassah University Hospital have addressed some of these points.

PREDICTING PTSD FROM EARLY RESPONSES TO TRAUMA

Success and failure in treatment should be weighed against the odds of spontaneous recovery. Given that 70-85% of any traumatized population are going to recover,[2,27] most forms of early treatment are likely to yield very positive results and, indeed, may accelerate recovery in those individuals who are likely to recover.[2] However, the extent to which early treatment is provided to most subjects at risk may determine the global effect of treatment in a given population. For example, the control group in Solomon et al.'s study of the Lebanon War was composed of combat veterans who had not had combat stress reaction and had not sought treatment during the year that followed the war. Yet, 16% of this group developed PTSD.[23] Given that the number of combat soldiers who do not have combat stress reactions largely exceeds that of combat stress reaction casualties, most cases of PTSD from a given war may come from a group that never gets treatment.

Yet even among survivors who are systematically followed, the clinical predictors of PTSD are problematic. In 1992[32] we reported a study of 16 survivors of a single terrorist attack, four of whom (25%) had PTSD 10 months after the incident. The Impact of Events Scale (IES)[33] was used as both predictor and continuous outcome measure. IES scores recorded immediately after the trauma were poorly correlated with those recorded 10 months later.

In a second study[34] 51 injured trauma survivors were interviewed 1 week and 6 months after a trauma. The incidence of PTSD was 25% ($n = 13$) and 12 of the 13 PTSD patients were correctly identified by having IES scores above 19 on the 1-week IES score (93% sensitivity). IES scores above 19, however, have erroneously identified 13 of 38 survivors who did not develop PTSD as being at higher risk for developing PTSD (66% specificity).

A third prospective study[35] examined 235 trauma survivors 1 week, 1 month, and 4 months after trauma. Structured clinical interviews identified PTSD at both 1 and 4 months, showing a prevalence of 26.8% ($n = 63$) 1 month after trauma and 17.4% ($n = 41$) at the 4-month assessment. Receiver Operator Characteristic analysis was used to assess the quality of psychometric instruments as predictors of PTSD (FIG. 1). The results indicate that all the questionnaires were better than chance at predicting PTSD. Measures of PTSD symptoms, such as the IES, were no better at predicting the disorder than were the more general state-anxiety and dissociation questionnaires. No difference in predictive value was found between questionnaires that were carried out at 1 week and those administered 1 month later. The negative predictive value (i.e., prediction of who will not get PTSD) of the IES and anxiety measures was better than their positive prediction. A clinician-administered interview (CAPS) was significantly better than self-reports in predicting PTSD.

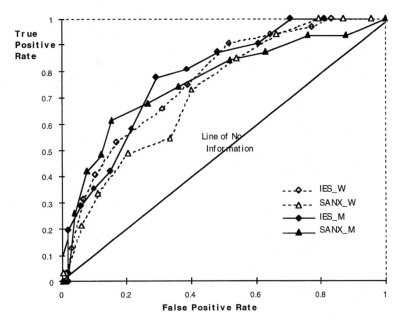

FIGURE 1. Predicting PTSD from early symptoms: Receiver operator characteristic curves. *Variables:* IES = Horowitz's Impact of Events Scale; SANX = Speilberger State Anxiety Inventory; W = 1 week after trauma; M = 1 month after trauma.

The foregoing data suggest that our ability to predict PTSD on the basis of early symptoms is limited. Most importantly, these results question the specificity of the relation between early PTSD-like symptoms that follow a trauma and the neurobiological processes that actually lead to PTSD.

VARIANCE OF CHRONIC PTSD SYMPTOMS EXPLAINED BY POSTEVENT VARIABLES

Peritraumatic Dissociation

Neurobiological theories suggest that PTSD may result from neuronal changes that are triggered by the traumatic event. These changes, however, may primarily occur in vulnerable individuals. Vulnerability factors include a yet unspecified genetic heritage,[36] prior traumatization, prior mental disorders, and an inappropriate rearing environment.[37] Abuse during childhood has been associated with dissociative disorders[38] and reduced hippocampal volume in adult survivors.[39] The latter may impair spatial recognition and orientation upon reexposure to stress in a way that mimics dissociation.

Dissociation during trauma (peritraumatic dissociation) has been associated with PTSD symptoms in survivors of the Oakland/Berkeley firestorm[40] and with chronic

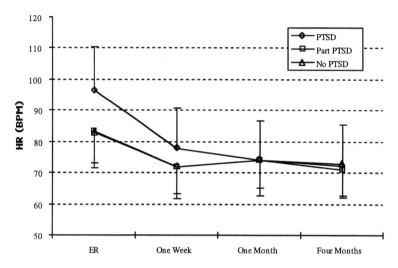

FIGURE 2. Heart rate response in recent trauma survivors versus time after trauma. *Variable:* ER = emergency room assessment.

PTSD in Vietnam combat veterans.[41] In the aforementioned prospective study,[34] peritraumatic dissociation was the best predictor of PTSD, explaining 29.4% of the variance in PTSD symptoms. Importantly, the contribution of peritraumatic dissociation to PTSD symptoms was not mediated by the intensity of early symptoms, suggesting a direct relation between this sequelae of earlier traumatization and PTSD. Early interventions may not be able to affect such a relationship.

Physiological Responses during Trauma

Another approach to the vulnerability-causation paradigm is through studies of early physiological responses to trauma. To the extent that such responses in subjects who develop PTSD exceed the effect of trauma intensity, they may be interpreted as reflecting prior vulnerability. Prior vulnerability is therefore reflected by amplification of the normal physiological response to stress.

Intense physiological responses to cues reminding of the trauma have been described in chronic PTSD.[42] In a follow-up study we recorded the heart rate (HR) of 86 trauma survivors on admission to the emergency room (ER) and 1-week, 1 month, and 4 months later. To reduce the variance in HR due to physical injury, only subjects with minor or no physical injuries were included (i.e., subjects who were sent back home directly from the ER). Twenty subjects (23.6%) had PTSD at the 4-month assessment (PTSD group), 22 (25.6%) met three of four PTSD diagnostic criteria (partial-PTSD group), and 44 had no PTSD. PTSD subjects had higher HR at the ER evaluation (95.45 ± 13.90 versus 83.44 ± 10.18 in partial PTSD and 83.00 ± 11.49 in individuals without PTSD; ANOVA $F(2,82) = 9.87$, $p < 0.001$) and 1 week after trauma, but not later (FIG. 2). Repeated measures ANOVA showed a significant

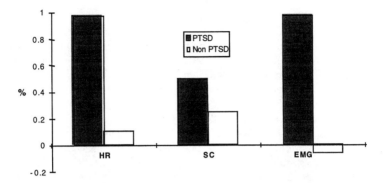

FIGURE 3. Response to traumatic imagery in PTSD 4 months after trauma (% of highest response) *Variables:* HR = heart rate; SC = skin conductance; EMG = orbicularis oculi electromyogram.

main effect of time ($p < .0001$) and a significant time by group interaction ($p < 0.003$). HR responses clearly differentiated PTSD from partial PTSD. The results remained significant when age, trauma severity, intensity of the immediate response to trauma, and peritraumatic dissociation were controlled. The results reflect elevated responsivity during stress in subjects who later develop PTSD. Importantly, such increased responsivity precedes the onset of the disorder and may predispose to it.

A CRITICAL POSTEVENT PERIOD?

Early treatment interventions may come too early or too late in the course of the response to trauma. The following psychophysiological studies illustrate the "timing" in which some typical responses of PTSD occur.

Responses to Mental Imagery

Increased physiological responses to mental imagery of the trauma have been described in chronic PTSD.[43,44] Yet, the extent to which such responses are present during the early stages of the disorder and the extent to which the presence of such responses differentiates PTSD from trauma survivors without PTSD are unknown. To address this question, heart rate (HR), skin conductance (SC), and frontalis electromyelographic (EMG) responses to mental imagery of the trauma were measured 4 months after trauma in 27 PTSD patients and 34 survivors without PTSD. Patients with PTSD showed higher responses to mental imagery of the trauma (FIG. 3).

Repeated endlessly in trauma survivors with PTSD, the link between physiological arousal and traumatic memories is reinforced with time. Beyond simple reinforcement, however, increased arousal on retrieving recollections of a trauma may interfere with the way in which such recollections are organized and stored in the brain.

Auditory Startle in Acute PTSD

Startle responses reflect neurophysiological mechanisms of stimulus evaluation, fear conditioning, habituation, and sensitization. Previous studies[45–48] have shown elevated HR and SC responses to loud tones and slower SC habituation in PTSD patients. The eyeblink startle reflex was assessed in several other studies,[49,50] and the results suggest that (1) the magnitude of the startle reflex in chronic PTSD is often similar to that of normal individuals; (2) the effects of fear enhancement on auditory startle in PTSD are similar to those observed in individuals without PTSD; and (3) contextual threat and chemical provocation are likely to enhance the response to startle in PTSD.

FIGURE 4 presents the results of a prospective study in which startle response was assessed 1 week, 1 month, and 4 months after trauma. Individuals who developed PTSD 4 months after trauma are compared with survivors without PTSD. The results show no difference between groups 1 week after the event and a progressive development of higher HR and eye blink responses (EMG) and of slower SC habituation in the PTSD group. This progression suggests that some neurophysiological characteristics of PTSD develop after trauma.

CONCLUSION AND FUTURE DIRECTIONS

Among the reasons for treatment failure in PTSD are the complex etiology of the disorder and the significant effect of constitutional factors, prior exposure, and prior mental illness. These factors may leave only a small proportion of the variance to be manipulated by treatment interventions. Prospective data just presented, however, suggest that some of the physiological particularities of chronic PTSD develop after trauma, leaving a "window of opportunity" for early interventions. Optimally, such interventions should address the mechanisms that lead to PTSD, yet is it often the case?

Traditionally, the etiology of PTSD has been construed in psychological terms, such as learned conditioning, generalization of avoidance, shattered cognitive assumptions, or development of inappropriate beliefs. This has led to psychological treatment for trauma survivors, the effectiveness of which must still be measured against the normal recovery curve in entire cohorts of survivors. The techniques of early psychological interventions are, nevertheless, congruent with the psychological theory of mental traumatization in that they do address the pathogenic processes (e.g., inappropriate generalization) rather then overt manifestations and symptoms.

In yet another formulation, PTSD results from the toxic effects of arousal on brain structures. Biological treatment designed to protect target organs from stress-induced injury may, therefore, help prevent the disorder. Current pharmacotherapy, however, does not directly address such processes, but rather the overt expression of the disorder, such as early anxiety or insomnia. In that sense, the pharmacological treatment that is currently offered to trauma survivors is incongruent with the hypothetical pathogenesis of PTSD. Moreover, the effect of pharmacological treatment on the course of most anxiety disorders is unclear. Despite substantial improvement with treatment, disorders such as panic disorder or obsessive-compulsive disorder often become chronic. By analogy, symptom-oriented pharmacotherapy may not prevent PTSD from becoming chronic.

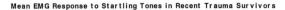

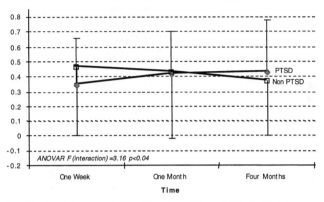

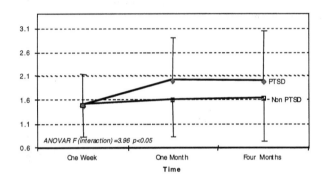

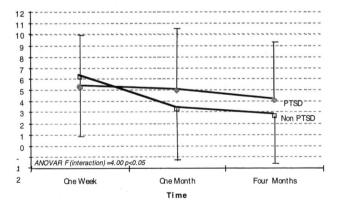

FIGURE 4. Startle response in trauma survivors.

Finally, the medical/disease model within which PTSD has been defined may overshadow an ecological understanding of PTSD, as an expected, yet unhappy consequence of violence and terror. Given the high prevalence of PTSD in the general population and among trauma survivors,[2] and given the substantial effect of genetic factors in determining PTSD symptoms,[34] we may wonder if PTSD is not an expression of our genetic heritage, which might have had some adaptive value. Indeed, the occurrence of a disabling condition in up to one third of human survivors of extreme events[27] would be incompatible with survival of the species. Hence, it may be true that in defining and treating PTSD we treat an expected yet undesirable consequence of violence and terror, namely, defeat and deterrence. Social defeat and chronic stress have been associated with hippocampal damage in primates[51] and analogous findings were reported in PTSD.[52] Moreover, defeat and deterrence could have played and may still play a significant role in imposing social dominance in some human societies. Identifying defeated and apprehended humans as having a mental disorder and providing help to victims of violence is an ethical choice and a major social achievement. Neurobiological models of PTSD, however, should explore both pathological and normal apprehension as a model for understanding and preventing PTSD.

ACKNOWLEDGMENTS

The research presented in this chapter was done with the greatest help and support of Tuvia Peri, Sara Freedman, Dalia Brandes, Euvgenia Gelpin, Nurit Inbar, and Tali Sahar from the Center for Traumatic Stress at Hadassah University Hospital in Jerusalem, and Roger K. Pitman and Scott P. Orr from Harvard Medical School/ Manchester VA Research Laboratory in Manchester, New Hampshire.

REFERENCES

1. ROTHBAUM, B. O. & E. B. FOA. 1983. Subtypes of posttraumatic stress disorder and duration of symptoms. *In* Posttraumatic Stress Disorder, DSM IV and Beyond. J. R. T. Davidson & E. B. Foa, Eds.: 23-35. American Psychiatric Press. Washington D.C.
2. KESSLER, R. C., A. SONNEGA, E. J. BROMET, M. HUGHES & C. B. NELSON. 1995. Posttraumatic stress disorder in the National Comorbidity Survey. Arch. Gen. Psychiatry **52:** 1048-1060.
3. SHALEV, A. Y., O. BONNE & S. ETH. 1996. Treatment of the post-traumatic stress disorder. Psychosom. Med. **58:** 165-182.
4. SOLOMON, S. D., E. T. GERRITY & A. M. MUFF. 1992. Efficacy of treatment for posttraumatic stress disorder. JAMA **268:** 633-638.
5. SHESTATZKI, M., D. GREENBERG & B. LERER. 1988. A controlled trial of phenelzine in posttraumatic stress disorder. Psychiatr. Res. **24:** 149-155.
6. FRANK, J. B., T. R. KOSTEN, E. L. GILLER & E. DAN. 1988. A randomized clinical trial of phenelzine and imipramine for posttraumatic stress disorder. Am. J. Psychiatry **145:** 1289-1291.
7. RIEST, C., C. D. KAUFFMAN & R. J. HAIER. 1976. A controlled trial of desipramine in 81 men with post traumatic stress disorder. Am. J. Psychiatry **146:** 513-516.
8. BRAUN, P., D. GREENBERG, H. DASBERG & B. LERER. 1990. Core symptoms of posttraumatic stress disorder unimproved by alprazolam treatment. J. Clin. Psychiatry **51:** 236-238.

9. DAVIDSON, J., H. KUDLER, R. SMITH, S. L. MAHORNEY, S. LIPPER, E. HAMMETT, W. B. SAUNDERS & J. O. J. CAVENAR. 1990. Treatment of posttraumatic stress disorder with amitriptyline and placebo. Arch. Gen. Psychiatry **47:** 259-266.

10. KOSTEN, T. R., J. B. FRANK, E. DAN *et al.* 1991. Pharmacotherapy for posttraumatic stress disorder using phenelzine or Imipramine. J. Nerv. Ment. Dis. **179:** 366-370.

11. DAVIDSON, J. R., H. S. KUDLER, W. B. SAUNDERS *et al.* 1993. Predicting response to amitriptyline in posttraumatic stress disorder. Am. J. Psychiatry **150:** 1024-1029.

12. VAN DER KOLK, B. A., D. DRYFUSS, M. MICHAELS *et al.* 1994. Fluoxetine in post traumatic stress disorder. J. Clin. Psychiatry **55:** 517-522.

13. PENISTON, E. G. 1986. EMG biofeedback assisted desensitization treatment for Vietnam combat veterans with post traumatic stress disorder. Clin. Biofeed Health **9:** 35-41.

14. RESICK, P. A., C. G. JORDAN, S. A. GIRELLI & C. K. HUTTER. 1988. A comparative outcome study of behavioral group therapy for sexual assault victims. Behavior-Therapy **19:** 385-401.

15. BROM, D., R. J. KLEBER & P. B. DEFARES. 1989. Brief psychotherapy for posttraumatic stress disorders. J. Consult. Clin. Psychol. **57:** 607-612.

16. KEANE, T. M., J. A. FAIRBANK, J. M. CADDEL & R. T. ZIMMERING. 1989. Implosive (flooding) therapy reduces symptoms of PTSD in Vietnam combat veterans. Behav. Ther. **20:** 245-260.

17. BOUDEWYNS, P. A., L. HYER, M. G. WOODS, W. R. HARRISON *et al.* 1990. PTSD among Vietnam veterans: An early look at treatment outcome using direct therapeutic exposure. J. Traumatic Stress **3:** 359-368.

18. FOA, E. B., B. O. ROTHBAUM, D. S. RIGGS & T. B. MURDOCK. 1991. Treatment of posttraumatic stress disorder in rape victims: A comparison between cognitive-behavioral procedures and counseling. J. Consult. Clin. Psychol. **59:** 715-723.

19. RESICK, P. A. & M. K. SCHNICKE. 1992. Cognitive processing therapy for sexual assault victims. J. Consult. Clin. Psychol. **60:** 748-756.

20. RICHARDS, D. A., K. LOVELL & I. M. MARKS. 1994. Post-traumatic stress disorder: Evaluation of a behavioral treatment program. J. Traumatic Stress **7:** 669-680.

21. KRYSTAL, J. H. 1996. Neurobiological Aspects of Dissociation and Trauma. Second World Conference of the International Society for Traumatic Stress, Jerusalem, June 9-14.

22. SOLOMON, Z. & R. BENBENISHTY. 1986. The role of proximity, immediacy, and expectancy in frontline treatment of combat stress reaction among Israelis in the Lebanon War. Am. J. Psychiatry **143:** 613-617.

23. SOLOMON, Z., M. WIESENBERG, J. SCHWARZWALD & M. MIKULINCER. 1987. Posttraumatic stress disorder among frontline soldiers with combat stress reaction: The 1982 Israeli experience. Am. J. Psychiatry **144:** 448-454.

24. BISSON, J. I. & M. P. DEAHL. 1994. Psychological debriefing and prevention of posttraumatic stress—More research is needed. Br. J. Psychiatry **165:** 717-720.

25. DEAHL, M. P., A. B. GILLHAM, J. THOMAS, M. M. SEARLE & M. SRINIVASAN. 1994. Psychological sequelae following the Gulf War: Factors associated with subsequent morbidity and the effectiveness of psychological debriefing. Br. J. Psychiatry **165:** 60-65.

26. BOURNE, P. G. 1978. Military psychiatry and the Viet Nam war in perspective. *In* The Psychology and Physiology of Stress. P. G. Bourne, Ed.: 219-236. Academic Press. New York, NY.

27. KULKA, R. A., W. E. SCHLENGER, J. A. FAIRBANK, R. L. HOUGH, B. K. JORDAN, C. R. MARMAR & D. S. WEISS. 1990. Trauma and the Vietnam War Generation: Report of Findings from the National Vietnam Veterans Readjustment Study. Brunner/Mazel. New York.

28. BROM, D., R. J. KLEBER & M. C. HOFMAN. 1993. Victims of traffic accidents: Incidence and prevention of post-traumatic stress disorder. J. Clin. Psychol. **49:** 131-140.

29. KENARDY, J. A., R. A. WEBSTER, T. J. LEWIN, V. J. CARR, P. L. HAZELL & G. L. CARTER. 1996. Stress debriefing and patterns of recovery following a natural disaster. J. Traumatic Stress **9:** 37-49.

30. GELPIN, E., T. PERI, O. BONNE, R. K. PITMAN & A. SHALEV. 1996. Treatment of early trauma survivors with benzodiazepines: A prospective study. J. Clin. Psychiatry **57:** 390-394.

31. HEBERT, M. A., M. POTEGAL, T. MOORE, A. R. EVENSON & J. L. MEYERHOFF. 1997. Diazepam enhances conditioned defeat in hamsters. Pharmacol. Biochem. Behav. *In* press.

32. SHALEV, A. 1992. Posttraumatic stress disorder among injured survivors of a terrorist attack: Predictive value of early intrusion and avoidance symptoms. J. Nerv. Ment. Dis. **180:** 505-509.

33. ZILBERG, N. J., D. S. WEISS & M. J. HOROWITZ. 1982. Impact of Event scale: A cross validation study and some empirical evidence supporting a conceptual model of stress response syndrome. J. Consult. Clin. Psychol. **50:** 407-414.

34. SHALEV, A. Y., T. PERI, L. CANNETI & S. SCHREIBER. 1996. Predictors of PTSD in recent trauma survivors: A prospective study. Am. J. Psychiatry **153:** 219-225.

35. SHALEV, A. Y., S. FREEDMAN, T. PERI, D. BRANDES & T. SAHAR. 1997. Predicting PTSD in civilian trauma survivors: Prospective evaluation of self report and clinician administered instruments. Br. J. Psychiatry, in press.

36. TRUE, W. R., J. RICE, S. A. EISEN, A. C. HEATH, J. GOLDBERG, M. J. LYONS & J. NOWAK. 1993. A twin study of genetic and environmental contributions to liability for posttraumatic stress symptoms. Arch. Gen. Psychiatry **50:** 257-264.

37. SHALEV, A. 1996. Stress versus traumatic stress: From acute homeostatic reaction to chronic psychopathology. *In* Traumatic Stress. The Effects of Overwhelming Life Experiences on Mind Body and Society. B. A. van der Kolk, A. C. McFarlane & L. Weisaeth, Eds.: 77-101. Guilford Press. New York, NY.

38. PUTNAM, F. W. & P. K. TRICKETT. 1993. Child sexual abuse: A model of chronic trauma. Psychiatry **56:** 82-95.

39. STEIN, M. B., C. HANNAH, C. KOVEROLA & B. MCCLARTY. 1995. Neuroanatomic and cognitive correlates of early abuse. Am. Psychiatr. Assoc. Syllabus Proc. Summary **148:** 113.

40. KOOPMAN, C., C. CLASSEN & D. SPIEGEL. 1994. Predictors of posttraumatic stress symptoms among survivors of the Oakland/Berkeley, Calif., firestorm. Am. J. Psychiatry **151:** 888-894.

41. MARMAR, C. R., D. S. WEISS, W. E. SCHLENGER, J. A. FAIRBANK, K. JORDAN, R. A. KULKA & R. L. HOUGH. 1994. Peritraumatic dissociation and posttraumatic stress in male Vietnam theater veterans. Am. J. Psychiatry **151:** 902-907.

42. SHALEV, A. Y. & Y. ROGEL-FUCHS. 1993. Psychophysiology of the post-traumatic stress disorder: From sulfur fumes to behavioral genetics. Psychosom. Med. **55:** 413-423.

43. PITMAN, R. K., S. P. ORR, D. F. FORGUE, J. B. DE JONG & J. M. CLAIBORN. 1987. Psychophysiology of PTSD imagery in Vietnam combat veterans. Arch. Gen. Psychiatry **44:** 970-975.

44. SHALEV, A. Y., S. P. ORR & R. K. PITMAN. 1993. Psychophysiologic assessment of traumatic imagery in Israeli civilian patients with post-traumatic stress disorder. Am. J. Psychiatry **150:** 620-624.

45. SHALEV, A. Y., S. P. ORR, T. PERI, S. SCHREIBER & R. K. PITMAN. 1992. Physiological responses to loud tones of Israeli post-traumatic stress disorder patients. Arch. Gen. Psychiatry **49:** 870-875.

46. ORR, S. P., N. LASKO, A. SHALEV & R. K. PITMAN. 1995. Physiologic responses to loud tones in Vietnam veterans with PTSD. J. Abnorm. Psychol. **104:** 75-82.

47. ORR, S. P., Z. SOLOMON, T. PERI, R. K. PITMAN & A. SHALEV. 1997. Physiological responses to loud tones in Israeli war veterans of the 1973 Yom Kippur War. Biol. Psychiatry **41:** 319-326.

48. SHALEV, A. Y., T. PERI, S. P. ORR, O. BONNE & R. K. PITMAN. 1997. Auditory startle responses in help seeking trauma survivors. Psychiatry Res. **69:** 1-7.

49. MORGAN, C. A., III, C. GRILLON, S. M. SOUTHWICK, L. NAGY, M. DAVIS., J. H. KRYSTAL & D. S. CHARNEY. 1995. Yohimbine facilitated acoustic startle in combat veterans with post-traumatic stress disorder. Psychopharmacology (Berlin) **117:** 466-471.

50. MORGAN, C. A., III, C. GRILLON, S. M. SOUTHWICK, M. DAVIS & D. S. CHARNEY. 1995. Fear-potentiated startle in post-traumatic stress disorder. Biol. Psychiatry **38:** 378-385.

51. UNO, H., R. TARARA, J. ELSE, M. SULEMAN & R. M. SAPOLSKY. 1989. Hippocampal damage associated with prolonged and fatal stress in primates. J. Neurosci. **9:** 1705-1711.

52. BREMNER, D., J. P. RANDALL, T. N. SCOTT, R. A. BRONEN, *et al.* 1995. MRI-based measurements of hippocampal volume in combat-related posttraumatic stress disorder. Am. J. Psychiatry **152:** 973-981.

Integrating Objective Indicators of Treatment Outcome in Posttraumatic Stress Disorder

MICHAEL G. GRIFFIN,[a] PALLAVI NISHITH,[a]
PATRICIA A. RESICK,[a] AND RACHEL YEHUDA [b]

[a]Department of Psychology
Center for Trauma Recovery
University of Missouri, St. Louis
St. Louis, Missouri 63121–4499

[b]Department of Psychiatry
Bronx VA Medical Center
Bronx, New York 10468

Psychophysiological and psychoendocrine studies of posttraumatic stress disorder (PTSD) have burgeoned in recent years as our appreciation for and understanding of the biological underpinnings of the disorder have increased. Not until the 1987 revision of the DSM III-R was a separate specific symptom cluster defined to identify physiological changes that are concomitant to the disorder. These include the "persistent symptoms of increased arousal" found in criterion D of DSM-III-R and more recently DSM-IV.[1] The emphasis on physiological manifestations in PTSD is the result of well-designed studies investigating psychophysiological alterations in subjects with PTSD. Curiously, physiological manifestations were some of the first symptoms noted by early investigators of posttrauma reactions. Kardiner,[2] writing from a psychodynamic perspective, described the biopsychological sequelae of combat trauma to include: severe startle response, a fixation on the traumatic event, general irritability, explosive aggressive reactions, muscle tension/spasms, and increased autonomic responses. Other early investigators of war-related trauma also identified a host of somatic ills in men immediately following combat experiences.[3] Often these symptoms went under the rubric of "operational fatigue" or "shell shock" and included such symptoms as inability to concentrate, emotional irritability, severe startle response, gastric upset, muscle tremors, and a general increase in arousal. Thus, the realization that underlying physiological changes are an essential component of the posttrauma response has been recognized for many years.

There is a general consensus among PTSD researchers that a biological approach holds genuine promise for a better understanding of the etiology and maintenance of the disorder. Furthermore, the establishment of biological parameters associated with the disorder allows objective assessment of the efficacy of treatment which in turn aids in generating more effective treatment approaches. We are now seeing evidence that "psychological treatments" can induce biological changes. For example, patients with obsessive-compulsive disorder who were treated successfully with exposure and response-prevention therapy showed significant changes in brain metabolic activity in regions associated with the disorder.[4,5] However, there is a dearth of information on changes in biological manifestations of PTSD following psychother-apeutic treatment. Many theorists have suggested that there is a dynamic interplay between the environment and the biological workings of the brain.[6] The biological study of treatment efficacy allows access to a window into this dynamic interplay.

Two of the primary biological approaches that hold promise for developing objective indicators for PTSD are psychophysiological and psychoendocrine assessments. In particular, psychophysiological measures including heart rate, electrodermal activity (e.g., skin conductance) and facial electromyogram (EMG), and the psychoendocrine challenge test, the low-dose dexamethasone suppression test (DST). These approaches are reviewed briefly, and pilot data from our laboratory using these approaches at pre- and posttreatment of sexual assault survivors are presented.

PSYCHOPHYSIOLOGICAL ALTERATIONS IN PTSD

The goal of psychophysiological studies is to noninvasively measure electrical events in the nervous system that reflect a particular psychological variable.[7] Most investigators employing a psychophysiological approach to the study of PTSD have used two basic strategies to assess autonomic reactivity. The first paradigm focuses on physiological responses to the presentation of specific reminders of the traumatic event, and the second approach examines reactivity to intense neutral stimuli in a startle paradigm. In the first paradigm, researchers generally either have presented standardized generic audiovisual cues such as combat sounds and movie clips or have used a personalized script-driven imagery procedure.[8] In the second paradigm, intense auditory stimuli were used in a few studies to examine startle responses and habituation to these stimuli following repeated presentations.[9] Results of most psychophysiological research are based on assessments of combat veterans with PTSD compared to non-PTSD combat veterans.

Pitman and Orr introduced a laboratory paradigm based on Lang's work[10] which shows that emotionally charged imagery elicits powerful autonomic responses. In the Pitman and Orr paradigm, short (~30 s) personalized scripts are generated for each individual based on their traumatic experiences as well as neutral scripts based on nontraumatic experiences. The scripts are recorded and played back to the subject while psychophysiological measures are recorded. They used this method with combat veterans from World War II and the Korean and Vietnam Wars. The results generalize across these different samples, and findings indicate that veterans diagnosed with PTSD have faster heart rate, greater skin conductance, and stronger facial EMG responses than do non-PTSD combat veterans.[8,11,12] Findings from this paradigm were extended to include survivors of terrorist attacks and motor vehicle accidents with PTSD for which the most reliable physiological discriminator was heart rate.[13,14] Interestingly, the differences in physiological responding are most notable for trauma-specific stimuli. Generally, research has not indicated differences between PTSD and non-PTSD subjects on autonomic measures during periods when nontrauma-related imagery are invoked in the laboratory.[8,11,12]

One use for psychophysiological measures is to aid in correctly diagnosing subjects who have PTSD from those who do not. Pitman and Orr and their coworkers calculated the sensitivity (true positives) and specificity (true negatives) of a PTSD diagnosis using multiple psychophysiological indices in their combat samples. Findings for diagnostic sensitivity range from 60–90% and for specificity from 80–100% across multiple studies. These findings suggest that psychophysiological assessment holds great promise for classifying individuals with PTSD objectively. However, there are only a few reports in the literature of this method being applied to the interpretation of treatment efficacy, and most of these studies are single case studies. Keane and Kaloupek[15] reported a decrease in heart rate during periods of combat imagery in a combat veteran with PTSD following exposure treatment. Fairbank and Keane[16] also found a reduction in physiological arousal following flooding in a Vietnam combat veteran. Two other studies show reduced physiologic responding to trauma-related imagery in combat veterans following exposure-based treatment.[17,18] Finally, a case study of an incest survivor, presumably with PTSD although not diagnosed as such, who was treated with implosive therapy found a decrease in skin conductance from pre- to posttherapy.[19] Recently, a new therapeutic approach, eye movement desensitization and reprocessing (EMDR), has been examined using psychophysiological measures before and after treatment. Findings again suggested a decrease in physiological arousal after treatment.[20–22] Studies examining psychophysiological changes pre- and posttreatment are summarized in TABLE 1. Note that most of these studies are a collection of case studies or studies with very small samples.

PSYCHOENDOCRINE ALTERATIONS IN PTSD

Interest in psychoendocrine changes in PTSD progressed from research on autonomic alterations in this disorder and increased understanding of the human stress response. The initial rationale behind the psychoendocrine approach was that PTSD is a stress response. This idea grew out of the general stress response literature first formulated by Selye.[23] He believed that stress would have lasting effects on an organism and that more severe and longer term stressors would have more serious biological consequences. The psychoendocrine approach emphasizes the simultaneous assessment of psychological states and hormonal activity.[24]

Selye[25] identified the systems in the body that respond to stress. Since that time, the hypothalamic-pituitary-adrenal (HPA) axis has become synonymous with the stress response system. The system is intimately involved in our immediate adaptation to a stressful situation, that is, the mobilization of resources to deal with a stressor. The HPA axis is an interdependent endocrine system that operates through a series of releasing factors and hormones. The basic operation of the system is straightforward: the hypothalamus releases corticotropin-releasing factor (CRF), which stimulates the pituitary to release adrenocorticotropic hormone (ACTH), which in turn stimulates the adrenal glands to secrete the glucocorticoid cortisol into the blood stream. Plasma cortisol then feeds back to the hypothalamus and produces a shutdown of the release of CRF that ultimately ends the release of cortisol. This system operates in a negative feedback fashion, because cortisol itself feeds back to shut down the release of any more cortisol. This appears to be a homeostatic response designed to protect the organism from long-term elevated levels of cortisol which are associated with a host of negative effects including cell death in the hippocampus,[26] increased risk of disease,[27] and even cognitive impairments.[28]

TABLE 1. Treatment Outcome Studies Using Psychphysiological Assessments

Treatment	Trauma	Biological DV	Change after Treatment	Significance	n	References
Exposure	Combat (Vietnam)	Heart rate	→	—	1	Keane & Kaloupek[15]
Exposure	Combat (Vietnam)	Heart rate	→	—	1	Fairbank & Keane[16]
Exposure	Incest	SCR	→	—	1	Rychtarik et al.[19]
		SCR	→	—		
		SCL	→	—		
Exposure	Combat (Vietnam)	HR	→	ns	51	Boudewyns & Hyer[17]
		SCL	→	ns		
		Frontalis EMG	→	ns		
Exposure	Various (Non Combat)	HR	→	—	3	Shalev et al.[18]
		SCL	↕	—		
		Frontalis EMG	→	—		
EMDR	Motor vehicle accident	Heart rate	↕	—	1	Montgomery & Ayllon[20]
		Systolic BP	→	—		
EMDR	Physical assault	Heart rate	→	—		
		Systolic BP	→	—		
EMDR	Various (noncombat)	Heart rate	→	ns	6	Montgomery & Ayllon[21]
		Systolic BP	→	ns		
EMDR	Various	Heart rate	→	<.001	23	Renfrey & Spates[22]

Abbreviations: EMDR = eye movement desentization and reprocessing; SCR = skin conductance response; SCL = skin conductance level; ns = nonsignificant.

Initial studies of combat veterans with PTSD indicated that they had lower than normal levels of 24-hour urinary free cortisol.[29,30] In order for cortisol to have a biological effect, it must be bound to a glucocorticoid receptor. Findings indicate an increased number of glucocorticoid receptors (upregulation) in lymphocytes of combat veterans with PTSD compared to normal controls.[31] This finding makes sense because typically there is an inverse relation between the concentration of an agonist (e.g., cortisol) and the number of receptors (e.g., glucocorticoid receptor). Yehuda *et al.*[31] also found that the number of glucocorticoid receptors was highly positively correlated with PTSD symptoms ($r = 0.73$). It has been argued that the increased number of glucocorticoid receptors allows for a more sensitive feedback response in the HPA axis to new stressors in subjects with PTSD, enabling these individuals to adapt more quickly to the new stressor. Intriguing preliminary findings from Resnick and Yehuda[32] in rape victims assessed immediately post-rape in hospital emergency rooms show that women with extensive trauma histories (i.e., exposure to multiple traumas) have a decreased output of cortisol compared to rape victims without prior trauma histories. These results support the notion of a supersensitive response in these women.

Results from baseline studies of PTSD in combat veterans lends credence to the view that there is dysregulation in the HPA axis characterized by low basal cortisol output and a supersensitive response to cortisol mediated by upregulation of glucocorticoid receptors. Another way that this system can be tested is through the use of an endocrine challenge such as the dexamethasone suppression test (DST).[33] Researchers originally hypothesized that subjects with PTSD would be DST nonsuppressors. In major depressive disorder, where this test was initially pioneered and has now been extensively studied, a general finding is that ~60% of patients diagnosed with major depressive disorder are DST nonsuppressors.[33,34] Several attempts to employ DST in combat veterans revealed no evidence of nonsuppression in PTSD subjects who did not also have comorbid major depression.[35,36]

Based on their earlier work, however, suggesting that the HPA axis was supersensitive in PTSD, Yehuda and colleagues[37] examined the proposition that subjects with PTSD would respond to dexamethasone with stronger negative feedback, eliciting a greater reduction in cortisol. Findings indicated an increased suppression of cortisol following administration of a low dose (0.5 mg) of dexamethasone in combat veterans with PTSD. In addition, examination of the means from previous DST studies, which were looking for cortisol nonsuppression, suggested *enhanced* suppression of cortisol.[31] These findings are opposite to what is typically found in major depression and therefore have implications for the differential diagnosis of PTSD from major depression.

The HPA results are generally suggestive of a supersensitive glucocorticoid system in PTSD subjects and may be useful in distinguishing PTSD from other disorders. In particular, low-dose DST appears to have utility as a biological marker for the disorder and as such would make an excellent objective indicator of treatment efficacy.

PRELIMINARY DATA

Data are presented from two preliminary investigations designed to incorporate biological measures into treatment outcome assessments. In Study 1 three subjects seeking treatment for rape-related PTSD were assessed with standard self-report and interview measures and were also assessed in a laboratory setting during which physiological measures of heart rate and skin conductance were collected during periods when the traumatic event was recalled. Assessments were conducted before and immediately after treatment (6 weeks later). Clinical data were analyzed using a single-case design statistical approach which allows the use of a statistical criterion to judge the significance of a change in score from pre-to posttreatment. This approach is superior to simply "eyeballing" the data, because objective criteria are used to judge a significant change.

In Study 2 a group of five subjects seeking treatment for rape-related PTSD were assessed with standard clinical instruments and were also administered low-dose DST (0.5 mg). Evaluation of their level of cortisol suppression following the DST will be tied to the clinical data.

STUDY 1. PSYCHOPHYSIOLOGICAL ASSESSMENT

Methods

Subjects

Subjects for this investigation were three treatment seekers who presented to our outpatient community mental health clinic. Subjects were referred from victim assistance agencies or mental health professionals or were self-referred. These subjects were part of a larger group of women who were recruited for evaluation of a cognitive processing therapy package designed by one of the authors (P.A.R.). We collected physiological data on them at pre-and posttreatment. These subjects were at least 1 year post-rape and met DSM-III-R criteria for diagnosis of PTSD. Other demographic information is presented in TABLE 2.

Assessment Instruments

Subjects were assessed with published clinical instruments that have sound psychometric properties including the Structured Clinical Interview for DSM-III-R–Nonpatient Version (SCID[38]); the Clinician-Administered PTSD scale (CAPS[39]); the Beck Depression Inventory (BDI[40]); the Beck Hopelessness Scale (BHS[41]); the PTSD Symptom Scale (PSS[42]); the Rape Aftermath Symptom Test (RAST[43]); the Coping Strategies Inventory (CSI[44]); and the Impact of Events Scale (IES[45]).

Apparatus. Laboratory assessments were conducted in an 8 × 10-foot room that was sound insulated and temperature and humidity controlled. Physiological measures of heart rate and nonspecific electrodermal responses (skin conductance response, SCR) were generated using a Coulbourn Instruments modular instruments system. A skin conductance response in excess of 0.1 μSiemens was counted as a valid response. Heart rate was calculated as beats per minute. Averages were calculated per phase for both physiological variables.

TABLE 2. Demographic and Self-Report Data from Study 1

	Subject		
Variable	A	B	C
Age	25	21	29
Race	White	White	White
Education (yr)	11	12	14
Income	10-20K	10-20K	20-30K
Marital status	M	M	S
Years post-rape	11	4	1

	Subject					
	Pretreatment			Posttreatment		
	A	B	C	A	B	C
PTSD-SS						
Reexperiencing	6	7	6	0	2	3
Avoidance	14	5	15	0	1	9
Arousal	17	16	11	1	2	6
Total Frequency	37	28	32	1	5	18
BDI	26	14	28	0	3	28
BHS	13	8	6	2	2	7
Coping Strategies Inventory						
Problem avoidance	27	17	26	12	13	20
Wishful thinking	34	33	35	13	16	29
Self-criticism	35	45	29	9	9	24
Self-worth	35	35	31	10	17	27
Rape Aftermath Symptom Test						
Global Distress	187	187	127	45	20	87
Impact of Events Scale						
Intrusion	23	33	27	0	4	20
Avoidance	34	19	30	0	0	19
Total	57	52	57	0	4	39

Procedure

Assessment Procedure. Assessments were conducted in the week prior to the start of treatment and then again within 1 week of the end of treatment. Subjects were asked to give informed consent and then were administered paper and pencil questionnaires and a laptop computer questionnaire consisting of a number of self-report scales.

Following completion of these instruments the laboratory assessment was begun. Subjects were seated in a comfortable armchair in the assessment room, and the physiological monitoring devices were attached from the Coulbourn modules. The assessment was begun approximately 5 minutes later to allow physiological readings to stabilize. There were five 5-minute phases to the laboratory assessment. The first phase was an initial resting baseline (B1) during which the interviewer left the subject alone in the room. After 5 minutes the interviewer returned and prompted the subject to talk about a neutral topic for the next 5-minute phase (N). At the end of the neutral phase the interviewer left again for a second baseline (B2). On returning, the interviewer prompted the subject to talk about the rape for the next 5-minute "trauma" phase (T). At the end of this period the interviewer again left for a final 5-minute baseline period (B3). Prior to the start of the talking phases (N&T) the interviewer gave the subject a prompt sheet with a list of topics to discuss during the phase. The interviewer instructed the subject that the interviewer would not be able to speak during the phase in order to record 5 minutes of the subject speaking.

Treatment Rationale and Procedure. The development and maintenance of PTSD have been conceptualized within the framework of information-processing theory.[46-51] This theory explains the organization and processing of information through the development of schemata. A schema is defined as a generic stored body of knowledge that interacts with the incoming information so that it influences how the information is encoded, comprehended, retrieved, and acted upon. It has been fairly well established in the social psychological literature that persons tend to subscribe to a just world belief, that good things happen to good people and bad things happen to bad people.[52] This belief probably serves a defensive function so that people feel less vulnerable to random negative events. The occurrence of a particularly negative event, such as rape, is schema-discrepant with this just world belief. Hollon and Garber[53] suggest that when an individual encounters new information that is inconsistent with preexisting beliefs or schemas, one of two things usually happens: assimilation or accommodation. Assimilation refers to the process whereby information is altered or distorted to fit (to be assimilated) into existing schemata. Accommodation, on the other hand, involves changing existing schemata to accept new, incompatible information.

Preexisting beliefs and events that occurred prior to the rape have a profound effect on how the traumatic event is processed. Early losses and traumas may result in negative schemas ("Bad things keep happening to me") that appear to be confirmed by the rape. In contrast, an overly sheltered childhood may result in an unrealistic just world schema ("as long as I follow the rules, nothing bad will ever happen to me") that may be shattered in the face of personal victimization. In acquaintance rape victims, assimilation is frequently observed when the victims blame themselves for being attacked or not resisting successfully, question whether the event was really a rape, or develop amnesia for all or part of the event. This is usually because an acquaintance rape is schema incongruent to preexisting rape-related beliefs which define rape as being committed by strangers. Accommodation, which is necessary for successful integration of the event, may not be successful for symptom reduction if the victim completely alters her view of the world in ways that prevent intimacy or trust and increase fear (overaccommodation).

McCann *et al.*[51] identified five areas that show a disruption in self-beliefs (assimilation) and other-beliefs (overaccommodation) as a result of victimization. These five areas are: safety, trust, power/control, esteem, and intimacy. PTSD is seen as resulting from an inability to integrate (via assimilation or accommodation) the traumatic event with prior beliefs and experiences, thus causing "stuck points"[54,55] in areas of self-blame, safety, trust, control, esteem, and intimacy. The goal in cognitive processing therapy[56] is to help the client integrate the event, with complete processing of emotions and accommodation of schemas, while maintaining a balanced perspective of the world (i.e., minimizing overaccommodation). When information is not processed adequately, intrusive recollections, flashbacks, and nightmares are likely to occur. These intrusive symptoms are associated with strong affective responses (fear, disgust, guilt, and anger), which then lead to escape and avoidance behavior such as avoiding situations that remind her of the event. Cognitive avoidance, refusing to accept what has occurred or to integrate the event into one's life experiences, prevents the extinction of strong affective responses (fear, guilt, disgust, and anger). Memories that have been encoded in rich detail because they were so schema discrepant[54] continue to elicit great affect when they are activated by stimuli in the environment. Fear cues, in particular, can generalize and create symptoms of chronic arousal and hyperactivity.

Cognitive processing therapy[56] focuses on the processing of trauma-related affect and the identification of stuck points.[57-62] These stuck points are then addressed and challenged, in 12 sessions of therapy across 6 weeks, in a systematic manner using education, exposure, and cognitive components to help the client integrate the trauma into her preexisting schemas. Education involves explaining information processing theory and the derivation of cognitive processing therapy from it. Exposure involves having the client write the rape account with all the sensory details and associated feelings. Cognitive therapy involves having her identify the faulty thinking patterns and challenge the automatic thoughts related to how she was interpreting the rape. The initial sessions focus on challenging the self-blame by the use of socratic questioning. The focus then shifts to the self and other beliefs in the five areas of safety, trust, control, esteem, and intimacy. The client works on rape-specific and current situation beliefs in each of these modules. She can see how the rape-specific beliefs are affecting her current functioning in the five areas and causing impairment in her social functioning. Cognitive therapy in successive sessions starts to translate into behavioral change, which further helps provide evidence against the maladaptive automatic beliefs and leads to a decrease in PTSD symptoms.

The specific content of the 12 1.5-hour weekly sessions of cognitive processing therapy have been described in detail elsewhere.[55] More information in the form of a treatment manual is also available to the interested reader.[56]

Self-Report Data Reduction. A statistical method for analyzing single case designs[63-65] was used for the self-report data of each subject. This approach is more quantitative than is visual inspection of the data and is useful when examining changes over time with relatively few data points. This approach relies on the reliability of an instrument to calculate a significant change over time. A more reliable instrument requires a smaller change to demonstrate that a treatment has produced a significant change. Raw scores from the various scales of interest were converted into ipsative Z-scores based on the mean and standard deviation of the scores pre- and posttreatment. A critical difference score was calculated for each variable based on its reliability and the number of comparisons to be made. The following formula was used to calculate the critical difference for a one-tailed test which was employed in the present study because we were only interested in changes in one direction:[65] critical difference

(CD) = 1.64 $[J(1 - r)]^{1/2}$, where J is the number of test points (J = 2) and r is the scale reliability. The reliability for each scale was obtained from published sources.

RESULTS

Demographic and clinical self-report descriptive data are presented in TABLE 2. Statistical analyses of the self-report data are presented in TABLE 3. Examination of these data clearly indicates that two of the subjects (A & B) responded very well to treatment. At posttreatment neither woman met diagnostic criteria for PTSD based on the CAPS. They showed clear decreases on all of the symptom measures at posttreatment with most decreases achieving statistical significance. These subjects were designated as ''PTSD-negative'' after treatment. Subject C showed more modest decreases on the self-report measures and she still met diagnostic criteria for PTSD at posttreatment. Subject C was designated as ''PTSD-positive'' following treatment. FIGURES 1 and 2 illustrate the changes in heart rate and skin conductance responses across the laboratory phases. These figures show clear changes on both of these measures in the PTSD-negative subjects, indicating a reduction in physiological arousal. The PTSD-positive subject, on the other hand, continued to show an elevated arousal response despite treatment. These data point to the utility of single case design statistics as a heuristically important way of examining treatment outcome data. This view is strengthened by psychophysiological data which indicate that subjects who were treatment responders showed a reduction in physiological arousal after treatment. This appears to be particularly true for the trauma-related segment of the laboratory assessment.

STUDY 2. PSYCHOENDOCRINE ASSESSMENT

Methods

Subjects

Subjects for this investigation were five treatment seekers who presented to our outpatient community mental health clinic. Subjects were referred from victim assistance agencies or mental health professionals or were self-referred. These subjects were part of a larger group of women who were recruited for evaluation of a cognitive processing therapy package designed by one of the authors (P.A.R.) and prolonged exposure which is described below. These subjects were at least 3 months post-rape and met DSM-III-R criteria for diagnosis of PTSD. Other demographic information is presented in TABLE 4.

Treatment Rationale and Procedure. Four subjects in this investigation were treated with cognitive processing therapy as previously discussed and one subject was treated with prolonged exposure. Prolonged exposure is a type of behavioral therapy that uses imaginal exposure and *in vivo* exposure techniques to help survivors process the emotional content of traumatic events. Imaginal exposure requires the survivor to relive the rape event in imagination. To do this, clients are instructed to imagine the rape as vividly as possible and describe the rape aloud. This process is

TABLE 3. Single Case Design Statistics from Study 1

Variable	Mean	SD	Reliability	Ipsative Z-Score		z diff	Crit Diff	p
				Pre z1	Post z2			
Subject A								
PTSD-SS								
Reexperiencing	7.4	4.50	0.66	−0.30	−1.64	1.34	1.35	ns
Avoidance	6.0	7.60	0.56	1.05	−0.78	1.83	1.53	0.05
Arousal	8.2	4.90	0.71	1.79	−1.47	3.26	1.25	0.05
Total Frequency	21.6	16.30	0.74	0.94	−1.26	2.20	1.18	0.05
BDI	8	9.30	0.65	1.93	−0.86	2.79	1.64	0.05
BHS	4.4	3.10	0.69	2.77	−0.79	3.56	1.54	0.05
Rape Aftermath Symptom Test								
Global distress	71.2	53.20	0.85	2.18	−0.49	2.67	0.90	0.05
Impact of Events Scale								
Intrusion	16.8	7.90	0.89	0.78	−2.12	2.90	0.77	0.05
Avoidance	10.8	10.80	0.79	2.14	−0.99	3.13	1.06	0.05
Total	27.6	17.60	0.87	1.67	−1.56	3.23	0.84	0.05
Subject B								
PTSD-SS								
Reexperiencing	7.4	4.50	0.66	−0.09	−1.2	1.11	1.35	ns
Avoidance	6.0	7.60	0.56	−0.13	−0.66	0.53	1.53	ns
Arousal	8.2	4.90	0.71	1.59	−1.26	2.85	1.25	0.05
Total Frequency	21.6	16.30	0.74	0.39	−1.02	1.41	1.18	0.05
BDI	8	9.30	0.65	0.65	−0.54	1.19	1.37	ns
BHS	4.4	3.10	0.69	1.15	−0.79	1.94	1.29	0.05
Rape Aftermath Symptom Test								
Global distress	71.2	53.20	0.85	2.18	−0.96	3.14	0.90	0.05
Impact of Events Scale								
Intrusion	16.8	7.90	0.89	2.05	−1.62	3.67	0.77	0.05
Avoidance	10.8	10.80	0.79	0.76	−0.99	1.75	1.06	0.05
Total	27.6	17.60	0.87	1.38	−1.34	2.72	0.84	0.05
Subject C								
PTSD-SS								
Reexperiencing	7.4	4.50	0.66	−0.30	−0.90	0.6	1.35	ns
Avoidance	6.0	7.60	0.56	1.18	0.39	0.79	1.53	ns
Arousal	8.2	4.90	0.71	0.57	−0.44	1.01	1.25	ns
Total Frequency	21.6	16.30	0.74	0.64	−0.22	0.86	1.18	ns
BDI	8	9.30	0.65	2.15	2.15	0	1.64	ns
BHS	4.4	3.10	0.69	0.50	0.82	−0.32	1.29	ns
Rape Aftermath Symptom Test								
Global distress	71.2	53.20	0.85	1.05	−0.3	1.35	0.89	0.05
Impact of Events Scale								
Intrusion	16.8	7.90	0.89	1.29	0.4	0.89	0.77	0.05
Avoidance	10.8	10.80	0.79	1.77	0.76	1.01	1.06	ns
Total	27.6	17.60	0.87	1.67	0.65	1.02	0.83	0.05

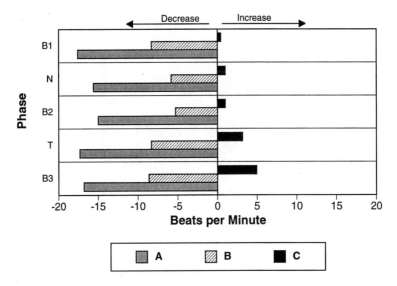

FIGURE 1. Heart rate change scores from pre- to posttreatment across the five laboratory phases.

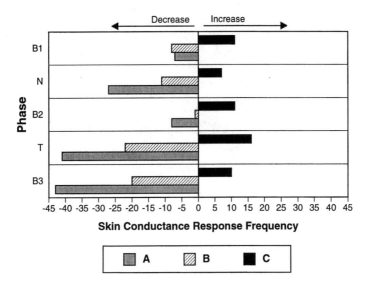

FIGURE 2. Skin conductance response (responses > 0.10 μSiemens) change scores from pre- to posttreatment across the five laboratory phases.

TABLE 4. Clinical Data at Pre- and Posttreatment from Study 2

	Clinical Data	Pretreatment	Posttreatment	3 Mo Posttreatment	9 Mo Posttreatment
Subject 1					
Treatment	CPT	PTSD	Yes	No	No	No
Age (yr)	23	Depression	No	No	No	No
Time post rape (mo)	84	CAPS (Sx)	3 ● 5 ● 4	0 ● 0 ● 1	0 ● 0 ● 1	1 ● 0 ● 1
Race	White	PSS (freq)	5 ● 12 ● 12 = 29	1 ● 0 ● 0 ● = 2	0 ● 1 ● 0 = 1	1 ● 0 ● 2 = 3
Education (yr)	15	BDI	14	4	2	7
Income	3	DES (%)	5.46	2.57	0.8	1.1
	PDEQ	29			
	Comorbidity	None			
	Lf Dx	Depression			
	Trauma Hx	Prior rape, domestic abuse			
	Drug Use	None	Alcohol (1)	None	None
Subject 2					
Treatment	CPT	PTSD	Yes	No	—	—
Age (yr)	22	Depression	No	No	—	—
Time post rape (mo)	16	CAPS (Sx)	3 ● 7 ● 6	1 ● 3 ● 1	—	—
Race	Asian	PSS (freq)	7 ● 17 ● 16 = 40	3 ● 3 ● 1 = 7	—	—
Education (yr)	16	BDI	34	7		
Income	1	DES (%)	25.2	12.7		
	PDEQ	26			
	Comorbidity	Panic Disorder			
	Lf Dx	Depression, Panic disorder, and Alcohol, cocaine, and Cannabis dependence			
	Trauma Hx	Close friend killed, criminal vict hx incl previous rape, domestic abuse			
	Drug Use	Tylenol (500 mg)	None		
Subject 3					
Treatment	PE	PTSD	Yes	No	No	—
Age (yr)	24	Depression	No	No	No	—
Time post rape (mo)	7	CAPS (Sx)	3 ● 4 ● 4	0 ● 1 ● 1	2 ● 1 ● 2	—
Race	White	PSS (freq)	7 ● 9 ● 15 = 31	1 ● 0 ● 0 = 1	3 ● 0 ● 4 = 7	—
Education (yr)	15	BDI	17	2	0	—
	DES (%)	26.5	9.86	12.7	—

Income	

Subject 4

	Value 1	Value 2
Treatment	CPT	
Age (yr)	32	
Time post rape (mo)	4	
Race	White	
Education (yr)	14	
Income	3	
PDEQ	12	
Comorbidity	None	
Lf Dx	None	
Trauma Hx	Previous rape, robbery, burglary	
Drug Use	Alcohol (5)	Alcohol (1)
PTSD	Yes	No
Depression	No	No
CAPS (Sx)	4 ● 4 ● 4	1 ● 1 ● 0
PSS (freq)	4 ● 5 ● 8 = 17	2 ● 2 ● 2 = 6
BDI	8	2
DES (%)	29.6	18.9
PDEQ	3	
Comorbidity	None	
Lf Dx	None	
Trauma Hx	Previous rape, domestic abuse, saw dead bodies	
Drug Use	Inderal (240 mg)	Alcohol (2), Marijuana (1/2 joint), Inderal (120mg)

Subject 5

	Value 1	Value 2
Treatment	CPT	
Age (yr)	24	
Time post rape (mo)	128	
Rare	White	
Education (yr)	15	
Income	3	
PTSD	Yes	No
Depression	No	No
CAPS (Sx)	3 ● 6 ● 4	1 ● 0 ● 1
PSS (freq)	10 ● 17 ● 14 = 41	2 ● 1 ● 2 = 5
BDI	33	
DES (%)	49.8	34.2
PDEQ	18	
Comorbidity	None	
Lf Dx	Depression	
Trauma Hx	Friend killed, attempted rape, domestic abuse, child sex abuse, natural disaster	
Drug Use	Alcohol (2), Nuprin (2)	Alcohol (2), BCP (Nortriptaline)

Note: See text for details and abbreviations.

repeated several times over a 60-minute period to reduce the client's anxiety and distress levels. *In vivo* exposure requires clients to confront anxiety-provoking situations in their lives that they have been avoiding since the rape. Focusing on situations that are realistically safe, clients are instructed to stay in the situation until anxiety levels decrease to manageable levels. The idea underlying prolonged exposure is that the avoidance behaviors associated with PTSD prevent the survivor from emotionally processing the rape and reinforce the fearful emotions experienced during the rape. Because of this, rape survivors continue to be fearful and anxious when remembering the rape or when they are in situations that remind them of the rape even if these situations are safe. Exposure techniques prevent the survivor from avoiding the rape memory and associated situations. Because they are no longer in real danger, their anxiety and fear eventually decrease and they can process the emotional content of the rape and manage everyday situations that had become associated with the rape. Foa and colleagues[66,67] propose that repeated reliving of the rape memories during prolonged exposure treatment decreases the anxiety associated with these memories through habituation and enables reevaluation of the meaning representations in the memory. This repeated reliving generates a more organized memory record that can be more readily integrated with existing schemas.

Assessment Instruments

Subjects were assessed with published clinical instruments that have sound psychometric properties including scales used in Study 1 which include the SCID, CAPS, BDI, and PSS. Additional psychometric scales administered for this assessment included the dissociative experiences scale (DES[68]); the Peritraumatic Dissociative Experiences Questionnaire (PDEQ[69]); and a trauma interview that assessed various lifetime traumatic events.

Procedure

Assessment Procedure. Assessments were conducted in the week prior to the start of treatment and then again immediately posttreatment with follow-ups for some of the subjects at 3 and 9 months posttreatment. Subjects were asked to give informed consent and then were administered paper and pencil questionnaires and a laptop computer questionnaire consisting of self-report scales.

DST Procedure. Baseline blood samples were drawn via venipuncture of the arm between 9:00 and 9:30 AM on the first day of the assessment. Subjects were given 0.5 mg of dexamethasone to take that evening at 11:00 PM. The next morning a follow-up blood sample was collected between 9:00 and 9:30 AM for all subjects. Blood was centrifuged within 30 minutes, and plasma was stored at −80°C until assays for cortisol concentration were performed. Cortisol and dexamethasone levels were determined in the laboratory of one of the authors (R.Y.). Dexamethasone levels were used to exclude subjects who had not taken dexamethasone as instructed.

RESULTS

Demographic and clinical self-report descriptive data are presented in TABLE 4. All of the subjects were diagnosed with PTSD prior to treatment and all of them recovered and were no longer meeting criteria for PTSD at all posttreatment assessments based on the CAPS interview. It is also notable that all five subjects had significant trauma histories. The data from the low-dose DST are presented in FIGURE 3. There were several types of responses to dexamethasone including those in two subjects (1 and 2) who continued to show supersuppression of cortisol even after successful treatment and two subjects who appeared to recover a more normal (moderate) level of suppression after receiving successful treatment (3 and 4). Finally, subject 5 did not display enhanced suppression of cortisol at any assessment even though she was diagnosed with PTSD at pretreatment. Examination of the clinical data revealed two possible patterns to the data between those subjects who continued to show supersuppression and those who showed normal suppression following successful treatment. TABLE 5 presents an interpretive summary of the clinical and biochemical data. Two patterns emerged from the data. First, subjects who continued to be supersuppressors after treatment were those who had a longer period of time since the rape ($\bar{x}$ = 50 months post rape) compared to those who returned to normal suppression ($\bar{x}$ = 5.5 months post rape). Second, supersuppressors were those subjects who scored in the high range on the PDEQ which indicates that they dissociated much more during the rape than did those who showed normal suppression.

These data are very preliminary but do suggest that time may be a factor in whether the biological alterations that may be produced by PTSD can be returned to the same levels as they were prior to exposure to the trauma. The suggestion is that there may be a critical period during which biological alterations are possible. If this window is missed, it may mean that the biological alterations become entrenched, and even successful treatment may not be able to fully reverse the effects.

Clearly more data are needed to move beyond the arena of speculation. The finding, that subject 5 who was diagnosed with PTSD prior to treatment yet did not show enhanced suppression, suggests that yet another pattern of responding is possible.

Implications

Taken together these preliminary data suggest that biological measures can generate information that will help to consolidate information that is derived from clinical assessments. In study 1, the psychophysiological findings clearly were in agreement with the statistical interpretation of the clinical data which indicated that two subjects responded well to treatment and were PTSD negative, whereas one subject did not show as much clinical improvement and remained PTSD positive. Psychophysiological measures appear to be very promising objective indicators of treatment response and can help to verify clinical impressions.

Biological measures can be helpful in the following areas related to treatment:

1. Objective indicators of treatment outcome. Development of reliable indicators of treatment response would benefit both the patient and the therapist.

2. Biological markers may be helpful in determining treatment strategy. For example, biological measures that can be assessed within therapy may allow an

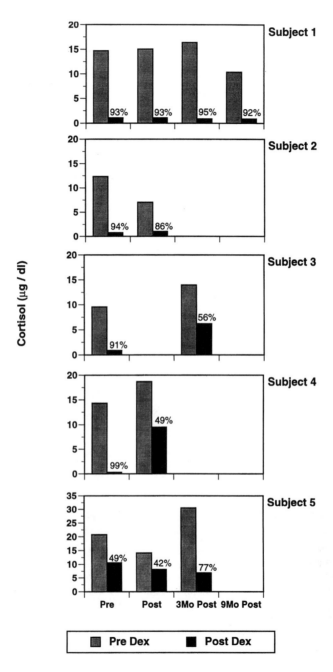

FIGURE 3. Biochemical data from the dexamethasone (DEX) suppression test. Percentages indicate the amount of suppression from baseline levels.

TABLE 5. Interpretive Summary of Dexamethasone Suppression Test Challenge

Subject	Pretreatment Suppression	Posttreatment Suppression	Time Post Rape (mo)	PTSD Pre/Post	Depression Pre/Post	DES	PDEQ	Trauma History	Comorbidity
1	+	+	84	±	-/-	-	+	+	-
2	+	+	16	±	-/-	-	+	+	+
3	+	-	6	±	-/-	-	-	+	-
4	+	-	4	±	-/-	-	-	+	-
5	-	-	128	±	-/-	+	+	+	-

evaluation of exactly where treatment begins to produce efficacy or relief from PTSD symptoms. Examination of biological variables may help determine which elements of the therapy are most advantageous for symptom reduction.

3. Discussion of biological alterations can be therapeutic for the client. This includes helping clients understand why they are having symptoms and normalizing their reactions. There may also be an added benefit of objectively demonstrating alterations in biological variables following treatment.

CONSIDERATIONS

1. PTSD subjects may differ on biological parameters prior to treatment or even prior to the traumatic event. The possibility of biological differences before exposure to trauma which are predisposing factors should not be discounted.

2. Treatment failures or nonresponders are an important part of the clinical picture and may reveal interesting information about biological variables.

3. How well will clients tolerate biological measures and will collection of biological measures have an impact on treatment? These questions are critical for understanding the role that therapy plays in altering biological variables.

4. Assessment of biological measures may eventually help us answer the question of whether psychological trauma per se alters biology. If so, can psychological therapy return the individuals biology back to pre-trauma conditions? This may ultimately be the most interesting question of all.

REFERENCES

1. AMERICAN PSYCHIATRIC ASSOCIATION. 1994. Diagnostic and Statistical Manual of Mental Disorders. 4th Ed. American Psychiatric Association. Washington, DC.
2. KARDINER, A. 1941. The Traumatic Neuroses of War. Paul B. Hoeber, Inc. New York.
3. GRINKER, R. R. & J. P. SPIEGEL. 1945. Men Under Stress. McGraw-Hill Book Co., Inc. New York.
4. BAXTER, L. R. *et al.* 1992. Caudate glucose metabolic rate changes with both drug and behavior therapy for obsessive-compulsive disorder. Arch. Gen. Psychiatry **49:** 681-689.
5. SCHWARTZ, J. M. *et al.* 1996. Systematic changes in cerebral glucose metabolic rate after successful behavior modification treatment of obsessive-compulsive disorder. Arch. Gen. Psychiatry **53:** 109-113.
6. VAN DER KOLK, B. A. 1994. The body keeps the score: Memory and the evolving psychobiology of posttraumatic stress. Harvard Rev. Psychiatry **1:** 253-265.
7. ORR, S. P. 1990. Psychophysiologic studies of posttraumatic stress disorder. *In* E. L. Giller Ed. Biological Assessment and Treatment of Posttraumatic Stress Disorder. 137-157. American Psychiatric Press. Washington, DC.
8. ORR, S. P. *et al.* 1993. Psychophysiological assessment of posttraumatic stress disorder imagery in World War II and Korean combat veterans. J. Abnorm. Psychol. **102:** 152-159.
9. SHALEV, A. Y. *et al.* 1992. Physiologic response to loud tones in Israeli patients with posttraumatic stress disorder. Arch. Gen. Psychiatry **49:** 870-875.
10. LANG, P. J. 1979. A bio-informational theory of emotional imagery. Psychophysiology **16:** 495-512.
11. PITMAN, R. K. *et al.* 1987. Psychophysiologic assessment of posttraumatic stress disorder imagery in Vietnam combat veterans. Arch. Gen. Psychiatry. **44:** 970-975.

12. PITMAN, R. K. *et al.* 1990. Psychophysiologic responses to combat imagery of Vietnam veterans with post-traumatic stress disorder versus other anxiety disorders. J. Abnorm. Psychol. **99:** 49-54.

13. SHALEV, A. Y., S. P. ORR & R. K. PITMAN. 1993. Psychophysiologic assessment of traumatic imagery in Israeli civilian patients with posttraumatic stress disorder. Am. J. Psychiatry **150:** 620-624.

14. BLANCHARD, E. B. *et al.* 1994. The psychophysiology of motor vehicle accident related posttraumatic stress disorder. Behav. Ther. **25:** 453-467.

15. KEANE, T. M. & D. KALOUPEK. 1982. Imaginal flooding in the treatment of a posttraumatic stress disorder. J. Consul. Psychol. **50:** 138-140.

16. FAIRBANK, J. A. & T. M. KEANE. 1982. Flooding for combat-related stress disorders: Assessment of anxiety reduction across traumatic memories. Behav. Ther. **13:** 499-510.

17. BOUDEWYNS, P. A. & L. HYER. 1990. Physiological response to combat memories and preliminary treatment outcome in Vietnam veteran PTSD patients treated with direct therapeutic exposure. Behav. Ther. **21:** 63-87.

18. SHALEV, A. Y., S. P. ORR & R. K. PITMAN. 1992. Psychophysiologic response during script-driven imagery as an outcome measure in post-traumatic stress disorder. J. Clin. Psychiatry **53:** 324-326.

19. RYCHTARIK, R. G. *et al.* 1984. Treatment of an incest victim with implosive therapy: A case study. Behav. Ther. **15:** 410-420.

20. MONTGOMERY, R. W. & T. AYLLON. 1994. Eye movement desensitization across images: A single case design. J. Behav. Ther. Exp. Psychiatry **25:** 23-28.

21. MONTGOMERY, R. W. & T. AYLLON. 1994. Eye movement desensitization across subjects: Subjective and physiological measures of treatment efficacy. J. Behav. Ther. Exp. Psychiatry **25:** 217-230.

22. RENFREY, G. & C. R. SPATES. 1994. Eye movement desensitization: A partial dismantling study. J. Behav. Ther. Exp. Psychiatry **25:** 231-239.

23. SELYE, H. 1956. The Stress of Life. McGraw-Hill. New York.

24. YEHUDA, R., E. L. GILLER & J. W. MASON. 1993. Psychoneuroendocrine assessment of posttraumatic stress disorder: Current progress and new directions. Prog. Neuropsychopharmacol. Biol. Psychiatry **17:** 541-550.

25. SELYE, H. 1936. Thymus and adrenals in the response of the organisms to injuries and intoxications. Br. J. Exp. Pathol. **17:** 234-246.

26. SAPOLSKY, R. M., L. C. KREY & B. S. MCEWEN. 1985. Prolonged glucocorticoid exposure reduces hippocampal neuron number. Implications for aging. J. Neurosci. **5:** 1221-1226.

27. MUNCK, A., P. M. GUYRE & N. J. HOLBROOK. 1984. Physiological functions of glucocorticoids in stress and their relation to pharmacological actions. Endocrinol. Rev. **93:** 9779-9783.

28. WOLKOWITZ, O. M. *et al.* 1990. Cognitive effects of corticosteroids. Am. J. Psychiatry **147:** 1297-1303.

29. MASON, J. W. *et al.* 1986. Urinary free-cortisol levels in post-traumatic stress disorder patients. J. Nerv. Ment. Dis. **174:** 145-149.

30. YEHUDA, R. *et al.* 1990. Low urinary cortisol excretion in PTSD. J. Nerv. Ment. Dis. **178:** 366-369.

31. YEHUDA, R. *et al.* 1991. Lymphocyte glucocorticoid receptor number in posttraumatic stress disorder. Am. J. Psychiatry **148:** 499-504.

32. RESNICK, H. S. & R. YEHUDA. 1993. Post-rape cortisol response associated with prior trauma history. Paper presented at the 9th annual meeting of the International Society for Traumatic Stress Studies, San Antonio, TX.

33. APA TASK FORCE ON LABORATORY TESTS IN PSYCHIATRY. 1987. The dexamethasone suppression test: An overview of its current status in psychiatry. Am. J. Psychiatry **144:** 1253-1262.

34. CARROLL, B. J. 1982. The dexamethasone suppression test for melancholia. Br. J. Psychiatry **140:** 292-304.

35. KUDLER, H. *et al.* 1987. The DST and post-traumatic stress disorder. Am. J. Psychiatry **144:** 1068-1071.

36. KOSTEN, T. R. *et al.* 1990. The dexamethasone suppression test and thyrotropin-releasing hormone stimulation test in posttraumatic stress disorder. Biol. Psychiatry **28:** 657-664.

37. YEHUDA, R. *et al.* 1993. Enhanced suppression of cortisol following dexamethasone administration in posttraumatic stress disorder. Am. J. Psychiatry **150:** 83-86.

38. SPITZER, R. L., J. B. W. WILLIAMS & M. GIBBON. 1987. Structured Clinical Interview for DSM-III-R SCID. Biometrics Research Department, New York State Psychiatric Institute. New York.

39. BLAKE, D. D. *et al.* 1990. A clinician rating scale for assessing current and lifetime PTSD: The CAPS-1. Behav. Ther. **18:** 187-188.

40. BECK, A. T. *et al.* 1961. An inventory for measuring depression. Arch. Gen. Psychiatry **4:** 561-571.

41. BECK, A. T. *et al.* 1974. The measurement of pessimism: The Hopelessness Scale. J. Consult. Clin. Psych. **42:** 861-865.

42. FOA, E. B. *et al.* 1993. Reliability and validity of a brief instrument for assessing posttraumatic stress disorder. J. Traumatic Stress **6:** 459-473.

43. KILPATRICK, D. J. 1988. Rape aftermath symptom test. *In* Dictionary of Behavioral Assessment Techniques: 366-367 M. Hersen & A. S. Bellack, Eds. Pergamon Press. Oxford.

44. TOBIN, D. L. *et al.* 1989. The hierarchical factor structure of the coping strategies inventory. Cognit. Ther. Res. **13:** 343-361.

45. HOROWITZ, M. J., N. WILNER & W. ALVAREZ. 1979. Impact of Event Scale: A measure of subjective distress. Psychosom. Med. **41:** 209-218.

46. CHEMTOB, C. *et al.* 1988. A cognitive action theory of post-traumatic stress disorder. *J. Anxiety Disord.* **2:** 253-275.

47. FOA, E. B., G. STEKETEE & B. O. ROTHBAUM. 1989. Behavioral/cognitive conceptualizations of post-traumatic stress disorder. Behav. Ther. **20:** 155-176.

48. HOROWITZ, M. J. 1976. Stress Response Syndromes. Jason Aronson. New York.

49. JONES, J. C. & D. H. BARLOW. 1990. The etiology of post-traumatic stress disorder. Clin. Psychol. Rev. **10:** 299-328.

50. MCCANN, I. L. & L. A. PEARLMAN. 1990. Psychological Trauma and the Adult Survivor: Theory, Therapy, and Transformation. Brunner/Mazel. New York.

51. MCCANN, I. L., D. K. SAKHEIM & D. J. ABRAHAMSON. 1988. Trauma and victimization: A model of psychological adaptation. Counsel Psychologist **16:** 531-594.

52. LERNER, M. J. & D. T. MILLER. 1978. Just world research and the attribution process: Looking back and ahead. Psychol. Bull. **85:** 1030-1051.

53. HOLLON, S. D. & J. GARBER. 1988. Cognitive therapy. *In* Social Cognition and Clinical Psychology: A Synthesis. L. Y. Abramson Ed.: 204-253. Guilford. New York.

54. RESICK, P. A. & M. K. SCHNICKE. 1990. Treating symptoms in adult victims of sexual assault. J. Interpers. Viol. **5:** 488-506.

55. RESICK, P. A. & M. K. SCHNICKE. 1992. Cognitive processing therapy for sexual assault victims. J. Consult. Clin. Psychol. **60:** 748-756.

56. RESICK, P. A. & M. K. SCHNICKE. 1993. Cognitive Processing Therapy for Rape Victims: A Treatment Manual. Sage Publications. Newbury Park, CA.

57. CALHOUN, K. S. & P. A. RESICK. 1993. Post-traumatic stress disorder. *In* Clinical Handbook of Psychological Disorders. D. H. Barlow, Ed.: 48-98. Guilford. New York.

58. ELLIS, L. F., L. D. BLACK & P. A. RESICK. 1992. Cognitive-behavioral treatment approaches for victims of crime. *In* Innovations in Clinical Practice: A Source Book. **11:** 23-38. Professional Resource Exchange. Sarasota, FL.

59. MECHANIC, M. B. & P. A. RESICK. 1994. An approach to treating posttraumatic stress disorder and depression. Paper presented at the 20th Annual Meeting of the National Association for Rural Mental Health, Des Moines, IA.

60. Resick, P. A. 1992. Cognitive treatment of a crime-related post-traumatic stress disorder. *In* Aggression and Violence throughout the Life Span. R. D. Peters, R. J. McMahon & V. L. Quincey, Eds.: 171–191. Sage. Newbury Park, CA.

61. Resick, P. A. 1994. Cognitive processing therapy CPT for rape-related PTSD and depression. Clin. Quart. **4:** 1–5.

62. Resick, P. A. & B. E. Gerth-Markaway. 1991. Clinical treatment of adult female victims of sexual assault. *In* Clinical Approaches to Sex Offenders and Their Victims. C. R. Hollin & K. Howells, Eds.: 261–284. Wiley. New York.

63. Nishith, P. *et al.* 1995. PTSD and major depression: Methodological and treatment considerations in a single case design. Behav. Ther. **26:** 319–335.

64. Mueser, K. T., P. R. Yarnold & D. W. Foy. 1991. Statistical analysis for single-case designs. Behav. Mod. **15:** 134–155.

65. Yarnold, P. R. 1988. Classical test theory methods for repeated measures N = 1 research designs. Educ. Psych. Meas. **48:** 913–919.

66. Dancu, C. V. & E. B. Foa. 1992. Posttraumatic stress disorder. *In* Comprehensive Casebook of Cognitive Therapy. A. Freeman & F. M. Dattilio, Eds.: 79–88. Plenum. New York.

67. Rothbaum, B. O. & E. B. Foa. 1992. Exposure therapy for rape victims with posttraumatic stress disorder. Behav. Ther. **15:** 219–222.

68. Bernstein, E. M. & F. W. Putnam. 1986. Development, reliability, and validity of a dissociation scale. J. Nerv. Ment. Dis. **174:** 727–735.

69. Marmar, C. R. *et al.* 1994. Peritraumatic dissociation and PTS in male Vietnam theater veterans. Am. J. Psychiatry **151:** 902–907.

Psychological Processes Related to Recovery from a Trauma and an Effective Treatment for PTSD

EDNA B. FOA

Allegheny University of the Health Sciences
3200 Henry Avenue
Philadelphia, Pennsylvania 19129

Many chapters in this volume discuss biological factors implicated in posttraumatic stress disorder (PTSD). I would like to focus on psychological factors that seem related to the etiology or maintenance of chronic PTSD. To this end I first present data to indicate that individuals differ in their ability to process a trauma successfully, discussing psychological factors that impede natural processing and thereby contribute to the development of chronic PTSD. I then discuss data demonstrating that psychosocial treatments, particularly cognitive behavioral treatments, are effective in reducing PTSD in female victims of assault. Finally, I discuss psychological factors that seem to mediate both the naturally occurring reduction in posttrauma disturbances and symptom reduction via treatment.

REACTION TO TRAUMA

Many studies have indicated that individuals differ in their ability to recover from a traumatic experience and that traumas differ in their likelihood to produce PTSD. For example, in a retrospective study of the prevalence of PTSD among a representative sample of women in the United States, 17.8% of aggravated assault victims and 12.4% of rape victims exhibited chronic PTSD. In contrast, PTSD was observed in only 3.4% of female victims of noncrime trauma.[1] Thus, female victims of assault are four to five times more likely to develop chronic PTSD than are female victims of noncrime traumas.

A similar picture has emerged from two prospective studies that we conducted with female victims of sexual and nonsexual assault.[2,3] In the first study, Rothbaum *et al.*[3] assessed weekly posttrauma reactions of 64 rape victims and 49 nonsexual assault victims, beginning within 2 weeks after the assault. The results of the first study are depicted in Figure 1.

As depicted in Figure 1, in the first assessment almost all rape victims (94%) had emotional disturbance severe enough to meet symptom criteria for PTSD. The percentage of victims with PTSD decreased gradually, but 3 months after the assault some victims seemed to have successfully processed the trauma and others did not: 47% of rape victims remained disturbed enough to meet diagnostic criteria for PTSD. A second, larger study compared the PTSD rate in 96 rape victims and 100 nonsexual assault victims yielding similar results.[2] Shortly after the assault 92% of rape victims and 74% of nonsexual assault victims met symptom criteria for PTSD at the first

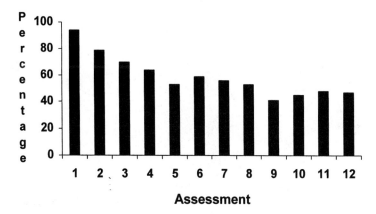

FIGURE 1. Percentage of rape with PTSD at 12 assessments.

assessment, about 2 weeks after the assault. Three months later, 47% of the former and 27% of the latter retained the PTSD diagnosis.

Thus, in both studies the number of victims who successfully processed the trauma increased with the passage of time, but the number of rape victims who failed to successfully process their rape experience was greater than the number who failed to process nonsexual assault. In fact, 6 months after the assault, 38% of rape victims versus 13% of nonsexual assault victims still met diagnostic criteria for PTSD.[2] The finding that many, but not all victims recover from their trauma points to the importance of identifying factors that determine whether individuals will process a trauma successfully or will fail to do so and hence develop chronic PTSD.

PSYCHOLOGICAL PROCESSES RELATED TO NATURAL RECOVERY

The Emotional Engagement Hypothesis

My starting point in the quest for understanding recovery processes is the emotional engagement hypothesis. Beginning with Janet and Freud[4,5] and continuing into present conceptualization,[6,7] trauma theorists have postulated that emotional engagement with traumatic memory is a necessary condition for successful processing of the event and resultant recovery. Conversely, deliberate avoidance of reminders of the trauma, or emotional withdrawal and dissociation, are thought to hinder recovery. Indeed, avoidance is included in numbing symptoms of posttraumatic stress disorder (PTSD) in DSM-IV.[8]

Despite the popularity of the emotional engagement hypothesis among trauma theorists, empirical studies of the relation between engagement and recovery have begun only recently, and the emerging results are supportive. For example, retrospective reports of dissociative experiences during trauma were related to the severity of PTSD later on.[9–11] Two prospective studies showed that dissociative symptoms

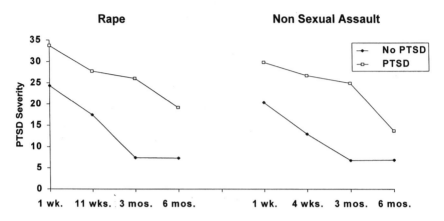

FIGURE 2. Severity of PTSD in female assault victims.

immediately after natural disasters were positively associated with PTSD symptom severity 7–9 months later.[12,13]

If a high level of dissociation is taken to indicate low emotional engagement, and if, as shown in the Foa and colleagues studies,[2,3] the presence of severe PTSD symptoms is the norm after an extreme trauma, then a peak in PTSD symptom severity *shortly* after the trauma could be seen as marking high emotional engagement. Conversely, a delay in the peak symptom severity can be interpreted as low emotional engagement. If these propositions are correct, then victims who exhibit the highest PTSD severity shortly after the trauma should show enhanced emotional processing and faster recovery than should victims with delayed peak symptom severity.

To explore this hypothesis we conducted two studies. In the first study, we utilized data from the second prospective discussed earlier.[2] As noted earlier, in this study sexual and nonsexual assault victims were assessed monthly up to 3 months, at which point some victims of each assault type had PTSD and others did not. The means of four groups (sexual and nonsexual assault victims, with and without PTSD 3 months postassault) are depicted in FIGURE 2.

Several interesting inferences can be drawn from the data. First, on the average, all four groups demonstrated some decline in PTSD severity over time. Second, rape induced more severe PTSD than did physical assault. Third, regardless of assault type, on the average, victims who exhibit more severe symptoms shortly after the trauma evidenced more severe symptoms later on. At first glance this latter finding contradicts the emotional engagement hypothesis. However, reanalysis of Rothbaum *et al.*'s[3] data which consisted of weekly assessment, thus allowing for more precise examination of the recovery patterns, revealed a more complex picture. To examine individual differences in patterns of reaction to trauma, Gilboa and Foa[14] adopted the methods of *individual growth modeling.*[15] In these methods, all individuals are postulated to share a common reaction pattern (growth model), whereas individuals' temporal reactions can differ in certain characteristics (growth parameters). Gilboa and Foa[14] examined four main characteristics of reaction to trauma: (1) magnitude

TABLE 1. Intercorrelation among Aspects of Emotional Reactions to Trauma

		1	2	3	4	5
1	Magnitude of initial reaction	–				
2	Magnitude of peak reaction	.90	–			
3	Time of peak reaction (in days)	–.21	.01	–		
4	Magnitude of reaction at 14 weeks	.55	.72	.36	–	
5	Rate of average weekly decline	–.14	–.34	–.49	–.76	–

of the initial reaction; (2) magnitude of the peak reaction; (3) delay of peak reaction; and (4) recovery rate. Of these the two most relevant to the engagement hypothesis are: first, the magnitude of the peak reaction, that is, the most intense reaction postassault, and second, the length of delay in peak reaction.

The emotional engagement hypothesis predicts that a delayed peak reaction will impede recovery whereas an immediate peak will enhance recovery. The intercorrelations among the individual growth parameters are presented in TABLE 1.

The first three variables in the correlation matrix, numbers 1 to 3, refer to characteristics of the emotional reaction; the last two variables, numbers 4 and 5, refer to outcome indices, namely, PTSD severity 14 weeks postassault and the rate of decline in PTSD severity. In contrast to the results of the group analysis presented earlier, this analysis indicates that the magnitude of the *peak* reaction predicted later PTSD severity better than did the magnitude of the *initial* reaction. The relevant correlations are .72 and .55, respectively. In addition, both the magnitude and the time of peak reaction were better predictors of the rate of symptom decline. The relevant correlations are –.34 and –.49 versus –.14, respectively.

To elucidate the relation between the delay in peak reaction and chronic psychopathology we included in the analysis only individuals whose peak reactions occurred within 6 weeks after the assault. This restriction guarantees that the correlation between delay and final assessment is not due to the temporal proximity between the assessment session at which peak reaction occurs and the final assessment because at least 8 weeks separate these two assessments. Longer delay of peak reaction in PTSD (as measured by days since the assault) was significantly related to depression as measured by the Beck Depression Inventory[16] and PTSD measures taken at the final assessment. FIGURE 3 depicts this association.

As would be predicted by the emotional engagement hypothesis, 14 weeks after the trauma, victims whose peak reaction occurred within the first 2 weeks exhibited less severe depression and PTSD than did victims whose peak reaction occurred between the second and sixth weeks. We will revisit the engagement hypothesis later, in the context of discussing treatment processes.

The Organization-Elaboration Hypothesis

Many trauma theorists also hold that traumatic memories are different from other types of memories and that recovery involves special processing efforts. Although

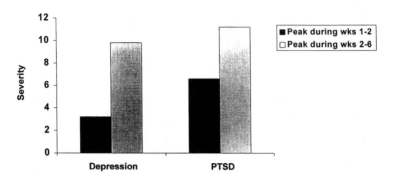

FIGURE 3. Time of peak reaction and persistent psychopathology.

research on traumatic memories is still in its beginning stages, the work of trauma experts such as Koss[17] and Pennebaker[18] implies the potential promise of studying trauma *narratives*. Clinical observations suggest that trauma narratives recounted by clients with chronic PTSD are characterized by an abundance of speech fillers, repetitions, and incomplete sentences; time and space in these narratives are disconnected; and thought utterances reflect confusion.

On the basis of studies on trauma narratives during treatment, Foa and Riggs[19] hypothesized that the natural process of recovery involves the organizing and streamlining of the traumatic memory. They further suggested that individuals who fail to organize this memory would exhibit more trauma-related disturbances. A related concept to narrative organization is narrative articulation. We hypothesized that the degree of articulation in rape narratives recounted by victims shortly after the assault would predict later PTSD.[20] Degree of articulation was determined by applying two indices of reading level to narratives of rape recounted by the victims about 2 weeks after the assault. The indices are: Reading Ease and Grade-School Level as determined by a computer program.[21] Consistent with the hypothesis, the correlation of PTSD with Reading Ease was −.63, and with Grade-School Level, .60. Interestingly, the correspondence correlations with severity of depression and anxiety were not significant, suggesting a specific relationship between level of processing the traumatic memory and PTSD. Later, in the context of treatment studies, I will come back to the hypothesis that organizing the trauma narrative is one of the mechanisms underlying successful processing.

Changes in Core Schemas

Another popular idea among trauma theorists is that the successful processing of a traumatic experience requires adjustments in core schemas, that is, beliefs about the world and about oneself.[6,22–24] For example, Janoff-Bulman[23] suggested that a traumatic experience violates the beliefs inherent in human beings that the world is benevolent and that the self is invulnerable. Accordingly, victims who had previously viewed themselves as invulnerable and extremely competent and had perceived their world as extremely safe would be more likely to show trauma-related disturbances than would victims who had not held such extreme positive beliefs. Results that contradict these observations come from studies indicating that multiple traumatic experiences and pre-trauma psychological disturbances increase the likelihood of PTSD.[25,26] Presumably individuals with such a history do not perceive themselves as extremely competent and the world as extremely safe. Rather, they are more likely to perceive the world as extremely dangerous and themselves as extremely incompetent.

In an attempt to reconcile these seeming contradictions, Foa and colleagues[7,19] suggested that it is not the holding of positive assumptions that render an individual less adept at processing a traumatic event, but rather the holding of an extremely rigid view. Accordingly, there may be two distinct and even opposite ways in which pre-trauma schemas can interfere with recovery: (1) when the trauma violates existing knowledge of oneself as extremely competent and of the world as extremely safe; (2) when the trauma primes existing knowledge of oneself as extremely incompetent and of the world as extremely dangerous. On the other hand, trauma victims whose life experiences have equipped them with rules of interpretation that allow finer discriminations of the degree of ''dangerousness'' and ''competence'' will be better able to process the trauma as a unique and unusual event, one that should not substantially change their evaluations of themselves and of the world. Data supporting the proposition that beliefs of one's competence and of how safe the world is are implicated in PTSD was reported by Foa.[2] Applying Janoff-Bulman's World Assumption Scale[23] and Resick's Personal Beliefs Scale[27] in the study described earlier of recent rape and nonsexual assault victims,[2] degree of self-esteem and perception of the world were assessed monthly, beginning about 2 weeks after the assault. As expected, individuals who had PTSD 3 months after the trauma exhibited a less positive view about the world and about themselves immediately after the trauma than did victims who recovered.

In summary, evidence suggests that the degree to which a victim is emotionally engaged with the traumatic memories, organizes and articulates the traumatic memory, and maintains a balanced view about the world and self determines whether he or she will recover or develop chronic disturbances.

THE EFFICACY OF COGNITIVE BEHAVIORAL THERAPY

Let us now move from the discussion of the psychopathology underlying PTSD and focus briefly on the efficacy of cognitive behavioral treatment. Two cognitive behavioral programs were used with PTSD with the introduction of the disorder into the DSM-III:[28] exposure therapy for Vietnam veterans[29] and stress inoculation training for rape victims.[30] With Vietnam veterans several reports demonstrated that variants of exposure therapy produced positive, although sometimes modest, improvement in chronic PTSD. The effects of stress inoculation training have not been studied systematically until recently.

Two studies were conducted by Foa and her colleagues comparing the efficacy of a manualized exposure treatment they have developed with that of stress inoculation training.[2,31] I will demonstrate the efficacy of these techniques by summarizing data from the latest complete study. Exposure treatment in this study consisted of four components: education about common reactions to trauma; breathing retraining; prolonged, repeated exposure to the trauma memory (reliving); and repeated *in vivo* exposure to situations the client is avoiding because of assault-related fear. Stress Inoculation Training included: relaxation training; thought stopping; guided self-dialogue; cognitive restructuring; covert modeling; and role playing (for more details see ref. 7). The efficacy of four conditions was compared: exposure treatment (PE), stress inoculation training (SIT), a combination of PE and SIT, and a wait list. Active treatments included nine 90-minute sessions conducted over 5 weeks.

Several indices of outcome have been used to compare the efficacy of the four conditions in Foa's study,[2] including a stringent index, defining responders as clients improved 50% or more in PTSD symptoms and who also had a normal score of depression and of general anxiety. Using this index, the number of responders in each treatment was calculated. Immediately after treatment, 46% of clients in the exposure therapy met this stringent criterion for responder status compared to 25% in the SIT group and 29% in the combined group. At follow-up all active groups were equivalent.

A comparison between clients who received exposure treatment and those who did not revealed that the former improved significantly more than the latter on all outcome indices. In contrast, clients who received Stress Inoculation Training did not differ significantly from those who did not. Thus, exposure therapy alone seems to be superior to both of the other two programs, especially when efficacy is assessed via a broad index of psychopathology. Effects size analyses corroborated this inference: on virtually all outcome measures, the group that received exposure therapy only exhibited larger effect sizes compared to the wait-list condition than did the other two groups.

Additional evidence for the efficacy of exposure treatment comes from an ongoing study conducted by Resick and her colleagues who compare exposure therapy with a treatment Resick developed and called cognitive processing therapy[32] (CPT; Resick, personal communication, 1996). CPT is a 12-session program that employs Ellis'[33] and Beck's[34] cognitive therapy to correct maladaptive cognitions of rape victims. This therapy also includes writing down the traumatic experience. Preliminary data from this study suggest that both treatments are highly and equally effective in ameliorating PTSD. I would like to suggest, however, that the superiority of exposure therapy lies in the ease with which therapists can be trained to deliver it. Cognitive Processing Therapy, like other versions of cognitive restructuring, requires extensive training and places considerable intellectual demands on the client. In contrast, exposure therapy is a relatively easy treatment to master.

In summary, exposure, Stress Inoculation Training, and Cognitive Processing Therapy are all effective in ameliorating PTSD. At present, evidence for the efficacy of exposure is more conclusive because this treatment has been studied by several research groups using different trauma populations. How can the efficacy of exposure therapy be explained?

PSYCHOLOGICAL PROCESSES RELATED TO OUTCOME OF COGNITIVE BEHAVIORAL THERAPY

The Emotional Engagement Hypothesis

From the outset, I suggest that we will best understand the success of this treatment if we construe it as encouraging the processes that are involved in natural recovery from a trauma and as correcting the two main erroneous cognitions that underlie PTSD, that is, "the world is extremely dangerous" and "I [the victim] am extremely incompetent."

Referring to the mechanisms involved in systematic desensitization, Lang[35] suggested that the affective component of imagined fear scenes "may be a key to the emotional processing which the therapy is designed to accomplish." In an attempt to articulate the concept of emotional processing, Foa and Kozak[36] suggested that anxiety disorders, including PTSD, can be viewed as representing cognitive fear structures that include pathological elements. Within this theoretical framework, treatment for anxiety disorders is construed as modifying the pathological elements underlying the disorder, and such modifications are thought to be the essence of emotional processing. It follows then that the therapeutic process can be viewed as involving the same mechanisms that underlie natural recovery from trauma, which were discussed earlier.

In considering the mechanisms underlying successful treatment for anxiety, Foa and Kozak[36] suggested that regardless of the type of therapeutic intervention used, two conditions are required for fear reduction. First, the fear structure needs to be activated by means of fear-relevant information, such as reliving the traumatic experience; if the fear structure is not accessed, it will not be available for modification. One can immediately recognize that the activation hypothesis is a version of the emotional engagement proposition introduced in the beginning of the paper. The second condition for emotional processing is the availability of corrective information that is incompatible with the pathological elements of the fear structure.

Foa and Kozak[36] identified three indicators of emotional processing that have been associated with successful outcome of exposure treatment. First, clients who improve with exposure therapy show fear on both physiological and self-report measures, which indicates that the fear structure has been activated. Second, their fear reactions decrease gradually while they are being confronted with feared images, objects, or situations. Third, their initial fear reaction at each exposure session decreases across successive sessions.

Several studies support the validity of these indicators.[37,38] Of particular relevance to PTSD is a study in which we demonstrated that fear activation, or emotional engagement, during treatment promotes successful outcome.[38] This study explored the relation between facial fear expression during the first session of reliving the assault, and improvement following treatment. The results are depicted in FIGURE 4.

As would be predicted by the emotional engagement hypothesis, clients who displayed more intense facial fear expressions during the first exposure session benefited more from treatment than did those who displayed less intense fear. Interestingly, clients who reported more anger prior to treatment displayed less fear during reliving of the trauma and benefited less from treatment than did clients who were

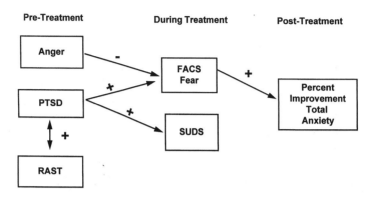

FIGURE 4. Predictive model of improvement with exposure therapy.

less angry. Foa[2] also reported that among recent assault victims, anger was found to impede natural recovery. Perhaps the relation between anger immediately after the trauma and later psychopathology is mediated by the failure of angry victims to engage emotionally with trauma-related fear. Thus, anger may be protective in the short run, but in the long run it seems to interfere with the well-being of the victim.

Support for both the emotional engagement and the habituation hypotheses comes from a study examining the patterns of subjective distress reported by clients during their recounting of the traumatic event in the context of exposure treatment.[39] Thirty-six female assault victims received treatment that involved repeated imaginal reliving of their traumatic experience and rated their distress at 10-minute intervals on a 0–100 Subjective Units of Distress (SUDs) scale. The average SUDs levels during each of six exposure sessions were submitted to cluster analysis. The results of cluster analysis are depicted in FIGURE 5.

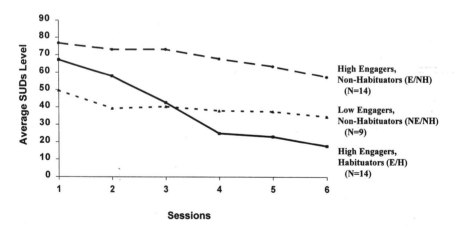

FIGURE 5. Average Subjective Units of Distress (SUDs) during trauma reliving within each cluster.

Three distinct clusters of clients emerged, differing with regard to their patterns of SUDs. The first cluster included clients who exhibited high distress in the first session and gradual decline over the remaining sessions; the second cluster included clients who exhibited high distress during the first session but did not show habituation over the course of treatment; finally, the third cluster included clients who exhibited only moderate distress during the first sessions and did not change over time.

As would be predicted by the engagement hypothesis, clients from the first group improved more after treatment than did clients belonging to the third group. Contrary to the engagement hypothesis, but consistent with the habituation hypothesis, clients belonging to the second group had inferior outcome to those from the first group. These results are consistent with the Gilboa and Foa[14] results from the individual growth modeling presented earlier. Thus, we have converging evidence from two kinds of studies, one examining natural recovery in recently assaulted victims and the other studying responses of clients with chronic PTSD during treatment. Both studies point to the influence of emotional engagement and of habituation on recovery.

The Organization-Elaboration Hypothesis

Earlier I suggested that successful processing of a traumatic event during natural recovery involves organizing and articulating the traumatic memory, and I discussed data demonstrating that victims with more articulated narratives exhibited less PTSD after their assault than did victims with less articulated narratives. I want to return to this hypothesis in the context of examining treatment processes.

As noted earlier, Foa and Riggs[19] proposed that memory records of traumatic events are more disorganized and more fragmented than are memory records of nontraumatic events. Similarly, Kilpatrick et al.[40] suggested that rape memories consist largely of representations of intense emotions, incomprehension, and confusion. Foa and Riggs[19] further suggested that the trauma memory records of victims with PTSD are especially disorganized and fragmented. It follows that successful treatment would result in more organized and less fragmented memories. Specifically, Foa et al.[41] hypothesized that repeated reliving of the traumatic event in the context of exposure therapy would produce changes in the trauma narrative and that these changes would be related to improvement after treatment. To test this hypotheses they developed a coding system and coded the first and last rape narratives during exposure treatment. They then compared the first and the last narrative on several dimensions. The results of this analysis are presented in FIGURE 6.

As depicted in FIGURE 6, proportionally less actions and dialogues, and more thoughts and feelings in general, and organized thoughts in particular, were expressed in the last narrative compared to the first one. These results are consistent with the hypothesis that successful treatment promotes organization of the traumatic memory. Also as hypothesized, the reduction in narrative fragmentation and increase in organization were highly correlated with reduction in trauma-related psychopathology, .73 and −.63, respectively.

Foa et al.'s[41] findings that trauma narratives became longer after successful therapy and included less concrete descriptions as well as the finding that symptom improvement was related to reduction in narrative fragmentation are consistent with Amir et

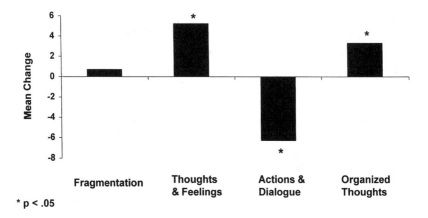

* p < .05

FIGURE 6. Change in mean utterances from first to last narratives.

al.'s[20] findings that victims whose trauma narratives were articulated well exhibited less PTSD. Thus, the two studies that investigated trauma narratives, one utilizing narratives of recent victims who have not been treated and the other examining narratives of chronically disturbed victims before and after therapy, converged to suggest that narrative organization is implicated in recovery from trauma.

Changes in Core Schemas

Foa and her colleagues[7,20] suggested that several cognitive modifications take place during treatment by repeated reliving of the trauma. First, the victim who, during repeated reliving of the trauma, experiences habituation of anxiety rather than the anticipated emotional breakdown will cease to interpret her symptoms as signs of incompetence. Second, repeated recounting of the trauma narrative reinforces discrimination between remembering the trauma and actually encountering it again and thereby promotes the notion that remembering itself is not dangerous. Third, prolonged exposure to the trauma memory promotes differentiation between the traumatic event and similar but safe events, thereby fostering the interpretation of the trauma as a unique event rather than as typical of a dangerous world. Fourth, repeated exposure to feared memories fosters an association between PTSD symptoms and mastery rather than incompetence. Finally, repeated reliving is thought to promote organization of the trauma narrative, thus facilitating integration of the traumatic experience into existing knowledge structures. These modifications directly correct the victim's perception that the world is entirely dangerous and the individual is entirely incompetent, the two dysfunctional cognitions that are thought to underlie PTSD.

In an attempt to account for the processes underlying the efficacy of Stress Inoculation Training, Foa and Jaycox[7] argued that the successful acquisition of anxiety management techniques has indirect effects on schemata of self and the world. Specifically, they proposed that the experience of oneself as being able to control

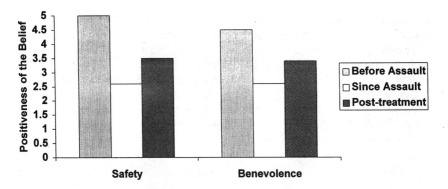

FIGURE 7. Beliefs about the world before trauma, before treatment, and after treatment.

the anxiety fosters a more positive self-image and the perception of oneself as a successful "coper," in turn, reduces the negative valence of potential future threats. If the victim perceives herself or himself as an "adequate coper," she or he will expect to be better able to avert potential dangers in the world. Finally, the increased perception of control over anxiety may allow the victim to tolerate the trauma memories for longer periods of time, thus fostering self-directed exposure and the resulting increased organization of trauma memory.

Preliminary results support the Foa and Jaycox[7] proposition that cognitive behavioral therapy induces change in world and self schemas. Female victims of assault who manifested chronic PTSD completed the Janoff-Bulman's World Assumption Scale[23] and Resick's Personal Beliefs and Reactions Scale[27] before and after 5 weeks of cognitive behavior therapy. In each of these assessment points, they were asked to indicate how positively they viewed the world and themselves both before the assault and at the time of the pretreatment interview. FIGURES 7 and 8 depict the results.

As is apparent from the data, cognitive behavioral therapy corrects pathological evaluations of oneself and of the world. Specifically, at the pretreatment assessment,

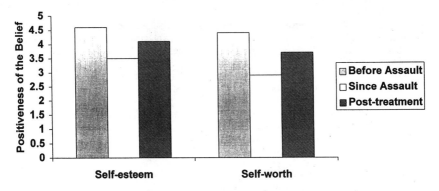

FIGURE 8. Beliefs about the self before trauma, before treatment, and after treatment.

clients indicated that their current perception of the world and of themselves was significantly less positive than their perception before the trauma. At the posttreatment assessment these perceptions were significantly more positive than those before treatment. These data suffer from the limitation inherent in employing self-report methods to study changes in core schemas and the limitation of inferring pre-trauma perception from retrospective inquiry. These limitations not withstanding, the investigation of natural recovery from a trauma and the study of treatment outcome converge to suggest that negative evaluations of the world and of oneself are associated with PTSD and that modification of these evaluations are related to recovery.

CONCLUSION

The three psychological factors involved in the successful processing of a traumatic event are: emotional engagement with the trauma memory; organization and articulation of the trauma narrative; and modification of basic core beliefs about the world and about oneself. All three factors were related to both natural recovery from a recent trauma and to a decrease of PTSD severity via cognitive behavioral therapy. No doubt there are other psychological processes that are involved in chronic PTSD, and these studies may require the development of new methods, as well as the use of existing ones. With increased knowledge about the biological and psychological factors involved in PTSD, we will be in a position to look at the relation between the two domains. The emotional engagement hypothesis currently constitutes a natural beginning for such a bridge.

REFERENCES

1. RESNICK, H. S., D. G. KILPATRICK, B. S. DANSKY, B. E. SAUNDERS & C. L. BEST. 1993. Prevalence of civilian trauma and posttraumatic stress disorder in a representative national sample of women. J. Consult. Clin. Psychol. **61:** 984–991.
2. FOA, E. B. 1995. Failure of emotional processing: Post trauma psychopathology. Paper presented at the World Congress of Behavioural & Cognitive Therapies, Copenhagen, Denmark.
3. ROTHBAUM, B. O., E. B. FOA, T. MURDOCK, D. S. RIGGS & W. WALSH. 1992. A prospective examination of post-traumatic stress disorder in rape victims. J. Traumatic Stress **5:** 455–475.
4. JANET, P. 1889. L'Automatisme Psychologique. Felix Alcan. Paris.
5. FREUD, S. 1973. The New Introductory Lectures in Psychoanalysis. Penguin. New York.
6. HOROWITZ, M. J. 1986. Stress Response Syndromes, 2nd Ed. Jason Aronson Inc. Northvale, NJ.
7. FOA, E. B. & L. H. JAYCOX. 1997. Cognitive-behavioral treatment of post-traumatic stress disorder. In Psychotherapeutic Frontiers: New Principles and Practices. D. Spiegel, Ed. American Psychiatric Press. Washington, DC. In press.
8. AMERICAN PSYCHIATRIC ASSOCIATION. 1994. Diagnostic and Statistical Manual of Mental Disorders, 4th Ed. Washington, DC.
9. BREMNER, J. D., S. SOUTHWICK, E. BRETT, A. FONTANA, R. ROSENHECK & D. S. CHARNEY. 1992. Dissociation and posttraumatic stress disorder in Vietnam combat veterans. *Am. J. Psychiatry* **149:** 328–332.
10. MARMAR, C. R., D. S. WEISS, W. E. SCHLENGER, J. A. FAIRBANK, B. K. JORDAN, R. A. KULKA & R. L. HOUGH. 1994. Peritraumatic dissociation and posttraumatic stress in male Vietnam theater veterans. Am. J. Psychiatry **151:** 902–907.

11. TICHENOR, V., C. R. MARMAR, D. S. WEISS, T. J. METZLER, & H. M. RONFELDT. 1996. The relationship of peritraumatic dissociation and posttraumatic stress: Findings in female Vietnam theater veterans. J. Consult. Clin. Psychol. **64:** 1054-1059.

12. CARDEÑA, E. & D. SPIEGEL. 1993. Dissociative reactions to the San Francisco Bay Area Earthquake of 1989. Am. J. Psychiatry **150:** 474-478.

13. KOOPMAN, C., C. CLASSEN & D. A. SPIEGEL. 1994. Predictors of posttraumatic stress symptoms among survivors of the Oakland/Berkeley, Calif., firestorm. Am. J. Psychiatry **151:** 888-894.

14. GILBOA, E. & E. B. FOA. 1996. Patterns of recovery after trauma: Individual differences and trauma characteristics. Unpublished observations.

15. WILLETT, J. B. & A. G. SAYER. 1994. Using covariance structure analysis to detect correlates and predictors of individual change over time. Psychol. Bull. **116:** 363-381.

16. BECK, A. T., C. H. WARD, M. MENDELSOHN, J. MOCK & J. ERBAUGH. 1961. An inventory for measuring depression. Arch. Gen. Psychiatry **4:** 561-571.

17. TROMP, S., M. P. KOSS, A. J. FIGUEREDO & M. THARAN. 1995. Are rape memories different? A comparison of rape, other unpleasant, and pleasant memories among employed women. J. Traumatic Stress **8:** 607-627.

18. HARBER, K. D. & J. W. PENNEBAKER. 1992. Overcoming traumatic memories. *In* The Handbook of Emotion and Memory: Research and Theory. S. Christianson, Ed.: 359-387. Lawrence Erlbaum Associates. NJ.

19. FOA, E. B. & D. S. RIGGS. 1993. Post-traumatic stress disorder in rape victims. *In* American Psychiatric Press Review of Psychiatry. J. Oldham, M. B. Riba & A. Tasman, Eds. Vol. 12: 273-303. American Psychiatric Press. Washington, DC.

20. AMIR, N., J. STAFFORD, M. S. FRESHMAN & E. B. FOA. 1997. Relationship between trauma narratives and symptoms in posttraumatic stress disorder. Submitted.

21. FLESCH, R. 1949. The Art of Readable Writing. Harper & Brothers Publishers. New York.

22. EPSTEIN, S. 1991. The self-concept, the traumatic neurosis, and the structure of personality. In Perspectives in Personality. D. Ozer, J. M. Healy & A. J. Stewart, Eds. Vol. 3, Part A: 63-98. Jessica Kingsley. London.

23. JANOFF-BULMAN, R. 1992. Shattered Assumptions: Towards a New Psychology of Trauma. The Free Press. New York.

24. MCCANN, I. L. & L. A. PEARLMAN. 1990. Psychological Trauma and the Adult Survivor: Theory, Therapy, and Transformation. Brunner/Mazel. New York.

25. BURGESS, A. W. & L. L. HOLMSTROM. 1978. Recovery from rape and prior life stress. Res. Nursing and Health **1:** 165-174.

26. RESICK, P. A. 1993. The psychological impact of rape. Special Section: Rape. J. Interpersonal Violence **8:** 223-255.

27. MECHANIC, M. B. & P. A. RESICK. 1993. The Personal Beliefs and Reactions Scale: Assessing Rape-Related Cognitive Schemata. Paper presented at the Meeting of International Society of Traumatic Stress Studies, San Antonio, TX.

28. AMERICAN PSYCHIATRIC ASSOCIATION. 1980. Diagnostic and Statistical Manual of Mental Disorders, 3rd Ed. Washington, DC.

29. KEANE, T. M., J. A. FAIRBANK, J. M. CADDELL & R. T., ZIMERING. 1989. Implosive (flooding) therapy reduces symptoms of PTSD in Vietnam combat veterans. Behav. Ther. **20:** 245-260.

30. KILPATRICK, D. G., L. J. VERONEN & P. A. RESICK. 1982. Psychological sequelae to rape: Assessment and treatment strategies. In Behavioral Medicine: Assessment and Treatment Strategies. D. M. Doleys, R. L. Meredity & A. R. Ciminero, Eds.: 473-497. Plenum Publishing Corporation. New York, NY.

31. FOA, E. B., B. O. ROTHBAUM, D. S. RIGGS & T. B. MURDOCK. 1991. Treatment of posttraumatic stress disorder in rape victims: A comparison between cognitive-behavioral procedures and counseling. J. Consult. Clin. Psychol. **59:** 715-723.

32. RESICK, P. A. & M. K. SCHNICKE. 1993. Cognitive Processing Therapy for Rape Victims. A Treatment Manual. Sage. California.

33. ELLIS, A. 1977. The basic clinical theory and rational-emotive therapy. *In* Handbook of Rational-Emotive Therapy, A. Ellis & R. Grieger, Eds.: 3-34. Springer. New York.
34. BECK, A. T., A. J. RUSH, B. F. SHAW & G. EMERY. 1979. Cognitive Therapy or Depression. Guilford Press. New York.
35. LANG, P. J. 1977. Imagery in therapy: An information processing analysis of fear. Behav. Ther. **8:** 862-886.
36. FOA, E. B. & M. J. KOZAK. 1986. Emotional processing of fear: Exposure to corrective information. Psychol. Bull. **99:** 20-35.
37. KOZAK, M. J., E. B. FOA, & G. STEKETEE. 1988. Process and outcome of exposure treatment with obsessive-compulsives: Psychophysiological indicators of emotional processing. Behav. Ther. **19:** 157-169.
38. FOA, E. B., D. S. RIGGS, E. D. MASSIE & M. YARCZOWER. 1995. The impact of fear activation and anger on the efficacy of exposure treatment for PTSD. Behav. Ther. **26:** 487-499.
39. JAYCOX, L. H., E. B. FOA & A. MORRAL. 1997. The influence of emotional engagement and habituation on outcome of exposure therapy for PTSD. In press.
40. KILPATRICK, D. G., H. S. RESNICK & J. R. FREEDY. 1992. Post-traumatic stress disorder field trial report: A comprehensive review of the initial result. Paper presented at the Annual Meeting of the American Psychiatric Association.
41. FOA, E. B., C. MOLNAR & L. CASHMAN. 1995. Change in rape narratives during exposure therapy for PTSD. J. Traumatic Stress **8:** 675-690.

PTSD in WWII Mustard Gas Test Participants

A Preliminary Report

PAULA P. SCHNURR,[a] JULIAN D. FORD,[a]
MATTHEW J. FRIEDMAN,[a] BONNIE L. GREEN,[b] AND
BRADLEY J. DAIN[c]

[a]*National Center for PTSD (116D)*
VA Medical and Regional Office Center
White River Junction, Vermont 05009

[b]*Department of Psychiatry*
Georgetown University Medical Center
211 Kober-Cogan Hall
Washington, DC

[c]*Department of Community and Family Medicine*
Dartmouth Medical School
Hanover, New Hampshire 03756

During World War II, the United States military conducted secret tests of the effectiveness of various strategies for protecting combatants against the effects of mustard gas and Lewisite, which cause blisters and other tissue damage and can be fatal. At least 4,000 men were extensively exposed to these agents[1] while participating in tests of protective clothing, either by being placed in a sealed room into which a chemical was introduced (a *chamber* test) or by traversing a contaminated area (a *field* test). Until recently, participants' experiences were not known because most had been sworn to secrecy and had kept their oath. When the testing became public knowledge in 1990, it appeared that many men had had significant medical and psychological problems as a result of participation and that their rights as human subjects had not been protected.

In 1992, the Department of Veterans Affairs (VA) began to allow compensation for cancers, ophthalmological problems, and respiratory problems that may have been caused by mustard gas. Psychiatric disorders were not included in the list despite the conclusion of an investigation by the National Academy of Sciences that posttraumatic stress disorder (PTSD) and other psychiatric disorders may have resulted from the gas exposure. The National Academy of Sciences also recommended that the VA study the issue. Following the Academy's recommendation, we assessed PTSD and other psychosocial outcomes in a sample of WWII mustard gas test participants.[2]

METHOD

We randomly sampled 250 Army and 250 Navy veterans from a registry developed for a mortality study of mustard gas test participants that is being conducted by the

VA's Office of Public Health and Environmental Hazards. Those alive as of October 1995 were considered to be the study population. Of the 500 men, 363 (72.6%) participated; 15% could not be located, 7.6% were ineligible or dead, 2.6% could not be scheduled, and 2% refused. Of those located and eligible, 93.8% participated.

At the time of study, participants' average age was 72 years. Almost all were White (98%), although 10% reported Hispanic ethnicity. Most were married (83%), were retired (78%), and had at least a high school education (64%).

Members of an experienced survey research team interviewed participants by telephone. The assessment battery included questions about: mustard gas test experiences; current and lifetime PTSD related to mustard gas; exposure to war zone trauma and other traumatic events; current health, well-being, and social support; and demographic background. Only results on PTSD prevalence and risk factors are presented here.

Mustard gas-related PTSD was assessed by the PTSD Checklist, which asks for ratings of the 17 DSM-IV PTSD symptoms on a 5-point scale. It has excellent convergence with a diagnosis based on structured clinical interview.[3] A symptom was scored as present if it was rated 3 or higher, indicating at least moderate levels (Weathers, personal communication, July 1996). Current PTSD prevalence indicates the percentage of men who met DSM-IV diagnostic criteria in the last month; lifetime prevalence indicates the percentage who ever had PTSD.

RESULTS

All of the analyses presented herein are preliminary. We used the chi-square test for comparisons between Army and Navy subgroups; Wilcoxin and Fisher's exact tests were used when indicated. Prevalence estimates for current and lifetime PTSD are presented with 95% confidence intervals in parentheses. Risk factors for current PTSD are presented as crude (unadjusted) odds ratios. The reference category for most variables is the group that did not have the factor, for example, not having volunteered for "volunteered." The reference category for timing of disclosure is "before 1991." There are small amounts of missing data for some variables. For several variables a sizable number of men, roughly 20 in each instance, replied "don't know." Rather than treat these men as having missing data, we included them as a separate category.

TABLE 1 presents information on the mustard gas test experiences of Army and Navy subgroups. The subgroups differed in many ways. Army veterans were more likely to have participated in a field test, whereas Navy veterans were more likely to have participated in a chamber test. Navy veterans were more likely than Army veterans to have a higher number of exposures, to have volunteered, to have experienced intense distress during the tests, to have been sworn to secrecy, and to have disclosed after the media exposure of the mustard gas story in 1990. Army veterans were more likely than Navy veterans to have experienced burns and loss of consciousness during the test.

The prevalence of current PTSD was 32% (27%, 37%) and the prevalence of lifetime PTSD was 37% (32%, 42%). Navy veterans were more likely than Army veterans to have current PTSD: prevalence was 37% (30%, 43%) in Navy veterans

TABLE 1. Characteristics of Mustard Gas Test Experiences by Branch of Service

	Army	Navy	Total
Participated in field test (% yes)	70.6	4.8	33.5***
Participated in chamber test (% yes)	58.0	98.4	80.3***
Volunteered for test (% yes)	71.3	87.1	79.9***
Total number of exposures**			
1–2	41.4	30.3	35.3
3–6	29.0	25.6	27.2
7+	19.8	38.0	29.7
Don't know	9.9	6.2	7.8
Felt life was in danger during test			
% Yes	19.3	21.4	20.4
% Don't know	5.4	10.4	8.1
Physical symptoms during testing (% yes)			
Eyes or skin burned	30.3	14.3	21.6**
Difficulty breathing	36.7	45.1	41.4
Nausea/vomiting	20.3	27.3	24.0
Failure to maintain consciousness	10.3	4.2	7.0*
Intense fear, helplessness, or horror during test	31.1	46.2	39.3***
Oath of secrecy/disclosure criminalized***			
% Yes	27.7	52.3	41.1
% Don't know	1.2	3.6	2.5
Timing of disclosure (%)***			
Up to 1990	60.0	57.4	58.6
1991 to present	9.7	24.4	17.7
Never disclosed	15.8	5.6	10.2
Don't know	14.6	12.7	13.5

* $p < 0.05$; ** $p < 0.01$; *** $p < 0.001$ for differences between Army and Navy subgroups.

and 26% (19%, 33%) in Army veterans ($p < 0.05$). Navy veterans also were more likely than Army veterans to have lifetime PTSD: prevalence was 44% (37%, 51%) in Navy veterans and 28% (21%, 35%) in Army veterans ($p < 0.01$). The mean number of current PTSD symptoms was 5.6 (SD 5.9) in both groups combined. On average, Navy veterans had 6.3 (SD 5.8) current symptoms and Army veterans had 4.7 (SD 6.0) current symptoms ($p < 0.05$).

TABLE 2 presents risk factors for current and lifetime PTSD. Navy veterans were more likely than Army veterans to have current and lifetime PTSD. Having volunteered was associated with a decreased likelihood of both outcomes. The risk of current and lifetime PTSD was increased by severity of traumatic exposure, as indicated by the number of exposures, feeling one's life was in danger, number of physical symptoms, and intense distress. Aspects of disclosure also were associated with the likelihood of PTSD. Risk of current and lifetime PTSD was increased among men who were sworn to secrecy or told that disclosure would be a criminal act, relative to those who were not. Having disclosed after the story became public knowledge was associated with increased risk of current PTSD.

TABLE 2. Risk Factors for Current and Lifetime PTSD

	Current		Lifetime	
	OR	95% CI	OR	95% CI
Branch of service				
Army	1.00		1.00	
Navy	1.65*	1.05, 2.59	2.06**	1.33, 3.21
Recruitment for test				
Did not volunteer	1.00		1.00	
Volunteered	.27***	.16, .47	.28***	.16, .48
Number of exposures				
1–2	1.00		1.00	
3–6	3.06***	1.70, 5.52	2.89***	1.63, 5.11
7+	2.06*	1.15, 3.71	2.27**	1.29, 3.99
Don't know	1.82	.74, 4.49	2.40*	1.02, 5.63
Felt life was in danger during test				
No	1.00		1.00	
Yes	5.68***	3.25, 9.90	5.00***	2.87, 8.69
Don't know	4.01***	1.82, 8.81	2.96**	1.36, 6.46
Physical symptoms during test (per sx)	2.95***	2.25, 3.88	3.40***	2.55, 4.53
Intense fear, helplessness, or horror during test				
No	1.00		1.00	
Yes	7.31***	4.45, 11.99	6.77***	4.21, 10.89
Oath of secrecy/disclosure criminalized				
No	1.00		1.00	
Yes	3.64***	2.28, 5.82	4.11***	2.60, 6.51
Don't know	2.00	.48, 8.34	2.69	.69, 10.42
Timing of disclosure				
Up to 1990	1.00		1.00	
1991 to present	2.04*	1.15, 3.62	1.65	.94, 2.90
Never disclosed	.64	.28, 1.47	.46	.20, 1.04
Don't know	.84	.42, 1.68	.60	.30, 1.19

Note: OR = odds ratio; CI = confidence interval. * $p < 0.05$; ** $p < 0.01$; *** $p < 0.001$.

DISCUSSION

We have shown that roughly one third of men who were exposed to mustard gas or Lewisite in secret tests during WWII developed PTSD. We also have shown that the likelihood of PTSD varies markedly as a function of individual differences in variables that capture participants' experiences before, during, and after the tests. Our results are generally consistent with both theory and other data on risk factors for PTSD, although some bear further scrutiny, for example, having never disclosed about the tests, which we would expect to increase the likelihood of PTSD, was nonsignificantly protective. We are conducting further analyses to better understand our findings and to explore the unique influences on PTSD prevalence that are associated with each risk factor.

REFERENCES

1. PECHURA, C. M. & D. P. RALL, Eds. 1993. Veterans at Risk: The Health Effects of Mustard Gas and Lewisite. National Academy Press. Washington, DC.
2. SCHNURR, P. P., M. J. FRIEDMAN & B. L. GREEN. 1996. Posttraumatic stress disorder among World War II mustard gas test participants. Milit. Med. **161:** 131-136.
3. WEATHERS, F. W., B. T. LITZ, D. S. HERMAN, J. A. HUSKA & T. M. KEANE. 1996. PTSD Checklist: Description, use, and psychometric properties. Submitted manuscript.

Relationship between Level of Spinal Cord Injury and Posttraumatic Stress Disorder Symptoms[a]

T. MARTIN BINKS,[b,c] CYNTHIA L. RADNITZ,[b,c,d]
ALBERTO I. MORAN,[b,c] AND
VINCENT VINCIGUERRA [b,c]

[b]Fairleigh Dickinson University
Teaneck, New Jersey 07666

[c]Department of Veterans Affairs Medical Center
Bronx, New York 10468

Previous studies of the prevalence of posttraumatic stress disorder (PTSD) among spinal cord injured (SCI) veterans found prevalence rates comparable to those obtained in other traumatized populations.[1] Additionally, the level of spinal cord injury was shown to be a predictor of PTSD diagnosis and symptom severity. Veterans with quadriplegia report less PTSD and a lesser degree of symptom severity than do both those with paraplegia and those who sustained traumatic injuries other than SCI.[2,3] The present study attempts to determine if there was a particular level of spinal cord injury that differentiated those with and those without PTSD.

METHODS

Subjects. Subjects were 105 veterans with spinal cord injury recruited from SCI services at three northeastern Veterans Affairs Medical Centers.

Measures. Mini-Mental Status Exam (MMSE): The MMSE is a brief measure of orientation, attention, concentration, and immediate recall designed to screen out those subjects who are not capable of understanding or answering accurately questions asked of them during the assessment procedure.[4]

The Clinician Administered PTSD Scale (CAPS): The CAPS is a rating scale that is administered as a structured interview to collect data relevant to obtaining PTSD severity scores and to making both current and lifetime PTSD diagnoses.[5]

Structured Clinical Interview for DSM III-R Patient Edition (SCID): The SCID is a structured interview designed to diagnose common psychiatric disorders using

[a]This project was supported by a grant from the American Association of Spinal Cord Injury Psychologists and Social Workers (to C.L.R.).

[d]Address for correspondence: Cynthia L. Radnitz, PhD, School of Psychology, Fairleigh Dickinson University, 1000 River Rd., Teaneck, NJ 07666.

criteria stipulated in the Diagnostic and Statistical Manual III-Revised.[6,7] The section relating to PTSD diagnosis (not commonly included with the interview) was obtained and used as an additional diagnostic tool with the CAPS.

Procedure. Trained research assistants approached subjects, explained the general nature of the study to them, and obtained informed consent. The MMSE was used to screen for cognitive impairment that might limit subjects' ability to participate. Subjects who scored above the cut score on the MMSE were administered the remaining questionnaires and interviews.

RESULTS AND DISCUSSION

Diagnoses of PTSD were made only in cases in which there was agreement between CAPS and SCID interviews. In evaluating various cut scores to determine which level of the spinal cord separated PTSD from non-PTSD subjects, it was found that only 1 of 62 with injuries above T1-T3 were diagnosed with current PTSD, whereas 10 of 45 with injuries below this level received diagnoses of current PTSD. For a lifetime diagnosis of PTSD, no apparent cutoff for level of injury could be identified. Level of injury significantly correlated with current PTSD severity (r (106) = -0.20, $p < 0.03$) but not with lifetime PTSD severity.

Point biserial correlations revealed that the level of injury was significantly related to the presence of the following current PTSD symptoms: recurrent intrusive recollections, recurrent and distressing dreams, flashbacks, distress in the presence of trauma-related stimuli, avoidance of thoughts and feelings related to the trauma, difficulty concentrating, and hypervigilence. PTSD symptoms not significantly correlated with level of injury included avoidance of trauma-related situations, psychogenic amnesia, anhedonia, detachment, restricted affect, sense of foreshortened future, sleep disturbance, irritability, exaggerated startle response, and physiological reactivity when exposed to events that resemble the trauma.

The findings suggest a relationship between level of spinal cord injury and current PTSD symptoms. More specifically, it appears that individuals with injuries above T1-T3 (high paraplegia/low quadriplegia) are less likely to be diagnosed with current PTSD than are those with injuries below this area. In addition, symptoms more specific to PTSD (i.e., intrusive recollections of the event) were related to level of injury, whereas those less specific were not. These findings are consistent with the idea that the peripheral nervous system plays an important role in PTSD symptoms.

REFERENCES

1. RADNITZ, C. L. *et al.* 1995. The prevalence of posttraumatic stress disorder in veterans with spinal cord injury. SCI Psychosocial Process **8:** 145-149.
2. RADNITZ, C. L. *et al.* 1996. A comparison of posttraumatic stress disorder in veterans with and without spinal cord injury. Submitted for publication.
3. RADNITZ, C. L. *et al.* 1996. Posttraumatic stress disorder in veterans with spinal cord injury: Trauma-related risk factors. Submitted for publication.
4. FOLSTEIN, M. F. *et al.* 1975. Mini-mental state: A practical method for grading the cognitive state of patients for the clinician. J. Psychiatric Res. **12:** 189-198.

5. BLAKE, D. *et al.* 1990. Clinician Administered PTSD Scale (CAPS). National Center for Post-Traumatic Stress Disorder. Behavioral Science Division-Boston.
6. AMERICAN PSYCHIATRIC ASSOCIATION 1987. Diagnostic and Statistical Manual of Mental Disorders. 3rd Ed., rev. Washington, DC.
7. SPITZER, R. L. *et al.* 1990. Structured Clinical Interview for DSM-III-R—Patient edition (SCID-P, Version 1.0). American Psychiatric Press. Washington, DC.

Acute Post-Rape Plasma Cortisol, Alcohol Use, and PTSD Symptom Profile among Recent Rape Victims

HEIDI S. RESNICK,[a,c] RACHEL YEHUDA,[b] AND
RON ACIERNO [a]

[a]National Crime Victims Research and Treatment Center
Medical University of South Carolina
171 Ashley Ave.
Charleston, South Carolina 29425–0742

[b]Bronx Veterans Administration Medical Center
Bronx, New York 10468

Our data from a sample of 37 rape victims indicated a significant interaction between a history of assault, rape stress characteristics, and initial post-rape plasma cortisol values.[1] Rape victims with an assault history had lower levels of post-rape cortisol, regardless of current rape stress characteristics, than did women for whom the recent rape was their first assault. This finding was consistent with previous studies of populations exposed to chronic stressors and may reflect downregulation of the cortisol system in response to chronic exposure to stress.[2] Among rape victims without an assault history, cortisol level was significantly higher in association with increased rape severity characteristics. It was hypothesized that this finding may indicate the onset of dysregulation at the time of event exposure among those not previously assaulted. In this study, only a history of assault was a significant predictor of the Structured Clinical Interview for DSM-III-R (SCID)-defined posttraumatic stress disorder (PTSD) at interviews conducted an average of 3 months post-rape.[3]

The present analyses of the same dataset focused on two primary questions: (1) What is the relation between reported alcohol use by the victim and post-rape cortisol, as a function of prior assault history? (2) Is there an association between initial cortisol levels and PTSD symptoms (as defined by a derived population-based SCL-90 PTSD cutoff score[4,5]) at 3 months post-rape? Given the pattern of interactions observed in the previous report, we hypothesized that patterns of association between alcohol use and cortisol and between cortisol and the PTSD cutoff score would differ in women with and without a prior assault history.

Demographic characteristics of this sample of young women have been described elsewhere.[1] Subjects were adult female victims of rape who reported the crime to police and who received forensic medical examinations within 72 hours post-rape. Forensic examination included questions about the victim's use of alcohol during or just before assault. Participants consented to the release of medical records, psychosocial follow-up interviews at 3 months post-rape, and analysis of blood samples for

[c]Tel: (803) 792–2945; fax: (803) 792–3388; e-mail: resnickh@musc.edu

433

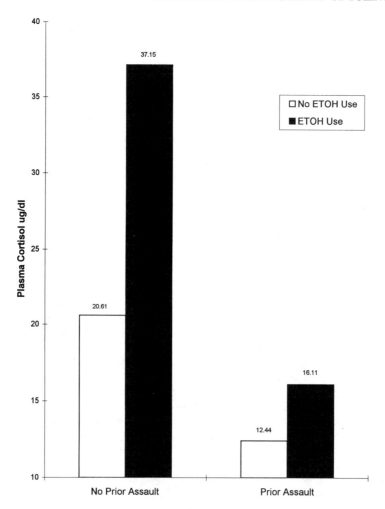

FIGURE 1. Plasma cortisol as a function of prior assault history and alcohol use ($n = 37$).

cortisol assays. Alcohol usage data were based on the total sample of 37 women. Data on the empirically derived crime-related PTSD symptom cutoff score[4,5] were based on a subset of 31 women who had completed this measure.

Self-Reported Alcohol Use. A total of 15 of 37 (41%) women reported alcohol use proximal to the time of assault. Reported alcohol use was not related to PTSD status based on the cutoff score described below. Cortisol was significantly negatively associated with time post-rape ($r = -.40$); therefore, all analyses included the number of hours post-rape as a covariate. A 2 (reported alcohol use) × 2 (prior history of assault) analysis of covariance (hours post-rape) using cortisol as the dependent measure was conducted. There were nonsignificant trend associations for the main

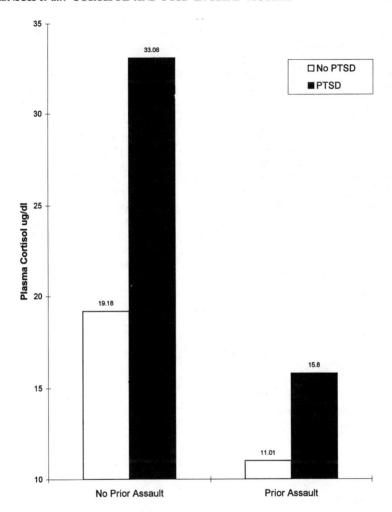

FIGURE 2. Plasma cortisol as a function of prior assault history and crime-related posttraumatic stress disorder (PTSD).

effect of alcohol use (alcohol use was associated with higher cortisol levels) ($F_{1,32}$ = 3.01, p = 0.09) and for the interaction of alcohol use and prior history of assault. (Among women with no prior history of rape, those using alcohol had higher plasma cortisol levels than did nonusers, whereas little difference was noted between users and nonusers in women with histories of assault ($F_{1,32}$ = 3.07, p = 0.09). There was a significant main effect for a history of assault ($F_{1,32}$ = 16.09, p = 0.001), with lower cortisol levels associated with a history of assault. The pattern of findings is displayed in FIGURE 1. Similar to our previously reported results then, elevated cortisol levels were observed in newly assaulted women. Elevated levels were particularly apparent in newly assaulted women who were using alcohol. Levels of cortisol were relatively low in women with histories of assault irrespective of alcohol use.

Crime Related PTSD Indicator Score. Of the 31 women completing the SCL-90 PTSD symptom scale, 22 (71%) met cutoff criteria for PTSD. A 2 (crime-related PTSD cutoff score) × 2 (history of assault) analysis of covariance (hours post-rape) using cortisol as the dependent measure was conducted. No significant interaction was noted between a history of assault and the PTSD cutoff score ($F_{1,26} = 0.46$, $p = 0.51$). As before, a main effect for a history of assault was noted ($F_{1,26} = 15.19$, $p < 0.005$), with cortisol levels lower among the prior history group. Moreover, a main effect was observed for the presence of crime-related PTSD in association with cortisol ($F_{1,26} = 6.22$, $p < 0.05$). Specifically, those who met the PTSD cutoff had a higher mean cortisol level. These data are displayed in FIGURE 2. Separate sets of correlations were conducted among the 11 women without a prior assault and among the 20 with a history between cortisol levels and each of the 28 symptoms. A p value of 0.002 was selected to determine statistical significance based on the number of tests conducted. Only the 11 women without a prior assault evinced significant positive correlations between cortisol and past-week 4-point severity ratings for items "Feeling afraid in open spaces or on the streets" ($r = .84$) and "Suddenly scared for no reason" ($r = .81$).

Data consistently indicated a different pattern of post-rape cortisol response among women with and those without a history of assault. Moreover, alcohol use appeared to be associated with higher levels of cortisol in women with no rape history. By contrast, cortisol levels were lower in both alcohol users and nonusers who had previously been victimized. Further investigation is needed, however, in which the time since last use of alcohol and long-term patterns of alcohol usage are controlled. Finally, PTSD symptom scale data indicated a possible association between elevated cortisol and PTSD symptom distress. This possibility should be explored in future studies with larger samples that control for assault history.

REFERENCES

1. RESNICK, H. S., R. YEHUDA, R. K. PITMAN & D. W. FOY. 1995. Effect of previous trauma on acute plasma cortisol level following rape. Am. J. Psychiatry 152: 1675-1677.
2. YEHUDA, R., E. L. GILLER, S. M. SOUTHWICK, M. T. LOWY & J. W. MASON. 1991. Hypothalamic-pituitary-adrenal dysfunction in posttraumatic stress disorder. Biol. Psychiatry 30: 1031-1048.
3. SPITZER, R. L., J. B. W. WILLIAMS & M. GIBBON. 1986. Structured Clinical Interview for DSM-III-R, Non-patient Version (SCID-NP). Biometric Research Department, New York State Psychiatric Institute. New York, NY.
4. SAUNDERS, B. E., C. M. ARATA & D. G. KILPATRICK. 1990. Development of a crime-related post-traumatic stress disorder scale for women within the symptom checklist-90-revised. J. Traumatic Stress 3: 439-448.
5. DEROGATIS, L. R. 1977. SCL-90: Administration, Scoring and Procedure Manual-I for the R(Revised) Version. John Hopkins University School of Medicine. Baltimore, MD.

The Acute Stress Response Following Motor Vehicle Accidents and Its Relation to PTSD

ALEXANDER C. McFARLANE,
MICHELLE ATCHISON, AND RACHEL YEHUDA

The University of Adelaide
Department of Psychiatry
The Queen Elizabeth Hospital
Woodville, South Australia

Mount Sinai School of Medicine
New York, New York

Bronx Veterans Affairs
Bronx, New York 10468

This study aimed to identify acute biological stress responses in trauma victims and to determine their contribution to the development of psychiatric illness, especially posttraumatic stress disorder (PTSD). Abnormalities of the hypothalamic-pituitary-adrenal (HPA) axis have been noted in PTSD, with evidence of heightened sensitivity in the negative feedback loop. However, it is not known if some abnormality of stress response occurs at the time of the traumatic event or if the disruption of the HPA axis develops during the course of the illness. An understanding of the acute stress response in accident victims who go on to develop PTSD may provide important information about biological vulnerability to psychiatric illness and may provide a marker of "at risk" individuals.[1]

The HPA axis is of particular interest because cortisol is one of the primary modulators of the stress response and both cortisol and ACTH modify the consolidation of memory. In PTSD, the laying down of memories of the trauma and their recall is a central component of the disorder. Therefore, abnormalities of this axis may provide critical information about the aetiological process in this disorder. The sensitisation of the HPA axis and suppression of the dexamethasone suppression test in PTSD appears to be one of the most specific neurobiological abnormalities in PTSD. The findings of this study has general theoretical importance about the etiology of PTSD from the perspective of whether this disorder is a continuum of a normative stress response or whether it is an atypical or abnormal stress response.

A question that has not been answered is whether these HPA abnormalities arise from an abnormal HPA response at the time of the trauma or whether they develop later in the course of the illness. An understanding of HPA responses at the time of trauma in individuals who later develop PTSD may give insight into biological vulnerabilities and perhaps allow identification of at risk individuals. The body of literature concerning HPA abnormalities in PTSD has concentrated on war veterans many years after the initial trauma, raising the strong possibility that intervening factors contribute to the HPA abnormalities. One small study has assessed acute cortisol levels in rape victims.[2] Acute cortisol responses did not predict the development of PTSD, but those subjects with a history of prior trauma showed attenuated cortisol responses and were at greater risk of developing PTSD. This raises the possibility that prior trauma may "sensitize" an individual's biological response to later trauma which leaves them at greater risk of PTSD. This study was only carried out on 26 subjects, and a larger number is needed to make more definitive statements. This is a central rational for conducting the proposed study.

METHOD

Subjects. The study group consisted of 40 individuals (30 males, 10 females) ranging in age from 15 to 77 years. They were recruited from a larger study of 200 motor vehicle accident victims who had been admitted for at least one night to a major teaching hospital. By law, all motor vehicle accident victims must have a blood sample taken for estimation of their alcohol level. Cortisol levels and lymphocyte glucocorticoid receptors were then determined by the hospitals pathology service.

Subjects were interviewed on the day following admission (Day 2), 10 days, and 6 months after the accident. During the Day 2 screening, after receiving appropriate consent, subjects were given the IES,[3] Brief SASRQ,[4] 36-item DSQ,[5] and a concentration questionnaire. The IES, SASRQ, and concentration measure were repeated on Day 10, along with the DISSI (Diagnostic Interview Schedule Screening Interview)[6] to account for preexisting psychiatric disorder. These measures were also repeated at a 6-month follow-up, in conjunction with the CAPS,[7] STAI–Anxiety,[8] Beck Depression Inventory,[9] and SIP.[10]

RESULTS

The 6-month follow-up of these subjects determined that seven had PTSD, seven from MDD and 12 had no disorder. The remainder of the subjects had a range of diagnoses and were excluded from analysis for this very reason. The mean of the time the accident occurred was 1330 hours, whilst the mean time a subjects blood sample was taken was 1400 hours. The serum cortisol results were examined for differences between these diagnostic grouping. Group means for cortisol results are presented in FIGURE 1. A one-way ANOVA showed that there was a difference in cortisol levels after the accident (F = 3.65, df = 2,25, $p < 0.05$). Post-hoc testing confirmed that the mean cortisol levels of subjects who had PTSD 6 months after the accident were significantly lower than those with MDD. This result were not significant when the effects of time the accident occurred and time the blood samples were taken were partialled out.

This result contrasts to the measures of psychological distress on Day 2, which had very little ability to predict the diagnostic outcome at 6 months (TABLE 1). There no differences on Day 2 between any of the diagnostic groups on either the IES or theSASRQ. On Day 10 the only significant difference on either of the measures of psychological distress was on the Flashback subscale of the SASRQ (F = 9.85, df = 2,25, $p < 0.001$). Post-hoc testing revealed that the PTSD group scored higher on this subscale than both the No diagnosis and MDD groups.

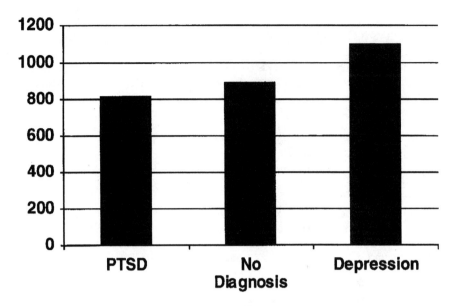

FIGURE 1. Cortisol means by diagnostic grouping.

TABLE 1. Mean and Standard Deviation of IES and SASRQ Subscale Scores on Day 2 across the Diagnostic Groups

	No Diagnosis		PTSD		MDD		p
	Mean	SD	Mean	SD	Mean	SD	
IES							
Avoidance	9.75	7.30	10.14	13.42	16.50	6.34	NS
Intrusion	12.67	5.05	12.66	5.05	17.33	9.58	NS
Total	22.41	8.14	20.71	14.87	33.83	13.21	NS
SASRQ							
Anxiety	3.92	1.83	4.29	3.25	5.33	2.58	NS
Dissociation	4.00	2.92	2.86	1.86	3.83	3.25	NS
Intrusion	1.25	0.97	1.43	1.13	1.67	1.63	NS
Avoidance	0.58	0.67	0.86	0.69	1.00	0.00	NS
Hyperarousal	2.58	1.68	2.57	2.15	3.17	1.94	NS
Flashback	0.08	0.29	0.57	0.98	1.00	1.10	NS

DISCUSSION

This study examined the acute psychological stress response and its relationship to the cortisol response amongst motor vehicle accident victims. Given the severity of the trauma in these subjects, all of whom were admitted to hospital for a minimum of 2 days, a significant rise in serum cortisols occurred. In this pilot study, the rise in serum cortisol was greatest in those with major depressive disorder, and lowest in the PTSD group. The no disorder group were in the mid-range. This is contrary to the idea that in PTSD there is an exaggerated acute stress response. These biological data are of particular note because of the absence of any significant differences between three subject groups on the psychological measures at 24 hours.

These data require replication. However, it suggests that the abnormalities of decreased hippocampal volume associated with PTSD may not be explained by an excessive cortisol response in these subjects at the time of the traumatic stressor. Secondly, it raises questions as to what has modified the cortisol response in these subjects. Resnick et al.'s[2] data suggests that prior traumatisation might be one issue modifying this vulnerability.

In contrast, the psychological stress response on Day 1 does not differentiate the PTSD subjects from those with major depression or no disorder. In particular, there were no differences in the dissociative symptoms recorded in the first 24 hours. This is in contrast to the differences that emerged by Day 10. These data suggest that PTSD may represent an abnormality of transition occurring in the immediate post traumatic period, rather than there being a significant difference in the psychological response. The neurohormonal response provoked by the traumatic stressor may be one important factor modulating this response. It also raises the question as to the relationship between these data and the enhanced negative feedback which has been identified by the work of Yehuda.

Further research into the relationship between the acute neurohormonal response to the stressor in PTSD is of particular interest in terms of prevention. The current psychological interventions which are offered do not appear to be particularly potent modifiers of the long-term course of the traumatic stress response. Better characterization of the acute stress response and investigation of its relationship to PTSD may provide other avenues for intervention.

REFERENCES

1. YEHUDA, R. & A. C. MCFARLANE. 1995. Conflict between current knowledge about posttraumatic stress disorder and its original conceptual basis. Am. J. Psychiatry **152:** 1705–1713.
2. RESNICK, H. S., R. YEHUDA, R. K. PITMAN & D. W. FOY. 1995. Effect of previous trauma on acute plasma cortisol level following rape. Am. J. Psychiatry **152:** 1675–1677.
3. HOROWITZ, M., B. A. WILZER W. ALVAREZ. 1979. Impact of Events Scale. Psychosom. Med. **41:** 209–218.
4. CARDENA, E., C. CLASSEN D. SPIEGEL. 1991. Stanford Acute Stress Reaction Questionnaire. Department of Psychiatry and Behavioural Sciences. Stanford Medical School.
5. ANDREWS, G., C. POLLOCK & G. STEWART. 1989. The determination of defense style by questionnaire. Arch. Gen. Psychiatry **46:** 455–460.
6. KOVESS, V. & L. FOURNIER. 1990. Social psychiatry and psychiatric epidemiology. J. Traumatic Stress **25:** 179–186.
7. BLAKE, D. D., F. W. WEATHERS, L. M. NAGY et al. 1993. A clinician rating scale for assessing current and lifetime PTSD: The CAPS-I. Behav. Ther. **18:** 187–188.
8. SPIELBERGER, C. 1978. State-Trait Anxiety Inventory. Florida State University. Tallahassee.

9. BECK, A. T. 1979. Beck Depression Inventory. The Psychological Corporation. Harcourt Brace Javanovich.
10. BERGNER, M., R. A. BOBBITT, W. B. CARTER & B. S. GILSON. 1981. The Sickness Impact Profile: Development and final revision of a health status measure. Med. Care **19:** 787–805.

Salivary Cortisol and PTSD Symptoms in Persian Gulf War Combatants

MICHAEL KELLNER,[a] DEWLEEN G. BAKER,[b] AND
RACHEL YEHUDA [a,c]

[a]Department of Psychiatry
Mount Sinai School of Medicine
Bronx Veterans Affairs Medical Center
Bronx, New York 10468

[b]Cincinnati Veterans Affairs Medical Center and
Department of Psychiatry
University of Cincinnati Medical Center
Cincinnati, Ohio 45220

Subjects with chronic posttraumatic stress disorder (PTSD) show a distinct profile of hypothalamic-pituitary-adrenocortical axis alterations characterized by diminished cortisol levels and stronger negative feedback inhibition.[1] So far, it is not clear if this endocrine regulation pattern represents a premorbid condition, an effect of trauma per se, or the consequence of former or ongoing PTSD symptoms. To address this issue, studies beginning closer to the traumatic event are needed. We examined the relationship between salivary cortisol concentrations and PTSD symptoms in Persian Gulf War combatants within 18 months of their homecoming.

METHODS

Eight nontreatment-seeking male soldiers (mean age 30.8 years, range 21-39), stationed at Ft. Knox, with Combat Exposure scores during Operation Desert Storm of 15-19 (mean 16.9) gave informed consent for this study. Subjects completed an Impact of Event Scale (IES) concerning Persian Gulf War experiences and gave a basal morning saliva sample at 8:00 AM. They were also asked to take 0.5 mg dexamethasone at 11:00 PM, and a postdexamethasone saliva sample was obtained at 8:00 AM the next day. Cortisol concentrations in saliva were determined radioimmunometrically as described previously.[2] Given the directional prediction, one-tailed statistical tests were performed.

[c]Address for correspondence: Dr. Rachel Yehuda, Psychiatry 116/A, Bronx VA Medical Center, 130 West Kingsbridge Rd., Bronx, NY 10468.

RESULTS

A negative correlation between basal morning saliva cortisol levels and IES scores was found (r = −0.57, F(1;6) = 3.0, p = 0.07). This was mostly due to the intrusion subscale (r = −0.67, F(1;6) = 4.9, p = 0.03), whereas the avoidance subscale was not correlated so closely (r = −0.46, F(1;6) = 1.6, p = 0.12).

After the exclusion of one subject, who obviously did not take the dexamethasone, mean cortisol suppression after dexamethasone was 90.1%. No significant correlations between the percent suppression of cortisol and any of the IES scores emerged (IES: r = 0.37, F(1;6) = 0.9, p = 0.19; intrusion subscore: r = 0.31, F(1;6) = 0.6, p = 0.22; avoidance subscore: r = 0.40, F(1;6) = 1.2, p = 0.16).

DISCUSSION

The data of this pilot field study show a significant negative correlation of intrusive PTSD symptoms and basal morning salivary cortisol levels. Similar correlations of category B symptoms of the Child Posttraumatic Stress Disorder Reaction Index and low salivary cortisol levels have been seen in adolescent survivors of an earthquake.[2] In contrast, low urinary cortisol excretion in Holocaust survivors has been linked to avoidance symptoms, as measured by the Clinician-Administered PTSD Scale, whereas no correlation with the intrusive subscale emerged.[3]

A hypersuppression of cortisol in the low dose dexamethasone suppression test was found in our subjects, as reported in chronic PTSD.[4] However, neither postdexamethasone cortisol levels nor the rate of cortisol suppression was clearly correlated with posttraumatic symptoms as measured by the IES.

The effect of trauma severity could not be tested in our small sample with very similar combat experience. Larger longitudinal studies with trauma survivors beginning as soon as possible after the traumatization are needed to further understand the impact of trauma severity, different symptom clusters, and long-term outcome on the neuroendocrine alterations in posttraumatic disorders.

REFERENCES

1. YEHUDA, R. *et al.* 1995. Hypothalamic-pituitary-adrenal functioning in post-traumatic stress disorder. Expanding the concept of the stress response spectrum. *In* Neurobiological and Clinical Consequences of Stress: From Normal Adaptation to PTSD. Lippincott-Raven Publishers. Philadelphia.
2. GOENJIAN, A. K. *et al.* 1996. Basal cortisol, dexamethasone suppression of cortisol, and MHPG in adolescents after the 1988 earthquake in Armenia. Am. J. Psychiatry **153:** 929–934.
3. YEHUDA, R. *et al.* 1995. Low urinary cortisol excretion in Holocaust survivors with posttraumatic stress disorder. Am. J. Psychiatry **152:** 982–986.
4. YEHUDA, R. *et al.* 1995. Dose-dependent changes in plasma cortisol and lymphocyte glucocorticoid receptors following dexamethasone administration in combat veterans with and without posttraumatic stress disorder. Arch. Gen. Psychiatry **52:** 583–593.

Behavioral and Plasma Cortisol Responses to Sodium Lactate Infusion in Posttraumatic Stress Disorder[a]

CARL F. JENSEN,[b] TIMOTHY W. KELLER,
ELAINE R. PESKIND, MILES E. McFALL,
RICHARD C. VEITH, DONALD MARTIN,
CHARLES W. WILKINSON, AND
MURRAY A. RASKIND

*Psychiatry Service and Geriatric
Research, Education and Clinical Center
VA Puget Sound Health Care System and
Department of Psychiatry and Behavioral Sciences
University of Washington School of Medicine
Seattle, Washington 98108*

Sodium lactate infusion has induced flashbacks accompanied by panic attacks in male combat veterans with concurrent posttraumatic stress disorder (PTSD) and panic disorder.[1] This study determined whether sodium lactate induces flashbacks or other intrusive PTSD symptoms in PTSD without comorbid panic disorder. Effects of sodium lactate on adrenocortical activity in PTSD also were estimated.

METHOD

Subjects. After written informed consent, subjects underwent standard structured diagnostic interviews. Seven PTSD subjects (45 ± 4 years [mean ± standard deviation]; 5 men, 2 women) had no history of diagnosable panic attacks in either the context of or separate from PTSD symptoms and had no other current psychiatric disorder. Six of seven PTSD subjects had experienced spontaneous flashbacks. Seven panic disorder subjects (39 ± 13 years; 4 men, 3 women) had no history of PTSD and no other current psychiatric disorder. Seven healthy control subjects (35 ± 8 years; 5 men, 2 women) had no current or past history of psychiatric disorder. All subjects were in good general health, had been free of drug or alcohol abuse for at least 9 months, and had been free of medications for at least 4 months.

[a] This work was supported by Department of Veterans Affairs and National Institutes of Health grant AG05136.

[b] Address for correspondence: Carl F. Jensen, MD, VA Puget Sound Health Care System, Mental Health Services (116A), 1660 S. Columbian Way, Seattle, WA 98108 (tel: (206)764-2063; fax (206)764-2573).

Procedures. After overnight fasting, intravenous catheters were placed in each arm at 9:00 AM. Thirty minutes later, 10 ml/kg of 0.5 M sodium lactate were administered over 20 minutes. Behavioral ratings and cardiovascular measures were obtained every 5 minutes. Blood samples for plasma cortisol were obtained before and after the infusion. Anxiety symptoms were assessed using the Acute Panic Inventory (API).[2] A "flashback" was defined as a sense of unreality accompanied by vivid images of a past traumatic situation as though it were actually present. Panic attack was defined as the abrupt onset of intense fear or discomfort, an increase in at least 4 API symptoms, and an increase of at least 2 and an achieved rating of at least 5 on the global anxiety scale. Mean arterial pressure (MAP) was calculated as 1/3 (systolic − diastolic) + diastolic. Plasma cortisol was determined by radioimmunoassay as described in a previous report from this laboratory.[3] Statistical analysis included ANOVA, chi-square test, and paired *t* tests.

RESULTS

PTSD symptoms occurred during lactate infusion in six of seven PTSD subjects but in no panic disorder or healthy subjects ($\chi^2 = 16.8$, $p < 0.001$) (TABLE 1). Flashbacks occurred in four PTSD subjects. They rated induced flashbacks as very similar to spontaneous flashbacks (10 point scale "sameness" rating = 8.3 ± 2.1). API scores increased significantly in all groups. Increases were substantially greater in PTSD and panic disorder groups than in healthy controls, but did not differ between PTSD and panic disorder groups (TABLE 2). Five of seven PTSD subjects (including all subjects experiencing flashbacks), four of seven panic disorder subjects, and no control subjects met a priori criteria for panic during lactate infusion.

Cortisol was lower in PTSD than in control subjects at the end of infusion and tended to be lower in PTSD than in panic disorder subjects at both time points (TABLE 2).

DISCUSSION

This study confirms that sodium lactate induces flashbacks in PTSD[1] and extends this observation to PTSD patients without comorbid panic disorder. Sodium lactate infusion induced flashbacks and other PTSD symptoms in both women and men and in subjects with both combat- and noncombat-related trauma. Although the number of PTSD subjects studied was small, these findings support the generalizability of the PTSD diagnostic criteria across gender and types of precipitant trauma. Despite no history of panic attacks either separate from or in the context of spontaneous PTSD symptoms, anxiety symptoms meeting a priori study criteria for panic accompanied induced flashbacks. Flashbacks and panic attacks may share a common pathophysiology or represent different interpretations of the same phenomenon. Alternatively, the API and the DSM-III-R panic criteria may not be sensitive to real differences between cognitive and autonomic anxiety symptoms occurring during a PTSD flashback and those occurring during panic attack. During a flashback, anxiety symptoms are an expected response to reexperiencing a life-threatening situation. Such anxiety

TABLE 1. PTSD Subjects: Demographic Variables, Etiologic Trauma, and Behavioral Responses to Sodium Lactate Infusion

Sex & Age	Trauma	Occurrence and Type of Induced PTSD Symptom	Similarity to Spontaneous Flashback or Other PTSD Symptom[a]	Content of Induced Flashback or Other PTSD Symptom	Panic Attack
M,48	Combat	Yes, flashback	6	"Chopper," grenades, under fire	Yes
M,42	Combat	Yes, flashback	10	Riot, buddy shot, feels paralyzed, fear	Yes
M,50	Combat	Yes, dissociation	7	"Went to open space"	No
M,44	Combat	Yes, intrusive memory	3	"Felt like combat"	No
M,38	Childhood trauma	No	Not applicable	Not applicable	Yes
F,46	Welding accident	Yes, flashback	9	Trapped in pipes, burning	Yes
F,49	Boating accident in which father died	Yes, flashback	Not applicable (no prior spontaneous flashback)	In cold water with drowning father	Yes

[a] Rated on 0–10 scale, 10 being like a severe, spontaneous flashback or other PTSD symptom.

TABLE 2. Acute Panic Inventory, Cardiovascular, and Plasma Cortisol Responses to Sodium Lactate Infusion

Measure	Controls ($n = 7$)	Panic ($n = 7$)	PTSD ($n = 7$)
API			
Baseline	0.3 ± 0.5	2.9 ± 3.6	2.4 ± 2.1
End infusion	3.7 ± 2.5^a	12.0 ± 7.2^a	$17.3 \pm 7.5^{a,b}$
Cortisol (μg/d)			
Baseline	8.9 ± 4.7	9.9 ± 5.2	4.6 ± 2.2
End infusion	9.8 ± 5.5	8.8 ± 3.9	$3.6 \pm 1.8^{c,d}$
Mean arterial pressure (mm Hg)			
Baseline	83.4 ± 7.3	90.3 ± 9.5	97.3 ± 14.1
End infusion	82.4 ± 7.9	93 ± 15.5	100.6 ± 18
Heart rate (beats/min)			
Baseline	55.6 ± 8.5	75.4 ± 10.1^b	63.1 ± 7.9
End infusion	88.7 ± 7.1^a	103.1 ± 25.7^a	97 ± 14.2^a

[a] Higher than baseline, $p < 0.01$, paired t test.
[b] Higher than controls, $p < 0.01$, ANOVA followed by Scheffe's test.
[c] Lower than controls, $p < 0.05$, ANOVA followed by Scheffe's test.
[d] Lower than baseline, $p \leq 0.05$, paired t test.

responses may be different from those occurring during a typical unexpected panic attack that lacks a precipitating threat of danger. Comparing responses to lactate and placebo in larger numbers of PTSD and panic disorder subjects using instruments sensitive to potential differences in anxiety symptom precipitants and perceptions between PTSD and panic disorder may clarify this issue.

Neuroendocrine results are consistent with previous studies suggesting decreased adrenocortical activity in PTSD.[4] Kellner *et al.*[5] recently demonstrated that sodium lactate infusion increases plasma concentrations of atrial natriuretic factor, a peptide that inhibits the adrenocorticotropin and cortisol responses to corticotropin-releasing hormone. Stimulation of atrial natriuretic factor by sodium lactate infusion is a potential explanation for the failure to observe a plasma cortisol response in the present study. These results provide rationale for further studies of neuroendocrine responses to sodium lactate in PTSD.

REFERENCES

1. RAINEY, J. M., A. ALEEM, A. ORTIZ, V. YERIGANI, R. POHL & R. BERCHOU. 1987. A laboratory procedure for the induction of flashbacks. Am. J. Psychiatry **144:** 1317–1319.
2. DILLON, D. J., J. M. GORMAN, M. R. LIEBOWITZ, A. J. FYER & D. F. KLEIN. 1987. Measurement of lactate-induced panic and anxiety. Psychiatry Res. **20:** 97–105.
3. RASKIND, M. A., E. R. PESKIND, R. C. VEITH, C. W. WILKINSON, D. FEDERIGHI & D. M. DORSA. 1990. Differential effects of aging on neuroendocrine responses to physostigmine in normal men. J. Clin. Endocrinol. Metab. **70:** 1420–1425.

4. YEHUDA, R., M. H. TEICHER, R. A. LEVENGOOD, R. L. TRESTMAN & L. J. SIEVER. 1994. Circadian regulation of basal cortisol levels in posttraumatic stress disorder. Ann. N.Y. Acad. Sci. **746:** 378–380.
5. KELLNER, M., L. HERZOG, A. YASSOURIDIS, F. HOLSBOER & K. WIEDERMANN. 1995. Possible role of atrial natriuretic hormone in pituitary-adrenocortical unresponsiveness in lactate-induced panic. Am. J. Psychiatry **152:** 1365–1367.

Cerebrospinal Fluid and Plasma β-Endorphin in Combat Veterans with Posttraumatic Stress Disorder[a]

DEWLEEN G. BAKER,[b,e] SCOTT A. WEST,[b]
DAVID N. ORTH,[c,d] KELLY HILL,[b]
WENDELL E. NICHOLSON,[c] NOSA N. EKHATOR,[b]
ANN BRUCE,[b] MATTHEW WORTMAN,[b]
PAUL E. KECK, JR.,[b] AND
THOMAS D. GERACIOTI, JR. [b]

[b]Cincinnati Veterans Affairs Medical Center and
Department of Psychiatry
University of Cincinnati College Medical Center
Cincinnati, Ohio 45220

[c]Departments of Medicine and
[d]Molecular Physiology and Biophysics
Vanderbilt University Medical Center
Nashville, Tennessee 37232-6303

Opioid-mediated analgesia develops in experimental animals after traumatic stress, and increased opioid-mediated analgesia has been observed in combat veterans with posttraumatic stress disorder (PTSD). These observations have led to the hypothesis that increased central nervous system (CNS) opioidergic activity exists in patients with PTSD. However, direct CNS data on opioid peptide concentrations and dynamics in patients with PTSD are lacking.

METHODS

We withdrew cerebrospinal fluid (CSF) via a flexible, indwelling subarachnoid catheter over a 6-hour period to determine hourly CSF concentrations of immunoreactive β-endorphin (irβEND) in 10 well-characterized combat veterans with PTSD and 9 matched normal volunteers. Blood was simultaneously withdrawn to obtain plasma for irβEND. PTSD symptom clusters, as measured by the Clinician Administered PTSD Scale (CAPS), were correlated with neuroendocrine data.

[a]This work was supported by VA Central Office Research Funds (T.D.G.).

[e]Address for correspondence: Dewleen G. Baker, MD, PTSD Unit-7E, Cincinnati VA Medical Center, 3200 Vine Street, Cincinnati, Ohio 45220 (tel: (513) 475-6386; fax: (513) 475-6387).

RESULTS

Mean CSF irβEND was significantly greater in patients with PTSD than in normals subjects (33.3 ± 4.4 vs 21.8 ± 2.5 pg/ml, [F (1, 17) = 4.49, $p < 0.05$ by ANOVA), and a negative correlation was noted between the irβEND and PTSD intrusive and avoidant symptoms of PTSD. No intergroup difference between plasma irβEND was found, and neither was there a significant correlation between CSF and plasma irβEND. Immunoreactive β-lipotropin (irβLPH) and proopiomelanocortin (irPOMC), the precursor of βEND, were much more plentiful than β-endorphin itself in human CSF, as has previously been reported.

CONCLUSION

Basal CSF irβEND concentrations are elevated in combat veterans with PTSD. It remains to be determined if the increased CNS opioid concentrations predate traumatic stress, thereby conferring a vulnerability to dissociative states and PTSD itself, or if they result from the trauma. The negative correlation between CSF irβEND and avoidant and intrusive symptoms suggests that CNS hypersecretion of opioids might constitute an adaptive response to traumatic experience. The lack of correlation between CSF and plasma irβEND precludes the use of plasma measurements to assess CNS opioid activity.

ACKNOWLEDGMENTS

We are indebted to Sean Stanton, Renee Hanna, and the Cincinnati VAMC Psychiatric Nursing Staff for their technical support and the Cincinnati VAMC Library Staff for their tireless assistance.

Urinary Catecholamine Excretion in Childhood Overanxious and Posttraumatic Stress Disorders[a]

MICHAEL D. DE BELLIS,[b,d] ANDREW S. BAUM,[c]
BORIS BIRMAHER,[b] AND NEAL D. RYAN [b]

[b]Department of Child & Adolescent Psychiatry
Western Psychiatric Institute and Clinic
University of Pittsburgh Medical Center
3811 O'Hara Street
Pittsburgh, Pennsylvania 15213

[c]Behavioral Medicine and Oncology
Pittsburgh Cancer Institute and
Department of Psychiatry and Psychology
University of Pittsburgh Medical Center
Pittsburgh, Pennsylvania 15213

Anxiety disorders including posttraumatic stress disorder (PTSD) are associated with catecholamine dysregulation.[1,2] Although there may be a genetic predisposition to anxiety disorders including PTSD,[3,4] PTSD has an exogenous origin, that is, a history of an intense overwhelming trauma. Trauma increases arousal, produces anxiety, increases responsiveness of locus coeruleus neurons to excitatory stimulation, increases norepinephrine turnover in specific brain regions associated with the regulation of reaction, memory, and emotion in experimental animals, activates the sympathetic nervous system, and causes biologic changes of the "fight or flight response" (reviewed by in refs. 2 and 5). Activation of the stress response can be measured by sampling concentrations of the catecholamines, norepinephrine, epinephrine, and dopamine excreted into urine.[6]

Behaviorally inhibited children have increased sympathetic tone.[4] Kagan et al.[4] hypothesized that the threshold of responsivity in limbic and hypothalamic structures to environmental unfamiliarity is tonically lower in these children. These children

[a]This work was supported in part by the 1994 Eli Lilly Pilot Research Award, "A Pilot Study of Urinary Catecholamine Excretion in Three Groups of Prepubescent Girls: Overanxious Disorder, Posttraumatic Stress Disorder, and Healthy Volunteers" (Principal Investigator: Michael D. De Bellis), the 1995 NARSAD Young Investigators Award, "Attention and Concentration in Maltreated Children with Posttraumatic Stress Disorder" (Principal Investigator: Michael D. De Bellis), and by National Institute of Mental Health grant MH 41712, "The Psychobiology of Depression in Children & Adolescents" (Principal Investigator: Neal D. Ryan).

[d]Address for correspondence: Michael D. De Bellis, MD, Department of Child & Adolescent Psychiatry, Western Psychiatric Institute and Clinic, University of Pittsburgh Medical Center, 3811 O'Hara Street, Pittsburgh, PA 15213 (tel: (412)624-2870; fax: (412)383-9527; e-mail: mddb+@pitt.edu).

are typically irritable as infants, shy and fearful as toddlers, and quiet, cautious, and introverted in grade school. Behaviorally inhibited children are at greater risk of developing anxiety disorders particularly, overanxious disorder, social phobia or avoidant disorder, and separation anxiety disorder.[7] Adult and childhood anxiety disorders are associated with increased sympathetic nervous system and norepinephrine activity.[1]

Like behaviorally inhibited children, combat veterans with PTSD have heightened sympathetic nervous system arousal and elevated 24-hour urinary excretion of catecholamines compared to controls.[2,5] There are little data on the psychobiology of childhood trauma. Child maltreatment is both a risk factor and a cause for PTSD as well as other psychiatric illnesses in adults and children. Psychobiological studies in sexually abused girls show dysregulation of stress response systems including higher 24-hour urinary catecholamine excretion.[6,8] These findings are similar to the psychobiology of adult PTSD.

The objective of this pilot investigation was to examine 24-hour urinary catecholamine excretion in children with: (1) overanxious disorder, (2) PTSD secondary to child maltreatment, and (3) controls. It was hypothesized that children with PTSD and overanxious disorder will manifest increased urinary catecholamine excretion when compared to controls, that is, endogenous and exogenous anxiety may have a final common pathway: permanent lowering of the threshold for arousal to unexpected environmental changes.

METHODS

Subjects. Child subjects with overanxious disorder ($n = 7$; 3 males aged 10.8 ± 1.5 years), PTSD ($n = 9$; 7 males aged 10.8 ± 2.0 years), and controls ($n = 14$; 7 males aged 10.9 ± 1.2 years) were recruited from the patient population at Western Psychiatric Institute and Clinic and local community mental health centers. Psychiatric assessment and diagnosis(es) were confirmed by the use of the K-SAD-E and P[9,10] as part of the initial psychiatric evaluation DSM III-R diagnosis(es). Symptoms of PTSD were assessed by psychiatric interview. Only PTSD resulting from child maltreatment defined as physical abuse, sexual abuse, or witnessing domestic and community violence was studied. Parents of subjects completed the Child Behavior Checklist,[11] the Child Depression Inventory,[12] and the Child Dissociative Checklist.[13] Comorbidity in the overanxious disorder group included two subjects with separation anxiety disorder and one with major depression. Trauma histories in the PTSD group were sexual abuse (5 of 9), physical and sexual abuse (2 of 9), physical abuse and witnessing violence (1 of 9), and physical abuse and neglect (1 of 9). The age of onset of maltreatment ranged from 3.5-8 years. Comorbidity in the PTSD group included two subjects with major depression, one with dysthymia, and one with adolescent onset conduct disorder. Healthy volunteers were recruited from control subjects through an ongoing study entitled, "The Psychobiology of Depression in Children and Adolescents" (Neal Ryan, Program Director) and had no Axis I diagnosis. No subject was taken off psychotropic medication in order to undergo this investigation. Mother(s) or guardian(s) was given written informed consent and subject(s) signed an assent form prior to participation. Confidentiality was maintained. Subjects received monetary compensation for participation.

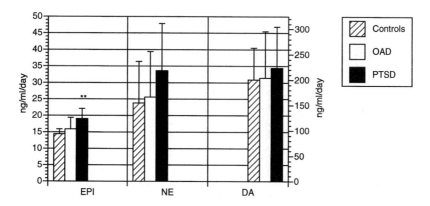

FIGURE 1. Means ± SD of 24-hour urinary catecholamine concentrations of epinephrine (EPI), norepinephrine (NE), and dopamine (DA) in control, overanxious (OAD), and PTSD children. ** F = 9.18, *p* < 0.001.

Exclusionary Criteria. These included: (1) The presence of a significant medical disorder, (2) the taking of any medications in the 2 weeks before 24-hour urine collection, (3) moderate obesity, (4) intelligence quotient below 70, (5) current substance abuse disorder, (6) enuresis, and (7) positive trauma history in subjects in the overanxious disorder and healthy volunteer subgroups.

Sample Collections. Subjects and their guardians were given detailed instructions concerning the weekend day collection of 24-hour urine specimens. Subjects followed a low monamine diet for 3 days before and on the day of collection. Urine specimens were refrigerated during the entire collection period in a sealed container. Aliquots were then frozen at −70°C until assayed.

Biochemical Measures. Biochemical analyses of urinary catecholamine concentrations were calculated as nanograms per milliliter excreted per 24 hours and determined with high performance liquid chromatography with electrochemical detection using standard methods.

Statistics. All data are presented as means ± standard deviation unless otherwise specified. Categorical data were examined with contingency table analysis. All data were tested for normality before using parametric tests. ANOVA was used to detect significant two-tailed differences at the *p* = 0.05 level. The Scheffe F- test was used to determine significant between-group comparisons.

RESULTS

Results of Urinary Catecholamine Excretion. Preliminary results show that PTSD subjects excreted statistically significantly greater concentrations of urinary epinephrine (per ml per day) than overanxious disorder and control subjects (F = 9.18 (2,27); *p* < 0.001; Scheffe F- test = 9.1; *p* < 0.05). Norepinephrine and dopamine concentrations did not differ between groups (FIG. 1).

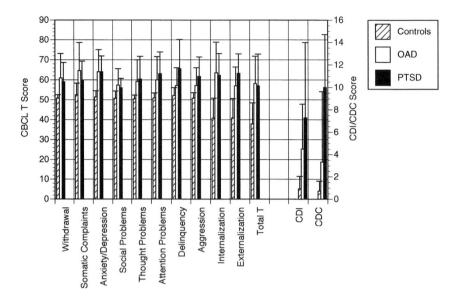

FIGURE 2. Means ± SD of Child Behavior Checklist (CBCL) T scores, Child Depression Inventory (CDI) scores, and Child Dissociative Checklist (CDC) scores in control, overanxious (OAD), and PTSD children.

Results of Psychological Profiles. On the Child Behavior Checklist, PTSD subjects had more symptoms of depression ($p < 0.01$), thought problems ($p < 0.05$), attention problems ($p < 0.01$), and aggressive and delinquent behaviors ($p < 0.05$) than did controls. Subjects with overanxious disorder had more symptoms of somatic complaints, anxiety and depression, and withdrawn behaviors than did controls ($p < 0.05$). Both the Internal and External T scores were elevated in PTSD and overanxious disorder subjects compared to controls.

PTSD subjects manifested more symptoms of depression on the Child Depression Inventory than did control subjects ($F = 6.54$ (2,24), $p < 0.01$). PTSD subjects also manifested more symptoms of dissociation on the Child Dissociative Checklist than did overanxious disorder and control subjects (Scheffe F- Test = 4.5 and 11.7, respectively; $p < 0.05$). PTSD subjects had more symptoms of items indicative of pathological dissociation such as dissociative amnesia, depersonalization, derealization, and identity alteration (FIG. 2).

DISCUSSION

Maltreated children with PTSD exhibited significantly greater concentrations of urinary epinephrine excretion than did overanxious disorder subjects or control children. Urinary catecholamine concentrations reflect plasma and peripheral sympathetic nervous system activity, tonic stimulation of the adrenal medulla, and metabolic breakdown of norepinephrine. Thus, these results support the hypothesis of hyperactivity of the catecholamine system in childhood PTSD, but not in nonmaltreated and nontraumatized children with anxiety disorders.

Patients with PTSD secondary to maltreatment were more likely to have more severe symptoms of internalizing and externalizing disorders than were anxious nontraumatized subjects or controls. PTSD subjects were also more likely to show symptoms of dissociation than were overanxious disorder or control subjects. Dissociative symptoms may be specific for trauma history.

Biological stress systems are neurobiological systems that significantly influence physical and cognitive development and emotional regulation. It is highly probable that many of the acute and chronic symptoms associated with trauma in childhood arise in conjunction with disturbances and dysregulation of these systems. Further investigations of the association of severe stress on the developing human are warranted.

REFERENCES

1. BLACK, B. 1993. Neurobiology of anxiety disorders. Child Adoles. Psychiatric Clin. N. Am. **2:** 749–762.
2. CHARNEY, D. S., A. Y. DEUTCH, J. H. KRYSTAL, S. M. SOUTHWICH & M. DAVIS. 1993. Psychobiological mechanisms of posttraumatic stress disorder. Arch. Gen. Psychiatry **50:** 294–305.
3. TRUE, W. R., J. RICE, S. A. EISEN, A. C. HEATH, J. GOLDBERG, M. J. LYONS & J. NOWAK. 1993. A twin study of genetic and environmental contributions to liability for posttraumatic stress symptoms. Arch. Gen. Psychiatry **50:** 257–264.
4. KAGAN, J., J. S. REZNICK & J. GIBBONS. 1988. Biological basis of childhood shyness. Science **240:** 167–171.
5. DE BELLIS, M. D. & F. W. PUTNAM. 1994. The psychobiology of childhood maltreatment. Child Adoles. Psychiatric Clin. N. Am. **3:** 663–677.
6. DE BELLIS, M. D., L. LEFTER, P. K. TRICKETT & F. W. PUTNAM. 1994. Urinary catecholamine excretion in sexually abused girls. J. Am. Acad. Child Adolesc. Psychiatry **33:** 320–327.
7. BIEDERMAN, J., J. F. ROSENBAUM, E. A. BOLDUC-MURPHY, S. V. FARAONE, J. CHALOFF, D. R. HIRSHFELD & J. KAGAN. 1993. Behavioral inhibition as a temperamental risk factor for anxiety disorders. Child Adolesc. Psychiatr. Clin. N. Am. **2:** 667–683.
8. DE BELLIS, M. D., G. P. CHROUSOS, L. D. DORN, L. BURKE, K. HELMERS, M. A. KLING, P. K. TRICKETT & F. W. PUTNAM. 1994. Hypothalamic-pituitary-adrenal axis dysregulation in sexually abused girls. J. Clin. Endocrinol. Metab. **78:** 249–255.
9. ORVASCHEL, H., J. PUIG-ANTICH, W. CHAMBERS, M. A. TABRIZI & R. JOHNSON. 1982. Retrospective assessment of prepubertal major depression with the Kiddie-SADS-E. J. Am. Acad. Child Adolesc. Psychiatry **21:** 392–397.
10. CHAMBERS, W. J., J. PUIG-ANTICH, M. HIRSCH, P. PAEZ, P. J. AMBROSINI, M. A. TABRIZI & M. DAVIS. 1985. The assessment of affective disorders in children and adolescents by semi-structured interview: Test-retest reliability KSADS present episode version. Arch. Gen. Psychiatry **42:** 696–702.
11. ACHENBACH, T. M. & C. S. EDELBROCK. 1983. Manual for the Child Behavior Checklist. Queen City Printers. Burlington, VT.
12. KOVACS, M. 1985. The Children's Depression Inventory (CDI). Psychopharmacol. Bull. **21:** 995–998.
13. PUTNAM, F. W. & G. PETERSON. 1994. Further validation of the Child Dissociative Checklist. Dissociation **7:** 204–211.

Psychoendocrinological Observations in Women with Chronic Pelvic Pain[a]

CHRISTINE HEIM,[b] ULRIKE EHLERT,
JOST REXHAUSEN, JÜRGEN P. HANKER, AND
DIRK H. HELLHAMMER

Center for Psychobiological and Psychosomatic Research
University of Trier
54286 Trier, Germany

Chronic pelvic pain (CPP) is a frequent gynecologic complaint accounting for many diagnostic laparoscopies performed in general hospitals. Numerous organic conditions can cause CPP such as endometriosis and adhesions. However, studies assessing the prevalence of organic disease in women with CPP yield an extreme variation in results, suggesting the absence of any organic correlate in many patients with CPP. (See ref. 1 for a review.) On the other hand, a constantly high prevalence of psychopathology has been reported in patients with CPP, especially with respect to depressive mood, anxiety, and somatization. (See ref. 2 for a review.) Recent studies revealed an enhanced prevalence of chronic stress and traumatic life events, particularly sexual and physical abuse, in women with CPP.[3-5] In summary, these results suggest that CPP might be a stress-related syndrome.

As stress is frequently associated with activation of the hypothalamic-pituitary-adrenal (HPA) axis, we recently explored psychoendocrinological features of women with CPP. Pain-free patients who underwent diagnostic laparoscopy because of infertility were recruited as controls. A high proportion of women with CPP had experienced sexual and/or physical abuse and fulfilled diagnostic criteria for posttraumatic stress disorder (PTSD) according to DSM-III-R criteria. Furthermore, women with CPP reported an enhanced total number of major life events, while these patients were typically not depressed. To assess HPA function, endocrine challenge tests were performed. In the corticotropin-releasing factor (CRF) stimulation test, women with CPP demonstrated normal basal and stimulated plasma ACTH levels, but blunted salivary cortisol responses compared to those in pain-free, infertile control subjects. In the low dose dexamethasone suppression test, patients with CPP had markedly lower salivary cortisol levels than did pain-free, infertile control subjects. However, in the presence of adrenocortical hyporeactivity, the latter result is inconclusive with respect to feedback sensitivity of the HPA axis. (See ref. 6 for a detailed description.)

[a]This research was supported by grant Eh 14311-1 from the Deutsche Forschungsgemeinschaft.

[b]Address for correspondence: Christine Heim, PhD, Department of Psychiatry and Behavioral Sciences, Emory University School of Medicine, 1639 Pierce Drive, Suite 4000, Atlanta, GA 30322 (tel: (404) 727-3719; fax: (404) 727-3233).

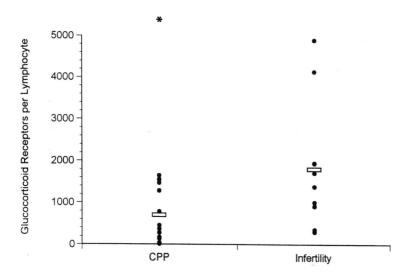

FIGURE 1. Number of glucocorticoid receptors per lymphocyte in women with chronic pelvic pain (CPP) and pain-free, infertile controls. *Open bars* represent group means. *$p < 0.05$ versus controls.

To further evaluate HPA function, we determined the number of glucocorticoid receptors (GR) in lymphocytes of women with CPP ($n = 14$) as compared to infertile, pain-free controls ($n = 11$) using a cytosolic radioligand binding assay. A specimen of whole blood was taken at 8 am by venipuncture, and mononuclear cells were separated in a Ficoll gradient. After incubation for 1.5 hours at 36°C in a 5% CO_2 atmosphere, the pure lymphocyte fraction was decanted from fixated monocytes. Lymphocytes were counted and stored at −196°C. The pellet was homogenized and ultracentrifuged at 226,000 g for 45 minutes. Aliquots were incubated overnight with 20 nmol of the specific ligand ^{3}H-RU28362 (plus 1,000 times excess RU28362 for the suppression of specific binding, respectively) at 4°C. Bound ligand was separated from free ligand by chromatography with Sephadex LH 20 over 1.5-ml columns. The amount of radioactivity was counted by scintillation, and specific binding was calculated. Mean GR number was statistically lower in women with CPP than in infertile controls (F = 6.20, $p = 0.02$). However, two outliers in the control group demonstrating relatively high GR levels might contribute to the effect, whereas GR number in women with CPP may be considered unchanged in comparison with that in most infertile patients (FIG. 1). Relatively low specific binding in both groups may reflect GR activation during the incubation step performed to eliminate monocytes which are known to contain a higher GR number than lymphocytes and, furthermore, become augmented relative to lymphocytes during stress.[7]

Despite a high prevalence of traumatic life events and PTSD, women with CPP demonstrate dysregulation of the HPA axis that partly parallels and partly differs from neuroendocrine correlates of PTSD.[8] Particularly, findings of normal pituitary responsiveness, but adrenocortical hyporeactivity in the CRF stimulation test as well as a decreased number of GR in lymphocytes are in contrast to the characteristics of PTSD. On the other hand, neuroendocrine alterations in women with CPP show a marked similarity to those in patients with bodily disorders such as fibromyalgia, chronic fatigue syndrome, rheumatoid arthritis, and asthma,[9-15] all of these disorders arguably being related to stress. From these results, we assume that hypocortisolism is not restricted to PTSD, but that it might play a role in the development of bodily disorders due to a lack of protective properties of the hormone on metabolism and immune function during stress. The lack of protective effects of cortisol might be especially expected if low cortisol levels are not counterbalanced by a compensatory upregulation of GR in target cells, but rather coincide with unchanged or decreased GR levels. Future studies should replicate our preliminary findings and furthermore assess GR characteristics in terms of affinity and receptor function. The mechanisms that contribute to the development of this specific HPA dysregulation may be heterogeneous and remain to be elucidated.

REFERENCES

1. STEEGE, J. F., A. L. STOUT & S. G. SOMKUTI. 1993. Obstet. Gynecol. Surv. **48:** 95-110.
2. ROSENTHAL, R. H. 1993. Obstet. Gynecol. Clin. North Am. **20:** 627-642.
3. HARROP-GRIFFITHS, J., W. KATON, E. WALKER, L. HOLM, J. RUSSO & L. HICKOCK. 1988. Obstet. Gynecol. **71:** 589-594.
4. RAPKIN, A. J., L. D. KAMES, L. DARKE, F. STAMPLER & B. D. NALIBOFF. 1990. Obstet. Gynecol. **76:** 92-96.
5. WALLING, M. K., M. W. O'HARA, R. C. REITER, A. K. MILBURN, G. LILLY & S. D. VINCENT. 1994. Obstet. Gynecol. **84:** 193-199.
6. HEIM, C., U. EHLERT, J. P. HANKER & D. H. HELLHAMMER. Submitted for publication.
7. DHABHAR, F. S., A. H. MILLER, B. S. McEWEN & R. L. SPENCER. 1995. J. Immunol. **154:** 5511-5527.
8. YEHUDA, R., E. GILLER, S. SOUTHWICK, M. LOWY & J. MASON. 1991. Biol. Psychiatry **30:** 1031-1048.
9. GRIEP, E. N., J. W. BOERSMA & E. R. DeKLOET. 1993. J. Rheumatol. **20:** 469-474.
10. CROFFORD, L. J., S. R. PILLEMER, K. KALOGERAS, J. M. CASH, D. MICHELSON, M. A. KLING, E. M. STERNBERG, P. W. GOLD, G. P. CHROUSOS & R. WILDER. 1994. Arthritis Rheum. **37:** 1583-1592.
11. DEMITRACK, M. A. 1993. *In* Chronic Fatigue and Related Immune Deficiency Syndromes. P. J. Goodnick & N. G. Klimas, Eds.: 45-66. American Psychiatric Press. Washington, DC.
12. SCHLAGHECKE, R., E. KORNLEY, J. WOLLENHAUPT & C. SPECKER. 1992. Arthritis Rheum. **35:** 740-744.
13. CHIKANZA, I. C., P. PETROU, G. P. CHROUSOS, G. KINGSLEY & G. P. PANAYI. 1992. Arthritis Rheum. **35:** 1281-1288.
14. SHER, E. R., Y. M. LEUNG & W. SURS. 1994. J. Clin. Invest. **93:** 33-39.
15. KRUGER, U. & H. SPIECKER. 1994. Pneumologie **48:** 793-789.

The Dexamethasone Suppression Test and Glucocorticoid Receptors in Borderline Personality Disorder

ROBERT GROSSMAN,[a] RACHEL YEHUDA, AND
LARRY SIEVER

Department of Psychiatry
Mount Sinai School of Medicine
New York, New York 10029

Some researchers have forwarded the provocative idea that borderline personality disorder (BPD) is best conceptualized as a "complex posttraumatic stress disorder."[1-4] The prevalence of trauma in patients with BPD is approximately 45-90%.[2-5] Trauma in BPD appears to be experienced more often during childhood or latency,[3,6,7] more frequently involves the patient's caregivers,[4,7-9] and is notable for its reported severity and duration.[3]

Phenomenologically, patients with BPD and those with chronic posttraumatic stress disorder (PTSD) display numerous areas of overlapping symptoms including: mood instability; hyperarousal and/or numbing of feelings; avoidance; dissociative symptoms; irritability; aggression; impulsivity; and high rates of substance abuse and suicide. Indeed, approximately 30% of BPD patients also meet diagnostic criteria for PTSD.[1] Given the prevalence of trauma in the history of individuals with BPD and the numerous areas of overlapping symptoms between BPD and PTSD, we have chosen to compare hypothalamic-pituitary-adrenal (HPA) axis alterations in these two disorders.

The HPA axis in PTSD has been studied through a variety of means. Daily cortisol production was assessed through 24-hour urinary cortisol secretion and repeated sampling of plasma cortisol sampling over the diurnal cycle. As compared to normal controls, PTSD subjects demonstrated both decreased 24-hour urinary cortisol secretion[10,11] and decreased average levels of plasma cortisol.[12,13] In the later study, chronobiological analysis of cortisol data revealed that subjects with PTSD had increased "signal to noise ratio" (amplitude of the coefficient of variation), implying more dynamically active cortisol release and stronger circadian cortisol rhythm (as reflected by the circadian quotient)[12,13] in PTSD than in normal controls and subjects with major depression.

In order for glucocorticoids to exert genomic effects, they must first couple with glucocorticoid receptors on the cell surface after which translocation to the cell nucleus can occur. Accompanying the aforementioned cortisol alterations is an increased number of lymphocyte glucocorticoid receptors in subjects with PTSD than in normal controls and subjects with major depressive disorder.[14,15] Glucocorticoid

[a] Address for correspondence: Robert Grossman, MD, Box 1230 Dept. of Psychiatry, Mount Sinai School of Medicine, 1 Gustave L. Levy Place, New York, NY 10029-6574 (tel: 212 824-8433).

receptors on peripheral lymphocytes are believed to reflect central glucocorticoid receptor (GR) density.[16,17] Additionally, subjects with PTSD, as compared to normal controls and combat veterans without PTSD, showed greater glucocorticoid receptor downregulation following administration of the synthetic steroid dexamethasone.[18]

The dexamethasone suppression test (DST) can also be used to assess HPA axis feedback sensitivity. For this test, an 8 AM blood sample is drawn for assay of plasma cortisol concentration. At 11 PM that night an oral dose of dexamethasone is administered. The usual effect of this exogenous glucocorticoid is a suppression of cortisol synthesis, which is reflected in an 8 AM assay for plasma cortisol the following morning. Metaanalysis of cortisol levels following the standard 1.0 mg DST in nondepressed subjects with PTSD was remarkable for an average cortisol value of 1.74 µg/dl, a value well below the standard cutoff of 5.0 µg/dl.[19] To better assess this apparent cortisol hypersuppression, a lower dose of dexamethasone, either 0.5 or 0.25 mg, was administered. In a 0.5 mg DST, combat veterans with PTSD showed enhanced suppression of cortisol compared to both combat-exposed veterans without PTSD and normal controls.[18,20] Taken together, the aforementioned findings indicate that subjects with PTSD have increased HPA axis negative feedback sensitivity.[19,21,22]

Prior findings on the standard 1.0 mg DST in BPD have been mixed. (For a review see Lehmayer et al.[23]) In five of seven studies the rate of nonsuppression was greater, whereas in two studies it did not differ from that of normal controls. Findings are difficult to interpret, for either many of the BPD subjects had concurrent major depression at the time of the challenge or this information was simply not collected. Of interest, however, is the finding that when comorbid BPD and major depression were documented, rates of nonsuppression did not differ from those of controls. In other words, the diagnosis of BPD decreased the rate of nonsuppression usually found in cases of major depression. In two studies of primary BPD, the rate of cortisol nonsuppression in subjects with low rates of major depression was 18% or less.[24,25] Reviewing authors concluded that subjects with BPD have low rates of nonsuppression, and nondepressed subjects with BPD are almost always suppressors.[23]

The preliminary results of the 0.5 mg DST and peripheral lymphocyte GR analyses in BPD patients are presented as a case series in order to focus on HPA axis alterations in BPD as related to trauma history. We ask the complex questions of which biological and behavioral/interpersonal patterns are unrelated to trauma history (BPD "trait markers"), which are the result of trauma exposure, and which are "state markers" for comorbid PTSD. The fact that BPD subjects with and without trauma histories can be studied, the overlap in BPD and PTSD symptoms, and the significant rate of comorbid PTSD make patients with BPD an ideal study population for evaluation of these unanswered questions. To date, this is the first study designed to evaluate the neurobiological role of trauma in BPD.

METHODS AND RESULTS

All subjects provided written informed consent before undergoing medical and psychiatric evaluation. All subjects were medically healthy and had not taken psychoactive medications for at least 10 weeks before their participation in the study. All subjects were free from substance/alcohol dependence, current major depression, and past or present psychotic or manic disorders. Axis I and II diagnoses were made using the Structured Clinical Interviews for DSM-IV. PTSD was diagnosed using the Clinician-Administered PTSD Scale.

Thirty milliliters of whole blood was obtained at 8 AM for GR and cortisol determination. Mononuclear cells were isolated using Ficoll-Hypaque within 1 hour. White blood cells were centrifuged at 300 g at 4°C, washed 4 times in Hanks' buffer solution, and pelleted for storage at −70°C. At 11 PM, subjects ingested 0.5 mg dexamethasone and were allowed nothing by mouth after midnight. Thirty milliliters of blood was again drawn at 8 AM the following morning.

Plasma cortisol levels were determined by radioimmunoassay (RIA) (Incstar Inc, Minneapolis, Minnesota) with inter- and intraassay coefficients of variation in our laboratory of 6.8 and 4.0%, respectively. Dexamethasone levels were also determined by RIA (IgG Corporation, Nashville, Tennessee) with inter- and intraassay coefficients of variation in our laboratory of 8.2 and 6.0%, respectively. As previously described, binding of lymphocyte GRs was measured with a cytosolic radioligand binding assay using tritiated dexamethasone. Inter- and intraassay coefficients of variation in our laboratory were 25.0 and 14.6%, respectively. The results are presented in TABLE 1.

DISCUSSION

Some interesting patterns may be discernible from this set of preliminary data. Subject 1 shows typical findings of a normal control without a history of sexual or physical abuse. Subject 1 has 21.1% cortisol suppression in response to the 0.5 mg DST. In our previous studies,[18] the mean cortisol suppression of the PTSD group was about 90% compared with about 73% for normal controls. The NC subject does not show glucocorticoid receptor downregulation 9 hours after 0.5 mg dexamethasone, which is also consistent with prior findings.[18]

Subjects 2 and 3 both have BPD, but neither reported a history of sexual or physical abuse. Both of these subjects showed marked cortisol suppression (hypersuppression) in response to the 0.5 mg DST (92.6 and 94.2%, respectively). This finding is of particular interest because it suggests that cortisol hypersuppression may exist in BPD regardless of trauma history. This particular subject has a response that would probably be viewed as nonsuppression. Indeed, approximately 10% of normal controls show nonsuppression on the standard DST, and this figure would be expected to be higher with the lower dose of dexamethasone used in this study.

Percent GR downregulation in subjects 2 and 3 was absent. There were no significant decreases in GR numbers before and after dexamethasone, a finding similar to that observed in normal control groups and combat veterans without PTSD in prior studies.

Subject 4 had BPD and also met diagnostic criteria for lifetime but not current PTSD. In addition to cortisol hypersuppression, this subject shows a 40% GR downregulation, similar to that observed in combat veterans with PTSD. Interestingly, the "trauma" endorsed by this subject was not a DSM-IV trauma, that is, it *did not* involve ". . . actual or threatened death or serious injury, or a threat to the physical integrity of self or others." Her "trauma" was that she was repeatedly teased by classmates during the sixth grade. This subject, however, did experience significant

TABLE 1. Trauma History, Diagnosis, and HPA Axis Measures

Subject #	Gender /Age	History of Sexual/ Physical Abuse	Normal Control	BPD	PTSD	8 AM Pre/Post DEX Cortisol μg/dl	Percent Cortisol Suppression	8 AM Pre/Post DEX GR # per Lymphocyte	Percent GR Change	8 AM DEX Level (ng/dl)
1	F/39	No	X			12.07/9.52	21.1	1752/2263	+29.10	46
2	F/30	No		X		5.97/0.44	92.6	1711/1775	+3.70	160
3	F/25	No		X		13.74/0.79	94.2	1911/1821	-4.70	55
4	F/24	No		X	Lifetime[a]	10.84/1.51	86.1	2851/1712	-40.0	70
5	F/25	Yes		X	Current	7.20/0.74	89.7	1890/116	-93.9	60

[a] DSM-IV Criteria A1 not met.

symptoms from clusters B, C, and D. Since patients with BPD often subjectively feel traumatized, the cortisol hypersuppression to dexamethasone may reflect this subjective experience even in the absence of a DSM-IV trauma.

Subject 5 meets diagnostic criteria for both BPD and current PTSD, with a history of both childhood sexual abuse and three rapes during her teenage years. This individual shows both cortisol hypersuppression and a strong GR downregulation. These findings too are consistent with earlier reported findings from our research on combat veterans with PTSD. These data from two subjects indicate that GR downregulation may be associated with PTSD symptoms. These data again compel a consideration of the subjective experience of trauma and PTSD in BPD.

Although these are only single case reports, we present these data to illustrate the approach that we are currently using to determine whether and to what extent the experiences of BPD and trauma survivors may overlap from a neurobiological perspective. We believe that this approach will ultimately allow us to draw conclusions about the complex interactions among biological vulnerability, developmental stressors, biological abnormalities, PTSD symptoms and characterlogical psychopathology.

REFERENCES

1. GUNDERSON, J. G. & A. N. SABO. 1993. The phenomenological and conceptual interface between borderline personality disorder and PTSD. Am. J. Psychiatry **150:** 19-27.
2. HERMAN, J. L. 1992. Trauma and Recovery. Basic Books. USA.
3. HERMAN, J. L., J. C. PERRY & B. A. VAN DER KOLK. 1989. Childhood trauma in borderline personality disorder. Am. J. Psychiatry **146:** 490-495.
4. OGATA, S. N., K. R. SILK, S. GOODRICH, N. E. LOHR, D. WESTEN & E. M. HILL. 1990. Childhood physical and sexual abuse in adult patients with borderline personality disorder. Am. J. Psychiatry **147:** 1008-1013.
5. VAN DER KOLK, B. A., C. PERRY & J. L. HERMAN. 1991. Childhood origins of self-destructive behavior. Am. J. Psychiatry **148:** 1665-1671.
6. ZANARINI, M. C., J. G. GUNDERSON, M. F. MARINO, E. O. SCHWARTZ & F. R. FRANKENBURG. 1989. Childhood experiences of borderline patients. Compr. Psychiatry **30:** 18-25.
7. WESTEN, D., P. LUDOLPH, B. MISLE, S. RUFFINS & M. J. BLOCK. 1990. Physical and sexual abuse in adolescent girls with borderline personality disorder. Am. J. Orthopsychiatry **60:** 55-66.
8. SHEARER, S. L., C. P. PETERS, M. S. QUAYTMAN & R. L. OGDEN. 1990. Frequency and correlates of childhood sexual and physical abuse histories in adult female borderline patients. Am. J. Psychiatry **147:** 214-216.
9. PARIS J. & H. ZWEIG-FRANK. 1992. A critical review of the role of childhood sexual abuse in the etiology of borderline personality disorder. Can. J. Psychiatry. **37:** 125-128.
10. YEHUDA, R., S. M. SOUTHWICK, G. NUSSBAUM, E. L. GILLER & J. W. MASON. 1990. Low urinary cortisol excretion in PTSD. J. Nerv. Ment. Dis. **178:** 366-369.
11. YEHUDA, R., S. M. SOUTHWICK, E. L. GILLER, X. MA & J. W. MASON. 1992. Urinary catecholamine excretion and severity of PTSD symptoms in Vietnam combat veterans. J. Nerv. Ment. Dis. **180:** 321-325.
12. YEHUDA, R., M. H. TEICHER, R. A. LEVENGOOD, R. L. TRESTMAN & L. J. SIEVER. 1994. Circadian regulation of basal cortisol levels in posttraumatic stress disorder. Ann. N.Y. Acad. Sci. **746:** 378-380.
13. YEHUDA, R., M. H. TEICHER, R. L. TRESTMAN, R. A. LEVENGOOD & L. J. SIEVER. 1995. Cortisol regulation in post-traumatic stress disorder: A chronobiological analysis. Submitted.

14. YEHUDA, R., M. T. LOWRY, S. M. SOUTHWICK, D. SHAFFER & E. L. GILLER. 1991. Lymphocyte glucocorticoid receptor number in posttraumatic stress disorder. Am. J. Psychiatry **148:** 499–504.

15. YEHUDA, R., D. BOISONEAU, J. W. MASON & E. L. GILLER. 1993. Relationship between lymphocyte glucocorticoid receptor number and urinary-free cortisol excretion in mood, anxiety, and psychotic disorder. Biol. Psychiatry **34:** 18–25.

16. LOWRY, M. T. 1990. Reserpine induced decrease in type I and II corticosteroid receptors in neuronal and lymphoid tissue of adrenalectomized rats. Neuroendocrinology **51:** 190–196.

17. LOWRY, M. T. 1989. Quantification of type I and II adrenal steroid receptors in neuronal, lymphoid, and pituitary tissues. Brain Res. **503:** 191–197.

18. YEHUDA, R., D. BOISONEAU, M. T. LOWRY & E. L. GILLER. 1995. Dose-response changes in plasma cortisol and lymphocyte glucocorticoid receptors following dexamethasone administration in combat veterans with and without posttraumatic stress disorder. Arch. Gen. Psychiatry **52:** 583–593.

19. YEHUDA, R., E. L. GILLER, S. M. SOUTHWICK, M. T. LOWRY & J. W. MASON. 1991. Hypothalamic-pituitary-adrenal dysfunction in posttraumatic stress disorder. Biol. Psychiatry **130:** 1031–1048.

20. YEHUDA, R., S. M. SOUTHWICK, J. H. KRYSTAL, D. BREMNER, D. S. CHARNEY & J. W. MASON. 1993. Enhanced suppression of cortisol following dexamethasone administration in posttraumatic stress disorder. Am. J. Psychiatry **150:** 83–86.

21. YEHUDA, R., E. L. GILLER, R. A. LEVENGOOD, S. M. SOUTHWICK & L. J. SIEVER. 1995. Hypothalamic-pituitary-adrenal functioning in PTSD: Expanding the concept of the stress response spectrum. *In* M. H. Friedman, D. S. Charney & A. Y. Deutch, Eds. Neurobiological and Clinical Consequences of Stress: From Normal Adaptation to PTSD. Raven Press. New York, NY.

22. YEHUDA, R., H. RESNICK, B. KAHANA & E. L. GILLER. 1993. Long-lasting hormonal alterations to extreme stress in humans: Normative or maladaptive? Psychosom. Med. **55:** 287–297.

23. LAHMEYER, H. W., C. F. REYNOLDS, D. J. KUPFER & R. KING. 1989. Biologic markers in borderline personality disorder: A review. J. Clin. Psychiatry **50:** 217–225.

24. NATHAN, R. S., P. H. SOLOFF, A. GEORGE *et al.* 1986. DST and TRH tests in borderline personality disorder. *In* Biological Psychiatry: Proceedings of the IVth World Congress of Biological Psychiatry. C. Shagass, R. G. Josiassen, B. H. Wagner *et al.*, Eds.: 564–565. Elsevier. New York.

25. SIEVER, L. H., F. F. COCCARO, H. KLAR *et al.* 1986. Biological markers in borderline and related personality disorders. *In* Biological Psychiatry: Proceedings of the IVth World Congress of Biological Psychiatry. C. Shagass, R. G. Josiassen, B. H. Wagner *et al.*, Eds.: 566–568. Elsevier. New York.

Enduring Effects of Early Abuse on Locomotor Activity, Sleep, and Circadian Rhythms[a]

CAROL A. GLOD,[b] MARTIN H. TEICHER,
CAROL R. HARTMAN, THOMAS HARAKAL, AND
CYNTHIA E. McGREENERY

Department of Psychiatry
Harvard Medical School
Developmental Biopsychiatry Research Program
McLean Hospital
and
College of Nursing
Northeastern University
Boston, Massachusetts 02115

The purpose of the present study was to ascertain the biobehavioral effects of early abuse on locomotor activity levels, sleep initiation and maintenance, and circadian rhythms. In particular, we sought to test the hypothesis that early abuse is associated with delayed sleep initiation and reduced sleep efficiency. Furthermore, we sought to determine if abused children with posttraumatic stress disorder (PTSD) differed from abused children without PTSD in their activity and sleep measures.

METHODS

Nineteen unmedicated prepubertal children with documented physical or sexual abuse were compared with 15 nonabused normal controls and 10 depressed children. All subjects received a complete semistructured diagnostic interview (K-SADS-E).[1] Motionlogger actigraphs (Ambulatory Monitoring, Inc, Ardsley, New York) collected activity data for 72 continuous hours in 1-minute epochs.

RESULTS

Nocturnal activity levels in abused children were twice as high as those in nonabused depressed or normal children.[2] Use of sleep estimation algorithms revealed

[a] This work was supported in part by MH48343, NR06807, and grants from the American and Massachusetts Nurses Foundation, and Sigma Theta Tau International.

[b] Address for correspondence: Carol A. Glod, R.N.C.S., Ph.D., Developmental Biopsychiatry Research Program, McLean Hospital, 115 Mill Street, Belmont, MA 02178 (tel: (617) 855-3325; fax: (617) 855-3712).

TABLE 1. Nocturnal and Diurnal Activity Parameters (mean ± SD) of Abused and Control Children

Measure	Controls (n = 15)	Abused Subjects (n = 19)	Abused Non-PTSD Subjects (n = 6)	Abused PTSD Subjects (n = 13)	Control vs Abused Subjects (p value)	PTSD vs Non-PTSD Subjects (p value)
Nocturnal activity[a]	52.6 ± 13.9	104.7 ± 51.3	129.9 ± 72.3	93.2 ± 36.2	0.001	NS
Sleep latency (min)	11.0 ± 8.8	33.9 ± 27.2	45.2 ± 28.0	28.8 ± 26.2	0.005	NS
Sleep efficiency	96.1 ± 1.6%	91.6 ± 5.1%	89.0 ± 5.8	92.8 ± 4.6	0.005	NS
Diurnal activity[a]	929.1 ± 153.9	1,016.2 ± 160.3	958.8 ± 232.5	1,042.7 ± 116.8	0.05	NS
Amplitude	582.1 ± 121.1	618.9 ± 103.3	549.8 ± 125.1	656.6 ± 69.4	NS	0.069
Relative amplitude	100.5 ± 9.4%	97.7 ± 7.6%	91.3 ± 4.4%	101.2 ± 6.6%	NS	0.01
Acrophase (min)	14:03 ± 00:44	14:41 ± 00:47	15:04 ± 00:27	14:36 ± 00:53	0.05	NS

[a] Counts/epoch.

that these disturbances stemmed from protracted sleep onset latency and diminished sleep efficiency (TABLE 1). Both physical and sexual abuse significantly disturbed sleep; however, physical abuse exerted a greater impact on sleep and nocturnal activity than did sexual abuse.[2] Neither PTSD nor depression exerted significant effects on sleep.

As seen in TABLE 1, abused children had elevated diurnal activity levels compared to normal controls.[3] Enhanced activity levels were largely due to those abused children with PTSD, who were 12% more active than normal.[3] Abused children with PTSD had a much greater relative circadian amplitude than did abused children without PTSD, whereas non-PTSD abused subjects had a peak in circadian activity rhythm 61 minutes later than that of normal volunteers (TABLE 1).[3]

The development of PTSD was strongly correlated with age at onset of abuse; earlier physical or sexual abuse was associated with a greater likelihood of PTSD. Overall, activity profiles of abused children with PTSD were similar to those observed in attention deficit hyperactivity disorder (ADHD). In this sample, 38% of children with PTSD versus 0% of abused children without PTSD met diagnostic criteria for ADHD. In contrast, abused children without PTSD had dysregulated activity profiles similar to those previously observed in depressed children.[4]

CONCLUSION

Quantitative assessment of circadian rest-activity levels and rhythms revealed significant differences in this sample of prepubertal abused and normal children. Abused children displayed more difficulty with sleep initiation and maintenance than did both normal and depressed controls. Abused children also displayed higher mean diurnal activity levels, largely in the subgroup with PTSD. Abused children with PTSD had robust and preserved circadian activity rhythms, whereas abused subjects without PTSD had dysregulated rhythms.

REFERENCES

1. ORVASCHEL, H. & J. PUIG-ANTICH. 1987. The Schedule for Affective Disorders and Schizophrenia for School-Age Children—Epidemologic Version (Kiddie-SADS-E). University of Pittsburgh. Pittsburgh, PA.
2. GLOD C. A., M. H. TEICHER, C. R. HARTMAN & T. HARAKAL. 1997. Increased nocturnal activity and impaired sleep maintenance in abused children. J. Am. Acad. Child. Adolesc. Psychiatry; in press.
3. GLOD, C. A. & M. H. TEICHER. 1996. Relationship between early abuse, posttraumatic stress disorder, and activity levels. J. Am. Acad. Child. Adolesc. Psychiatry **34:** 1384-1393.
4. TEICHER, M. H. *et al.* 1993. Locomotor activity in depressed children and adolescents. J. Am. Acad. Child. Adolesc. Psychiatry **32:** 760-769.

Neurological Status of Combat Veterans and Adult Survivors of Sexual Abuse PTSD[a]

TAMARA V. GURVITS, MARK W. GILBERTSON,
NATASHA B. LASKO, SCOTT P. ORR, AND
ROGER K. PITMAN

Department of Psychiatry
Harvard Medical School
Boston, Massachusetts

Research Service
VA Medical Center
Manchester, New Hampshire 03103

So-called "soft" neurological signs (NSS) have been used as an instrument for investigation of organic brain dysfunction in psychiatric disorders including schizophrenia[1,3,5-7] and obsessive-compulsive disorder.[4] NSS are generally considered to reflect immaturities in development of language, motor coordination, or perception.[6]

Despite a growing literature on the status of NSS in the foregoing disorders, little has been published on the presence of NSS in posttraumatic stress disorder (PTSD). A few reports examining traumatized children/adolescents suggested an increased incidence of nonspecific NSS (in the absence of known head trauma) in these individuals. These studies, however, did not specifically examine the role of PTSD.

We previously demonstrated a statistically significant increase of NSS in Vietnam combat veterans with PTSD.[2] Using a more precise methodology, the present study examines NSS in PTSD and non-PTSD participants and explores the hypothesis that participants with PTSD will have greater neurological impairment and compromised developmental history in independent samples in which the nature of the traumatic experience and gender differs. This study examined two groups of traumatized individuals, male Vietnam combat veterans and adult female survivors of childhood sexual abuse.

METHOD

The first group was comprised of 42 male Vietnam combat veterans, 26 with current PTSD and 16 with no lifetime PTSD (non-PTSD). Mean (SD) age was 50.0 years (3.9) for the PTSD group and 49.0 (3.2) for the non-PTSD group. Mean (SD) education level was 14.0 years (3.0) for the PTSD group and 15.7 (2.3) for the non-PTSD group.

[a] This research was supported by a VA Research Career Development Award (T.V.G.).

TABLE 1. Percentage of Vietnam Combat Veterans with PTSD and Controls Positive for Selective Items of Neuropsychiatric History

Item	PTSD	Control
History of:		
26. Delay of walk	14.3	0
28. Attention deficit	33.3	14.3
29. Motor hyperactivity	20.00	0
30. Learning problems	16.0	7.1
31. (reading, writing, arithmetic)	16.0	0
34. Repeated grades	36.0	7.1
Percent of subjects with positive items	60.0	24.4
Mean number of positive items	1.64	0.64
19–21. Head injury with loss of consciousness	36.0	24.4
Family History of:		
73. Learning disorders	27.2	7.1
102. Alcohol abuse life-time	75.0	42.8
117. Drug abuse life-time	54.2	42.8
Family History of Substance Abuse:		
127. Alcohol abuse father	62.5	35.7
128. Alcohol abuse mother	75.0	23.0
129. Alcohol abuse siblings	70.8	7.1
137. Drug abuse siblings	16.7	0
Past History of Abuse:		
158. Witness of abuse	29.2	14.3
159. Was abused as a child	33.3	14.3
163. Sexual abuse	12.6	7.1

The second group was comprised of 35 adult female survivors of childhood sexual abuse, 13 with current PTSD, 9 with no lifetime PTSD (non-PTSD), and 12 with past and/or partial PTSD (PP). Mean (SD) age was 42.8 years (8.0) for the PTSD group, 44.2 (8.5) for the non-PTSD group, and 39.9 (8.9) for the PP group. Mean (SD) education level was 15.2 (1.7), 15.1 (2.3), and 14.1 years (2.1), respectively, in the three groups.

The Structured Clinical Interview for DSM-IV (SCID) and the Clinician-Administered PTSD Scale (CAPS) were administered to establish the diagnostic status for each participant (PTSD vs non-PTSD).

Each participant underwent a videotaped neurological examination of 58 soft neurological signs, each scored on a predefined 0–3 scale. A standardized neuropsychiatric history was taken with special attention given to developmental problems, CNS insults, and family history of neurological impairment and substance abuse. In addition, an abbreviated Wechsler Adult Intelligence Scale-Revised (WAIS-R) was administered to each participant.

TABLE 2. Percentage of Adult Survivors of Sexual Abuse Females Positive for Selective Items of Neuropsychiatric History

Item	PTSD	Control	Past/Partial
20-24. Pathology prenatal	100	17	43
History of:			
27. Delay of talk	14	0	8
28. Attention deficit	25	0	45
29. Motor hyperactivity	17	0	27
30. Learning problems	25	10	25
31. (reading, writing, arithmetic)	31	10	25
34. Repeated grades	8	0	17
36. Enuresis	31	0	20
Number of subjects with positive items	62	30	58
19. Head injury with loss of consciousness	31	10	17
102. Alcohol abuse life-time	46	30	42
117. Drug abuse life-time	38	30	17
Family History of Substance Abuse:			
127. Alcohol abuse father	62	60	89
128. Alcohol abuse mother	54	20	45
129. Alcohol abuse siblings	78	40	100
137. Drug abuse siblings	45	20	55
Past History of Physical Abuse:			
158. Witness of abuse	58	50	45
159. Was abused as a child	83	40	45

RESULTS

1. Mean (SD) NSS scores for the combat groups were 29.3 (10.0) for PTSD and 17.6 (6.6) for non-PTSD group; t = (40) = 4.2, p = 0.0002. Mean (SD) NSS scores in the sexual abuse groups were 28.9 (14.0) for PTSD and 14.6 (5.2) for non-PTSD participants; t = (16.2) = 3.1, p = 0.004. Mean NSS scores for the PP group were 17.4 (5.4). PTSD versus PP p = 0.02; Tukey's PTSD > PP, non-PTSD, F (2.8) 7.0, p = 0.003.

The most significant differences were found in performance of the copy figure (cube) and in the fist-palm-side test (motor sequence).

2. Handedness: PTSD participants were more often not right-hand dominant compared to non-PTSD participants: combat, 23% versus 12.5%; sexual abuse, 23.1% versus 11%, respectively, and 42% of PP participants. These differences, however, were not statistically significant.

3. Past developmental history in both PTSD groups was compromised relative to participants with no history of PTSD. In combat groups, positive history was

identified in 58% of PTSD versus 21% of non-PTSD participants, $p = 0.03$; in sexual abuse groups, in 62% of PTSD versus 11% of non-PTSD participants, and 75% of PP participants, $p = 0.01$.

4. Family history was remarkable for heavy alcohol abuse in 76% of combat PTSD versus 43% of non-PTSD participants, $p = 0.04$; in sexual abuse groups, 100% of PTSD versus 11% of non-PTSD participants, and 67% of PP participants, $p = 0.0001$.

5. Childhood physical abuse was identified in 35% of combat PTSD versus 14% of non-PTSD participants, 82% of sexual abuse PTSD versus 44% of non-PTSD participants, and 58% of PP participants.

6. Combat veterans with PTSD demonstrated an estimated mean IQ of 105.3 (13.1) compared with a mean of 119.2 (11.2) in non-PTSD combat veterans (t (35) = 3.28, $p = 0.002$). Total NSS score and IQ were significantly correlated ($r = -0.48$, $p = 0.003$).

SUMMARY

We found higher levels of positive soft neurological signs in PTSD participants than in participants who also experienced similar trauma but did not develop PTSD. This finding was replicated in two samples, that is, Vietnam combat veterans and adult female survivors of childhood sexual abuse, despite differences in gender, age, nature of trauma, and period of life when the trauma occurred. Past developmental history of participants and a substance abuse history of first-degree relatives also differentiated PTSD from non-PTSD groups in both combat and sexual abuse samples. Evidence for neurological impairment and compromised developmental history raises the possibility of pretrauma impairment as a risk factor for the development of PTSD.

REFERENCES

1. Cox, S. M. & A. M. Ludwig. 1979. Neurological soft signs and psychopathology. I. Findings in schizophrenia. J. Nerv. Ment. Disord. **167:** 161-165.
2. Gurvits, T. G., N. B. Lasko, S. C. Schachter, A. A. Kuhne, S. P. Orr & R. K. Pitman. 1993. Neurological status of Vietnam veterans with chronic post-traumatic stress disorder. J. Neuropsychiatry Clin. Neurosci. **5:** 183-188.
3. Heinrichs, D. W. & R. W. Buchanan. 1988. The significance and meaning of neurological signs in schizophrenia. Am. J. Psychiatry **145:** 11-18.
4. Hollander, E., E. Schiffman, B. Cohen *et al.* 1990. Signs of central nervous system dysfunction in obsessive-compulsive disorder. Arch. Gen. Psychiatry **47:** 27-32.
5. King, D. J., A. Wilson, S. J. Cooper *et al.* 1991. The clinical correlates of neurological soft signs in chronic schizophrenia. Br. J. Psychiatry **158:** 770-775.
6. Nasrallah, H. A., J. Tippin & M. McCalley-Whitters. 1983. Neurological soft signs in manic patients: A comparison with schizophrenic and control groups. J. Affective Disord. **5:** 45-50.
7. Quitkin, F., A. Fifkin & D. F. Klein. 1976. Neurologic soft signs in schizophrenic and character disorders. Arch. Gen. Psychiatry **33:** 845-853.

Source Monitoring in PTSD

JULIA GOLIER,[a] PHILIP HARVEY, ANN STEINER,
AND RACHEL YEHUDA

Department of Psychiatry
Bronx VA Medical Center
116A, 130 West Kingsbridge Road
Bronx, New York 10468

Department of Psychiatry
Mount Sinai School of Medicine
New York, New York 10029

The cognitive symptoms of posttraumatic stress disorder (PTSD) in general and the reexperiencing symptoms in particular may result from a failure to correctly identify the source of traumatic memories. For instance, the reexperiencing symptoms, such as flashbacks or intrusive thoughts, consist of retrieved memory information that is incorrectly interpreted as currently taking place. A consistent tendency towards confusion of information from different sources could also lead to anticipatory anxiety. Thus, poor ability to monitor the source of information in memory could correlate with the presence of PTSD. The goal of this study was to examine whether the symptoms of PTSD can be conceptualized as a special case of source monitoring failure. *Source monitoring* refers to the set of processes involved in making attributions about the origins of knowledge or memories.[1] The spatial and temporal context in which the memory was acquired and the modalities in which it was received are among the characteristics of the source. According to the source monitoring model, the source of a memory is attributed to it through a decision-making process performed during remembering.[1] The present study examines the hypothesis that PTSD symptoms should correlate with poor source monitoring and also examines the influence of general versus personally relevant traumatic information on performance.

METHODS

Fourteen male Vietnam combat veterans were selected from consecutive admissions to the PTSD Unit at the Bronx VA Hospital. Subjects were administered the Structured Clinical Interview for DSM-III-R, the Clinician Administered PTSD Scale (CAPS), and self-report questionnaires. To meet PTSD criteria, subjects had to have a Mississippi Scale for Combat-related PTSD score greater than 107. (Thirteen met

---

[a] Address for correspondence: Julia Golier, 116A, Bronx VA Medical Center, 130 West Kingsbridge Road, Bronx, NY 10468.

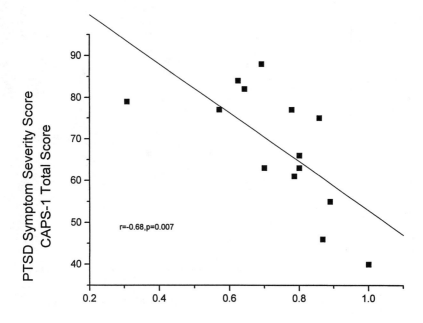

FIGURE 1. Symptom severity and source monitoring for nonspecific trauma words.

PTSD criteria by CAPS interview.) Subjects with psychotic, neurologic, or primary substance abuse disorders were excluded.

Source Monitoring Procedure. Three types of stimuli were used: neutral words, nonspecific combat trauma words, and personally relevant combat trauma words. For the neutral condition, 24 of the 100 most common words in English were used. The same words were used in all three monitoring conditions and were randomized across the conditions. The personally relevant trauma words were derived from a written description of the military events that veterans recalled as most traumatic to them. From these narratives, 10 or more concrete nouns describing aspects of the trauma were selected and mixed in with a pool of words selected from other veterans' narratives. Subjects were asked to "Rank order these words from most to least personally relevant to you." The 24 most relevant words were used as "personally relevant" stimuli. The 24 "nonspecific" trauma words were drawn from a single veteran's narrative and used for all subjects. Words that coincided with an individual veteran's relevant words were replaced.

Subjects were presented words in separate conditions: Say vs Think, Say vs Listen, and Think vs Listen. "Say" words, written on an index card, were read aloud by the subject. "Listen" words were read aloud by a research assistant. "Think" words were shown on an index card; subjects were instructed to "Imagine yourself saying this word out loud." Words were presented in an alternating format at a one word per two second pace. At the end of each test, subjects were asked to identify

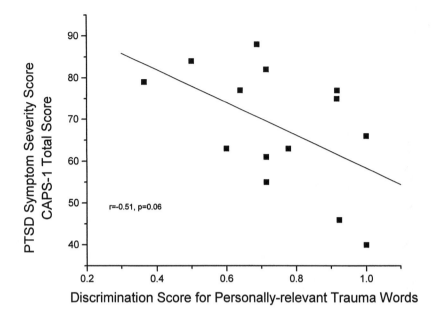

FIGURE 2. Symptom severity and source monitoring for personally relevant trauma words.

the source of the word by discriminating it from the words from the other source and an equal number of recognition foils. The "Discrimination Ratio," the number of words correctly attributed to their source, divided by the total number of words correctly identified as "old," was used as the dependent variable. Because of the small number of subjects, data were collapsed across conditions and are presented as a discrimination ratio for each type of information. A ratio of .50 is random.

RESULTS

The mean age of the veterans was 47.4 ± 2.8 years, education level was 13.0 ± 1.9 years, Mississippi score was 134.6 ± 16.2, the Combat Exposure Scale (CES) score was 32.9 ± 9.1, and the CAPS total was 68.8 ± 19.9. The mean discrimination ratio for neutral words was 0.62 ± 0.18, for nonspecific trauma words 0.74 ± 0.17, and for personally relevant trauma words 0.75 ± 0.19. A repeated measures ANOVA reveals significant differences in performance across stimuli type (F = 3.7, df = 2/26, $p = 0.04$). Post-hoc analyses show that source monitoring for both personally relevant and nonspecific trauma words were significantly greater than that for neutral words. PTSD severity (CAPS total) did not correlate with source monitoring for neutral words but did correlate for nonspecific trauma and personally relevant words ($r = 0.68$, $p = 0.007$ and $r = 0.51$, $p = 0.06$, respectively; FIGS. 1 and 2). The CES did not correlate with source monitoring for any of the types of stimuli.

DISCUSSION

This pilot study of combat veterans with PTSD found that their performance in the source monitoring of neutral stimuli is very poor compared to that of normal subjects in previous studies.[2] Personally relevant aspects of the individual's trauma history were monitored better than was neutral information. Nonspecific trauma information was equally facilitated, suggesting that the personal meaning of the information may be less important in its effect on cognitive processes than its generally traumatic nature. Facilitation by trauma-relevant information is consistent with findings of enhanced memory for trauma-related information in PTSD subjects in other paradigms.[3] Poor source monitoring of trauma-relevant stimuli was associated with symptom severity, but not the degree of trauma exposure. It may be that trauma-relevant stimuli increase arousal and performance, but in the most symptomatic cause excessive arousal and impaired performance. In the absence of a control for "pure emotional" words it is not clear if the facilitative effect is due to the traumatic nature of the words. Additionally, work is underway to recruit combat controls to assess the specificity of these findings to PTSD.

REFERENCES

1. JOHNSON, M. K. & C. L. RAYE. 1981. Reality monitoring. Psychol. Rev. **88:** 67-85.
2. HAHROUDI, S. & L. D. CHROSNIAK & M. K. JOHNSON. 1989. Aging and source monitoring. Psychology and Aging. **4:** 106-112.
3. ZEITLIN, S. B. & R. J. McNALLY. 1991. Implicit and explicit memory bias for threat in post-traumatic stress disorder. Behav. Res. Ther. **29:** 451-457.

Neuropsychological Assessment of Vietnam Combat Veterans with and without PTSD

MARK W. GILBERTSON, TAMARA V. GURVITS,
NATASHA B. LASKO, AND ROGER K. PITMAN

Research Service
VA Medical Center
Manchester, New Hampshire 03103

Department of Psychiatry
Harvard Medical School
Boston, Massachusetts

Neuropsychological investigations of individuals with posttraumatic stress disorder (PTSD) have suggested both global and specific impairments in performance on standardized tests of memory.[1,2] Given the well-established relation between recent memory impairment and hippocampal regions of the brain,[3] these findings are of great interest and consistent with reports of diminished hippocampal volume in this disorder.[4-6] Most studies of neuropsychological function in PTSD have only examined PTSD in the context of a normal control population and have been unable to determine whether deficits are associated specifically with the development of PTSD or reflect a general response to trauma exposure. The current investigation reports the results of a study assessing attention, memory, visuospatial skills, and executive (frontal lobe) function in PTSD in which trauma-exposed non-PTSD individuals serve as a control.

METHODS

Participants consisted of 33 male Vietnam combat veterans. Following administration of the Structured Clinical Interview for DSM-III-R, participants were classified into PTSD ($n = 19$) and non-PTSD ($n = 14$) groups. Subjects meeting criteria for bipolar or psychotic disorder or alcohol/substance abuse or dependence within the last year were excluded. Also excluded were participants with a history of gross head trauma or neurological impairment. All subjects were free of psychotropic medications for at least 2 weeks before examination. A battery of standardized neuropsychological tests was administered, the components of which are listed in TABLE 1. In addition, subjects completed the Clinician-Administered PTSD Scale (CAPS), Combat Exposure Scale (CES), and Michigan Alcoholism Screening Test (MAST) for severity of past substance abuse. Demographic and psychometric data are presented in TABLE 2.

TABLE 1. Neuropsychological Data Group Differences: PTSD vs Non-PTSD

	PTSD (n = 19)	Non-PTSD (n = 14)	t	p
WAIS-R Estimated IQ	105.7 ± 13.8	119.2 ± 11.3	3.0	.0048
WAIS-R Digit Span	9.3 ± 1.3	12.3 ± 2.1	4.8	.0001
Trail Making Test				
A	38.8 ± 13.7	33.7 ± 12.7	1.1	.2837
B	95.2 ± 31.7	66.7 ± 21.9	2.8	.0082
Adjusted (B/A)	2.7 ± 1.14	2.2 ± 1.0	1.4	.1583
Symbol Digit Modalities	42.8 ± 8.4	53.0 ± 8.2	3.4	.0018
Wechsler Memory Scale				
General Index	96.1 ± 12.3	114.6 ± 11.2	4.5	.0001
Verbal Index	96.6 ± 9.9	111.2 ± 10.3	4.1	.0003
Visual Index	98.5 ± 16.7	114.5 ± 8.9	3.5	.0014
Delayed Recall Index	95.6 ± 14.4	112.6 ± 8.7	3.9	.0004
Rey-Osterreith Complex Figure				
Copy	33.6 ± 3.4	35.4 ± 0.9	2.2	.0387
Immediate Recall	20.5 ± 7.8	18.4 ± 7.9	0.8	.4578
Delayed Recall	19.7 ± 7.3	17.3 ± 8.5	0.9	.3846
Wisconsin Card Sort				
Categories	4.2 ± 2.2	5.5 ± 1.4	2.1	.0487
Perseverative Error %	24.6 ± 19.4	10.9 ± 7.4	2.8	.0087

TABLE 2. Demographics and Psychometrics

	PTSD (n = 19)	Non-PTSD (n = 14)	t	p
Age	46.4 ± 2.8	49.1 ± 3.0	2.7	.0122
Education	14.2 ± 3.3	15.7 ± 2.1	1.6	.1294
Age in Vietnam	19.6 ± 2.2	22.7 ± 3.4	3.2	.0034
Combat Tour (mo.)	11.9 ± 4.5	11.4 ± 5.5	0.3	.7962
CES	31.4 ± 8.0	16.9 ± 9.8	4.3	.0002
CAPS	71.7 ± 19.8	6.4 ± 9.5	12.6	.0001
MAST	17.5 ± 15.6	3.2 ± 4.5	3.2	.0070

Abbreviations: CES = Combat Exposure Scale; CAPS = Clinician-Administered PTSD Scale; MAST = Michigan Alcoholism Screening Test.

RESULTS

Neuropsychological test results are shown in TABLE 1, revealing that PTSD subjects demonstrated poorer performance across most neurocognitive domains. However, a stepwise discriminant analysis including all neuropsychological variables identified attention (WAIS-R Digit Span; partial $r^2 = 0.47$, $p = 0.0001$) and memory (WMS-R General; partial $r^2 = 0.27$, $p = 0.003$) as the only significant independent factors predicting group membership. These two variables accounted for 61% of group difference variance (Wilks' Lambda = 0.39, $p = 0.0001$). Impairments in both attention and memory were highly related to increased PTSD severity as measured by the CAPS ($r = .62$, $p = 0.0001$ and $r = 0.61$, p = 0.0002, respectively). Attentional impairment (as measured by WAIS-R Digit Span) was also significantly related to combat exposure ($r = -0.65$, $p = 0.0001$). Of interest, however, was the failure to find a significant relation between memory performance and combat exposure ($r = 0.24$, $p = 0.18$). A series of analyses of covariance were performed, which revealed that differences in memory performance between PTSD and non-PTSD groups were maintained even when controlling for the effects of attention (F = 8.3, $p = 0.0074$), IQ (F = 7.6, $p = 0.0098$), and MAST (F = 9.6, $p = 0.0052$).

DISCUSSION

We assessed neuropsychological function in Vietnam combat veterans with and without PTSD. While PTSD subjects demonstrated poorer performance on most neurocognitive tasks, this may have, in part, reflected the effects of attentional disturbance. The emergence of attention as a key neuropsychological impairment is not surprising given its role as a DSM-III-R criterion for PTSD. However, memory impairment also emerged as a key factor which could not be explained by the secondary effects of attention, IQ, or substance use. These results support the specific relevance of memory function in PTSD and are consistent with reports of diminished hippocampal volume in this disorder. Although speculative, the specific absence of a relation between memory impairment and degree of combat exposure suggests that memory function may serve as a premorbid vulnerability factor in the development of PTSD rather than as a sole outcome of traumatic exposure per se. These findings are consistent with recent reports suggesting premorbid IQ as a PTSD risk[7] and perhaps indicate that memory may be a more specific manifestation of this vulnerability. The results further suggest that combat-exposed non-PTSD subjects were characterized by above average memory abilities rather than PTSD subjects showing impaired memory. This suggests the hypothesis that superior memory system and hippocampal function may protect against the development of chronic PTSD.

REFERENCES

1. YEHUDA, R. *et al.* 1995. Learning and memory in combat veterans with posttraumatic stress disorder. Am. J. Psychiatry **152:** 137–139.
2. BREMNER, J. D. *et al.* 1993. Deficits in short-term memory in posttraumatic stress disorder. Am. J. Psychiatry **150:** 1015–1019.

3. SQUIRE, L. R. 1986. Mechanisms of memory. Science **232:** 1612-1619.
4. GURVITS, T. V. *et al.* 1997. Magnetic resonance imaging study of hippocampal volume in chronic, combat-related post-traumatic stress disorder. Biol. Psychiatry. In press.
5. BREMNER, J. D. *et al.* 1995. MRI-based measurement of hippocampal volume in patients with combat-related posttraumatic stress disorder. Am. J. Psychiatry **152:** 973-981.
6. STEIN, M. B. *et al.* 1995. Neuroanatomic and cognitive correlates of early abuse. Am. Psychiatr. Assoc. Syllabus Proc. Summary **148:** 113.
7. MACKLIN, M. L. *et al.* 1996. Pre-combat IQ is a vulnerability factor for post traumatic stress disorder. Presented at the 12th Annual Meeting of the International Society for Traumatic Stress Studies. Boston, MA, June 12, 1996.

Application of Computer Methods in the Diagnosis of Posttraumatic Memory Impairment and Changes in Interhemispheric Functional Asymmetry

S. B. TSVETOVSKY [a]

Institute of Traumatology and Orthopaedics
Frunze str. 17
630091 Novosibirsk, Russia

The ability to perceive, process information, and respond correctly to it is affected by both injury and stress caused by the pain syndrome and the circumstances of trauma. Mild head trauma is a model of this situation. To estimate the character and degree of impairments and their dynamics during treatment, computer neuropsychological tests were developed. At relatively short-term examinations they permitted the acquisition of the quantitative characteristics of perception and memory, velocity of neural processes, attention and fatigability, as well as the state of interhemispheric functional brain asymmetry in perceiving and processing nonverbal and verbal visual information.

Tachistoscopic methods were used to test the velocity of response to verbal or nonverbal visual stimuli of the right and left visual hemifield. Programs control the ratio of probability of the appearance of target stimuli, previously reported to the patient, and nontarget stimuli, as well as the equal probability of stimuli exposition in the right and left visual field, that is, addressing the right or left hemisphere. The velocities of reactions to target and irrelevant stimuli are analyzed separately. The mean velocities of reactions, their dispersion, and trend indicators are analyzed, characterizing attention, fatigability, or training. The number and character of mistakes (gaps or false alarms) that the patient makes in the exposition of stimuli in each visual field are defined. The asymmetry coefficients for velocity of responses to target and nontarget stimuli and the ratio of these velocities for each visual field (hemispheres) are calculated. The number and character of mistakes and the differences in the velocities of responses to target and nontarget stimuli reflect the ability to retain and the method of recognition defined by hemisphere specialization. The change in size of target stimuli sets allows us to estimate the velocity of memory access.

In addition to tachistoscopy, special tests were used to estimate operative memory, that is, the ability to retain targeted processing of initially perceived material. Test patients had to deal with consecutively shown pairs of numbers and to recall results

[a]Tel: ++7-(3832)-244-752; fax ++7(3832)-245-570; e-mail: root@niito.nsk.su

after the series ended. Along with a formalized quantitative characteristic of operative memory volume, tests define the indicators of proactive and retroactive interference. In some cases, other tests of short-term memory were used, particularly those of visuospatial memory, and also tests of intellectual activity effectiveness, in which a leading role belongs to either the left or the right hemisphere. For this, tasks on spatial imagination and composing sentences of "unordered" groups of words were used.

The notion of the norm was obtained by examining 162 healthy persons; 134 patients with mild head trauma were examined. In brain concussion, changes in velocity, attention, working capacity, and asymmetry instability registered during the acute period were very informative. In mild cases, when the main factor was stress, most patients had faster responses to testing on days 3-8 than on day 1. The increased instability was more pronounced in responses to stimuli in the right visual field (left hemisphere). Mistakes in recognition became moderately more frequent; however, interhemispheric differences in the types of mistake varied from the norm, with more "false alarms" from the right hemisphere and more "gaps" from the left hemisphere. In the healthy control group, repeat testing in analogous terms revealed less variability in response velocities and complex indicators of interhemispheric asymmetry. In more severe lesions the slow responses did not recover fast. During testing responses often slowed down, indicating fast fatigability or deficit arbitrary attention regulation. The number of mistakes of both types increased significantly. The asymmetry indicators of responses on target and nontarget stimuli varied and differed from the norm. The most invariant in the norm asymmetry manifestations, namely, the hemisphere difference in velocity ratios of the "yes" and "no" responses, varied. In the norm, differences between faster responses to target stimuli and slower ones to nontarget are more pronounced for responses from the right hemisphere than from the left. When the velocity of target stimuli response for the right hemisphere exceeded the velocity of the nontarget response. More frequent than the norm was the general slowing down of responses to target stimuli, the choice difficulty. Responses were more delayed with the increase in target stimuli set size, which shows a slowing down in comparison with information held in memory. The operative memory volume decreased with the increase in proactive interference. In focal lesions of the brain, sharp asymmetry deviations from the norm, memory impairment, and information processing productivity were observed.

Abnormal Cerebral Laterality in Posttraumatic Stress Disorder

FRIEDEMANN GERHARDS,[a,c] RACHEL YEHUDA,[b,d]
MORAN SHOHAM,[a] AND DIRK H. HELLHAMMER [a,e]

[a]Center for Psychobiological and Psychosomatic Research
University of Trier
Gebaeude D, D-54286 Trier, Germany

[b]Mount Sinai Medical School
Psychiatry 116/A
Bronx Veterans Affairs Hospital
New York, New York 10468

Different studies[1,2] have shown evidence of an augmented startle probe reflex in persons with posttraumatic stress disorder (PTSD). In normal subjects a potentiation of the startle probe reflex amplitude has been observed under conditions of negative emotional arousal[3,4] or during shock anticipation.[5] Under conditions without shock anticipation (lack of anticipatory anxiety), the startle response was greater and of shorter latency when the acoustic startle probe stimulus was delivered to the left ear (i.e., right cerebral hemisphere) as opposed to the right ear,[5] whereas under conditions of shock anticipation the right-left difference was in the opposite direction (significant interaction "condition x ear"). These findings suggest that the normally observed right hemispheric dominance of the startle response gets lost under stress; instead, a left hemispheric dominance develops. Other results are in line with this interpretation of a stress-induced abnormal cerebral laterality: under stress the normally observed left hemispheric advantage in processing verbal stimuli gives way to a right hemispheric advantage.[6,7]

Concerning these data it can be hypothesized that subjects with PTSD may show an abnormal cerebral laterality. The hypothesis is supported by data on auditory functions in PTSD subjects[8] showing a more pronounced asymmetry in performance scores for right versus left ear stimulation in PTSD subjects than in controls. Data on auditory probe-evoked potential attenuation as an index of hemispheric activity reported by Schiffer et al.[9] also hint at an abnormal or altered cerebral laterality in PTSD: subjects with a history of childhood trauma were reported to show a significant left dominant asymmetry during neutral memory, which markedly shifted to the right during unpleasant memory, whereas control subjects without childhood trauma did not display a significant asymmetry during either task or a significant shift between tasks.

The present investigation was designed as a pilot study to test the hypothesis of abnormal or altered cerebral laterality in PTSD. Two functions that are dominated

[c]Tel: (+49) 651-9472456; fax: (+49) 651-9462458; e-mail: GERHARDS@UNI-TRIER.DE
[d]Tel: (718) 584-9000; fax: (718) 364 3576; e-mail: YEHUDA.RACHEL@BRONX.VA.GOV
[e]Tel: (+49) 651-2012928; fax: (+49) 651-2012934; e-mail: HELLHAMM@UNI-TRIER.DE

by the right or left cerebral hemisphere in normal right-handed subjects (processing of facially expressed emotions and of verbal stimuli) were investigated. Because both PTSD and cerebral laterality seem to be related to alexithymia,[10,11] the degree of alexithymia was assessed as well.

METHOD

Subjects

Twenty-four male patients of the Mount Sinai Medical School and 24 healthy male (German) persons took part in the study. Among the patients, 19 had a diagnosis of PTSD; the remaining five persons were diagnosed as having a mental disorder other than PTSD.

Procedure and Instruments

All patients took part in two experiments; 14 healthy subjects participated in Experiment I and the remaining 10 took part in Experiment II. In Experiment I, one emotionally neutral face and one face expressing a basic emotion were presented simultaneously (exposition time 150 ms) in subsequent trials. In half the trials the neutral item was presented to the left visual half field (VHF) and the emotional one to the right VHF; in the remaining trials the arrangement was inverse. For each trial, subjects had to decide (by pressing a response key) on which side the emotional face had been presented. In Experiment II a syllable (consonant vowel consonant, cvc; letters arranged horizontally in the conventional manner) was initially presented for 500 ms at the center of a computer monitor. The initial stimulus was followed by the exposition (150 ms) of two vertically arranged syllables (cvc) in capital letters, one of them being presented in the left and the other in the right VHF. In half the trials the left syllable and in the remaining half the right syllable was identical to the one presented before centrally. For each trial, subjects had to decide (by pressing a response key) whether syllable identity was given on the right or the left side. For both experiments the number of hits and the mean reaction time for hits were assessed for target stimulus presentation in the left and right VHF separately. Asymmetry scores for hits and reaction time were computed with the formula: $(R - L)/(R + L)$ or $(L - R)/(R + L)$. A positive score indicates a right hemispheric dominance in processing of facially expressed emotions and a left hemispheric dominance in processing verbal stimuli. Alexithymia was assessed by the 20-item Toronto Alexithymia Scale[12] in the patient groups and in those healthy controls who took part in Experiment I.

RESULTS

The asymmetry scores from Experiment I and II of the PTSD subjects as well as the scores for alexithymia were compared with those of the patients with a diagnosis other than PTSD and with those of the healthy controls nonparametrically (Mann-

Whitney U tests). For processing of facially expressed emotions, there was a tendentiously significant difference between PTSD subjects and healthy controls in reaction time asymmetry (Md: .01 vs −.01; $p = 10$, two-tailed). Whereas the control subjects showed the expected right hemispheric advantage (14.4 ms), PTSD subjects showed a left hemispheric advantage (19.3 ms). There were no significant differences for processing of facially expressed emotions between patients with and those without PTSD. For processing verbal stimuli no significant differences were noted between PTSD subjects and other patients or healthy controls.

Analyses of the data for alexithymia showed significantly higher scores ($p <$ 0.001) in PTSD subjects than in healthy controls (Md: 63 vs 46); the scores of patients with and those without PTSD (Md = 64) were comparable. Correlational analyses (Spearman) on the relation of cerebral laterality and alexithymia revealed that a high degree of alexithymia was associated with a low degree of right hemispheric dominance or even a high degree of left hemispheric dominance (reaction time asymmetry) in processing emotional faces ($R = 0.37$, $p = 0.056$). This correlation was especially high for PTSD subjects ($R = 0.69$, $p = 0.01$). The correlation of alexithymia and the asymmetry scores for processing of verbal stimuli was not significant.

DISCUSSION

The results of the present pilot study are consistent with the hypothesis of an abnormal or altered cerebral laterality in PTSD. In contrast to healthy controls, who showed the expected right hemispheric advantage in processing emotional stimuli, subjects with PTSD showed an abnormal left hemispheric advantage. Additionally, subjects with PTSD showed a much higher degree of alexithymia than did healthy controls. In PTSD subjects the degree of the abnormal functional asymmetry was particularly strongly associated with alexithymia. This finding is consistent with results on conjugate lateral eye movements and alexithymia,[11] suggesting an association of alexithymia with left cerebral lateralization.

Because subjects with a mental disorder other than PTSD were comparable to the PTSD group with respect to cerebral laterality, it is questionable whether abnormal laterality is specific for PTSD. It is well known, for example, that patients with depression show an abnormal pattern of cerebral laterality. Because the diagnoses of the patients without PTSD in this study are unknown and because it is unclear to what extent the PTSD patients might have a comorbid depression, this question cannot be answered from the present study. Further research with well-defined groups is needed.

REFERENCES

1. ORR, S. P. *et al.* 1995. Physiologic responses to loud tones in Vietnam veterans with posttraumatic stress disorder. J. Abnorm. Psychol. **104:** 75–82.
2. SHALEV, A. Y. *et al.* 1992. Physiologic responses to loud tones in Israeli patients with posttraumatic stress disorder. Arch. Gen. Psychiatry **49:** 870–875.
3. BRADLEY, M. M. *et al.* 1991. Startle and emotion: Lateral acoustic probes and the bilateral blink. Psychophysiology **28:** 285–295.

4. COOK, E. W. *et al.* 1991. Affective individual differences and startle reflex modulation. J. Abnorm. Psychol. **100:** 5-13.
5. GRILLON, C. & M. DAVIS. 1995. Acoustic startle and anticipatory anxiety in humans: Effects of monoaural right and left ear stimulation. Psychophysiology **32:** 155-161.
6. ASBJORNSEN, A. *et al.* 1992. Manipulation of subjects level of arousal in dichotic listening. Brain Cognit. **19:** 183-194.
7. GRUZELIER, J. & M. PHELAN. 1991. Stress induced reversal of a lexical divided visual-field asymmetry accompanied by retarded electrodermal habituation. Int. J. Psychophysiol. **11:** 269-276.
8. SHALEV, A. *et al.* 1988. Audiological evaluation of nonalcoholic, drug-free posttraumatic stress disorder patients. Biol. Psychiatry **24:** 522-530.
9. SCHIFFER, F. *et al.* 1995. Evoked potential evidence for right brain activity during the recall of traumatic memories. J. Neuropsychiatry Clin. Neurosci. **7:** 169-175.
10. KRYSTAL, J. H. *et al.* 1986. Assessment of alexithymia in posttraumatic stress disorder and somatic illness: Introduction of a reliable measure. Psychosom. Med. **48:** 84-94.
11. PARKER, J. D. *et al.* 1992. Relationship between conjugate lateral eye movements and alexithymia. Psychother. Psychosom. **57:** 94-101.
12. BAGBY, R. M. *et al.* 1994. The twenty-item Toronto Alexithymia Scale—I. Item selection and cross validation of the factor structure. J. Psychosom. Res. **38:** 23-32.

Startle Deficits in Women with Sexual Assault-Related PTSD

C. A. MORGAN, III, C. GRILLON, H. LUBIN, AND
S. M. SOUTHWICK

Yale University
and
National Center for PTSD
VA Connecticut Medical Center
950 Campbell Ave.
West Haven, CT 06516

The startle reflex, a cross-species response to intense stimuli with abrupt onset, is characterized by considerable plasticity and behavioral flexibility that can be exploited to assess various cognitive, attentional, and sensory processes.[1] In recent years, a growing number of studies have reported on the eye-blink component of the startle response in combat veterans with posttraumatic stress disorder (PTSD).[2-7] However, the extent to which the neurobiologic alterations described in veterans with PTSD can be extended to other populations is currently unknown.

This investigation was designed to assess the acoustic startle response in treatment-seeking women with sexual assault-related PTSD. In this study the eye-blink response was recorded from both eyes because of evidence that lateralized deficits may exist in subjects with PTSD.[8,9]

METHODS

Subjects. Thirteen female civilian subjects with sexual assault-related PTSD (mean age 38.1, SD 7.5) and 16 healthy female civilian comparison subjects (mean age 37.6, SD 10.5) were recruited for this study. Each subject with PTSD met full symptom criteria for PTSD per Structured Clinical Interview for DSM-III-R diagnosis (SCID). Patients with PTSD were also administered the Mississippi PTSD Symptom Scale for civilian trauma.[10] In addition, all subjects were administered the Speilberger State/Trait Anxiety Inventory (STAI).[11]

Startle Testing. The acoustic stimuli were bursts of white noise delivered binaurally through headphones. There were three types of trial: two pulse-alone trials (40-ms duration bursts or white noise at 92 dB[A] and 102 dB[A]) and a prepulse + pulse trial (a 30-ms duration 70 dB[A] white noise delivered 120 ms before the onset of a 40-ms duration 102 dB[A] pulse). The orbicularis oculi electromyographic (EMG) activity was recorded with two disk electrodes (Ag/AgCl) placed below each eye.

RESULTS

TABLE 1 presents magnitude startle data in women with PTSD and in the comparison group. The magnitude of startle to the *first* startle stimulus was asymmetrically

TABLE 1. Mean Magnitude (μV) and Standard Error of Startle in Traumatized Women with PTSD and in the Comparison Group

Group		First	Block 1 92 dB	Block 1 102 dB	Block 2 92 dB	Block 2 102 dB
Comparison Group						
	Left	210.6	64.9	103.2	49.9	93.5
		(38.5)	(21.4)	(28.6)	(16.6)	(23.3)
	Right	214.4	68.6	115.2	53.9	93.0
		(42.8)	(23.8)	(33.1)	(24.5)	(17.9)
PTSD Group						
	Left	229.8	134.4	227.6	77.9	177.4
		(35.1)	(26.8)	(34.4)	(21.1)	(37.3)
	Right	178.7	103.2	166.3	58.2	147.9
		(33.2)	(19.0)	(25.6)	(12.3)	(31.3)

TABLE 2. Results of the Four-Way Interaction (Group $\times$ Eye $\times$ Block $\times$ Intensity of the Magnitude) Startle Data

Effects	df	E	p
Group	1,27	2.8	NS
Group $\times$ Eye	1,27	7.7	0.01
Group $\times$ Block	1,27	6.0	0.02
Group $\times$ Intensity	1,27	6.7	0.01
Group $\times$ Eye $\times$ Block	1,27	8.5	0.007
Group $\times$ Eye $\times$ Intensity	1,27	3.7	0.06
Group $\times$ Block $\times$ Intensity	1,27	0.5	NS
Group $\times$ Eye $\times$ Block $\times$ Intensity	1,27	6.6	0.01

distributed in the PTSD subjects but not in the comparison subjects. This was reflected by a significant Group X Eye of Recording interaction ($F(1,27) = 4.3$, $p < 0.04$) which was due to the greater magnitude of startle over the left eye than the right eye in PTSD subjects only (PTSD: $F(1,12) = 6.0$, $p < 0.03$; comparison subjects: NS).

TABLE 2 shows the results of the four-way ANOVA of the magnitude startle data. Although the overall magnitude of startle was not significantly greater in PTSD subjects than in comparison subjects, significant group differences were reflected by several significant interactions with the factor group, including four-way interaction.

These interactions were due to the fact that the magnitude of startle was lateralized (left > right) in PTSD patients ($F(1,12) = 7.79$, $p < 0.01$) but not in comparison ($F(1,16) = 0.002$) subjects. As a result, the magnitude of startle was greater in the PTSD group than in the comparison group over the left eye than the right. In addition, this laterality was affected by the intensity of the startle stimulus and the block of stimulus delivery. It tended to be greater after the more intense startle stimulus and in block 1. Posthoc group comparison for each trial in each block indicated that startle magnitude was greater in PTSD patients than in comparison subjects only over the left eye in response to the 102-dB startle stimuli in blocks 1 (t(27) = 2.8, $p < 0.009$) and 2 (t(27) = 2.0, $p < 0.05$) and in response to the 92-dB startle stimuli in block 1 (t(27) = 2.0, $p < 0.05$). The prepulse inhibition effect was not lateralized and did not differ significantly between the two groups.

Effects of Time since Trauma. The patient group demonstrated a bimodal distribution in the time elapsed since the index trauma (range 2-6 years and 10-27 years). Individuals whose index trauma fell within the last 6 years (mean = 3.73, SD 1.97 years) were identified as the "recent" trauma group, and they were compared to the "long-standing" trauma group whose index trauma occurred more than 10 years (mean = 16.16 years, SD 6.17 years) prior to testing. The two groups did not significantly differ in age (recent trauma group: 38.8 years, SD 8.3 years; long-standing trauma group: 37.6 years, SD, 7.3 years).

The two PTSD groups were compared using the same ANOVAs as just described. There was a differential group asymmetry of the magnitude of startle to the *first* pulse-alone trial (Group X Eye of Recording: F(1,11) = 5.6, $p < 0.03$). This interaction was due to the greater magnitude of startle over the left eye (272.4 µV, SE 47.7 µV) than the right (182.0 µV, SE 44.6 µV) in the recent but not the long-standing trauma group (180.1 µV, SE 48.2 µV vs 174.9 µV, SE 54.3 µV). There was also a trend for the magnitude of eye blink recorded during the two blocks of pulse-alone trials to be differentially distributed over the two eyes in the recent and long-standing trauma groups (Group X Eye of Recording: F(1,11) = 3.0, $p = 0.11$). In the recent trauma group, the overall magnitude of eye blink was significantly greater over the left eye (175.2 µV, SE 48.1 µV) than the right (120.2 µV, SE 54.3 µV) eye (t(6) = 2.5, $p < 0.04$). In the long-standing trauma group, no significant difference was noted between the left (129.9 µV, SE 31.0 µV) and the right (117.4 µV, SE 28.1 µV) eye.

When compared to the comparison group, only the recent trauma group showed significant differences in startle reactivity. A differential group asymmetry of eye-blink magnitude was noted (first trial: F(1,21) = 8.7, $p < 0.008$; two blocks of trials: F(1,21) = 10.8, $p < 0.003$). Although the overall magnitude of startle tended to be greater in the recent trauma group than in the comparison group (F(1,21) = 2.6, $p = 0.12$), a greater difference was found over the left eye (t(21) = 2.1, $p < 0.04$).

DISCUSSION

This study provides the first objective evidence of acoustic startle deficits in women with PTSD. In addition, these findings add to the growing body of evidence for exaggerated acoustic startle in PTSD and suggest that some similarities in pathophysiology may exist in women and men with the disorder. The significantly greater startle responses over the left eye than the right in PTSD subjects suggest a laterality effect. Bremner *et al.*[23,24] reported decreased *right* hippocampal volume in male veterans with PTSD and decreased *left* hippocampal volume in civilian women with PTSD.

Coover and Levine[12] reported that lesions of the rat hippocampus may lead to an increase in startle. Therefore, it is conceivable that the exaggerated startle seen over the *left* eye in women with PTSD may be due to left-sided hippocampal deficits, the effects of which on the startle response are exhibited through the ipsilaterally innervated (cranial nerve VII) left orbicularis oculi muscle.

Preclinical investigations in the rat indicate that unconditioned sensitization of the startle response can be observed for a long time following shock administration.[13] The amygdala is critically involved in shock sensitization of startle.[14] In a subgroup of individuals with PTSD, repeated exposure to trauma or a single intense trauma may sensitize startle. Startle sensitization, however, should dissipate with time after the traumatic event. In aplysia, short-term sensitization generally fades within 1 hour, but severe or repeated intense stress leads to more durable increases in reactivity.[15] This model may hold true in humans and is supported by findings of increased startle in the PTSD subjects of the "recent" than of the "long-standing" trauma group.

REFERENCES

1. DAVIS, M. 1984. The mammalian startle response. *In* Neural Mechanisms of Startle Behavior. R. C. Eaton, Ed.: 287–351. Plenum Press. New York.
2. SHALEV, A. Y., S. P. ORR, T. PERI, S. SCHREIBER & R. K. PITMAN. 1992. Physiologic responses to loud tones in Israeli patients with posttraumatic stress disorder. Arch. Gen. Psychiatry **49:** 870–875.
3. BUTLER, R. W., D. L. BRAFF, J. L. RAUSCH, M. A. JENKINS, J. SPROCK & M. A. GEYER. 1990. Physiological evidence of exaggerated startle response in a subgroup of Vietnam veterans with combat related PTSD. Am. J. Psychiatry **147:** 1308–1312.
4. GRILLON, C., C. A. MORGAN, III, M. DAVIS & D. S. CHARNEY. 1996. Baseline startle and prepulse inhibition in Vietnam combat veterans with PTSD. Psychiatry Res. **64:** 169–178.
5. ORR, S. P., R. K. PITMAN & A. Y. SHALEV. 1995. Physiologic responses to loud tones in Vietnam veterans with posttraumatic stress disorder. J. Abnorm. Psychol. **104:** 75–82.
6. ORNITZ, E. M. & R. S. PYNOOS. 1989. Startle modulation in children with posttraumatic stress disorder. Am. J. Psychiatry **146:** 866–870.
7. MORGAN, C. A., C. GRILLON, M. DAVIS, S. M. SOUTHWICK & D. S. CHARNEY. 1996. Exaggerated acoustic startle in Desert Storm Veterans with post traumatic stress disorder. Am. J. Psychiatry **153:** 64–68.
8. BREMNER, J. D., P. RANDALL, T. M. SCOTT, R. A. BRONEN, J. P. SEIBYL, S. M. SOUTHWICK, R. C. DELANEY, G. MCCARTHY, D. S. CHARNEY & R. B. INNIS. 1995. MRI-based measurement of hippocampal volume in combat-related posttraumatic stress disorder. Am. J. Psychiatry **152:** 973–981.
9. BREMNER, J. D., P. RANDALL, E. VERMETTEN, L. STAIB, R. A. BRONEN, S. CAPELLI, G. MCCARTHY, R. B. INNIS & D. S. CHARNEY. 1996. MRI-based measurement of hippocampal volume in posttraumatic stress disorder related to childhood physical and sexual abuse: A preliminary report. Biol. Psychiatry, in press.
10. KEANE, T. M., J. M. CADDELL & K. L. TAYLOR. 1988. Mississippi Scale for combat-related posttraumatic stress disorder: Three studies in reliability and validity. J. Consult. Clin. Psychol. **56:** 85–90.
11. SPEILBERGER, C. D. 1983. Manual for the State-Trait Anxiety Inventory. Consulting Psychologist Press. Palo Alto, CA.
12. COOVER, G. D. & S. LEVINE. 1972. Auditory startle response of hippocampectomized rats. Physiol. Behav. **9:** 75–78.

13. HITCHCOCK, J. M., C. B. SANANES & M. DAVIS. 1989. Sensitization of the startle reflex by footshock: Blockade by lesions of the central nucleus of the amygdala or its efferent pathway to the brainstem. Behav. Neurosci, **103:** 509-518.
14. SANANES, C. B. & M. DAVIS. 1992. *N*-Methyl-D-Aspartate lesions of the lateral and basolateral nuclei of the amygdala block fear-potentiated startle and shock sensitization of startle. Behav. Neurosci, **106:** 72-80.
15. GOELET, P. & E. R. KANDEL. 1986. Tracking the flow of learned information from membrane receptors to genome. TINS **9:** 492-499.

Psychophysiologic Assessment of PTSD in Adult Females Sexually Abused during Childhood[a]

SCOTT P. ORR, NATASHA B. LASKO,
LINDA J. METZGER, NANCY J. BERRY,
CARYL E. AHERN, AND ROGER K. PITMAN

Veterans Affairs Research Service
228 Maple Street, 2nd Floor
Manchester, New Hampshire 03103

Department of Psychiatry
Harvard Medical School
Boston, Massachusetts 02115

Previous studies have shown that individuals with posttraumatic stress disorder (PTSD) have heightened physiologic responses to cues reminiscent of traumatic experiences compared to individuals who never had PTSD.[1,2] The present study used psychophysiology to measure adult females' emotional responses during imagery of personal childhood sexual abuse experiences.

METHODS

Seventy-one women able to recount two or more penetrative episodes of sexual abuse prior to age 13 were classified via the Structured Clinical Interview for DSM-III-R[3] into Current ($n = 29$), Lifetime ($n = 24$), or Never ($n = 18$) PTSD groups. Information on whether abuse memories were recovered or continuous was also obtained. Using a script-driven imagery technique,[4,5] participants were asked to imagine personal and hypothetical experiences as vividly as possible while heart rate (HR), skin conductance (SC), and lateral frontalis (LF) and corrugator (C) electromyograms (EMGs) were recorded. Response scores were calculated for each physiologic dependent variable by subtracting the preceding baseline value from the mean level during imagery. Scripts were rated by experts for event severity on 0-12 scales. A discriminant function derived from the HR, SC, and LF-EMG responses during personal traumatic imagery of previously studied individuals ($n = 96$) with and without PTSD[4-7] was used to classify physiologic responses of participants.

[a]This project was supported by Department of Veterans Affairs Merit Review grants (to S. O. and R. P.) and National Institute of Mental Health grant RO1MH48559-01A2.

RESULTS

The Current group scored higher on measures of PTSD symptoms and general psychopathology, had higher expert-rated severities for the abuse experiences, and had higher resting HR levels than those of the Never group. MANOVA revealed a significant group difference for averaged physiologic (HR, SC, LF-EMG, and C-EMG) responses during abuse imagery ($F(4,66) = 3.3$, $p = 0.02$, Roy's Greatest Root) but not during nonabuse stressful imagery ($F(4,66) < 1$). The Current group produced larger HR responses during abuse imagery than those of the Lifetime and Never groups and larger C-EMG responses than those of the Never group. Responses of the Lifetime group tended to fall between those of the Current and Never groups. Resting levels and response magnitudes of medicated and unmedicated Current PTSD participants did not differ. Application of the discriminant function to the HR, SC, and LF-EMG responses (average of two abuse experiences) resulted in 19 of 29 Current (sensitivity = 66%), 10 of 24 Lifetime, and 4 of 18 Never (specificity = 78%) participants being classified as "physiologic responders." The numbers of individuals classified as physiologic responders differed significantly across groups (chi-square = 8.7, $df = 2$, $p = 0.01$). Within the Current PTSD group, responders had higher Clinician-Administered PTSD Scale scores (M = 63.2) than nonresponders (M = 41.0; $t(23) = 2.4$, $p = 0.03$, $n = 25$).

Seventeen participants (10 Current, 6 Lifetime, and 1 Never) had recovered sexual abuse memories. The relation between memory continuity and PTSD status was marginally significant (chi-square = 5.1, $df = 2$, $p = 0.08$). Among PTSD participants, those with recovered memories reported significantly more symptoms than did those with continuous memories on the Impact of Event (M = 50.4 vs M = 33.2, $t(27) = 2.5$, $p = 0.02$) and Mississippi (M = 129.4 vs M = 112.8, $t(27) = 2.0$, $p = .05$) Scales. Magnitudes of physiologic responses during personal abuse imagery did not differ between the two subgroups.

CONCLUSIONS

Women with current PTSD resulting from childhood sexual abuse had higher resting HR levels and showed larger physiologic responses during imagery of their abuse experiences than did women who never had PTSD. These findings are consistent with those from previous psychophysiologic studies of PTSD, provide validation for the PTSD diagnosis in individuals who experienced sexual abuse during childhood, and support the pathogenic role of these experiences. Nearly half the participants with lifetime PTSD continued to have heightened physiologic responses despite only mild symptoms, suggesting that symptomatic remission does not necessarily involve extinction of the conditioned emotional response to reminders of the traumatic event. The results also suggest that PTSD associated with continuous or recovered memories is comparable.

REFERENCES

1. ORR, S. P. 1994. An overview of psychophysiological studies of PTSD. PTSD Res. Q. **5:** 1–7.

2. KEANE, T. M., L. C. KOLB, D. G. KALOUPEK, S. P. ORR, R. G. THOMAS, F. HSIEH & P. LAVORI. 1997. Results of a multisite clinical trial on the psychophysiological assessment of posttraumatic stress disorder. Submitted.
3. SPITZER, R. L., J. B. WILLIAMS, M. GIBBON & M. B. FIRST. 1990. Structured Clinical Interview for DSM-III-R—Non-Patient Edition (SCID-NP, Version 1.0). American Psychiatric Press. Washington, DC.
4. ORR, S. P., R. K. PITMAN, N. B. LASKO & L. R. HERZ. 1993. Psychophysiologic assessment of posttraumatic stress disorder imagery in World War II and Korean combat veterans. J. Abnorm. Psychol. **102:** 152-159.
5. PITMAN, R. K., S. P. ORR, D. F. FORGUE, J. B. DE JONG & J. M. CLAIBORN. 1987. Psychophysiologic assessment of posttraumatic stress disorder imagery in Vietnam combat veterans. Arch. Gen. Psychiatry **44:** 970-975.
6. PITMAN, R. K., S. P. ORR, D. F. FORGUE, B. ALTMAN, J. B. DE JONG & L. R. HERZ. 1990. Psychophysiologic responses to combat imagery of Vietnam veterans with post-traumatic stress disorder versus other anxiety disorders. J. Abnorm. Psychol. **99:** 49-54.
7. SHALEV, A. Y., S. P. ORR & R. K. PITMAN. 1993. Psychophysiologic assessment of traumatic imagery in Israeli civilian post-traumatic stress disorder patients. Am. J. Psychiatry **150:** 620-624.

Interest of Events-Related Potentials in Assessment of Posttraumatic Stress Disorder

M. BOUDARENE AND M. TIMSIT-BERTHIER [a]

Laboratoire de Psychophysiologie Cognitive Appliquee
84 rue du Pr Mahaim
Liège 4000, Belgium

The aim of the current study was to assess posttraumatic stress disorder (PTSD) using conjointly P300 and contingent negative variation (CNV). These events-related potentials (ERPs) are obtained in recording EEG from subjects submitted to cognitive tasks. They are related to both cognitive and emotional factors; more precisely, P300 is related to "context updating" and to working memory,[1] whereas CNV is influenced by attention, motivation, and motor preparation.[2] Moreover, they are modulated by cholinergic, GABAergic, and noradrenergic systems[3,4] that are also implied in the frontal defense system.[5]

These ERPs have been studied extensively in schizophrenia and depression (reviewed in ref. 4), but still now, few publications have been dedicated to stress processes.[6–9]

METHODOLOGY

Subjects

Nineteen patients (10 females) aged 40 ± 9 years with PTSD according to DSM-IV criteria were tested at least 10 months after their traumatic events. Thirty-five paid subjects (18 females) aged 40 ± 10 years selected on the basis of life events scale score served as controls. They were submitted to life events (Amiel-Lebigre) scale, Spielberger Anxiety Scale (STAI), and Plutchik and Van Praag Depression Scale (PVP) testing. According to their scores on life events scale, they were split into two subgroups, group A (17 subjects, 9 females, aged 38 ± 10 years) with numerous life events (impact score >200) and group B (18 subjects, 9 females, aged 42 ± 10 years) without life events (impact score <200).

Neurophysiological Assessment

P300. Subjects listened to a series of tone bursts occurring every 1,000 ms. The tones were either "low" (800 Hz) and "standard" (80%) or either "high" (1,470

[a]Tel: 32/4/254/77/18-19; fax: 32/4/254/77/18.

TABLE 1. Comparison between PTSD Group and Two Control Groups

A. Psychological Data

	PTSD (n = 19)	Group A (n = 18)	Group B (n = 17)	Difference (F. Test, DF = 2)
Anxiety state (Spielberger)	59 ± 13	34 ± 8	28 ± 6	p = 0.0001
Anxiety trait (Spielberger)	60 ± 8	36 ± 11	34 ± 7	p = 0.0001
Depression (Plutchik-Van Praag)	35 ± 16	14 ± 7	4 ± 4	p = 0.0001

B. Behavioral and Neurophysiological Data

	PTSD (n = 19)	Group A (n = 18)	Group B (n = 17)	Difference (F. Test, DF = 2)
R. Time CNV	446 ± 179	250 ± 57	232 ± 36	p = 0.0001
P3 Ampl. (P3a Fz)	6 ± 4	12 ± 6	9 ± 4	p = 0.0004
(P3b Fz)	7 ± 6	15 ± 6	11 ± 4	p = 0.0001
CNV Ampl. Cz				
Early	6 ± 5	11 ± 6	14 ± 7	p = 0.0009
Late	8 ± 4	16 ± 7	20 ± 6	p = 0.0001

Hz) and "target" (20%). The subject's task was to respond to targets by pressing a button. The EEG was recorded from Fz, Cz, and Pz, referred to linked earlobes, and was sampled for 1 second beginning 100 ms prior to the onset of the tone, at a rate of 1,024 Hz. Only the free-artefacted cortical responses evoked by the well-discriminated tones were averaged and analyzed (30 trials). Amplitude and latency of P3a and P3b were measured between 230 and 600 ms after the target stimulus. Reaction time and the number of correct responses were also measured.

Contingent Negative Variation (CNV). Subjects were submitted to a warning stimulus (S1 = 1,000 Hz, 50-ms duration tone) followed 1 second later by light flashes (S2) that the subject had to stop by pushing a button. Stimuli presentations were separated by pseudorandom intertrial intervals ranging from 7 to 25 seconds. Subjects were instructed to keep their eyes closed during all ERP recording sessions to minimize eyes artefact. The EEG was recorded from Fz and Cz referred to linked earlobes, sampled for 4 seconds, beginning 100 ms prior to S1, at a rate of 256 Hz and averaged (32 trials). Both early (500-700 ms after S1) and late (800-1,000 ms after S1) CNV components were measured. Reaction time was also measured.

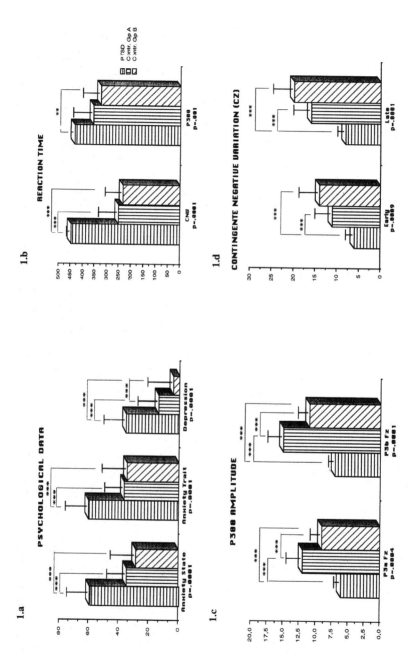

FIGURE 1. (a) In all psychological data, PTSD shows higher results than those of the two control groups. **(b)** In CNV paradigm, PTSD patients display a longer reaction time than do control subjects. **(c)** P300 amplitudes are the smallest in the PTSD group, whereas they are highest in control group A. **(d)** PTSD group displays the lowest CNV amplitude.

Data Analysis

Separate one-way analyses of variance (patients vs A and B controls) were computed for psychological data, reaction time, P3a and P3b amplitudes and latencies, and early and late CNV amplitude.

RESULTS

PTSD patients displayed the highest scores on the anxiety and depressive scales. Moreover, they had longer reaction times and lower CNV and P300 amplitude than did control subjects. These differences are illustrated by TABLE 1 and FIGURE 1. Interestingly, controls with numerous life events (group A) displayed the highest P300 amplitude.

DISCUSSION AND CONCLUSION

PTSD, as generalized anxiety and a subgroup of depressive disorders, exhibited a slow reaction time and a decreased ERP amplitude (P300 as well as CNV). These results may be related to the lack of motivational and emotional involvement in experimental protocols and fit well with the predominance of avoidance and numbing symptoms that characterize this disease.[10]

As CNV and P300 amplitudes are modulated by frontal noradrenergic processes related to the cerebral defense system,[5] such data could imply a weakness of catecholaminergic system mobilization in PTSD. Conversely, data from controls submitted to numerous life events suggest catecholaminergic hyperreactivity associated with hyperarousal. These data can be compared to those of in controls who displayed a very high CNV amplitude immediately after acute stress.[6]

CNV and P300 may be useful in assessing the dynamics of the cerebral defense system after stressful events.

REFERENCES

1. DONCHIN, E. & M. G. H. COLES. 1988. Is the P300 component a manifestation of context updating? *In* Behavioral and Brain Sciences. Vol. 11, No. 3. Cambridge University Press.
2. TECCE, J. J. & L. CATTANACH. 1993. Contingent negative variation (CNV). *In* Electroencephalography: Basic Principles, Clinical Applications and Related Fields, 3rd Ed. E. Nierdermeyer & F. Lopes da Silva, Eds. Williams & Wilkins. Baltimore.
3. MARCZYNSKI, T. J. 1993. Neurochemical interpretations of cortical slow potentials as they relate to cognitive processes and a parsimonious model of mammalian brain. *In* Slow Potentials Changes in the Human Brain. W. C. Mc Callum & S. H. Curry, Eds. Plenum Press. New York.
4. BIRBAUMER, N., T. ELBERT, A. CANAVAN & B. ROCKSTROH. 1990. Slow potentials of the cerebral cortex and behaviour. Physiol. Rev. **70:** 1-41.
5. SKINNER, J. E. 1985. The regulation of cardiac vulnerability by the cerebral defense system. J. Am. Coll. Cardiol. **5:** 88B-94B.
6. GLANZMANN P. & W. D. FROEHLICH. 1984. Anxiety, stress and contingent negative variation reconsidered. Ann. N.Y. Acad. Sci. **425:** 578-584.

7. Mc FARLANE, A. C., D. L. WEBER & C. R. CLARK. 1993. Abnormal stimulus in posttraumatic stress disorder. Biol. Psychiatry **34:** 311–320.
8. TIMSIT-BERTHIER, M. 1993. Contingent negative variation and its relationships to arousal and stress in psychopathology. *In* Slow Potential Changes in the Human Brain. W. C. Mc Callum & S. H. Curry, Eds. Plenum Press. New York.
9. CHARLES, G., M. HANSENNE, M. ANSSEAU, W. PITCHOT, R. MACHOWSKI, M. SCHITTECATE & J. WILMOTTE. 1995. P300 in posttraumatic stress disorder. Biol. Psychiatr. Neuropsychobiol. **32:** 72–74.
10. FOA, E. B., D. S. RIGGS & B. S. GERSHUNY. 1995. Arousal, numbing, and intrusion: Symptom structure of PTSD following assault. Am. J. Psychiatry **152:** 1.
11. ROCKSTROH, B. & W. C. Mc CALLUM. 1993. Theories and Significance of SPs. *In* Slow Potentials Changes in the Human Brain. W. C. Mc Callum & S. H. Curry, Eds. Plenum Press. New York.
12. TIMSIT-BERTHIER, M. & M. BOUDARENE. 1996. Effects of Natural Stressors on ERPs (CNV and P300). Presented at the 6th International Conference on Cognitive Neurosis (ICON IV). Azilomar, May–June, 1996.

Evidence for Diminished P3 Amplitudes in PTSD[a]

LINDA J. METZGER, SCOTT P. ORR,
NATASHA B. LASKO, NANCY J. BERRY, AND
ROGER K. PITMAN

Department of Psychiatry
Harvard Medical School
Boston, Massachusetts 02115

Research Service
VA Medical Center
Manchester, New Hampshire 03103

Abnormal auditory event-related brain potentials (ERPs) have been demonstrated in two different posttraumatic stress disorder (PTSD) populations. In the context of a three-tone "oddball" task, a mixed trauma group with PTSD had delayed N2 latencies and smaller P3 amplitudes to target and distractor tones compared to matched controls and were slower to make button-press responses to target tones.[1] The finding of smaller P3 amplitudes to target tones was replicated in assault victims with PTSD using a two-tone oddball paradigm, but other potential ERP or performance abnormalities were not explored.[2] Reduced P3 amplitude is the most robust ERP abnormality reported for clinical populations and has been interpreted as reflecting a deficit in the amount of attentional resources allocated during stimulus evaluation and memory updating processes. It has been proposed that this ERP abnormality in PTSD may index the disturbed concentration found in this disorder.[1] The goal of the present research was to examine the generalizability of abnormal ERPs in PTSD by attempting to extend these findings to Vietnam combat veterans and women sexually abused during childhood.

METHOD

Participants were 35 Vietnam combat veterans (PTSD = 25; non-PTSD = 10) and 17 women sexually abused during childhood (PTSD = 9; non-PTSD = 8). Sixteen of the veterans with PTSD were on a psychotropic medication. Because medication has sometimes been shown to normalize ERPs in other clinical disorders, data from these participants (med-PTSD) were analyzed separately. Data from individuals with comorbid panic disorder were not included on the basis of findings of larger P3 amplitudes in this clinical group. All participants underwent a structured diagnostic interview and psychometric testing and completed the auditory "oddball" task[3] which

[a] This research was supported by National Institute of Mental Health postdoctoral Research Fellowship Award 5F32MH10315 and RO1 Award (RO1MH48559) and by VA Merit Review Grants.

requires the detection of infrequent target tones embedded in a series of equally infrequent distractor and frequent common tones. Reaction time to targets (measured via button press) and the numbers of correct responses and false alarms were recorded.

Electroencephalographic activity was recorded from the midline frontal (Fz), central (Cz), and parietal (Pz) sites. Peak and latency measures for the ERP components N1, P2, and P3 were determined from each participant's averaged waveforms, and N2 measures from target-common and distractor-common difference waveforms, for each tone using an automated scoring program.

RESULTS

Age, psychometric, and behavioral data are presented in TABLE 1. There were no group differences in the speed or accuracy of behavioral responses to target stimuli, indicating that the PTSD and non-PTSD groups performed the task comparably well.

All group ERP effects were limited to P3 amplitude differences at Pz. As evident in FIGURE 1, veteran groups differed in their P3 amplitude to target tones ($F (2, 32) = 3.2, p = 0.05$); planned pairwise comparisons indicated significantly ($p < 0.05$) smaller P3 amplitudes in PTSD (M = 7.5, SD = 4.1) than in both med-PTSD (M = 12.4, SD = 6.3) and non-PTSD (M = 13.6, SD = 5.2) veterans. Similarly, for the women sexually abused during childhood, P3 amplitudes to target tones were smaller ($t (15) = 1.7, p = 0.05$; one-tailed) in the PTSD (M = 15.0, SD = 5.3) than in the non-PTSD group ($M = 19.3$, SD = 4.9). Women with PTSD (M = 10.3, SD = 4.4) also had significantly smaller P3 amplitudes to distractor tones compared to women without PTSD (M = 14.7, SD = 5.2; $t (15) = -1.9, p = 0.04$; one-tailed).

DISCUSSION

Present findings replicated diminished P3 amplitudes in two additional PTSD populations. Vietnam combat veterans and women sexually abused during childhood with PTSD had smaller parietal P3 amplitudes to target tones compared to trauma-matched participants without PTSD. The women with PTSD also had significantly smaller parietal P3 amplitudes to distractor tones. The present studies did not replicate findings of longer N2 latencies and reaction times as observed in a mixed trauma group with PTSD.[1] The findings of diminished P3 amplitudes across PTSD trauma populations suggest the existence of a general information processing abnormality in this disorder and may reflect attention or concentration difficulties. The absence of ERP differences between medicated PTSD veterans and non-PTSD veterans, despite the paradoxically higher levels of self-reported PTSD symptoms in this group, suggests that medication may normalize ERPs and possibly restore some cognitive functions. Future studies should employ more cognitively demanding tasks in search of a behavioral or performance correlate of reduced P3 amplitude. Additionally, alternative explanations for this ERP abnormality that consider possible underlying emotional, motivational, or neuropsychological deficits should be explored.

TABLE 1. Group Mean (SD) Age, Psychometric, and Performance Data, with Statistical Results

Vietnam Veterans	Non-PTSD (n, n = 10)		PTSD (P, n = 9)		Med-PTSD (M, n = 16)		F	df	p	Tukey's Tests[a]
Age (yr)	50.9	(3.2)	47.7	(3.7)	46.9	(2.5)	5.7	2,32	.008	N > P,M
Total CAPS Score	7.4	(9.4)	61.6	(18.2)	73.5	(20.5)	45.2	2,29	.0001	N < P,M
Mississippi Scale	67.8	(18.3)	112.4	(19.5)	127.2	(16.4)	38.4	2,32	.0001	N < P < M
Reaction time to targets (ms)	541	(153)	457	(93)	472	(111)	1.2	2,30	.30	—
Correct responses to target stimuli	38.4	(4.6)	39.1	(2.3)	39.7	(0.6)	<1	2,28	ns	—
Incorrect responses to distractor stimuli	1.2	(1.7)	1.3	(1.5)	1.7	(2.6)	<1	2,28	ns	—
Incorrect responses to common stimuli	2.9	(3.7)	6.8	(13.5)	4.9	(7.7)	<1	2,28	ns	—

Women Sexually Abused during Childhood	Non-PTSD (n = 8)		PTSD (n = 9)		T	df	p
Age (yr)	34.1	(7.6)	39.2	(10.8)	1.1	15	.28
Total CAPS score	14.0	(18.2)	47.2	(16.5)	3.9	15	.001
Mississippi Scale	57.3	(39.2)	103.5	(25.1)	2.8	14	.01
Reaction time to targets (ms)	469	(79.1)	489	(102.7)	<1	15	ns
Correct responses to target stimuli	40.0	(0)	39.6	(.7)	1.7	15	.11
Incorrect responses to distractor stimuli	.3	(.5)	1.6	(2.7)	1.4	15	.19
Incorrect responses to common stimuli	.8	(.7)	.4	(1.1)	<1	15	ns

[a] Letters indicate group comparisons for which p < .05.

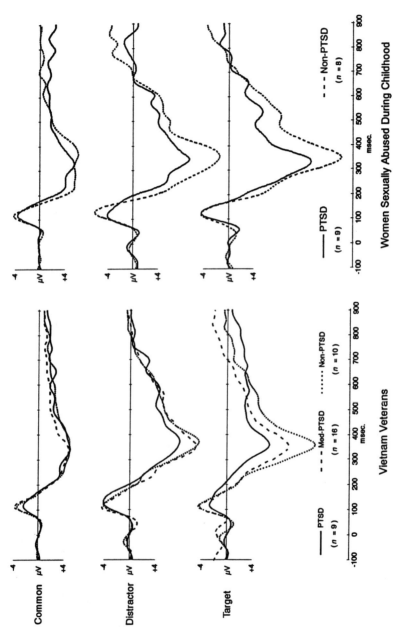

FIGURE 1. Group grand average waveforms at the parietal (Pz) site.

REFERENCES

1. McFarlane A. C., D. L. Weber & C. R. Clark. 1993. Abnormal stimulus processing in post-traumatic stress disorder. Biol. Psychiatry **34:** 311-320.
2. Charles, G., M. Hansenne, M. Ansseau, W. Pitchot, R. Machowski, M. Schittecatte & J. Wilmotte. 1995. P300 in posttraumatic stress disorder. Neuropsychobiology **32:** 72-74.
3. Pfefferbaum A., J. M. Ford, B. G. Wenegrat, W. T. Roth & B. S. Kopell. 1984. Clinical application of the P3 component of event-related potentials. I. Normal aging. Electroencephal. Clin. Neurophysiol. **59:** 85-103.

Electrophysiology of Combat-Related PTSD

JOHN KOUNIOS,[a,c] BRETT LITZ,[b]
DANNY KALOUPEK,[b] DAVID RIGGS,[b] JEFF KNIGHT,[b]
FRANK WEATHERS,[b] JANE E. ANDERSON,[b] AND
TERENCE KEANE [b]

[a]Department of Psychology
University of Pennsylvania
3815 Walnut St.
Philadelphia, Pennsylvania 19104–6196

[b]National Center for PTSD
Boston Veterans Affairs Medical Center (116B-2)
150 S. Huntington Ave.
Boston, Massachusetts 02130

One technique that has been applied to the study of posttraumatic stress disorder (PTSD) is the measurement of event-related brain potentials (ERPs).[1] ERPs are measured by scalp-electrode recordings of a subject's electroencephalogram during performance of a task involving discrete stimulus and/or response events. Segments of the electroencephalogram following presentations of members of a class of stimuli are averaged, yielding a wave depicting the brain's average electrical response to that stimulus class. Analyzing the temporal information given by the positive and negative deflections of such a wave and the spatial information provided by an array of electrodes distributed across the scalp yields valuable neurophysiological and functional-anatomical information.[2]

We explored the neurophysiology of PTSD by measuring ERPs while patients and control subjects viewed threatening and relatively nonthreatening words. In particular, we examined differences between patients and controls that could elucidate whether PTSD is best characterized as an exaggerated neural response specifically to trauma-related stimuli or a general disorder characterized by aberrant brain responses to all stimuli.

Sixteen male, right-handed, native English-speaking, Vietnam-era combat veterans participated. Eight were diagnosed with PTSD; the others were well-adjusted veterans (WAV). ERPs were measured with 64 tin electrodes mounted in an elastic cap (referenced to the left mastoid). The stimuli were a sequence of words displayed on a monitor. There were three blocks of words, each consisting of 45 "trauma" words (related to combat experiences in Vietnam, e.g., grenade), 45 comparatively neutral "nontrauma" words (related to school experiences, e.g., pencil), and 18

[c]Address for correspondence: John Kounios, Ph.D., Department of Psychology, University of Pennsylvania, 3815 Walnut St., Philadelphia, PA 19104-6196 (tel: (215)573-5767; e-mail: jkounios @cattell.psych.upenn.edu).

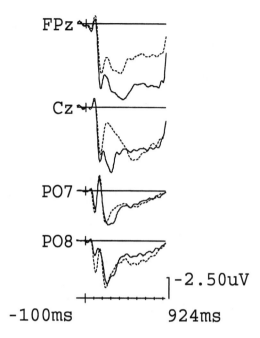

FIGURE 1. Event-related brain potentials (ERPs) for PTSD and WAV subjects averaged across blocks and stimulus types (with negative voltages plotted up; time from left to right; PTSD ERPs as *solid lines;* WAVs as *dashed lines.*

infrequent target food words (e.g., bread), all intermixed in random order. The three blocks used the same trauma and neutral words intermixed with new food words (in a new random order).

Subjects fixated at a "+" sign at the center of the screen. On each trial, this fixation mark was replaced by a word for 2,000 ms. This was followed by the reinstatement of the fixation mark for 2,000 ms. followed by the next word, etc. Their task was to press a button with the index finger of their right hand whenever the displayed word was a type of food and to do nothing if the word was not a food.

Subjects' EEG's were amplified (50,000×), digitized at 250 Hz, and recorded continuously. ERPs were computed by averaging (separately for each block and type of stimulus) 1,048-ms segments of artifact-free EEG beginning 100 ms prior to stimulus onset. The results reported focus on major differences between the ERPs of PTSD and WAV participants in response to the trauma and nontrauma stimuli.

One finding concerns an early positive deflection in the ERP peaking at 120 ms (i.e., P1) and focused bilaterally over left (PO7) and right (PO8) parietooccipital electrode sites. FIGURE 1 shows this deflection averaged across blocks and stimulus types (with negative voltages plotted up; time from left to right; PTSD ERPs as solid lines, WAVs as dashed). Although the amplitude of this component was not reliably influenced by repetition or stimulus types, there was a clear difference between the PTSD patients and WAVs. Specifically, P1 amplitude did not differ reliably across groups over the left posterior cortex (site PO7), but it was diminished over the homologous right hemisphere area (PO8) for the PTSD patients relative to the WAVs.

P1 has been the focus of studies of attention in normal subjects which suggest that this wave is generated in ventrolateral extrastriate cortex (probably the fusiform gyrus) and is associated with a gain-control mechanism that regulates the amount of visual information passed along to inferotemporal cortex.[3] Accordingly, the present finding suggests that visual information transmission to inferotemporal cortical centers responsible for higher visual function is attenuated in PTSD patients, but only in the right hemisphere.

A second finding is of a difference in the ERPs measured over prefrontal cortex. As FIGURE 1 shows, the prefrontal ERPs (at midline site Fpz) of PTSD patients were shifted to the positive relative to those of the WAV controls (with no significant difference between trauma and nontrauma stimuli). Such slow, tonic, DC-like shifts have become a focus of interest in recent years and are thought to reflect changes in the firing thresholds of large-scale neuronal networks. In particular, some evidence suggests that such positive shifts may reflect neuronal hyperpolarization (i.e., reduced excitability), whereas negative shifts represent neuronal depolarization (i.e., increased excitability).[4] Such results are important to the study of PTSD, because prefrontal cortex has been implicated in the control, suppression, and coordination of emotion (e.g., via inhibitory inputs to limbic and temporal areas), and because prefrontal deficiency has been suggested as playing a role in PTSD.[5]

This study also revealed a striking brain response in the 250-350-ms time window. As FIGURE 1 shows, subjects with PTSD yielded a distinct positive peak circa 300 ms (''P300tr'') in the ERP where the WAV participants yielded a negative trough. This peak was broadly distributed, with a maximum near vertex site Cz. There were no consistent stimulus effects in this time window. Previous ERP studies of emotion in normal subjects found (and mislabeled) positive deflections in this time window, although these studies all found larger deflections for emotional stimuli than for neutral stimuli.[6] This result suggests that the PTSD subjects were reacting strongly to all the words, irrespective of their associations with traumatic experiences, whereas the WAVs were reacting weakly to all the words, irrespective of their associations. This suggests that PTSD can be characterized by a heightened neurophysiological response to all such stimuli, at least in a context in which threat-related stimuli appear frequently, and that WAVs, despite their traumatic experiences, do not have PTSD because (at least in such threatening situations) they can suppress this response to all stimuli.

These results demonstrate three abnormalities associated with PTSD. First, the attentuated right-hemisphere P1 suggests an adaptive strategy to limit perceptual input to downstream processors in the same hemisphere (which is known to play a special role in emotional processing and autonomic arousal). Second, the positive shift at prefrontal sites indicates a different tonic level of cortical excitability over an area of the brain known to be involved in the suppression and control of emotion. And third, the newly identified P300tr component suggests an exaggerated emotional response by PTSD patients. Conversely, this P300tr was suppressed to all stimuli in WAV subjects. This suggests that future studies of the neurophysiology of PTSD examine the responses of individuals who have had traumatic experiences but do not have PTSD. Such individuals may also be ''abnormal,'' albeit in an adaptive fashion that permits them to escape the consequences of emotional trauma.

REFERENCES

1. (a) PAIGE, S. R., G. M. REID, M. G. ALLEN & J. E. O. NEWTON 1990. Psychophysiological correlates of posttraumatic stress disorder in Vietnam veterans. Biol. Psychiatry **27:** 419–430.
   (b) MCFARLANE, A. C., D. L. WEBER & C. R. CLARK. 1993. Abnormal stimulus processing in posttraumatic stress disorder. Biol. Psychiatry **34:** 311–320.
   (c) CHARLES, G., M. HANSENNE, M. ANSEAU, W. PITCHOT, R. MACHOWSKI, M. SCHITTECATTE & J. WILMOTTE. 1995. P300 in posttraumatic stress disorder. Neuropsychobiology **32:** 72–74.
2. HILLYARD, S. A. & T. W. PICTON. 1987. Electrophysiology of cognition. *In* Handbook of Physiology: Section 1. Neurophysiology. F. Plum, Ed.: 519–584. American Physiological Society. New York.
3. (a) MANGUN, G. R., S. A. HILLYARD & S. A. LUCK. 1993. Electrocortical substrates of visual selective attention. *In* Attention and Performance XIV. D. E. Meyer & S. Kornblum, Eds.: 219–243. The MIT. Cambridge, MA.
   (b) HEINZE, H. J., G. R. MANGUN, W. BURCHERT, H. HINRICHS, M. SCHOLZ, T. F. MUENTE, A. GOES, M. SCHERG, S. JOHANNES, H. HUNDESHAGEN, M. S. GAZZANIGA & S. A. HILLYARD. 1994. Combined spatial and temporal imaging of brain activity during visual selective attention in humans. Nature **372:** 543–546.
4. MCCALLUM, W. C. & S. H. CURRY (Eds.). 1993. Slow Potential Changes in the Human Brain. Plenum. New York.
5. (a) DAVIDSON, R. J. & S. K. SUTTON. 1995. Affective neuroscience: The emergence of a discipline. Curr. Opin. Neurobiol. **5:** 217–224.
   (b) LE DOUX, J. E. 1994. Emotion, memory, and the brain. Sci. Am. **270:** 50–57.
6. (a) STORMARK, K. M., H. NORDBY & K. HUGDAHL. 1995. Attentional shifts to emotionally charged cues: Behavioral and ERP data. Cognit. Emotion **9:** 507–523.
   (b) JOHNSTON, V. S., M. H. BURLESON & D. R. MILLER. 1987. Emotional value and late positive components of ERPs. *In* Current Trends in Event-Related Potential Research. R. Johnson, Jr., J. W. Rohrbaugh & R. Parasuraman, Eds.: 198–203. Elsevier. Amsterdam.
   (c) YEE, C. M. & G. A. MILLER. 1987. Affective valence and information processing. *In* Current Trends in Event-Related Potential Research. R. Johnson, Jr., J. W. Rohrbaugh & R. Parasuraman, Eds.: 300–307. Elsevier. Amsterdam.

Electrophysiological Abnormalities in PTSD

JEFFREY DAVID LEWINE,[a,b,e] JOSE M. CANIVE,[c]
WILLIAM W. ORRISON, JR.,[a,d] CHRIS J. EDGAR,[b]
SHERRI L. PROVENCAL,[b] JOHN T. DAVIS,
KIM PAULSON, DAVID GRAEBER,[c]
BRIAN ROBERTS,[c] PATRICIO R. ESCALONA,[c] AND
LAWRENCE CALAIS

*The New Mexico Institute of Neuroimaging and
Departments of [a]Radiology, [b]Psychology,
[c]Psychiatry, and [d]Neurology
Albuquerque Veterans Affairs Medical Center
and
University of New Mexico
2100 Ridgecrest Drive, SE
Albuquerque, New Mexico 87108*

Paige and colleagues[1] previously found patients with posttraumatic stress disorder (PTSD) to demonstrate abnormal sensory gating as assessed by the auditory evoked potential. Tone pips elicit an auditory event-related potential characterized by several components including a vertex negative component at 100 ms poststimulus (N100) and a vertex positive component at 200 ms (P200). In control subjects, the amplitude of both N100 and P200 increases as a function of tone intensity, even for tones as loud as 100 dB. Paige and colleagues found that many PTSD patients show the normal augmentation pattern for N100, but a reducing pattern for P200 in which the response to loud sounds is actually smaller than that to intermediate intensity sounds. This study sought to replicate and extend this work by combining EEG measurements with magnetoencephalographic (MEG) measurements. MEG involves measurement of the magnetic field generated by intracellular neuronal currents.[2] Using dipole modeling procedures, MEG can clarify the neuronal structures involved in the generation and modulation of N100 and P200 responses. Basic concepts in EEG and MEG are shown in FIGURE 1.

METHODS

Subjects. Forty-two outpatients with combat-related PTSD were evaluated along with 20 control subjects without neurological or psychiatric problems. All subjects were male, and the PTSD and normal control groups were matched on average age

[e]Tel: (801) 581-4583; fax: (801) 581-2414; e-mail: lewine@doug.med.utah.edu

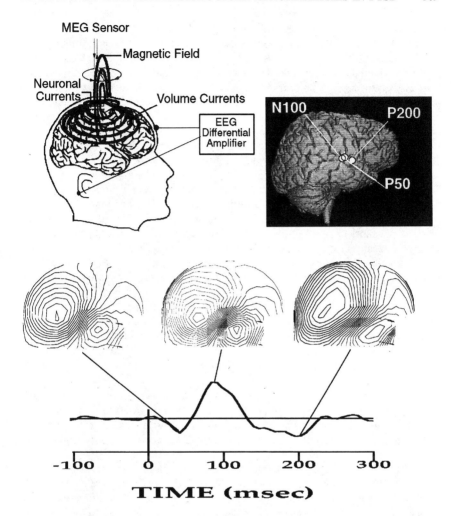

FIGURE 1. *Basic concepts in magnetoencephalography (MEG) and EEG.* Neuronal currents generate a surrounding magnetic field and extracellular volume currents. Magnetoencephalography used special superconducting sensors to measure temporal changes in the magnetic field. Extracellular volume currents cause electrical potential gradients at the scalp surface. These are measured in electroencephalography by differential amplifiers connected to electrodes attached to the scalp surface. When tones are presented repeatedly and epochs of MEG/ EEG data are averaged, time-locked event-related signals can be extracted. The pattern of electromagnetic activity at each instant in time provides clues to the location of the relevant neuronal generators. In MEG, the field pattern is often characterized by an area of emerging magnetic flux (*dark lines* on contour maps) and entering magnetic flux (*lighter lines*). Mathematical modeling of the field pattern allows for localization of active areas on magnetic resonance images and three-dimensional-surfaced rendered pictures.

(±5 years). The PTSD diagnosis was based on the Structured Clinical Interview for DSM-III-R (SCID). PTSD patients were also administered the Clinical Administered PTSD Scale (CAPS) and the Mississippi Scale for Combat Related PTSD. Exclusionary criteria included previous head trauma, gross neurological dysfunction, hearing loss, concurrent alcohol or drug abuse or dependence, or borderline or antisocial personality. All subjects were free of gross neurological dysfunction and had a 6-month abstinent period if they had past diagnoses of an alcohol or substance abuse or dependence disorder.

EEG/MEG. EEG data were collected using an electrode cap with placements at 10-20 locations. Data were collected referenced to the right mastoid and then re-referenced off-line to linked mastoids. MEG was collected simultaneously with the EEG using a 122-channel whole head biomagnetometer. Data were collected with a bandpass of 0.1-100 hz. During an experiment, one hundred and ten 2,000-hz tone pips (50-ms duration) were presented in random, blocked order (22 tones of a particular intensity per block) at each of the following intensities: 65.0, 72.5, 80, 87.5, and 95 dB. The intensity of the P200 response at Cz (EEG) was determined, and the slope of the function relating response magnitude to sound intensity was determined. A positive slope was classified as an augmenting pattern and a negative slope as a reducing pattern. Some subjects demonstrated poor auditory responses, and slopes could not be determined reliably. MEG data were analyzed to determine if the augmentation versus reduction reflected differences in the pattern of the magnitude of cortical response or the ampliotopic organization of the cortex.

RESULTS

As shown in FIGURE 2, 95% of the control subjects showed the expected augmentation pattern, whereas only 31% of the PTSD subjects showed this pattern. Eight PTSD patients (15%) showed poor auditory responses overall, and 21 (50%) showed a reducing pattern. MEG demonstrated the P200 component to have its origin in the auditory association cortex. For augmenters, as sound intensity increased, there was generally an increase in the dipole moment, indicating an increasing level of cortical activation. There was also a tendency for the source to become more superficial, a result believed to reflect ampliotopic organization of secondary auditory areas. For subjects with a reducing pattern, the reduction mostly reflected decreased cortical activation rather than an abnormality in ampliotopic organization.

No significant correlation was noted between auditory response patterns and age or severity of PTSD as measured by CAPS and Mississippi scores. There was no significant relationship with other comorbid factors. Several of the patients studied here demonstrate white matter lesions on magnetic resonance imaging (MRI). Interestingly, no significant relation was noted between physiological abnormalities and gross MRI abnormalities, a finding that suggests that the two reflect different pathophysiological processes.

DISCUSSION

The present experiments demonstrate significant neurophysiolgical abnormalities in patients with PTSD. The physiological data replicate and extend previous observa-

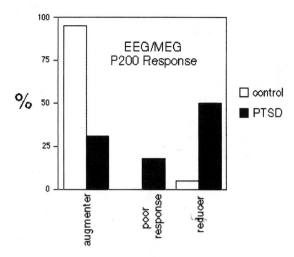

FIGURE 2. *Auditory reactivity patterns.* Data are from 42 patients with combat-related PTSD and 20 control subjects. The vast majority of control subjects demonstrate an augmentation pattern in which louder sounds elicit larger responses. Less than half the PTSD patients showed this pattern. Several had poor auditory responses to all sounds, and 50% showed a reducing pattern in which the response to the loudest sound was smaller than that to intermediate sounds.

tions by Paige and coworkers. An important aspect of the data is that PTSD subjects generally demonstrated a normal augmentation pattern for the N100 response. This, combined with the MEG localization of the P200 response to auditory association cortex, indicates that the reducing effect reflects a decrease in the activation of the auditory association cortex. High intensity sounds provide appropriate activation of primary cortex, but the system undergoes a sensory overload with information being blocked from reaching higher cortical areas.

The neural mechanisms that regulate sensory gating have yet to be fully defined, but it is likely that limbic structures play an important role in cortical gating. Several investigators have shown that PTSD subjects demonstrate reduced hippocampal volumes. We are currently exploring the correlation between hippocampal volume and auditory gating to determine if these are linked phenomena. If so, PTSD symptoms of mnemonic dysfunction and hyperarousal and sensitivity would be demonstrated to reflect a common neurobiological pathway.

REFERENCES

1. PAIGE, S. R., G. M. REID, M. G. ALLEN & J. O. NEWTON. 1990. Psychophysiological correlates of post-traumatic stress disorder in Vietnam veterans. Biol. Psychiatry **27:** 419–430.
2. LEWINE, J. D. & W. W. ORRISON, JR. 1995. Magnetoencephalography and magnetic source imaging. *In* Functional Brain Imaging. W. W. Orrison, Jr., J. D. Lewine, J. A. Sanders & M. F. Hartshorne, Eds.: 369–417. Mosby-Year Book Inc. St. Louis, MO.

MRI Reveals Gross Structural Abnormalities in PTSD

JOSE M. CANIVE,[c,e] JEFFREY DAVID LEWINE,[a,b]
WILLIAM W. ORRISON, JR.,[a,d] CHRIS J. EDGAR,[b]
SHERRI L. PROVENCAL,[b] JOHN T. DAVIS,
KIM PAULSON, DAVID GRAEBER,[c]
BRIAN ROBERTS,[c] PATRICIO R. ESCALONA,[c] AND
LAWRENCE CALAIS

*The New Mexico Institute of Neuroimaging and
Departments of [a]Radiology, [b]Psychology,
[c]Psychiatry, and [d]Neurology
Albuquerque Veterans Affairs Medical Center and
University of New Mexico
2100 Ridgecrest Drive, SE
Albuquerque, New Mexico 87108*

Whereas posttraumatic stress disorder (PTSD) was once believed to be mostly psychogenic in nature, evidence of specific neurobiological correlates is growing. In a wide range of clinical conditions, including schizophrenia, dementia, and autism, assessment of brain anatomy via magnetic resonance imaging (MRI) has proven fruitful in elucidating neurobiological correlates. To date, MRI investigations of the PTSD brain have used T1-weighted pulse sequences that allow volumetric measurements of the hippocampal formation.[1] Available data indicate a reduction of hippocampal volume in the PTSD brain, a finding that seems likely to be related to behaviorally observed alterations in mnemonic functions. However, in considering the overall behavioral manifestations of PTSD and also in trying to do better neurobiological subtyping of this diverse disorder, it may be that hypothesis-driven evaluation of just the hippocampal formation has caused investigators to overlook other significant alterations in brain structure. To determine if patients with PTSD show MRI abnormalities beyond reduced hippocampal volumes, this study obtained magnetic resonance images from a large population of PTSD outpatients, using several different imaging protocols.

METHODS

Subjects. Forty-two outpatients with combat-related PTSD were evaluated along with 20 control subjects without neurological or psychiatric problems. All subjects were male, and the PTSD, normal control, and depression groups were matched on

[e]Tel: (801) 581-4583; fax: (801) 581-2414; e-mail: lewine@doug.med.utah.edu

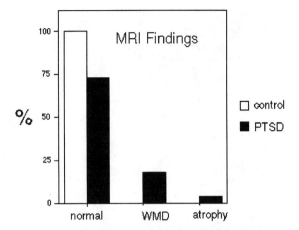

FIGURE 1. *MRI abnormalities in PTSD.* Magnetic resonance imaging results in 42 patients with PTSD and 20 normal control subjects. All control subjects had normal MR examinations. Eight patients with PTSD demonstrated white matter disease (WMD). This typically consisted of one or more focal areas of increased signal intensity on FLAIR images. Two patients showed excessive cortical atrophy.

average age (±5 years). The PTSD diagnosis was based on the Structured Clinical Interview for DSM-III-R (SCID). PTSD patients were also administered the Clinical Administered PTSD Scale (CAPS) and the Mississippi Scale for Combat Related PTSD. Exclusionary criteria included previous head trauma, gross neurological dysfunction, hearing loss, concurrent alcohol or drug abuse or dependence, or borderline or antisocial personality. All subjects were required to have a 6-month abstinent period if they had past diagnoses of an alcohol or substance abuse or dependence disorder. Subjects were excluded if any history of or current psychotic features were present.

Magnetic Resonance Imaging. Subject to machine availability, MRI was performed using either a 1.5 Tesla whole-body imaging system (Edge, Picker International) or a 0.23T open-design imaging system (Outlook, Picker-Nordstar). Prior to study, all subjects filled out a metal screening form and a Human Research Review Committee (HRRC)-approved consent form. Image quality on the low field system was sufficiently high that images from the two systems could not be distinguished easily, with prior work by our group indicating that both systems are fully adequate for identifying even subtle neuroanatomical anomalies. T1-weighted, 1.5-mm contiguous sagittal images were acquired as were T2-weighted axial images. Additional axial images were acquired using a fluid attenuated inversion recovery (FLAIR) pulse sequence. All image sets were evaluated by two neuroradiologists blind to the clinical status of the subjects.

RESULTS

As summarized in FIGURE 1, none of the normal control subjects demonstrated gross abnormalities on MR examination. Two patients with PTSD showed excessive

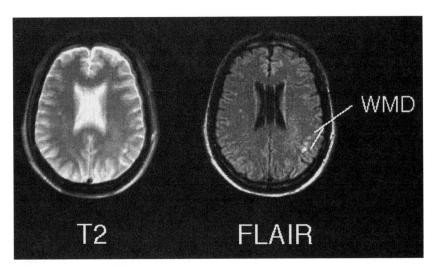

FIGURE 2. *White matter disease (WMD) in PTSD.* The patient was a 51-year-old with PTSD and a history of alcohol abuse, diabetes, and hypertension. MRI shows punctate WMD. In many cases it is difficult to identify subtle white matter abnormalities on T2-weighted images, because the cerebrospinal fluid (CSF) appears bright. In contrast, the FLAIR sequence causes suppression of the CSF signal, with white matter lesions remaining bright.

cortical atrophy and eight showed focal white matter lesions. White matter lesions were of one of two types, involving either periventricular regions or regions near the white/gray cortical junction. No significant correlations were noted between the presence of MR abnormalities and PTSD comorbid factors, including depression or a history of alcohol abuse. Also, correlation with severity of illness was lacking, as assessed by scores on the CAPS and Mississippi test batteries.

An important observation is that many of these white matter lesions could not easily be identified on standard T1 or T2 weighted images. That is, most of the identifications of white matter disease were made using FLAIR images in which signal from the cerebrospinal fluid is suppressed with white matter lesions appearing bright white on the images. An example is shown in FIGURE 2.

DISCUSSION

The incidence of gross abnormalities in the MRI of patients with PTSD is higher than that found in a neurologically normal population. The most significant finding is the presence of focal white matter lesions in PTSD. One problem in the study of PTSD is its high comorbidity with depression and alcohol abuse. Some investigators previously reported white matter changes in depression, but the lesions seen in our PTSD patients are much larger than those previously reported in depression. A review of the available literature on white matter changes in alcohol abuse also shows that there may be white matter findings for this group, out published reports refer to nonspecific diffuse changes and/or decreased white matter volume, a picture that is very different from the focal lesions seen in this study. On the one hand, it is surprising that a high prevalence of white matter lesions has not been reported in previous MR investigations of PTSD, but this most likely reflects a failure of past investigators to use the FLAIR imaging sequence. The finding of cortical atrophy in two PTSD patients is also of interest, but this, unlike the white matter changes, is probably a mere reflection of comorbidity with alcohol abuse or depression.

At present, the exact neurobiological mechanisms involved in the generation of these white matter lesions is unclear, but they may be a product of chronic stress and arousal. Because the present sample size was relatively small, we have not yet been able to determine if there are specific behavioral and neuropsychological correlates of the reported lesions, although this seems likely.

REFERENCES

1. BREMNER, J. D. *et al.* 1995. MRI-based measurements of hippocampal volume in patients with combat-related post traumatic stress disorder. Am. J. Psychiatry **152:** 973-981.

Reduced Hippocampal Volume and N-Acetyl Aspartate in Posttraumatic Stress Disorder

N. SCHUFF, C. R. MARMAR, D. S. WEISS,
T. C. NEYLAN, F. SCHOENFELD, G. FEIN, AND
M. W. WEINER

Magnetic Resonance Unit
Radiology and Psychiatry Services
Department of Veterans Affairs Medical Center
and
Departments of Radiology, Neurology, and Psychiatry
University of California, San Francisco
San Francisco, California 94121

Several earlier studies reported reduced hippocampal volume in combat veterans[1,2] and childhood sexual abuse victims[3,4] with posttraumatic stress disorder (PTSD). These volume changes were found in the right[1] left,[3,4] and both[2] hippocampi. A potential complicating factor in these reports is the effect of alcohol abuse, common in PTSD,[5] which causes atrophy of brain structures including the hippocampus.[6] Proton magnetic resonance spectroscopy (^{1}HMRS) or [1]HMR spectroscopic imaging (MRSI) detects the amino acid N-acetyl aspartate (NAA) which is found only in neurons and absent in glia.[7] Therefore, changes in NAA are thought to reflect changes in neuron viability and density. Previous work from this and other laboratories demonstrated that changes in NAA are detected in neurodegenerative diseases without accompanying changes in tissue volume or other morphological characteristics as detected by MRI. For example, in temporal lobe epilepsy, decreased NAA occurs in the seizure focus, in the absence of atrophy detected by MRI.[8] Similarly, in Alzheimer's disease, decreased NAA is independent of tissue atrophy.[9] Therefore, it has been proposed that NAA is a more sensitive measure of neuron loss than MRI. The goal of this small pilot study was to test the hypothesis that hippocampal NAA (measured by ^{1}H MRSI) is decreased in PTSD and that the decrease of NAA is greater than the decrease of hippocampal volume (measured by MRI).

METHODS

Subjects. Seven Vietnam veterans, 6 males and 1 female, with chronic combat-related PTSD were studied (mean age 48.0 [SD = 2.0; range 45–51]; 3 African American, 3 Caucasian, 1 Asian/Pacific Islander; average educational attainment = 14.6 years). All subjects had the MRI examination and five successfully completed ^{1}H MRSI. Subjects were eligible for the study if they were male or female veterans with combat-related PTSD whose war zone service was verified by military discharge

516

TABLE 1. Right Hippocampal Volume and NAA/(Cho + Cr) Ratio (means ± SE) in PTSD and Control Subjects

	PTSD	Control	% Difference	Effect Size	P Value
Volume (mm³)	3,279 ± 128	3,488 ± 95	−6.0	0.71	0.31
NAA/(Cho + Cr)	0.67 ± 0.03	0.82 ± 0.03	−18.2	2.12	0.06

records. Subjects were excluded if they met lifetime criteria for schizophrenia, bipolar affective disorder, or alcohol and/or substance abuse or dependence in the past 3 months. They were also excluded for imaging if they reported being claustrophobic, were at risk for seizures in the magnet, had evidence of ferrous magnetic objects in eyes, head, or body including shrapnel, or required life support monitoring. Women veterans were excluded if they were pregnant or not using reliable of contraception. Comorbid diagnoses (from Structured Clinical Interview [SCID][10]: 4 of 7 lifetime alcohol dependence; 6 of 7 lifetime major depressive episode; 1 of 7 current major depressive episode; 3 of 7 lifetime substance abuse; 1 of 7 simple phobia, 1 of 7 somatoform pain disorder, 2 of 7 paranoid personality disorder, and 1 of 7 schizoid personality disorder). Data from seven control subjects with mean age 42.4 (SD = 6.0; range 36-56) who were being recruited as controls for a study of temporal lobe epilepsy were used.

MRI and ^{1}H MRSI. Subjects were scanned with a 1.5-T Vision MR system (Siemens Inc., Iselin, New Jersey) using a volumetric magnetization prepared rapid gradient echo sequence (MP-RAGE , TR/TE = 10/4 ms, 15° flip angle, ROI 250 × 250 × 230 mm³, matrix 256 × 256 × 164). This resulted in 164 T_1-weighted images of 1.4-mm slice thickness with 1.0 × 1.0 mm² inplane resolution oriented orthogonal to the long axis of the hippocampus. Boundaries of the hippocampal region were outlined based on these images using software developed here (G. Fein) and following the method of Watson *et al.*[11]

After MRI, ^{1}H MRSI data were acquired from a 15-mm thick and typically 80 × 100 mm² wide volume of interest oriented parallel to the long axis of the hippocampus. The ^{1}H MRSI parameters (TR/TE = 1800/140 ms, 24 × 24 phase encoding) resulted in a nominal MRSI volume element (voxel) size of approximately 1.5 ml. MR spectra were extracted from voxels located in the head, body, and tail of the right and left hippocampus and the signal intensities of NAA, choline (Cho), and creatine (Cr) were derived from fitting the corresponding resonance peak areas. The peak ratio NAA/(Cho+Cr) was used for primary analysis to compensate for atrophy effects within voxels.

Statistical Analysis. One-way ANOVA was used to compare hippocampal volume and metabolite ratios between groups.

RESULTS AND DISCUSSION

TABLE 1 and FIGURE 1 demonstrate that right hippocampal volume (not corrected for intracranial volume) was reduced 6% in PTSD subjects compared with controls,

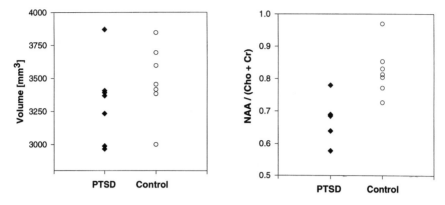

FIGURE 1. Scatter plot of volume (*left*) and NAA/(Cho+Cr) (*right*) from right hippocampus in PTSD and control subjects.

similar to one previous report.[1] Right NAA/(Cho+Cr) was reduced 18% in PTSD versus control subjects. FIGURE 1 demonstrates little overlap in the distributions of PTSD subjects and controls. A single PTSD subject had high NAA/(Cho+Cr) and that subject had a very large head and hippocampus. Changes of the left hippocampus were in the same direction, but NAA/(Cho+Cr) was only decreased by 6.6%. The 18% reduction of right hippocampal NAA/(Cho+Cr) compares with a 27% reduction in temporal lobe epilepsy[8] and a 30% reduction in Alzheimer's disease.[12]

In this sample, mean hippocampal volume and NAA/(Cho+Cr) of the nonalcoholic combat veteran subjects were virtually the same as those of the alcoholic subjects, suggesting that hippocampal changes were due to PTSD and not alcohol. The finding that the change in hippocampal NAA/(Cho+Cr) was considerably greater than the change in volume suggests that NAA may be a more sensitive measure of hippocampal change in PTSD. However, because the controls were nonveterans, without a history of alcohol abuse, these pilot results do not firmly establish that PTSD is responsible for the observed hippocampal differences. Future studies must be performed to carefully distinguish the effects of PTSD from those of alcohol.

These findings add weight to previous MRI studies suggesting reduction of hippocampal volume in PTSD. It is not clear if trauma exposure alone, combat-related PTSD, or comorbid substance abuse is responsible for hippocampal atrophy or alternatively if reduced hippocampal size is a premorbid condition, predisposing to the development of PTSD. Previous findings of altered hypothalamic pituitary axis function,[13] particularly increased lymphocyte glucocorticoid receptors,[14] raise the possibility that reduced hippocampal size is a consequence of posttraumatic glucocorticoid induced injury.

Finally, these findings from hippocampus may have treatment implications. The hippocampus may play an important role in both the acquisition and extinction of fear responses.[15] Animal data suggest that hippocampal lesioning may interfere with habituation or extinction of conditioned fear responses.[16] From this one could conclude that in combat related PTSD widely used treatments such as prolonged exposure, which depend on habituation of trauma-related conditioned fear responses, may be less effective than cognitive reprocessing or social skills training which depend less on habituation. Among chronic cases of combat-related PTSD, those veterans with hippocampal atrophy may be less responsive to psychologic treatments, such as prolonged exposure, which rely upon habituation, and may benefit more from pharmacotherapy. Further investigation using MRI and ¹H MRSI to measure the volume and metabolites in the hippocampus and other brain structures may be important for diagnosis, prognosis, and therapeutic management of PTSD.

ACKNOWLEDGMENTS

We gratefully acknowledge the efforts of Mrs. Katheryn Wentworth who was in charge of recruiting the patients and of Mr. Sean Steinman who performed MRI/MRSI acquisition. We are thankful to Dr. Diane Amend for the measurement of hippocampal volumes.

REFERENCES

1. BREMNER, J. D., P. RANDALL, T. M. SCOTT, R. A. BRONEN, J. P. & SEIBYL, S. M. SOUTHWICK, R. C. DELANEY, G. MCCARTHY, D. S. CHARNEY & R. B. INNIS. 1995. MRI-based measurement of hippocampal volume in patients with combat-related post-traumatic stress disorder. Am. J. Psychiatry **152:** 973-981.
2. GURVITS, T. V., M. E. SHENTON, H. HOKAMA, H. OHTA, N. B. LASKO, S. P. ORR, R. KIKINIS, F. A. JOLESZ, R. W. MCCARLEY & R. K. PITMAN. 1996. Magnetic resonance imaging study of hippocampal volume in chronic, combat-related post-traumatic stress disorder. Biol. Psychiatry **40:** 1091-1099.
3. BREMNER, J. D., P. RANDALL E. VERMETTEN, L. STAIB, R. A. BRONEN, C. MAZURE, S. CAPELLI, G. MCCARTHY, R. B. INNIS & D. S. CHARNEY. 1997. MRI-based measurement of hippocampal volume in posttraumatic stress disorder related to childhood physical and sexual abuse-A preliminary report. Biol. Psychiatry **41:** 23-32.
4. STEIN, M. B., C. KOVEROLA, C. HANNA, M. G. TORCHIA, V. VAERUM & B. MCCLARTY. 1996. Memory and hippocampal volume in adult female survivors of childhood sexual abuse. Submitted.
5. FONTANA, A., R. ROSENHECK & H. SPENCER. 1990. The first progress report on the Department of Veterans Affairs PTSD clinical teams program. West Haven, CT. Northeast Program Evaluation Center.
6. SULLIVAN, E. V., L. MARSH, D. H. MATHALON, K. O. LIM & A. PFEFFERBAUM. 1995. Anterior hippocampal volume deficits in nonamnesic, aging chronic alcoholics. Alcohol Clin. Exp. Res. **19:** 110-122.
7. BIRKEN, D. L. & W. H. OLDENDORF. 1989. *N*-Acetyl-L-aspartic acid: A literature review of a compound prominent in ¹H-NMR spectroscopic studies of brain. Neurosci. Biobehav. Rev. **13:** 23-31.
8. ENDE, G., K. D. LAXER, R. KNOWLTON, G. B. MATSON & M. W. WEINER. 1995. Quantitative ¹H MRSI shows bilateral metabolite changes in unilateral TLE patients with and without hippocampal atrophy. Proc. Soc. Magnetic Resonance **144:** (Abstr.).
9. MACKAY, S., F. EZEKIEL, V. D. SCLAFANI, J. GERSON, D. J. MEYERHOFF, D. NORMAN, G. FEIN & M. W. WEINER. 1996. Combining MRI segmentation and ¹H MR spectroscopic imaging in the study of Alzheimer's disease, subcortical ischemic vascular dementia and elderly controls. Radiology **198:** 537-545; Schuff, N. *et al.* Unpublished results.

10. Spitzer, R. L., J. B. Williams, M. Gibbon & M. B. First. 1992. The Structured Clinical Interview for DSM-III-R (SCID). I. History, rationale, and description. Arch. Gen. Psychiatry **49:** 624-629.

11. Watson, C., F. Andermann, P. Gloor, M. Jones-Gotman, T. Peters, A. Evans, A. Olivier, D. Melanson & G. Leroux. 1992. Anatomic basis of amygdaloid and hippocampal volume measurement by magnetic resonance imaging. Neurology, **42:** 1743-1750.

12. Schuff, N., R. Knowlton, D. L. Amend, D. J. Meyerhoff, J. L. Tanabe, G. Fein & M. W. Weiner. 1996. Changes of NAA in Alzheimer's disease are more prominent in hippocampus than in cortical gray matter: A ^{1}H MR spectroscopic imaging study. Proc. Int. Soc. Magnetic Resonance Med. **4:** 308 (Abstr.).

13. Yehuda, R., S. M. Southwick, J. H. Krystal, D. Bremner, D. S. Charney & J. W. Mason. 1993. Enhanced suppression of cortisol following dexamethasone administration in posttraumatic stress disorder. Am. J. Psychiatry **150:** 83-86.

14. Yehuda, R., D. Boisoneau, M. T. Lowy & E. L. Giller, Jr. 1995. Dose-response changes in plasma cortisol and lymphocyte glucocorticoid receptors following dexamethasone administration in combat veterans with and without posttraumatic stress disorder. Arch. Gen. Psychiatry **52:** 583-593.

15. W. A. Falls & M. Davis. 1995. Behavioral and physiological analysis of fear inhibition: Extinction and conditioned inhibition. *In* Neurobiological and Clinical Consequences of Stress: From Normal Adaptation to Post-traumatic Stress Disorder. M. J. Friedman, D. S. Charney & A. Y. Deutch, Eds.: 177. Lippincott-Raven. Philadelphia.

16. Schmaltz, L. W. & J. Theios. 1972. Acquisition and extinction of a classically conditioned response in hippocampectomized rabbits (*Oryctolagus cuniculus*). J. Comp. Physiol. Psychol. **79:** 328-333.

A Positron Emission Tomographic Study of Symptom Provocation in PTSD

LISA M. SHIN,[a,g] RICHARD J. McNALLY,[a]
STEPHEN M. KOSSLYN,[a,b] WILLIAM L. THOMPSON,[a]
SCOTT L. RAUCH,[c] NATHANIEL M. ALPERT,[d]
LINDA J. METZGER,[e] NATASHA B. LASKO,[e]
SCOTT P. ORR,[e,f] AND ROGER K. PITMAN [e,f]

[a]Department of Psychology
Harvard University
Cambridge, Massachusetts 02138

[b]Department of Neurology
Massachussetts General Hospital
Boston, Massachusetts 02114

[c]Department of Radiology and Psychiatry
Massachusetts General Hospital and
Harvard Medical School
Boston, Massachusetts 02114

[d]Department of Radiology,
Massachusetts General Hospital
Boston, Massachusetts 02114

[e]VA Research Service
Manchester, New Hampshire 03103

[f]Harvard Medical School
Boston, Massachusetts

The purpose of this study was to elucidate the mediating functional neuroanatomy of posttraumatic stress disorder (PTSD) symptoms. Recently, Rauch and colleagues[1] used script-driven imagery and positron emission tomography (PET) to measure regional cerebral blood flow (rCBF) in eight individuals with PTSD. In separate scans, subjects imagined traumatic and neutral events. In the traumatic imagery condition, relative to control conditions, increased rCBF was found in several right-sided limbic, paralimbic, and visual areas, including amygdala, orbitofrontal cortex, insular cortex, anterior temporal pole, anterior cingulate cortex, and secondary visual cortex. Decreased rCBF occurred in Broca's area. In the current study, we sought

[g]Address for correspondence: Lisa M. Shin, Department of Psychology, Harvard University, William James Hall, 33 Kirkland Street, Cambridge, MA 02138 (tel: (617) 496-2991; fax (617) 496-3122, email:ls@wjh.harvard.edu).

to replicate these results and to determine whether similar rCBF increases occur in trauma-exposed individuals without PTSD.

METHODS

Subjects were 15 right-handed women with histories of childhood sexual abuse, 8 with PTSD (as determined by the Clinician Administered PTSD Scale[2]) and 7 without PTSD. Additional subjects remain to be tested. The PTSD subjects were screened as physiologically responsive to traumatic imagery, and control subjects were screened as physiologically nonresponsive to traumatic imagery. The PTSD and control groups were similar in age and years of education. None of the subjects was taking psychoactive medication at the time of testing.

Prior to the scanning session, each subject prepared written descriptions of both neutral and traumatic autobiographical events. These scripts were prepared (according to the guidelines of Pitman *et al.*[3]) and tape recorded for playback in the PET scanner. Each script served to prompt imagery of the relevant autobiographical event and was always presented to the subject immediately before commencement of PET scanning.

Each subject participated in three conditions: traumatic, neutral, and teeth clenching. During the traumatic and neutral conditions, subjects imagined traumatic and neutral autobiographical events, respectively. In the teeth-clenching condition, subjects imagined the same neutral events while clenching their teeth. We used statistical parametric mapping (SPM)[4] to compare the blood flow images collected in the traumatic condition with those collected in the neutral and teeth-clenching control conditions. This process yielded Z-score images, which were inspected for foci of activation. We employed a Z-score threshold of 2.58 ($p < 0.005$, uncorrected for multiple comparisons) for foci of activation in a priori regions of interest (amygdala, orbitofrontal cortex, insular cortex, anterior temporal poles, anterior cingulate cortex, visual cortex, and Broca's area). This Z-score threshold was raised to 3.09 ($p < 0.001$, uncorrected for multiple comparisons) for foci of activation in regions about which we had no a priori prediction. Detailed descriptions of PET procedures and data analytic techniques used in our laboratory have been published previously.[1,5]

Subjects' heart rate and blood pressure were recorded in all conditions. After each scan, subjects rated the intensity of the various emotions (e.g., fear, anger, sadness, guilt, and disgust) that they experienced during imagery.

RESULTS

Because this dataset is not currently complete, the following results should be considered strictly preliminary. The PTSD subjects had significantly higher heart rate responses in the traumatic condition than did control subjects. In the PTSD group, ratings of fear, anger, sadness, guilt, and disgust were significantly higher in the traumatic condition than in the neutral condition. In the control group, ratings of fear, sadness, and disgust were significantly higher in the traumatic condition than in the neutral condition. In the PTSD group, rCBF increases were found in the following regions during the traumatic versus control conditions: orbitofrontal cortex, and anterior temporal poles. Also in the PTSD group, rCBF decreases were found in Broca's area, middle frontal gyri, inferior and middle temporal gyri, inferior parietal lobule, and fusiform gyrus. In the control group, rCBF increases were found in the following regions during the traumatic versus control conditions: orbitofrontal cortex, anterior cingulate cortex, anterior temporal poles, insular cortex, superior temporal gyrus, and inferior, medial, and superior frontal gyri. Also in the control group, rCBF decreases were found in primary and secondary visual cortex, visual association cortex, and inferior parietal lobule.

CONCLUSIONS

The preliminary results from our PTSD group are consistent with the findings of a previous symptom provocation study of PTSD[1] and further suggest that paralimbic regions mediate emotional responses to imagery of traumatic events in individuals with PTSD. However, preliminary results from our control group suggest that some paralimbic regions may mediate relatively normal emotional responses to imagery of traumatic events and may not be associated with a current diagnosis of PTSD.

REFERENCES

1. RAUCH, S. L., B. A. VAN DER KOLK, R. E. FISLER, N. M. ALPERT, S. P. ORR, C. R. SAVAGE, A. J. FISCHMAN, M. A. JENIKE & R. K. PITMAN. 1996. A symptom provocation study of posttraumatic stress disorder using positron emission tomography and script-driven imagery. Arch. Gen. Psychiatry **53:** 380–387.
2. BLAKE, D. D., F. W. WEATHERS, L. M. NAGY, D. G. KALOUPEK, G. KLAUMINZEV & T. M. KEANE. 1990. Rating scale for assessing current and lifetime PTSD: The CAPS-I. Behav. Therapist **13:** 187–188.
3. PITMAN, R. K., S. P. ORR, D. F. FORGUE, J. B. DE JONG & J. M. CLAIBORN. 1987. Psychophysiologic assessment of posttraumatic stress disorder imagery in Vietnam combat veterans. Arch. Gen. Psychiatry **44:** 970–975.
4. FRISTON, K. J., C. D. FRITH, P. F. LIDDLE & R. S. J. FRAKOWIAK. 1991. Comparing functional (PET) images: The assessment of significant change. J. Cereb. Blood Flow Metab. **11:** 690–699.
5. RAUCH S. L., M. A. JENIKE, N. M. ALPERT, L. BAER, H. C. R. BREITER, C. R. SAVAGE & A. J. FISCHMAN. 1994. Regional cerebral blood flow measured during symptom provocation in obsessive-compulsive disorder using oxygen 15-labeled carbon dioxide and positron emission tomography. Arch. Gen. Psychiatry **51:** 62–70.

VEPs and AEPs: Mapping of Occlusive Lesions in Cerebral Vessels

SERGEY LYTAEV AND SERGEY SHEVCHENKO

Military-Medical Academy
6 Lebedev
St. Petersburg, 194175, Russia

The recording of cerebral evoked potentials (EPs) has had a rich history. At the same time, the neuromapper computer produced in the last 10 years increased the possibility of looking into a living brain. These advances were the basis for neuroimaging, neurovisualization, and neuromapping studies. On the one hand, the results of such studies are contradictory, but on the other, these methods are relatively inexpensive compared to computerized tomography, magnetic resonance imaging (or tomography), positron emission tomography, and the like, and they are totally noninvasive.[2–7]

The present study estimates the diagnostic significance of EP mapping and the functional significance of the cortical structure in vascular lesions.

METHODS

Nine patients with acute cerebral blood circulation disorders according to ischemic type in the left internal carotid artery basin and eight patients with disorders in the right internal carotid artery were examined. Verification of the level and distribution of the cerebral artery lesions was carried out by angiography and ultrasonic dopplerography, but objectivization of pathomorphologic cerebral changes was shown by CT. EPs were recorded with the computer neuromapper "brain surveyor" in the 19th monopolar sites by system 10/20. Visual and auditory stimulation was applied. Successive cerebral maps were estimated by changing the analyzed epoch at intervals of 100–1,000 ms, and discriminant analysis (BMDP 7M) was performed (according to criteria of F statistics, $F > 1.0$)[1] and compared with data in a control group of healthy subjects ($n = 16$). Patients were examined at the neurosurgery clinic before hospitalization within 1–3 weeks after the stroke.

RESULTS AND DISCUSSION

From the position of structure formation of evoked responses, stroke at the middle brain artery basin was considered the lesion of the temporal-sincipital cortex of a hemisphere. The results of recording and analysis of visual EPs (VEPs) showed that the main disorders in the response structures occurred 100 ms after the moment of signaling. Ischemic lesions of the left temporal-sincipital cortex are accompanied by generalized lengthening of peak latency (PL) and by a reduction of component

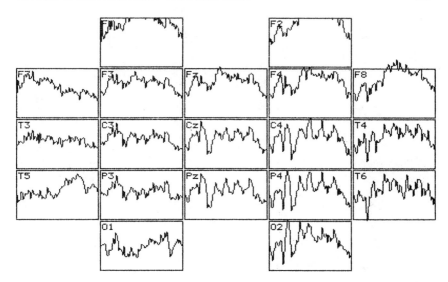

FIGURE 1. Distribution of VEPs in a patient with left-sided ischemic stroke. Epoch = 1,000 ms.

amplitude N150 with a maximum in sites C3 (F = 38.1) and F4 (F = 13.7). Blood supply disorders in the symmetrical areas (from the right) have similar but more limited changes only in the anterior cerebral departments with a maximum in the left frontal site (F = 22.2).

At an interval of 200–300 ms, left vascular temporal-sincipital ischemia is characterized by VEP amplitude reduction throughout the cerebral areas as well as the sincipital ones, with a maximum at site C3 (F = 16.4). Vascular lesions of symmetrical cerebral areas do not differ from the control indicators.

Ischemic stroke significantly influenced the latest waves of VEPs. A generalized increase in wave amplitude N750 with a maximum difference in the left occipital lobe (F = 11.5) with a left blood supply disorder and, in contrast, in the right occipital lobe (F = 8.1) with a right blood supply disorder was recorded.

The latest estimated VEP component N900 in left-sided vascular ischemia is accompanied by increased amplitude at site C4 (F = 4.3) and F4 (F = 5.3), whereas a right vascular lesion is characterized by shortening of PL in the cortex lobe. Distribution of VEPs in a patient with left-sided ischemic stroke is shown in FIGURE 1. The significant visual reduction of amplitude N150 is seen on the side of the damaged hemisphere and even in the frontal cortex of the intact hemisphere of the brain (sites 02, P4, and C4).

Recording and analysis of auditory EP (AEP) topomaps have shown that a left-sided blood supply disorder on simple rhythmic stimulation is accompanied by simplification of the amplitude of the earliest analyzed component (N18) in the frontal cortex from the left (F = 6.0) and from the right (F = 6.6) and also in the sinciput (F = 4.3) and in the central site (F = 4.6) of the healthy hemisphere. Relevant loading (activation of the patient's attention) contributes to the increased amplitude in the

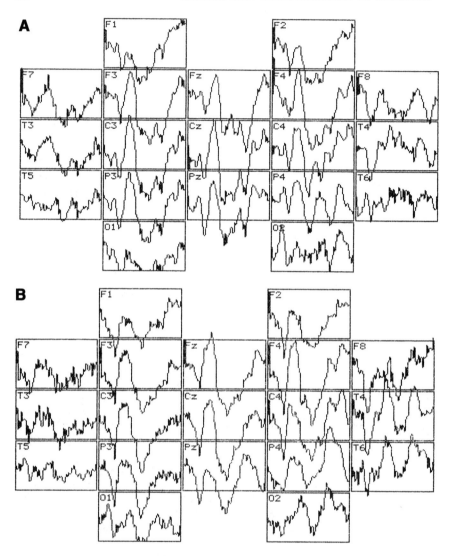

FIGURE 2. Distribution of AEPs in a patient with right-sided ischemic stroke in rhythmic sound stimulation (**A**) and in a test to attract the subjective attention (**B**). Epoch = 400 ms.

vertex (F = 5.0), in site C4 (F = 6.8), and also in the left sinciput (F = 6.0). In this disease the main indicator between samples is the rise in amplitude in the damaged sinciput and in the vertex. Left-sided lesions regardless of the type of stimulation do not produce different values from those of the control group (F <4.0).

Left-sided vascular pathology in rhythmic sound stimulation for wave N90 is characterized by indices similar to control ones. The object signal selecting test for wave N90 contributes to PL lengthening over all points of registration and to increased amplitude especially on the lesion side in site F3 (F =10.6). Component N145 is reduced in the frontal areas from both left (F = 5.1) and right (F = 4.7). The significant PL increase is maintained throughout the cerebral cortex (F >4.0).

Right-sided temporal and sincipital ischemia under rhythmic sound stimulation does not influence parameter N145, but it contributes to the tendency to amplitude increasing N90 over all points of recording, with a maximum in the left frontal cortex (F = 5.1). Perception of the object irritants is characterized by amplitude increasing N90 in the vertex (F = 19.3) and also on sites P3 (F = 8.3) and C4 (F = 8.1). (PL is also increased [F >4.0].) Amplitude N145 does not practically differ from the values of the control group, but at the same time PL is lengthened in Cz (F = 5.2) and F4 (F = 6.3).

Left-sided vascular pathology of the temporal and sincipital cortex under rhythmic sound stimulation does not influence parameter N250, whereas PL N350 in the damaged hemisphere is lengthened (sites P3, F = 4.5, and C3, F = 4.7) and its amplitude is increased in C3 (F = 4.3) and F3 (F = 5.8). In the sample with useful signal selecting, wave N350 does not change, but in wave N250 PL is increased in the central and frontal branches of both hemispheres.

In right-sided vascular ischemia under rhythmic sound stimulation, PL N250 is minimized in the area of the lesion and its amplitude is reduced in the symmetrical point of a healthy hemisphere (branch P3, F = 13.0) (FIG. 2). Amplitude N350 is increased in the left sincipital site (F = 8.1) (FIG. 2). Relevant stimulation also contributes to the rise in amplitude of the latest components especially on the side of lesion P4, C4, T4, and F4 (FIG. 2). In addition, lengthening of PL N250 is seen in C4 (F = 1.2) and 1 Cz (F = 6.2) and also of PL N350 in F3 (F = 6.9).

Thus, analysis of EP topomaps of brain permitted us to establish the following patterns:

1. In visual stimulation, significant decay and reduction of practically all waves on the side of the ischemic stroke are visible. At the same time, increased bioelectrical activity of the intact hemisphere of the brain is recorded mainly at an interval of 400–1,000 ms.

2. Auditory stimulation is accompanied by more significant variability in the formation of auditory EPs. In rhythmic sound stimulation the component reduction in the damaged area is less marked. At the same time, the generalized neocortex activity is increased. In contrast, in the test to attract the patient's attention, the EP amplitude rise is recorded in the ischemic area with conservation of increased activity over all points registering attraction of the patient's attention.

REFERENCES

1. BMDP USER'S DIGEST. 1987. M. A. Mill, Ed. University of California Press. Los Angeles, CA.
2. BRANDEIS, D. & D. LEHMANN 1986. Event-related potentials of the brain and cognitive processes: Approaches and applications. Neuropsychologia 21: 151–168.
3. DUFFY, F. H. 1986. Topographic Mapping of Brain Electric Activity. Butterworth. London.
4. GEVINS, A. S. & A. REMOND, Eds. 1987. Methods of Analysis of Brain Electrical and Magnetic Signals. Elsevier. Amsterdam.

5. HARI, R. 1990. The neuromagnetic method in the study of the human auditory cortex. Adv. Audiol. **6:** 222–282.
6. NAATANEN, R. & T. PICTON. 1987. The N1 wave of the human electric and magnetic response to sound: A review and analysis of the component structure. Psychophysiology **24:** 375–425.
7. SHAGASS, C. & R. A. ROEMER, Eds. 1986. Brain Electrical Potentials and Psychopathology. Elsevier. Amsterdam.

Posttraumatic Stress and Depression

A Neurochemical Anatomy of the Learned Helplessness Animal Model

FREDERICK PETTY,[a] GERALD L. KRAMER,
JIANHUA WU, AND LORI L. DAVIS

*Veterans Affairs Medical Center and
Department of Psychiatry
University of Texas Southwestern Medical School
Dallas, Texas 75216*

Learned helplessness (LH) is a behavioral depression, or maladaptive response, resulting from exposure to inescapable stress. Since LH represents an adverse reaction to severe stress, it may prove useful in understanding the psychobiology of posttraumatic stress disorder (PTSD). Because stress has multiple effects on multiple neurotransmitter systems, identifying those that are functionally related to maladaptive outcome is done by the behavioral test involved in the LH model (FIGS. 1 and 2).

We have used techniques of *in vivo* microdialysis, intracerebral microinjection,[1] neurotransmitter release from tissue slices, and quantitative autoradiography to develop a neuronal map for LH.[2] The initial cortical response to stress is increased dopamine (DA) release in medial prefrontal cortex (mPFC). Increased DA release in mPFC, in turn, leads to increased release of serotonin (5-HT),[3] and rats that go on to develop LH have greater 5-HT release, leading to intraneuronal 5-HT depletion in mPFC.[4] Treatments that prevent LH have in common the prevention of 5-HT depletion in mPFC. Imipramine, or 5-HT, injected into mPFC reverse LH. Thus, 5-HT may be the key neurotransmitter involved in the development and maintenance of LH in mPFC.[5] The amino acid neurotransmitters γ-aminobutyric acid (GABA) and glutamate modulate LH in mPFC, because GABA microinjection prevents LH and glutamate microinjection causes LH in naive nonstressed rats.

We hypothesize a link from the mPFC via the entorhinal cortex (GABA locus) to the hippocampus. GABA plays a key role in hippocampus, because microinjection of GABA both prevents and reverses LH, microinjection of the GABA$_A$ receptor blocker bicuculine causes LH if microinjected into naive animals,[6] and microinjection of diazepam into hippocampus before stress prevents LH. Also, maintenance of adequate norepinephrine in hippocampus is essential to homeostasis and to prevention of deleterious stress effects.[7] Microinjection of imipramine into hippocampus before stress exposure protects from LH development, but it will not reverse stress effects if injected after stress. Also, 5-HT$_2$ receptors have decreased density in hippocampus of rats that do not develop LH after stress. Stable ''long-term'' LH behavior showed

---

[a] Address for correspondence: Frederick Petty, PhD, MD, Mental Health Clinic 116A, Veterans Affairs Medical Center, Dallas, TX 75216 (tel: (214)376-5451; fax: (214)372-7086; e-mail: petty.frederick@dallas.va.gov).

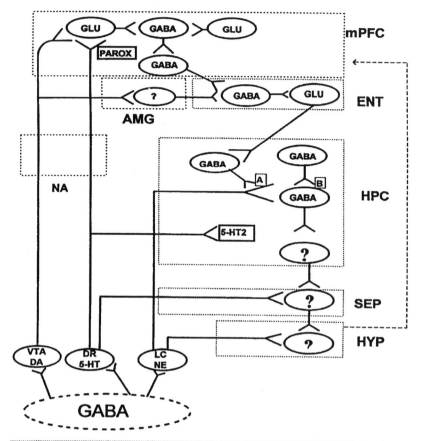

ABBREVIATIONS: gamma-aminobutyric acid (GABA); glutamate (GLU); medial prefrontal cortex (mPFC); amygdala (AMG); entorhinal cortex (ENT); hippocampus (HPC); nucleus accumbens (NA); septum (SEP); hypothalamus (HYP); ventral tegmental area (VTA); dopamine (DA); dorsal raphe (DR); serotonin (5-HT); locus ceruleus (LC); norepinephrine (NE)

FIGURE 1. Hypothetical neuronal network in the learned helplessness animal model.

increased norepinephrine release in hippocampus during mild re-stress; stressed, but nonhelpless rats were similar to controls.[8] Therefore, 5-HT, norepinephrine, GABA interaction hippocampus may preserve normal, nonhelpless homeostasis.

A norepinephrine locus in hypothalamus correlates with LH behavior in this brain region, where the neuroendocrine effects of stress are manifest.

We hypothesize that LH itself is stressful and that a "feedback" loop to mPFC maintains this behavior beyond the time of the acute stress response. Learned helplessness involves multiple regions of the limbic system and multiple neurotransmitters.

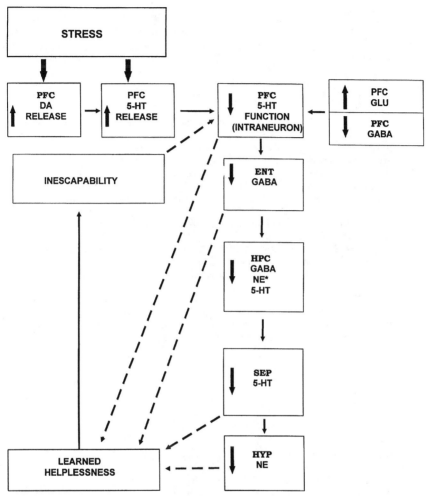

ABBREVIATIONS: dopamine (**DA**); serotonin (**5-HT**); prefrontal cortex (**PFC**); glutamate (**GLU**); gamma aminobutyric acid (**GABA**); entorhinal cortex (**ENT**); hippocampus (**HPC**); septum (**SEP**); acetylcholine (**ACH**); norepinephrine (**NE**); hypothalamus (**HYP**); *NE sensitized to re-stress in **HPC**

FIGURE 2. From stress to learned helplessness.

In summary, LH is a behavioral depression[9] resulting from exposure to inescapable stress and may provide a convenient animal model for some aspects of PTSD, perhaps more so for acute than for chronic PTSD. Learned helplessness involves multiple neurotransmitters including norepinephrine, serotonin, dopamine, GABA, and glutamate. Learned helplessness may be conceptualized as a limbic system disorder, with different brain regions involved in different aspects of the development and maintenance of the maladaptive stress response. Medial prefrontal cortex, hippocampus, septum, and hypothalamus are known to be involved in LH, and amygdala and nucleus accumbens are being studied. Sensitization of the neurochemical stress responses in helpless rats may explain the biological basis of the stress sensitization seen in PTSD.

REFERENCES

1. PETTY, F. *et al.* 1980. Regional aspects of the prevention of learned helplessness by desipramine. Life Sci. **26:** 1447–1452.
2. SHERMAN, A. D. *et al.* 1980. Neurochemical basis of the action of antidepressants on learned helplessness. Behav. Neural Biol. **30:** 119–134.
3. PETTY, F. *et al.* 1993. Learned helplessness and *in vivo* hippocampal norepinephrine release. Pharmacol. Biochem. Behav. **46:** 231–235.
4. PETTY, F. *et al.* 1992. Prevention of learned helplessness: *In vivo* correlation with cortical serotonin. Pharmacol. Biochem. Behav. **43:** 361–367.
5. PETTY, F. *et al.* 1981. GABAergic modulation of learned helplessness. Pharmacol. Biochem. Behav. **15:** 567–570.
6. PETTY, F. *et al.* 1994. Does learned helplessness induction by haloperidol involve serotonin mediation? Pharmacol. Biochem. & Behav. **48:** 671–676.
7. PETTY, F. *et al.* Learned helplessness sensitizes hippocampal norepinephrine to mild re-stress. Biol. Psychiatry **35:** 903–908.
8. SHERMAN, A. D. *et al.* 1982. Specificity of the learned helplessness model of depression. Pharmacol. Biochem. Behav. **16:** 449–454.
9. SHERMAN, A. D. *et al.* 1982. Additivity of neurochemical changes produced by learned helplessness and imipramine. Behav. Neural. Biol **35:** 344–353.

Psychophysiologic Parameters of Traumatic Stress Disorder in Rats[a]

T. GARRICK,[b] N. MORROW,[b] S. ETH,[c]
D. MARCIANO,[b] AND A. SHALEV [d]

[b]West Los Angeles VA Medical Center
Los Angeles, California

[c]St. Vincent's Hospital
New York, New York

[d]Hadassah University Hospital
Jerusalem, Israel

The acoustic startle reflex in humans and animals has been shown to accommodate to the repeated administration of loud noises, so that the subject orients to the sound but ceases to startle (startle habituation).[1] Humans who have diagnosable posttraumatic stress disorder (PTSD) resulting from a variety of stressors have both an exagerrated startle[2] as well as nonhabituation of the autonomic components of startle response. Patients with other types of anxiety disorders, however, show the usual pattern of startle habituation. Thus, the absence of startle habituation may be a specific biological marker of PTSD.[1]

We developed and tested the following paradigm in an attempt to develop an animal model of PTSD. We chose rats as the animal, electric tail shock administered in a confined space as the trauma, and acoustic startle habituation as the diagnostic marker of PTSD. This model depends on hyperarousal as an indicator of PTSD, because subjective symptoms of the disorder (e.g., reexperiencing phenomena) cannot be determined in the rat. The complete dataset from these studies will be reported elsewhere.

MATERIALS AND METHODS

Subjects were Sprague-Dawley rats weighing approximately 275 g. Institutional Review Board approval was obtained for the performance of these procedures on animal subjects. The startle apparatus was described previously.[3] The startle signals were acquired by computer and subsequently analyzed using analysis software (Dadisp, DSP Corporation, Cambridge, Massachusetts) programmed to quantify the peak amplitude and peak latency occurring subsequent to startle stimuli. Intermittent tail shock was performed as described previously: the rat was loosely restrained in a plexiglas tube inside a sound-attenuated, ventilated, illuminated box. Electrodes were taped to the tail that extended out the end of the tube. A constant current shock

[a]This work was supported by the Department of Veterans Affairs, Psychiatry and Research Services, Merit Review Research Program, West Los Angeles, California.

generator (Lafayette Instrument Co., Lafayette, Indiana) provided intermittent shocks (5-s 1-ma unpredictable tail shocks, average 1/min) controlled by a Commodore microcomputer.

PROCEDURES

Pretrauma Baseline Testing. In the first phase of the experiment, each subject was tested for baseline startle reactivity to assess pretrauma differences in startle reactivity and to generate a biological measurement baseline against which each subsequent test could be compared. Each subject was placed in the startle measurement apparatus and presented with a series of 150 startle-eliciting bursts of white noise (intensity 125 dB SPL; 0 ms rise-fall time; duration 10 ms) at 6-second intervals. Data were collected as already noted.

Trauma Induction. In the second phase of the experiment, experimental subjects were exposed to a 3-day course of traumatic shock. On day 1, subjects received 30 tail shocks with a variable interval (VI), average 1/minute schedule, and were then returned to their home cage. On day 2 after being placed in the same plexiglas cage for 8 minutes, subjects received 5 additional tail shocks VI 6-minute average. On day 3, subjects were placed in the shock chamber without any electric shock for 30 minutes. Control animals were placed through the same procedures without any electric shock delivery.

Startle Testing. In the third phase of the experiment all subjects were tested for startle reactivity over time. This startle testing, as described above, was performed before experimental (or control) procedures (day 0) and then for 6 days in the 8 days following termination of startle (days 1, 4, 5, 6, 7, and 8, skipping weekend days), and then weekly thereafter for 1 month. Subjects were tested for startle reactivity before stress inoculation.

Data Analysis. Because subjects characteristically showed reactions exceeding 0.5 V in the first few startle presentations, early startle reactions were not included in the average amplitudes analyzed. The startle for each animal was thus the raw amplitude measure (in V) averaged from trial 5 through 150.

For data analysis, all posttrauma startle trials were averaged to obtain an average startle reaction for each rat. One-way analyses of variance were used to determine cumulative group differences over posttrauma startle trials. Repeated analyses of variance (ANOVA-R) were used to ascertain within group differences over individual startle trials. Posthoc comparisons were made using Tukey's protected t test. In the prepost study, a t test was used to determine group differences in the pretrauma startle trial.

Data are presented as both raw scores and change from percentage pretrauma baseline measurement period. Criteria for the presence of PTSD-like stress disorder were operationally defined: startle responses greater than 2 standard deviations above the mean for prestartle trials were used to differentiate a PTSD-like stress disorder from non-PTSD-like animals.

RESULTS

Pretrauma Startle Reactivity. Prior to trauma induction, no significant group differences in startle reactivity were noted (mean [+SEM] volts: control = 0.25 ± 0.016; experimental = 0.22 ± 0.018, n = 31 in each group).

Posttrauma Startle Reactivity. Experimental subjects: As noted in pilot experiments, the experimental (traumatized) subjects demonstrated two divergent responses and were divided into stress-disordered rats (n = 9) and nonstress-disordered rats (n = 22), the former having startle reactivity at least 2 standard deviations higher than the latter in the poststartle period as just described.

Following trauma induction, rats exposed to tail shock had significantly greater startle reactivity (F(2,555) = 36.43, p < 0.001) than did control animals. Posthoc comparisons indicated that startle reactivity in stress-disordered rats was significantly elevated over that of nonstress-disordered rats and control animals. Nonstress-disordered rats also had greater average startle reactivity than did control rats. In stress-disordered rats (n = 9), posttrauma startle reactivity across all nine startle trials was consistently elevated over pretrauma trials (F(9,8) = 5.279, p < 0.0001). Overall, posttrauma measures represented a 236% increase over pretrauma levels (significantly greater than those of both control and nonstress-disordered experimental groups, p < 0.0001).

In contrast, increased startle reactivity in nonstress-disordered rats was not consistently elevated across posttrauma startle trials. Most of these animals (n = 22) demonstrated a pattern resembling that of control subjects. After trauma, using repeated measures analysis of variance to assess for differences at each time point, only three of nine posttrauma time periods (2, 8, and 9) were significantly elevated from basal levels.

Control Subjects. Control subjects (n = 31) demonstrated minimal change in startle amplitude over time. On the first day of startle testing, average amplitude was 0.25 ± 0.01 V for startle numbers 5–150. Startle reactivity in control animals was not significantly elevated over pretrauma startle values. Average startle amplitude for the subsequent nine trials over 3 weeks was 0.26 ± 0.007 V. No control rats were classified as stress disordered, as none of these rats exhibited startle reactivity greater than 2 SDs above pretrauma startle values.

On posthoc analysis, significant differences in pretrauma startle reactivity were noted between the stress-disordered rats and the other two groups. Pretrauma baseline testing in the stress-disordered group was half that of either of the other two groups (0.124 ± 0.013; p < 0.01). During the pretrauma baseline testing, nonstress-disordered experimental animals demonstrated an average amplitude of 0.23 ± 0.022, no different from that of the control group.

Startle latency was equivalent in all subjects; 70–80% of all startle peaks occurred in less than 100 ms following the onset of the startle stimulus.

DISCUSSION

These studies present a reliable technique for assessing the traumatic effect of stress in rats as measured by nonhabituation of startle responses over time. Using a prolonged session of startle-eliciting acoustic stimuli, control rats rapidly and consistently habituated without persistently high startle reactions. Subjects traumatized with intermittent tail shock over a brief period (with two brief reinforcement sessions) demonstrated two patterns. One, resembling the control subjects, consisted of rapid habituation to startle in the first session and a similar response in subsequent startle trials. The second demonstrated a pattern akin to the nonhabituation described in PTSD patients,[1] in which the animal failed to habituate to startle stimuli. This was particularly striking because subjects were exposed to many startle-eliciting stimuli over several trials of several weeks' duration. The responses in each animal were normalized to their own pretrauma startle response, thus providing a longitudinally reliable picture of the development of startle nonhabituation over time. The number of animals developing the PTSD-type pattern of startle hyperactivity was similar to that reported in humans, at about 29%.[2] Interestingly, this group also demonstrated lower baseline startle amplitudes when tested before stress inoculation.

The uniqueness of this animal modeling system is its focus on nonhabituation of startle in the absence of trauma-related cues. It is the continued hyperarousal in the absence of specific cues, typified by nonhabituation of the startle reactions,[1] that more accurately reflects the clinical situation. This is not a fear-conditioning or inescapable shock (IES) paradigm as used previously to model PTSD.[4] The IES model is one of experimental depression, usually using foot shock and a shuttle box learning paradigm. The inescapable nature of the shock is not dissimilar, but our protocol is not paired to a learning task and contains startle reactivity, which has not been a feature of IES. The testing situation does not use a fear-potentiated startle reaction.[5] Subjects are in a small plastic restraining cage with electrodes taped to their tail in the induction phase and are freely moving in a plastic box with a wire top for startle testing. The startle situation is different from the condition in which the animals were traumatized.

The current model satisfies most of Yehuda's recently proposed criteria for an animal model, most particularly the long-lasting nature of the effect as well as the fact that only a subset of animals develop the syndrome.[6] It is unclear at this time whether changes in shock intensity, volume, or timing in the stress paradigm will affect the number of subjects developing nonhabituation of their startle reactions.

SUMMARY

Nonhabituation of the acoustic startle response is used to identify rat subjects with altered alarm responses subsequent to trauma exposure. Subjects ($n = 31$) were exposed to 30 minutes of intermittent tail shock on 2 days followed by exposure to the apparatus on the third day. Twenty-nine percent of traumatized rats developed nonhabituation of startle over the subsequent 3 weeks of testing. No control rats developed nonhabituation of startle reactions over a similar time period. These data suggest that this system represents a more accurate representation of clinical PTSD than do other animal models.

REFERENCES

1. SHALEV, A. Y., S. P. ORR, T. PERI, S. SCHREIBER & R. K. PITMAN. 1992. Physiologic responses to loud tones in Israeli patients with post traumatic stress disorder. Arch. Gen. Psychiatry **49:** 870-875.
2. SHORE, J. H., W. M. VOLLMER & E. L. TATUM. 1989. Community patterns of postraumatic stress disorders. J. Nerv. Ment. Dis. **177:** 681-685.
3. LEITNER, D. S. 1986. Alterations in other sensory modalities accompanying stress analgesia as measured by startle reflex modification. Ann. N.Y. Acad. Sci. **467:** 82-91.
4. OTTENWELLER, J. E., B. H. NATELSON, D. L. PITMAN & S. D. DRASTAL. 1989. Adrenocortical and behavioral responses to repeated stressors: Toward an animal model of chronic stress and stress-related mental illness. Biol. Psychiatry **26:** 829-841.
5. DAVIS, M. & D. ASTRACHAN. 1978. Conditioned fear and startle magnitude: Effects of different footshocks or backshock intensities used in training. J. Exp. Psych. Anim. Behav. Processes **4:** 95-103.
6. YEHUDA, R. & S. M. ANTELMAN. 1993. Criteria for rationally evaluating animal models of posttraumatic stress disorder. Biol. Psychiatry **33:** 479-486.

Serotonergic Modulation of Learned Helplessness

FREDERICK PETTY,[a] GERALD L. KRAMER, AND
JIANHUA WU

Veterans Affairs Medical Center and
Department of Psychiatry
University of Texas Southwestern Medical School
Dallas, Texas 75216

Selective serotonin reuptake inhibitors (SSRIs) have shown clinical utility in the treatment of posttraumatic stress disorder (PTSD), suggesting that serotonin (5-HT) may be implicated in the neurochemical pathophysiology of this disorder. Learned helplessness (LH) is a stress-induced behavioral deficit that may serve as an animal model for some aspects of PTSD. Learned helplessness is reversed by SSRIs and by the 5-HT$_{1A}$ receptor agonists 8-OH-DPAT and ipsapirone.[1] In naive rats, 5-HT depletion causes LH-like behavior, and this behavior is reversed by subsequent antidepressant treatment.[2] Microinjection and microdialysis experiments support a key role for 5-HT in the development and maintenance of LH, particularly in the medial prefrontal cortex.[3,4] The relation between LH and 5-HT receptors and the 5-HT transporter has not been extensively studied.[5] Chronic treatment with the antidepressant imipramine decreases the density of 5-HT$_{1A}$ and 5-HT$_2$ receptors and 5-HT transporter sites in the cortex and hippocampus. We therefore undertook the present study using quantitative autoradiography.

Standard behavioral procedures were used with inescapable tailshock stress. Shuttlebox testing 1 day later allowed assignment of rats into LH and nonhelpless (NH) groups. Controls included restrained (nonshocked) and tested (TC) and naive, nonhandled controls (NC). Quantitative autoradiography was performed using standard procedures, for the 5-HT$_{1A}$ receptor using [^{3}H] 8-OH-DPAT, for the 5-HT$_2$ receptor using [^{3}H] ketanserin, and for the 5-HT uptake site using [^{3}H] paroxetine. Brain regions studied included medial prefrontal cortex, dorsal hippocampus, septum, hypothalamus, and amygdala.

For 5-HT$_{1A}$ receptors, there were no significant group differences in the density of [^{3}H] 8-OH-DPAT in any area examined (Figs. 1 to 3). receptors, there was significantly lower [^{3}H] ketanserin density in the dorsal hippocampus of NH rats and in the hypothalamus and amygdala of LH rats compared to TC or NC rats; however, in the latter two regions, LH was not significantly different from NH. For 5-HT uptake sites, medial prefrontal cortex density of [^{3}H] paroxetine sites in LH rats was significantly lower than that of controls, but not NH groups.

[a] Address for correspondence: Frederick Petty, PhD, MD, Mental Health Clinic, VAMC−116A, 4500 South Lancaster Road, Dallas, TX 75216 (tel: (214)376-5451; fax: (214)372-7086; e-mail: petty.frederick@dallas.va.gov).

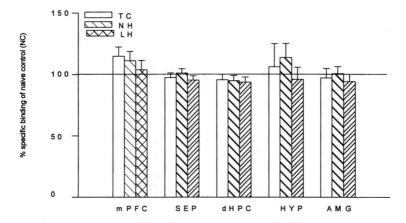

FIGURE 1. Values represent mean specific binding (uncorrected for batch differences) of [³H] 8-OH-DPAT (% of NC ± SEM). Abbreviations: mPFC = medial prefrontal cortex; SEP = septum; dHPC = dorsal hippocampus; HYP = hypothalamus; AMG = amygdala; TC = tested control; NH = nonhelpless; LH = learned helpless.

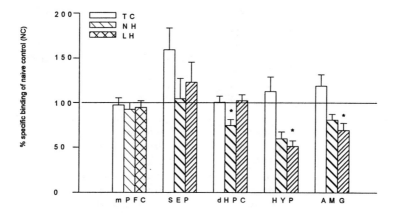

FIGURE 2. Values represent mean specific binding (uncorrected for batch differences) of [³H] ketanserin (% of NC ± SEM). Abbreviations: mPFC = medial prefrontal cortex; SEP = septum; dHPC = dorsal hippocampus; HYP = hypothalamus; AMG = amygdala; TC = tested control; NH = nonhelpless; LH = learned helpless. *$p < 0.05$ compared to NC or TC.

TC rats had escape latencies comparable to those of NH rats, demonstrating that restraint without tailshock does not induce LH behavior. TC rats had densities of receptor similar to those of NC, indicating that changes in receptor densities in LH and NH were not due to effects of restraint stress or of the footshock and motor stress involved in shuttlebox testing.

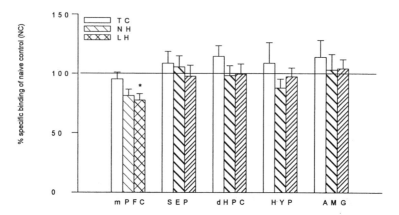

FIGURE 3. Values represent mean specific binding (uncorrected for batch differences) of [^{3}H] paroxetine (% of NC ± SEM). Abbreviations: mPFC = medial prefrontal cortex; SEP = septum; dHPC = dorsal hippocampus; HYP = hypothalamus; AMG = amygdala; TC = tested control; NH = nonhelpless; LH = learned helpless. *$p < 0.05$ compared to nonhandled controls (NC).

A major finding was the differential pattern of response of 5-HT$_2$ receptors. In dorsal hippocampus, 5-HT$_2$ receptor density decreased in NH rats, but remained unchanged in LH rats. In contrast to dorsal hippocampus, 5-HT$_2$ receptor density was decreased in the amygdala and hypothalamus of both LH and NH rats. Previous research shows that treatment of rats with chronic, but not acute imipramine decreases the number of 5-HT$_2$ receptors in hippocampus, and a single dose of the 5-HT$_2$ receptor antagonist methysergide prevents the induction of LH behavior. Thus, a decrease of 5-HT$_2$ receptor densities in dorsal hippocampus of NH rats may correlate with resistance to the development of LH. The decrease in 5-HT$_2$ receptor densities in the amygdala and hypothalamus appeared to be a response to inescapable stress per se and not a functional correlate of LH behavior.

The density of 5-HT transport sites in the medial prefrontal cortex was lower in both LH and NH rats, but more so in LH. Both LH and NH rats received comparable exposure to inescapable stress, but had different behavioral responses. Thus, the decrease or downregulation of 5-HT transport sites was not a functional correlate of the behavioral consequences of inescapable stress, but rather to a nonspecific stress effect. However, although the decrease in 5-HT transport sites may be the result of inescapable stress, the degree of this decrease may possibly influence the reuptake of 5-HT into neurons and subsequently influence or maintain LH behavior.[6]

In summary, our data indicate that 5-HT$_{1A}$ receptors may not be functionally related to the development of LH, at least at the terminal fields. The 5-HT transport mechanisms in the medial prefrontal cortex and the 5-HT$_2$ receptors in the amygdala and hypothalamus may reflect an inescapable stress effect rather than maladaptive coping mechanisms. Finally, the dorsal hippocampus 5-HT$_2$ receptors may play a crucial role in the prevention of or resistance to the maladaptive stress response termed "learned helplessness."

REFERENCES

1. PETTY, F. *et al.* 1994. *In vivo* serotonin release and learned helplessness. Psychiatry Res. **52:** 285-293.
2. SHERMAN, A. D. *et al.* 1980. Neurochemical basis of the action of antidepressants on learned helplessness. Behav. Neural. Biol. **30:** 119-134.
3. PETTY, F. *et al.* 1992. Prevention of learned helplessness: *In vivo* correlation with cortical serotonin. Pharmacol. Biochem. Behav. **43:** 361-367.
4. SHERMAN, A. D. *et al.* 1982. Additivity of neurochemical changes in learned helplessness and imipramine. Behav. Neural. Biol. **35:** 344-353.
5. EDWARDS, E. *et al.* 1991. 5-HT$_{1B}$ receptors in an animal model of depression. Neuropharmacology **30:** 101-105.
6. EDWARDS, E. *et al.* 1991. Modulation of [^{3}H] paroxetine binding to the 5-hydroxytryptamine uptake site in an animal model of depression. J. Neurochem. **56:** 1581-1586.

Effects of Isolation-Rearing on Acoustic Startle and Pre-Pulse Inhibition in Wistar and Fawn Hooded Rats

F. S. HALL,[a] S. HUANG, AND G. FONG

Laboratory of Clinical Studies/DICBR
National Institute on Alcohol Abuse and Alcoholism
Bethesda, Maryland 20892

Isolation-rearing of rats induces a variety of behavioral changes including impaired prepulse inhibition of acoustic startle[1] and may potentiate acoustic startle (F.S.H., unpublished observations). Similar effects were reported for several psychiatric conditions, including posttraumatic stress disorder (PTSD).[2] These behavioral changes in rats are associated with concomitant upregulation of presynaptic dopamine function and enhanced responses to dopamine agonists.[3] One important question that has not yet been addressed is whether animals of different genetic backgrounds vary in sensitivity to the effects of early social deprivation. The present experiment examines the potential interaction between genetic and experiential effects on acoustic startle and pre-pulse inhibition (PPI) using Wistar and Fawn Hooded rats, to identify possible predisposing factors to augmentation of startle and impairment of PPI. Fawn Hooded rats have impaired serotonin function,[4] as do isolation-reared rats.[5] Under some conditions Fawn Hooded rats are also hyperactive (F.S.H., unpublished observation) which may indicate that they have enhanced dopamine function as well.

METHODS

Subjects were Fawn Hooded (National Cancer Institute, Frederick, Maryland) and Wistar (Charles River, Frederick, Maryland) male rats received on postnatal day 21 and randomly divided into rearing conditions, socially reared versus isolation-reared. After 8 weeks of housing, Fawn Hooded rats ($n = 5$ isolation-reared, $n = 8$ socially reared) and Wistar ($n = 9$ isolation-reared, $n = 8$ socially reared) were tested for acoustic startle and PPI using a San Diego instruments startle chamber (SRLAB). Subjects were singly placed in the startle chambers and allowed to habituate to a background noise of 70 dB for 5 minutes. Thereafter, multiple trials were conducted with subjects exposed to either a startle stimulus of 120 dB or a startle stimulus preceded by a prepulse stimulus of 90 dB.

[a] Address for correspondence: Dr. F. S. Hall, NIH/NIAAA, Bldg. 10, Room 3C-207, Bethesda, MD 20892.

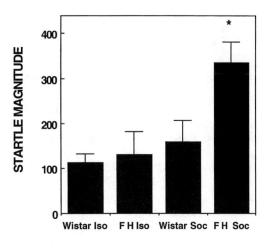

FIGURE 1. Posthabituation average acoustic startle values in Wistar and Fawn Hooded (FH), socially reared (SOC), and isolation-reared (ISO) rats. *Significant posthoc difference between strains of SOC rats ($p < 0.05$).

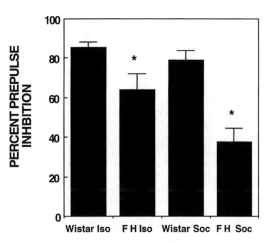

FIGURE 2. Posthabituation average percent prepulse inhibition of acoustic startle in Wistar and Fawn Hooded (FH), socially reared (SOC), and isolation-reared (ISO) rats. *Significant posthoc difference between strains of SOC and ISO rats ($p < 0.05$).

RESULTS

All subjects exhibited pronounced habituation of acoustic startle during the first few trials after which stable startle values were maintained for the rest of the testing period. Fawn Hooded socially reared rats exhibited greatly enhanced startle values compared to the other three groups in the first three trials and after habituation. This is readily apparent in the average startle data (average of all trials after the first two startle trials; STRAIN × REAR $F[1,26] = 4.39$, $p < 0.05$; FIG. 1).

Fawn Hooded rats exhibited diminished PPI compared to Wistar rats (STRAIN: $F[1,26] = 36.70$, $p < 0.0001$; FIG. 2). There was a strong trend towards greater impairment in Fawn Hooded socially reared rats; although this did not reach statistical significance (STRAIN × REAR; F[1,26] = 3.66, $p < 0.07$), it did result in socially reared rats having lower PPI values overall (REAR: F[1,26] = 9.95, $p < 0.005$).

CONCLUSIONS

Contrary to expectations from the effects of isolation-rearing in other strains of rats, socially reared Fawn Hooded rats had greater startle responses than did the other three groups that did not differ from each other. Furthermore, Fawn Hooded rats had impaired PPI compared to Wistar rats, and this impairment was greater in socially reared Fawn Hooded rats. Although PPI did not differ in isolation-reared and socially reared Wistar rats, this may have been due to a ceiling effect. Even though the greater impairment of PPI in socially reared Fawn Hooded rats was contrary to expectations, the data strongly support the role of social experience and genetic background in these functions. They may indicate that Fawn Hooded rats have potentiated dopaminergic function, related to impaired PPI, as well as impaired serotonergic function, and they may constitute an animal model of predisposition to PTSD. Data further suggest that in rats that tend to have enhanced acoustic startle or prepulse inhibition of acoustic startle, early social environment plays a crucial role in the expression of those changes, albeit in an unexpected manner.

REFERENCES

1. GEYER, M. A., L. S. WILKINSON, T. HUMBY & T. W. ROBBINS. 1993. Isolation rearing of rats produces a deficit in prepulse inhibition of acoustic startle similar to that in schizophrenia. Biol. Psychiatry **34:** 361-372.
2. MORGAN, C. A., C. GRILLON, S. M. SOUTHWICK, M. DAVIS & D. S. CHARNEY. 1995. Fear-potentiated startle in posttraumatic stress disorder. Biol. Psychiatry **38:** 378-385.
3. JONES, G. H., C. A. MARSDEN & T. W. ROBBINS. 1990. Increased sensitivity to amphetamine and reward-related stimuli following social isolation in rats: Possible disruption of dopamine-dependent mechanisms. Psychopharmacology **102:** 364-372.
4. REZVANI, A. H., D. H. OVERSTREET & D. S. JANOWSKY. 1990. Genetic serotonin deficiency and alcohol preference in the fawn hooded rats. Alcohol Alcoholism **25:** 573-575.
5. JONES, G. H., T. D. HERNANDEZ, D. A. KENDALL, C. A. MARSDEN & T. W. ROBBINS. 1992. Dopaminergic and serotonergic function following isolation-rearing in rats: A study of behavioral responses and post-mortem and *in vivo* neurochemistry. Pharm. Biochem. Behav. **43:** 17-35.

Neurobiological Alterations in Adult Nonhuman Primates Exposed to Unpredictable Early Rearing

Relevance to Posttraumatic Stress Disorder[a]

ERIC L. P. SMITH,[b] JEREMY D. COPLAN,[c] RONALD
C. TROST,[b] BRUCE A. SCHARF,[d] AND
LEONARD A. ROSENBLUM[b]

[b]Primate Behavior Laboratory
Department of Psychiatry
State University of New York–Health Science Center at Brooklyn
Brooklyn, New York 11203

[c]Department of Psychiatry
Columbia University College of Physicians and Surgeons
New York, New York 10032

[d]Division of Laboratory Animal Resources
State University of New York—Health Science Center at Brooklyn
Brooklyn, New York 11203

There is growing recognition that particular types of early experience, perhaps interacting with genetic predisposition, can play a critical role in the shaping of an integrated organismic pattern of behavioral, monoaminergic, and neuropeptidergic sequelae that in some contexts may be considered pathological. Through the investigation of differentially reared nonhuman primates,[1,2] we have attempted to address the complex relationship between early experiential factors and subsequent long-term susceptibility to anxiety and affective disorders. In our laboratory, mother-infant dyads of bonnet macaques (*Macaca radiata*) of genetically random backgrounds are exposed to environments that vary in the effort required to obtain daily rations and in the predictability of that requirement. These "foraging demands" are imposed for several months when infants are between 2 and 6 months of age. No food deprivation is involved in these procedures. Low foraging demand (LFD) is comparable to *ad libitum* feeding, whereas high foraging demand (HFD) may require several hours per day to obtain full rations. Variable foraging demand (VFD) is simply the semimonthly alternation of the LFD and HFD conditions.

When mothers are exposed to these circumstances, infants in the VFD condition ('VFDs') subsequently and for years afterwards show striking behavioral differences from infants who have been raised under either consistently low or consistently high foraging demand conditions.[1,2] The VFD effects may include apparent depressive episodes, diminished autonomous functioning, increased timidity, and decreased ex-

[a]This work was supported by National Institute of Mental Health grants MH-42545 and MH-15965.

ploratory behavior when challenged. This cluster of behaviors resembles that of genetically high-reactive macaques[3] and of the young children called "behaviorally inhibited to the unfamiliar."[4]

NEUROHUMORAL EFFECTS OF ADVERSE REARING

In previous studies,[2,5] VFDs exhibited anxious- and depressive-like behaviors and demonstrated noradrenergic and serotonergic differences from control animals. In current studies, VFDs were again compared neurochemically to HFD- and LFD-reared subjects. Inasmuch as assay values for HFDs and LFDs did not differ, they were combined for these analyses. Cisternal cerebrospinal fluid (CSF) concentrations of corticotropin-releasing factor (CRF),[6] somatostatin (SOM), and 5-hydroxyindole-acetic acid (5-HIAA) were significantly elevated in VFDs ($n = 14$) compared to non-VFDs ($n = 14$), whereas CSF cortisol concentrations were significantly lower. Homovanillic acid (HVA) concentrations in VFDs also were marginally elevated, but this finding warrants caution pending further investigation. In the VFDs, CSF CRF was significantly correlated with CSF SOM ($r = 0.74$), CSF 5-HIAA ($r = 0.72$), and CSF HVA ($r = 0.80$). By contrast, in the non-VFDs, only CSF SOM correlated with CSF CRF, an effect carried solely by one high HFD outlier. No significant relationship was found between CSF cortisol and CSF CRF either across all subjects or within groups, a finding consistent with the suggested dissociation of the primate hypothalamic-pituitary-adrenal (HPA) axis and central CRF system.[7]

CLONIDINE CHALLENGE, CRF, AND GROWTH HORMONE RESPONSE

In humans, blunting of the growth hormone response to the alpha$_2$-adrenoceptor agonist clonidine has proven to be among the most specific and reliable biological markers for a range of anxiety and mood disorders. We tested 21 bonnet macaques for response to clonidine while under ketamine anesthesia. Growth hormone levels were determined from periodically sampled blood taken concurrently with the cloni-dine administration regimen. Baseline CSF CRF concentrations were available for 7 of these subjects. All but one had a history of variable foraging demand while with their mothers, but none had been exposed to these conditions for at least 3 years. Data from these subjects are shown in FIGURE 1, in which subjects are grouped by high and low CSF CRF baseline concentrations. As found by others,[8] baseline growth hormone levels (at the zero time point) did not appear affected by capture or anesthesia in either group. However, animals with higher baseline CSF CRF concentrations showed significantly less growth hormone secretion in response to the range of clonidine doses employed than did subjects with lower CSF CRF concentrations.

FIGURE 2 presents the correlation between baseline CSF CRF and plasma growth hormone response 30 minutes after administration of the intermediate clonidine dose (at the 60-minute point in FIG. 1; cumulative dose = 0.1 mg/kg). This was the point of maximum separation of growth hormone response between the high- and low-CRF groups. A strong inverse linear relation between the monkeys' baseline CSF CRF levels and their growth hormone response to clonidine is apparent.

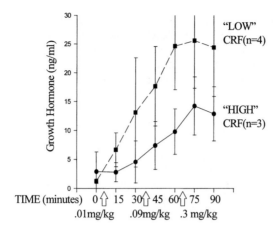

FIGURE 1. Effect of increasing clonidine dose on plasma growth hormone levels in bonnet macaques grouped by baseline level of corticotropin-releasing factor (CRF) in cisternal cerebrospinal fluid. Blood was sampled every 15 minutes. Zero time point marks the first blood withdrawal, 30 minutes after initial ketamine injection and approximately 90 minutes after capture; first clonidine dose was given intravenously immediately afterward. Subsequent doses of clonidine followed blood sampling at 30 and 60 minutes *(arrows).*

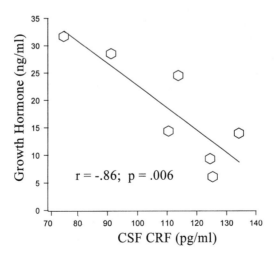

FIGURE 2. Correlation between baseline levels of corticotropin-releasing factor (CRF) in cisternal cerebrospinal fluid (CSF) and plasma growth hormone response to clonidine determined from blood sampled at the session's 60-minute point (0.1 mg/kg cumulative clonidine dose; see FIG. 1). Each point represents one subject.

In summary, our data indicate that even relatively brief maternal exposure to the variable foraging regimen resulted in persistent neurobiological effects in the offspring in the absence of material privation or exceptional effort requirements. As in posttraumatic stress disorder (PTSD), HPA axis function as reflected by CSF cortisol appears reduced in the VFD-reared subjects despite increased CSF CRF concentrations. In addition, there was a clear negative correlation between growth hormone response to clonidine and baseline cisternal CSF CRF concentrations. Thus, adverse early rearing can promote a wide-ranging, well-defined, and long-lasting behavioral and neurochemical syndrome, one component of which is a blunting of noradrenergic responsivity, as demonstrated by reduced growth hormone release to clonidine challenge. Moreover, the strong correlation between central CSF levels and growth hormone response suggests mediation of this effect by CRF in these adversely reared primates, whose seemingly paradoxical CRF/cortisol relation mirrors that found in PTSD.

ACKNOWLEDGMENTS

The authors wish to acknowledge the contributions of Michael W. Andrews, Steven Friedman, Jack M. Gorman, Charles B. Nemeroff, and Michael J. Owens to the fundamental work associated with the current material. The comments of S. R. B. Weiss are also gratefully acknowledged, as is the significant technical support of Siobhán Noland, Antoinette Rookard, and Douglas Rosenblum.

REFERENCES

1. ANDREWS, M. W. & L. A. ROSENBLUM. 1994. The development of affiliative and agonistic social patterns in differentially reared monkeys. Child Dev. **65:** 1398-1404.
2. ROSENBLUM, L. A. & G. S. PAULLY. 1984. The effects of varying environmental demands on maternal and infant behavior. Child Dev. **55:** 305-314.
3. SUOMI, S. J. et al. 1978. Effects of imipramine treatment separation-induced social disorder in rhesus monkeys. Arch. Gen Psychiatry **35:** 321-325.
4. KAGAN, J. et al. 1987. The physiology and psychology of behavioral inhibition in children. Child Dev. **58:** 1459-1473.
5. ROSENBLUM, L. A. et al. 1994. Adverse early experiences affect noradrenergic and serotonergic functioning in adult primates. Biol. Psychiatry **35:** 221-227.
6. COPLAN, J. D. et al. 1996. Persistent elevations of cerebrospinal fluid concentrations of corticotropin-releasing factor in adult nonhuman primates exposed to early-life stressors: Implications for the pathophysiology of mood and anxiety disorders. Proc. Natl. Acad. Sci. USA **93:** 1619-1623.
7. KALIN, N. H. et al. 1987. A diurnal rhythm in cerebrospinal fluid corticotropin-releasing hormone different from the rhythm of pituitary-adrenal activity. Brain Res. **426:** 385-391.
8. BLANK, M. et al. 1983. Effects of capture and venipuncture on serum levels of prolactin, growth hormone and cortisol in outdoor compound-housed female rhesus monkeys (*M. mulatta*). Acta Endocrinol. **102:** 190-195.

Index of Contributors